Innovations in Rhinoplasty

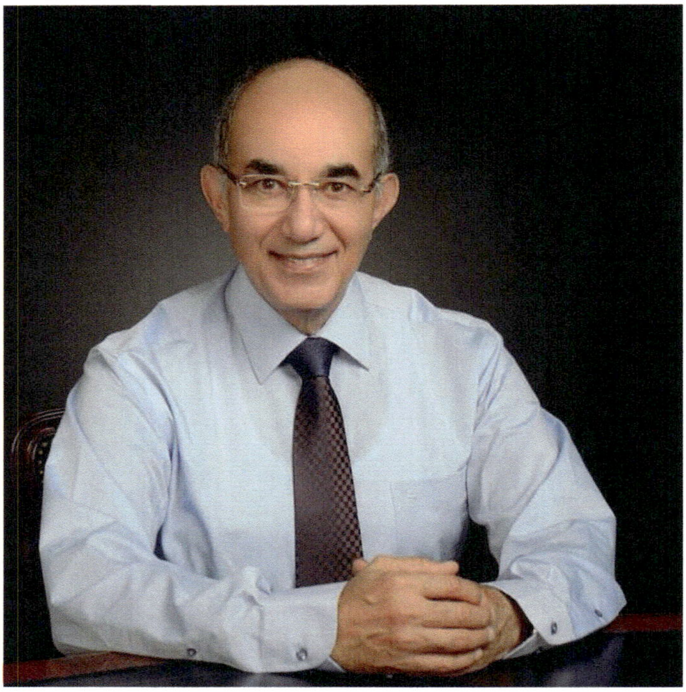

Motaz H. A. Shafy

Innovations in Rhinoplasty

Anatomy, Photography and Surgical Techniques

Springer

Motaz H. A. Shafy
Consultant E.N.T.
and Rhinoplasty Surgeon
Shafy Center
Giza, Egypt

ISBN 978-3-030-94572-5 ISBN 978-3-030-94573-2 (eBook)
https://doi.org/10.1007/978-3-030-94573-2

This Springer imprint is published by the registered company Springer Nature Switzerland AG
The registered company address is: Gewerbestrasse 11, 6330 Cham, Switzerland

Preface

Rhinoplasty is one of the most challenging aesthetic surgeries. The nose is a complex three-dimensional (3D) structure. Sound knowledge of the anatomy and physiology of the nose is essential for a successful outcome. The various anatomical structures of the nose **must maintain their accurate three-dimensional relations to each other** for the best **physiological and aesthetic** results.

Innovative Approach to Nasal Anatomy

Studying the three-dimensional structure of the nose has led to a **better understanding** of the well-known basic anatomy and the **discovery of new anatomical** structures and the revelation of new anatomical areas.

New anatomical structures, i.e., the **Inferior Vestibular Band** and the **Vestibular Septum** are described and proved histologically.

The accurate definitions of the lower lateral crurae have led to describing the **fourth wall** in the lower third of the nose.

The three-Dimensional Anatomical Studies revealed soft folds and weak areas within and around the four-walled lower thirds of the nose.

The physiology of nasal respiration is better understood and the surgical techniques are improved.

Definitions and Terminology

Precise definitions and accurate terminology are imperative for a **clear understanding** and **detailed description** of the anatomy.

Definitions

Each component structure of the nose is defined anatomically by its exact **location**, **description** and **boundaries**. As well as describing the location, the size, shape and consistency of each component, its exact course and relation with the surrounding structures are defined.

Terminology

The given name to each structure **must correspond to the anatomical definition**. This avoids confusion. Loose and inaccurate terms are kept away.

Precise definitions and accurate terminology provide the best ground for easy and full detailed description of anatomy.

Examples of terminology

- The **medial**, **middle** and **lateral curae** of the lower lateral cartilage are **precisely identified** by defining the **medial** and **lateral genua** that divides them. This enables the **full description of the body** of each crus, its **location**, **course** and **relations** with their surrounding structures.
- Differentiations are made between the **alar cartilages** and the **alae nasi**. The first are the lower lateral cartilages, which is a preferable term, while the latter are the two wing-like structures on the sides of the lower third of the nose.
- The **Nasal Lobule** is an attractive and widely used term to describe the surfaces of the nasal tip, supratip or infra-tip areas of the nose. The nasal lobule is **not an anatomical structure**. This term lacks accurate anatomical definition and, therefore, cannot be used in the detailed anatomical description. A lobule does not have a body with a certain shape, size and consistency nor does it have defined boundaries and relations to other structures.

Nasal Attachments to the Face

The upper third of the nose has a **solid bony attachment** to the face via its bony pyramid. The **middle third,** i.e., midvault, represented by the upper lateral cartilage, is attached to the margins of the bony opening via **two tough fixed fibrous membranes**.

The **lower third** has a soft mobile attachment to **orbicularis oris muscle** of the upper lip via the alae nasi and the Inferior Vestibular Band (newly discovered structure). This is called the **nasal base**. In order to understand the anatomical details of this important attachment area, surgeons must be well oriented to the **anatomy of the orbicularis oris muscle**, its relation to the **nasal base** and the skin that covers this junctional area. The nasal base includes the alar base, vestibular floor and caudal cartilaginous septum.

In the midline, the columella is attached to the filtrum of the upper lip. The cartilaginous septum is attached to the palatine process of the maxilla and the bony septum is attached to the sphenoid and ethmoid bones.

The Four Walls of the Lower Third of the Nose

The nose is transformed at its lower third from a **three-walled** pyramidal structure into **two separate four-walled chambers**. A **fourth anterior** wall is now present in each chamber that is made by **the middle crus**.

The two chambers are lined by skin internally and externally. They are separated by the membranous septum and the columella. The two double-walled chambers are conjoined in one four-walled chamber that takes a **rounded** rather than **rectangular** appearance for **aesthetic** and **functional** purposes. The two anterior walls, i.e., the two middle crurae, are integrated to make the **nasal tip**.

The two skin layered walls contain the firm structures of the lower third, i.e., the lower lateral cartilages, caudal cartilaginous septum, the inferior vestibular bands and the alae nasi. These firm structures occupy and support only parts of the four walls, i.e., the four walls of the lower thirds of the nose, unlike the upper two-thirds, are not totally solid motionless tubes. They have the advantages of being mobile and have a better aesthetic contribution to the nose.

The Thirteen Weak and Soft Areas in the Nasal Walls

Between the firm structures in the walls of the lower third of the nose, there are weak and soft areas. They are imperative for nasal aesthetics and kinetic movements of the lower third. These movements are essential for facial expressions and the physiology of nasal respiration. A total of **eleven weak and soft areas** are present in the nasal walls.

Examples of these weak and soft areas are the weak triangle, the soft triangle and the membranous septum. They are present at the junctional areas of the lower third of the nose, i.e., with the midvault superiorly and with the upper lip inferiorly.

The Nasal Valves and The Physiology of Nasal Respiration

Mobility of the lower third is achieved by the **small muscles of the nose**. These movements are necessary for **facial expressions** and the regulation of **nasal respiration**. The **locations**, **definitions** and **functions** of the **nasal valves**, and hence the **physiology of nasal respiration**, are studied in full detail in order to secure the nasal airways while performing Rhinoplasty.

Accurate anatomical and physiological definitions of the external and internal nasal valves.

The Seven Types of Nasal Skin and Surgical Significance

There are **seven** histologically different areas of skin that covers the nose. The **skin** and **subdermal tissues** are variable from one area of the nose to the other. The **skin** varies from being thick, thin, greasy, hair-bearing or non-hair-bearing. The **subdermal tissues** may be loose, tight, full of fat, areolar connective tissues or totally absent.

The surgical management of the skin in each area of the nose varies according to its histological structure. Location of external **skin incisions**, **undermining** and **defatting** are all essential techniques in achieving better aesthetic results with no apparent external scars.

The Surgical Significance of Nasal Base Attachments to the Orbicularis Oris

The base of the lower third of the nose has three major components:

i. The Alar Base.
ii. The Vestibular Floors.
iii. The Nasal sill bands which are part of the Inferior Vestibular Bands IVB (newly described anatomical structure).

All three components of the nasal base are attached to the Orbicularis Oris, muscle and its covering skin.

This is an important junctional area. Understanding the detailed anatomy of this area is the main foundation for accurate nasal and alar base surgeries.

Anatomical Variations of the Nose

Noses are like fingerprints, and they vary from one person to the other in different ethnic groups and from one side of the nose to the other; variations are in the different components in the nose, i.e., the upper two-thirds, lower third and the skin are displayed with illustration and photographs.

Rhinoplasty Photography

Photographic Assessment and Standardization

A totally **new look at photography** is detailed in this text. A separate section is allocated for this purpose.

The main purposes of the photography are **medicolegal documentation** and **pre- and post-operative assessment**.

Photographs may highlight certain anatomical areas that are overlooked or could not be seen at the time of clinical examination.

It cannot be emphasized strongly enough the vital importance of the role of photography.

- **Pre-operative assessment**
  Some anatomical areas may either be overlooked or could not be seen at the time of clinical examination. As well as the four standard views, there are four newly introduced specialized views that aim at the four surgical anatomical subdivisions of the nose.
  The newly introduced specialized views provide a more accurate pre-operative diagnosis that leads to well-targeted, precise and shorter time in surgery and more predictable results.
  Failing to study pre-operative photographs deprives the surgeon of a very important source of information. Photographs may be the only way of seeing certain deformity or defect. The outcome is less confidence in proceeding for surgery, prolonged time of surgery and less predictable results.
- **Intraoperative guide**
  The display of patient's photographs in front of the surgeon intraoperatively is of great help to monitor the progress of surgery.
- **Post-operative Assessment**
  Follow-up of patients photographically is a continuing educational process in the short and long terms. Great deal of lessons are learned from the different stages of patient's photographs.
  Patients may underestimate, do not appreciate or even forget the changes in their noses. Many of them are surprised by their looks before surgeries. "Did I look like this?" surprisingly most of them as even a few months after surgery.
- **Research**
- **A simple Approach to patient photography**
  Many surgeons have the idea that photography is a complicated procedure that needs a qualified photographer and expensive equipment.
  Photographic equipment, techniques and setup are aimed at being as **simple** as possible without compromising the basic clinical photographic IMI (Institute of Medical Illustrators) recommendations. Any surgeon or competent assistant will be able to take high-quality photographs of his **own patients** in his **own practice**.
  (a) **Equipment**: The main triad for equipment is the **Camera**, the **Lens** and the **Flash**.
  Several choices are suggested for selecting **good-quality equipment** that produces **high-quality photographs**. They all are quite **easy to use** at an affordable price.
  (b) **The Setup**: It is surprisingly how small is the area needed for the photographic setup. Only **a 2 × 1.5 m area** is all that is necessary.
  (c) **Standardization of photography**: Understanding the photographic terminology and the methods to achieve standardization are all discussed in simple terms.

(d) **Photographic views**
- **The standard views**: These are the well-known four views, **Frontal** (Anterior), **Oblique**, **Lateral** and **Basal views**.
- **The specialized views**: These are four newly introduced views that aim at visualizing each of the four specific anatomical areas of the nose. The specialized views are as follows: **Overhead, Direct Dorsal, Backward Tilting and Nasal Aperture Views**.
- **The method** of taking each view includes the setup, orientation of the patient and camera, the camera view, lens focus, lens aperture and finally the area and number of photographs taken.

(e) **Photographic Assessment**
The **aims and benefits** of each view are analyzed. The **naso-facial relationships** are best seen in the **standard** views, while the **specific anatomical areas** are best shown in the **specialized views**.

(f) **Tables**: The views and the assessment process of the views are displayed in Microsoft Word tables. These tables include all the details in a simplified way so that facts can easily be seen at a glance. They work as a checklist.

(g) **Filing**: Methods for filing and backing up digital images.

Surgical Techniques

Closed Versus Open Rhinoplasty

An academic approach anatomically, physiologically and aesthetically is made. They are two different approaches for two different objectives. The role of each approach is clearly defined.

The Surgical Difficulties of Rhinoplasty

Rhinoplasty is not an easy operation. Not every surgeon is prepared to perform Rhinoplasty and not every patient with a deformed nose is prepared for Rhinoplasty.

There are surgical difficulties that are unique to this type of surgery.

The technical difficulties start from the **pre-operative assessment** both clinically and photographically to the actual **procedure** and finally to the idiosyncrasies of some **results**.

The management of these difficulties is discussed in order to minimize pre-operative misjudgments, intraoperative misfortunes, post-operative complications and idiosyncratic results.

The Importance of Psychology of the Patient and the Surgeon

Rhinoplasty is associated with varying degrees of emotional and psychological impact on the patients.

Rhinoplasty patients go through **five psychological stages** which are described in full detail. These stages are as follows:

1. Stage of discontent.
2. Stage of decision.
3. Stage of action.
4. Immediate post-operative stage.
5. Stage of facing reality.

The surgeons' attitude throughout the different stages is a definite help for better patients' choice and management.

The Four Anatomical Areas of the Nose

There are four **anatomically** different areas of the nose. Each area has a different structure and a different clinical presentation. Each area requires **its own surgical technique**. These areas are as follows:

1. The **Frontolateral Walls** including the nasal tip.
2. The **Medial Wall** including the nasal septum and columella.
3. The **Bony Pyramid** and **Midvault**.
4. The **Nasal Base**.

Clinical assessment starts with inspection and palpation of the clinical four areas of the nose.

Rhinoplasty: Four Surgeries in One

Rhinoplasty is not a single operation. It is rather **Four different operations,** one for each of the four areas of the nose. The four surgeries must complement each other to finally produce a well-integrated, attractive and functional nose. These four surgeries include the following areas:

(1) The **Frontolateral Walls**.
(2) The **Medial Wall** including the columella and nasal septum.
(3) The **Bony Pyramid and the Midvault**.
(4) The **Nasal Base**.

Each of the four areas requires different **surgical techniques**. A single Rhinoplasty may include one, two, three or all of the four areas of the nose.

Clinical Varieties of Rhinoplasty

People seeking Rhinoplasty have different aesthetic conditions according to the structure of their noses. Each of these conditions requires a different surgical approach and different considerations.

The conditions that surgeons commonly see are as follows:

1. The Large Nose.
2. The Bulky Nose.
3. The Crooked Nose.
4. The Deviated Nose.
5. The Fractured Nose.
6. Secondary Rhinoplasty.
7. Finesse Rhinoplasty.
8. Ethnic noses.
9. Children.
10. Special clinical conditions.
    - Developmental and congenital anomalies.
    - Sliding tips.
    - Large Alae Nasio.

Giza, Egypt Motaz H. A. Shafy

Acknowledgements

I would like to acknowledge and give special thanks to the following people without whom the following textbook and atlas would not have been possible. As a medical professional, I see surgery, specifically rhinoplasty, as a work of art as well as a scientific endeavor. Every artist has their muse, or inspiration; for me, this person was Mr. Tony R. Bull, F.R.C.S. Consultant E.N.T. Surgeon who was my mentor at the Royal National Throat, Nose and Ear Hospital in London. Mr. Bull's creative approach, passion and devotion toward the field of rhinoplasty were what inspired me to develop my own innovative surgical techniques. Mr. Bull was also one of the people who has seen my early work and encouraged me to take my research further turning it from a research article to a full-fledged book.

I would also like to thank my great friend and colleague, Mr. Bahir Skinner A.B.I.P.P, Medical Photographer, for his professional advice regarding medical photography and other technical details.

Furthermore, I would like to show my gratitude toward Elia Anis Ishaak, M.Sc. Ph.D. Professor of Pathology, and Solafa Amin AbdulAziz, MD Professor of Pathology, who work at Cairo University for their help in the histology of the Inferior Vestibular Bands and the Vestibular Septum.

Additionally, I am thankful to Dr. Mohamed Saad Lotfy, CEO of Viral Media, his team and Engineer Roshdy Al Bahlool, B.S.C. from Monofia University of Egypt, for their technical expertise in conducting the medical artistic illustrations evidenced in this book.

Moreover, I would like to thank Dr. Soliman Fakeeh and Dr. Mazen Fakeeh for providing their hospital's facilities, including their O.R. and pathology department, where I conducted my ear, nose and throat surgeries.

I would like to thank Easel M. Monton, R.N.B.S.N. for her diligent efforts in her secretarial assistance.

I would like to thank Ms. Elizabeth Pope, Editor at Springer, for her professional guidance regarding the writing and reviewing of this book taking it to new heights.

Last, but not least, I would like to give a special thanks to my family, without whose support this book would not have been possible.

Introduction

This is a comprehensive textbook that covers all aspects of Rhinoplasty in which there is a totally innovative approach to anatomy, photography and surgical techniques.

Rhinoplasty has a totally different concept and approach from all other aesthetic surgeries. The nose is like a fingerprint, and every nose on this planet is different. Even the two sides of the same nose are different. Each nose has its own individualized surgery. The same nose may have a different operation in different individuals according to their height, body build, social background, personal preference, ethnicity and gender. That is why **not every competent surgeon is readily prepared to perform Rhinoplasty and not every individual with a deformed nose is readily prepared to have Rhinoplasty**.

Patients must be ready physically, mentally, psychologically and emotionally.

Surgeons must have the knowledge and the ability to think in three dimensions. There is an element of artistry and fine motor skills. Surgeons must have the talent, right attitude and well balanced mentally and emotionally.

With the right aptitude, surgeons quickly learn assessment methods, i.e., clinically, psychologically and photographically.

The appreciation of the three-dimensional nasal anatomy and physiology is an essential basic start for surgeons.

The three-dimensional study of nasal anatomy has led to the discovery of new anatomical structures, a clearer understanding of the four-walled lower third and finally the weak areas and soft folds in the nasal walls.

In-depth knowledge of the histological structure of the seven types of nasal skin has promoted surgeries of nasal tip and alar base.

Detailed knowledge of the anatomy of the junctional area between the nasal base and the Orbicularis Oris was essential to promote alar base surgery.

The nose is like a fingerprint and every person has his own individual nasal print. The study of the wide variations in the anatomy of the nose boosts the clinical sense of surgeons.

Photography is an invaluable source of knowledge. **Photographic Anatomy** is a new concept of correlating each part of the nose with the corresponding anatomical component.

The **standard views** are insufficient generalized outlook to the nose and face. They were promoted by adding further standard views. New **Specialized views** for each part of the nose have expanded knowledge.

High-standard photographic technique is made simple. The surgeon or even a well-trained assistant is capable of taking the photographs. **Equipments** are not necessarily expensive. **The setup** is as small as 1.5 × 2 m, i.e., at a corner of a normal practice.

The innovative preservation surgery to the frontolateral walls and alar base has made surgical techniques simpler. The surgery takes a shorter time and the same individual image is maintained, i.e., the same nasal print.

Contents

Part I

Clinical Varieties of Rhinoplasty

1 A Guide to the Three-Dimensional Visualization and Examination of the Nose

Abstract

Rhinoplasty is one of the most challenging aesthetic surgeries. The nose is a complex three-dimensional structure. Sound knowledge of the anatomy and physiology of the nose is essential for successful rhinoplasty. All anatomical structures of the nose must maintain their accurate three-dimensional relations to each other for the best physiological and aesthetic results. An innovative method of understanding the three-dimensional anatomy of the nose is introduced. The following are general guidance that helps in understanding the three-dimensional anatomy:

1. **Basic anatomical knowledge**: These must be clearly known to the surgeon.
2. **Accurate anatomical definitions**: Going through the different anatomical parts of the nose especially the lower there was a severe lack of definition of the medial, middle and lateral crurae. Other structures like the inferior vestibular bands, membranous septum, weak triangle and soft triangles needed to be clearly described in order to have the full picture of the three-dimensional structure of the nose.
3. **The four subdivisions of the nose: For easy** understanding, the nose is subdivided into four main areas:
   i. The Frontolateral Walls.
   ii. The Medial Wall.
   iii. The Bony Pyramid.
   iv. The Alar Base.
4. **Clinical examination method:** Both **inspections** and **palpation** must be encouraged by using one or two fingers of the bare ungloved hands. External and internal parts of the nose, i.e., bimanually, are examined accurately. New clinical tests are introduced to enhance the ability for three-dimensional tactile sensation of nasal anatomy.
5. **Photography** is an essential tool in seeing what the normal eyes of the surgeon may miss during a clinical examination. The newly introduced specialized photographs of four different parts of the nose have made this possible.
6. **Imagination**: Surgeons must be capable of developing a sense of imagination. They should continue to work on this ability throughout their professional career. This will greatly improve their abilities to understand the three-dimensional anatomy of the nose.

Keyword

3 dimensional visualization of the nose

The nose is a three-dimensional organ that protrudes out of the middle third of the face.

Anatomical facts about the nose are mainly derived from the direct dissection of chemically prepared or fresh cadavers. These facts are reaffirmed during live surgeries.

M. H. A. Shafy, *Innovations in Rhinoplasty*,
https://doi.org/10.1007/978-3-030-94573-2_1

1.1 The Significance of Maintaining the Nasal Three Dimensions

The lower third of the nose has an additional unique source of anatomical information. Its structural components have certain three-dimensional relationships. These relationships are maintained in their position in free space in order to keep the shapes as well as the functions of these parts of the nose in a constantly stable condition.

Control of all the inspired and expired air starts and ends at this important entrance to the respiratory system of the body. Structures in this gateway are governed by delicate muscles that harmoniously work to control the physiology of nasal respiration.

1.2 Difficulties of Studying the Three-Dimensional Anatomy

It is not easy to see and understand clearly the relation between the different structures of the nose in free space, i.e., the three-dimensional anatomy. The classic method of cadaveric dissection or intraoperative dissection is insufficient to provide a full three-dimensional picture in the surgeon's mind.

Cadaveric study of the nasal anatomy has its clear advantages. In the case of the lower third of the nose, there are certain drawbacks.

The nose of a cadaver collapses and deforms within a few hours of death. Tissues, therefore, lose their exact inter-structural three-dimensional relationship in free space. This is due to the following:

i. Loss of the facial muscular tone.
ii. Loss of the binding effects of the inter-structural yellow elastic tissues, bands and ligaments.
iii. The texture of the main supportive structures is lost at death and by the effects of chemical preparation.

1.3 Guide for the Three-Dimensional Study of Nasal Anatomy

It is important for the surgeon to clinically examine and visualize the three-dimensional structure of the patient's nose.

The following recommendations will significantly make pre-operative diagnosis and planning for surgery more accurate. Surgery will be well-targeted and precise and post-operative results will be greatly improved.

1.3.1 Knowledge and Definitions of Anatomical Parts of the Nose

1.3.1.1 The Basic Anatomical Facts

The first rule of understanding the three-dimensional anatomy is to have sound **knowledge** of the basic anatomical and clinical anatomical facts. Tactile support of this knowledge is achieved by surgical experience that includes a wide range of clinical exposure to the various aesthetic and functional surgical techniques.

1.3.1.2 Accurate Anatomical Definitions

Accurate definitions are essential for the different structures of the nose especially those of the lower third.

A series of accurate definitions are introduced, e.g., the angles and the borders of the weak and flat triangles, nasal base, Inferior Vestibular Bands and medial and lateral genua of the lower lateral cartilages.

1.3.1.3 Surgical Anatomical Subdivisions of the Nose

The nose is further subdivided into four inter-related anatomical areas:

i. The **Frontolateral Walls**, which are made of the lower lateral cartilages and the alae nasi.

ii. The **Medial Wall** which includes the **nasal septum** and the **columella.**
iii. The **Bony Pyramid** and **Midvault.**
iv. The **Nasal Base,** i.e., the **inferior wall** which includes the vestibular floors, the flat triangles and the alar base.

The basic anatomy of each of these areas is studied in full detail. Facts are then added to each other, until the final full three-dimensional picture becomes clear and complete.

1.3.2 Clinical Examination

1.3.2.1 Live Clinical Assessment

The structures of the lower third of the nose are all subcutaneous. They can be palpated externally and/or internally, i.e., vestibularyl or bimanually. These structures, therefore, are readily available for clinical assessment.

Inspection

A great deal of information is gained from studying the surface anatomy by inspection. Inspection includes patients in the clinic and in the operating room.

Each and every person has a unique nose that differs from other noses, like a fingerprint. The whole world is an **open free museum** for our eyes to observe. There are **wide varieties of noses of different ages, sexes and ethnic origins**. This is an endless, rich and comprehensive source of knowledge.

Palpation

Palpation is another valuable source of information. One may start with his own nose, then clinically palpate the patient's noses in the clinic and under anesthesia in the operating room.

By the time, this practical routine progressively improves the tactile clinical abilities of the surgeon.

One or two fingers may be used to palpate the bony pyramid, midvault, lower lateral cartilages, columella, septum, soft areas as well as any defects or grafts. **Ungloved Bare hands** are better for fine palpation. On the **External nasal surface, intranasal** and **bimanual** palpation is made to feel the thickness of the walls and the structures between them, e.g., columella, alae nasi and the nasal tip.

Clinical Tests

A new **clinical test,** i.e., the **rim-sill test** is introduced to clarify the surface anatomy of structures that have different textures and consistencies. A blunt probe is used at the boundaries of the nasal sills and alar margins to demonstrate the rim-sill folds.

1.3.3 Photography

Photography is an important tool in studying the three-dimensional relations of nasal structures.

Standard views as well as the newly introduced **specialized views** are vitally important to boost the three-dimensional imagination of the nose (details on Photographic Chapter).

1.3.4 Imagination

The surgeon must have, or be capable of, creating and developing a sense of imagination. He must continue to work on this ability throughout his professional career. Understanding the anatomy of the lower lateral cartilages, for example, is almost impossible by post-mortem or intraoperative dissection only. Describing their shapes while standing as a live three-dimensional structure in free space is only possible by using our imagination. It is the only way to visualize and describe the curves and folds of each cartilage, as well as the shape they make together in the formation of the nasal tip.

Imagination is the most strongly needed quality to study and understand the anatomy of the lower third of the nose.

1.4 Conclusion

In order to enhance the ability to visualize the three-dimensional anatomy of the nose, a complete comprehensive study is made in the **four directions** in each case:

i. Command of the **basic anatomical knowledge**.
ii. Meticulous **clinical assessment**, inspection, palpation and special tests.
iii. **Photography**.
iv. The continuous use of the sense of **imagination**.

The three-dimensional study of the nose has made it possible to accurately describe the **anatomy of the lower third of the nose**. It becomes possible to precisely **define the beginning and end** of each of the **lower lateral crurae**. The anatomical **weak and soft areas** in the walls of the lower third of the nose are clearly seen and described. It was possible to discover **new anatomical areas** which otherwise could not be seen by the usual dissection methods.

2 Innovative Approach to Anatomy of the External Nose

Abstract

The external nose is a pyramidal structure that gracefully protrudes out in the middle of the face. As well as studying the **detailed anatomy** of the nose it is imperative to have a full understanding of its bony attachment to the facial skeleton, soft tissue **attachments to the bony skeleton and the upper lip**. The nature and **types of skin** that covers different parts of the nose must be clearly studied.

Keywords

Gross anatomy of the external nose · Anatomy of the upper two-thirds of the nose · Anatomy of the Nasal Septum · Anatomy of the lower third of the nose · The four walled structure of the lower third · The weak and soft areas in the walls of the nose · Nasal attachment to the orbicularis oris · Skin cover of the nose · The nasal bones · The frontal processes of the maxillae · The vertical lacrimal crest · The key stone area · The fibrous membrane · Stability and support of the bony pyramid · Bilateral maxillary asymmetry · The membranous septum "The weak area of the nose" · The mobile tip and the sliding tip · The four walled structure of the lower third of the nose · The columella · The medial curae · The lateral crus · The alae nasi · The alar grooves · The middle crurae · Medial genu · Lateral genu · The vestibular floor · The nasal base · The soft triangle · The flat triangle

The external nose is a pyramidal structure that gracefully protrudes out in the middle of the face. As well as studying the **detailed anatomy** of the nose it is imperative to have a full understanding of its bony attachment to the facial skeleton, soft tissue **attachments to the bony skeleton and the upper lip**. The nature and **types of skin** that covers different parts of the nose must be clearly studied.

<u>The Upper Two-Thirds and the Lower Third.</u>

The upper two-thirds of the nose is totally different from the lower third, both **anatomically** and **physiologically**.

The **upper two-thirds** is a pyramidal three-walled osteocartilaginous structure. It is totally **solid** and **immobile**.

The **lower third** of the nose is made of **two conjoined soft cartilaginous and fibrofatty tissues**. Each side of the lower third of the nose is characterized by having a **fourth anterior wall** which is made by the body of the middle crus.

In contradistinction to the upper two-thirds, the walls of the lower third have varying degrees of **active movements** by the small muscles of the nose. These movements are essential for the

M. H. A. Shafy, *Innovations in Rhinoplasty*,
https://doi.org/10.1007/978-3-030-94573-2_2

physiology of the nasal respiration, facial expression and shock absorption against injury.

As a result of evolution of the fourth wall in the lower third of the nose, gaps appear within its walls and at the junction between the upper two-thirds and lower third of the nose. Other gaps are present at the junction between the nasal base and the upper lip. These gaps are filled with the weak and soft areas of the nose. Examples of these areas are the weak triangle and the soft triangles.

There are **two new anatomical structures** that are studied and proved histologically. They are introduced and described in full details. These are the **Inferior Vestibular Bands** and the **Vestibular septum**.

Studying the anatomy of the nose therefore includes the following:

I. Gross Anatomy of the External Nose.
II. Anatomy of the upper two-thirds of the nose.
III. Anatomy of the Nasal Septum.
IV. Anatomy of the lower third of the nose which includes:
   1. Understanding the Four Walled Structure of the lower third.
   2. Anatomy of the Four Walls.
V. The Weak and Soft areas in the Walls of the Nose.
VI. Nasal attachment to the Orbicularis Oris.
VII. Skin cover of the nose.
VIII. Histological studies of New Anatomical Structures.

2.1 Gross Anatomy of the External Nose

The external nose is a pyramidal structure which gracefully protrudes out of the middle of the face. It is generally composed of four parts.

2.1.1 The Four Components of the External Nose

2.1.1.1 The Fixed Bony Part

This is a part of the facial bony skeleton and is made of the **nasal bones** and the **nasal processes of the maxillae** and the **nasal processes of the frontal bone**.

2.1.1.2 The Fixed Cartilaginous Part

This part of the nose is made of the **upper lateral cartilage** together with the **quadrilateral cartilage** of the nasal septum as one unit. The **solid fixation** of this cartilaginous unit comes from its firm attachment to the bony part i.e., between the upper lateral cartilages, the nasal bones as well as between the cartilaginous and bony septum.

2.1.1.3 The Relatively Mobile Cartilaginous Part

This part is made of the **two lower lateral cartilages**. The relative mobility of this part of the nose is the result of two main factors:

(a) The relative loose attachments to the fixed cartilaginous part i.e., to the upper lateral cartilage and cartilaginous septum. There are three areas of attachments between these parts i.e., the junction between the fixed and mobile cartilages of the nose. These areas are:
   i. The overlapping of the two lateral crura over the lower border of the upper lateral cartilage at the scroll area.
   ii. The bands and ligaments in the weak triangle between the anterior septal angle and middle crurae.
   iii. The membranous septum which is a loose midline structure that joins the caudal margin of the septum to the medial crurae of the lower lateral cartilages.

(b) The effect of the depressor septi muscles which are attached to the inferior borders of the medial crura and to the caudal septal cartilage.

2.1.1.4 The Actively Mobile Fibro-Fatty Part

This part is made of both of **the alae nasi**. The alae nasi are two relatively independent outwards protrusions on the sidewalls of the nose. They are attached to the nose via the alar muscle layer **superiorly**, while **posteriorly** they are attached to the upper lip via their underlying deep layer of the Orbicularis Oris.

Externally their attachment to the nose appears as the **superior alar grooves** and to the **lip** as the **posterior alar grooves**.

2.1.2 The Bony Opening of the Nose

The bony component of the external nose is made of the nasal bones and the nasal and the palatine processes of the maxillary bones (Fig. 2.1). The bony opening of the nose is in the form of a pear or inverted **heart shaped**. The **narrow** end is upwards and is made by the two nasal bones. The **wide** end is made by the thin sharp curved margin of the nasal processes of the maxillary bones. They both end inferiorly by sharing in the formation of the anterior nasal spine.

The nasal spine is part of the palatine process of the maxillary bone. The latter forms part of the floor of the nasal cavity.

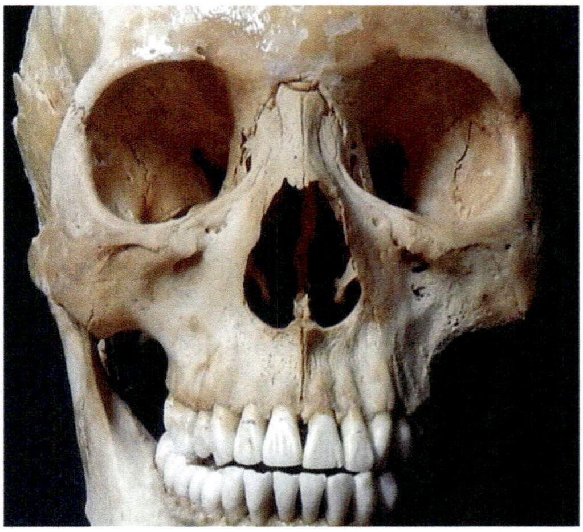

Fig. 2.1 The bony opening of the nose

2.1.3 Attachments of the External Nose to the Face

The **soft tissues of the nose** are attached to the face via its **skeletal** and **soft tissue** structures as follows.

2.1.3.1 Skeletal Attachments

i. The superior border of the upper lateral cartilage is attached to the **nasal bones** in a unique firm attachment.
ii. There is a **tough fibrous membrane** that communicates the curved margin of the **nasal process of the maxilla** to the postero-superior margin of the **lateral crus**.
iii. The skin of the **vestibular floor** is attached to the anterior margin of the **palatine process** of the maxilla till it reaches the **anterior nasal spine**.

2.1.3.2 Soft Tissue Attachments

The posterior margins of the alae nasi and the nasal sill bands are attached to the upper lip with its underlying muscles. It is very significant for the alae nasi to be attached to the upper lip and not to the cheek skin so that they will **not** droop-down with age or protrude forwards and recede backwards with the increase and decrease of the cheek fat as the body weight increases or decreases.

Furthermore the upper lip is a much more **firm** and **stable** base for the nose. The deep muscle layer of the **Orbicularis Oris** provides the alae nasi with muscle fibers for their movements which is useful for facial expressions and nasal respiration.

2.2 Anatomy of the Upper Two-Thirds of the Nose

The upper two-thirds of the nose is further subdivided into two components, the bony pyramid and the cartilaginous midvault.

They both are firmly attached to each other to make an almost one unit. The upper two-thirds has two main characteristics i.e., they are three-walled structure and have firmly fixed and immobile walls.

2.2.1 Anatomy of the Bony Pyramid

The bony pyramid of the nose is structured and built up by a **single bone** and **two pairs of bones**. The single bone is the **nasal part of the frontal bone** that makes the nasal root superior. It articulates with a pair of **nasal bones** and **frontal processes of the maxillae** that make the dorsum and sidewalls of the bony pyramid successively.

2.2.1.1 Nasal Bony Attachments to the Face

The external nose has a bony base that stems from the face i.e., the frontal processes and the palatine processes of maxillary bones. Their inferior sharp margins make a pear-shaped opening. The narrow side of the opening is superior while the wide part is inferior. The palatine processes share in the formation of the anterior nasal spine.

2.2.1.2 Definition of the Bony Pyramid

The nasal bony pyramid is the prominent bony part of the nose that derives its base from the bodies of maxillae at the facial surface and ends at its summit that makes the bony dorsum. It usually constitutes the upper third of the nose in adults.

The nasal bony pyramid is not the equivalent of the nasal bones. The nasal bones are only part of the bony pyramid which share in the formation of its dorsum.

2.2.1.3 Anatomical Components of the Bony Pyramid

The Nasal Part of the Frontal Bone

The nasal part of the frontal bone is quite a thick and compact part of the frontal bone. It is comparable with the mastoid bone in its thickness and consistency. It lies between the two supraorbital margins. It has a **thick inferior cirrated nasal notch** that **articulates with** the **nasal bones**, the frontal processes of the maxillae and the lacrimal bones successively from before, backwards and laterally.

The posterior half of the inferior cirrated margin projects behind i.e., inside the center of the nasal bones and the nasal processes of the maxillae. It shares in **supporting the dorsum of the nose**. Both sides end up making the **nasal spine** which has minimal contribution to the nasal septum.

<u>Surgical Significances:</u>

The most important surgical anatomical fact about the nasal part of the frontal bone is that it is **quite thick** and **compact**. It lies at the bottom of the **nasion** or the **nasofrontal** angle.

Surgically this location is met with in two situations:

i. **Flat nasofrontal angle:**

These cases may be associated with a high dorsum or a nasal hump. Reduction of the nasofrontal angle needs extensive **bone work**. The bone is gradually reduced using a special nasofrontal rasp or a chisel.

ii. **Superior osteotomies:**

On performing an external osteotomy, a too high osteotomy is both difficult and of little aesthetic gain. A superior osteotomy is better done below the nasofrontal suture at the level of the inner canthus of the eye and the palpable lacrimal tubercle just next to it.

The Nasal Bones

There are two nasal bones which are mainly oblong in shape. Not only they vary in size but also vary in their shapes. Both nasal bones meet to articulate with each other in the midline.

Both nasal bones are **thick superiorly** and laterally while their **inferior free borders** are very thin. The **Procerus muscles** are attached to the periostrum of the most inferior parts of the anterior surfaces of the nasal bones.

The nasal bones make a small contribution to the bony septum internally (Posteriorly) which is called the **vertical crest.**

The nasal bones articulate laterally with the frontal processes of the maxillae and superiorly with the nasal part of the frontal bone.

Surgical Significances:

i. The nasal bones have a **concavo-convex shape** in their profile appearance i.e., the upper half is concave near the nasofrontal angle while the lower half is convex (Fig. 2.2). On reducing a nasal hump, not only the whole hump has to be reduced but also the naturally convex lower half of the nasal bones. They need to be reduced to become at the same level with the upper half of the nasal bones otherwise a residual hump may remain post-operatively. Removal of the nasal hump will lead to an open roof deformity, which will be closed by lateral osteotomies and medialisation of the lateral walls of the bony pyramid.

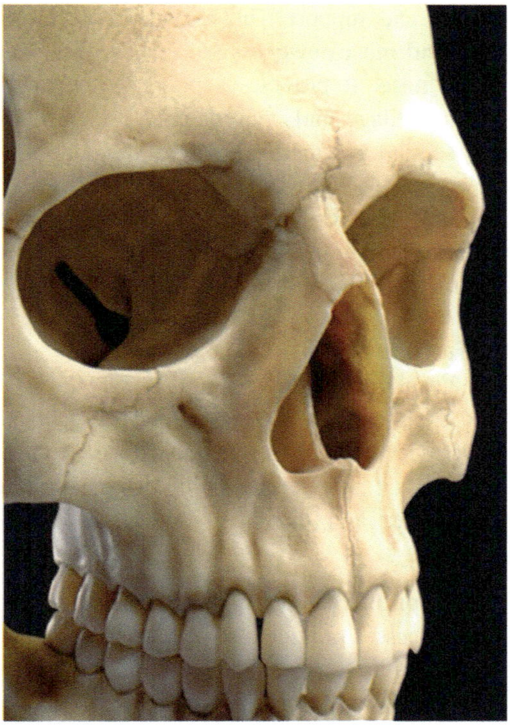

Fig. 2.2 The right frontal process of maxilla and right nasal bone

ii. The nasal bones **do not reach the base of the bony pyramid**. A lateral osteotomy therefore is not made at the posterior margin of the nasal bone. The line of lateral osteotomy is rather made at the **root of the frontal process of the maxilla flush with the anterior surface of the body of the maxilla**.

iii. All bones of the nasal pyramid are **thick at their attachment lines to the face** i.e., **laterally** and **superiorly**. They become **thinner** as they reach their free margins **inferiorly**.

The Frontal Processes of the Maxillae

Each frontal process projects posterosuperiorly, from the body of the maxilla between the nasal bone anteriorly and the lacrimal bone posteriorly. Superiorly it articulates with the nasal part of the frontal bone. It has a thin free margin inferiorly (Fig. 2.2).

The Beginning of the Frontal Process:

The beginning of the frontal process of the maxilla is of particular surgical importance. It emerges and protrudes forwards, from the maxillary body. This is the exact location of the root of the bony nasal pyramid and the accurate site for lateral osteotomy.

The External (lateral) Surface of the Frontal Process:

There are two important anatomical landmarks on this surface:

i. **The Vertical Lacrimal Crest:**

   The external surface is subdivided into a mainly **wide nasal** and a **narrow orbital** surfaces by a vertical ridge called the **vertical lacrimal crest**. The latter continues to become the **inferior orbital margin**.

   The orbital surface has a groove that shares with the lacrimal bone in making the lacrimal fossa, while the nasal surface makes the main body of the base of the bony pyramid of the nose.

ii. **The Tubercle:**

   At the top of the lacrimal crest is a **palpable tubercle** which is a guide to the lacrimal sac.

The sac itself is farther inside the orbit (Fig. 2.2).

Surgical significances:

On performing lateral osteotomies, the osteotomy line starts inferiorly **at the angle between the anterior surface of body of the maxilla** and its **frontal process**. Osteotomy then continues **upwards** and **medially**, just outside, and following the inferior orbital margin and the **orbital crest** till it reaches, and ends, at the **palpable tubercle**. These landmarks are, and should be, palpated at all times during osteotomy.

The **lacrimal sac** is usually quite inside the osteotomy line. It is quite uncommon to injure the lacrimal sac.

Fortunately, even with a little knowledge of the anatomy of the area, an osteotome or a chisel that follows the angle between the body of the maxillary bone and the forwardly protruding frontal process of the maxilla seems quite a safe dictum.

The Internal (Medial) Surface of the Frontal Process:

The internal surface of the frontal process of the maxilla shares in the formation of the lateral nasal wall. It makes the anterior limit of the ethmoid air cells and the middle concha.

2.2.1.4 Inferior Attachments of the Bony Pyramid

The Key Stone Area

The **nasal bones** overlap the superior margin of the upper lateral cartilage in variable degrees. They are firmly attached to each other.

Care must be taken to avoid trauma to this attachment while **rasping a bony hump**. The rasping procedure **should not be vertical**, but must be in an **oblique** fashion in order to avoid disruption of this overlap.

The Fibrous Membrane

There is a dense fibrous membrane which attaches the lower free margin of the **frontal process of the maxilla** to:

- The posterior margin of the **upper lateral cartilage** and
- The **lateral crus** of the lower cartilage.

The membrane has three or four small sesamoid cartilages inside. It has a **free lower margin** that can be **palpated** by the tip of one's little finger when introduced inside the nose. It is felt as a distinct tough margin that can be traced from its origin near the lateral crus till the root of the anterior nasal spine.

This tough membrane makes the **floor of the muscular triangle** i.e., the **hinge area**.

2.2.1.5 Stability and Support of the Bony Pyramid

Should the bony pyramid be only made of the two nasal bones, it would have been a very fragile structure that cannot withstand even the mildest trauma. In fact the nasal bones are the weakest of the pyramidal bones and the commonest to be broken in accidental trauma. The main task of the multiple bones in the structure of the nasal bony pyramid is to provide strength, stability and support. The bony pyramid **is the main and most powerful support to the whole of the nose**. It provides support to the upper lateral cartilage and consequently the cartilaginous septum and the lower lateral cartilages.

Stabilizing Factors of the Nasal Bony Pyramid

Strength and support of the nasal bony pyramid are provided by the following two structures.

The Facial Bones

The Nasal Part of the Frontal Bone

This is quite a thick, compact and strong bone that provides a **superior support** to the root of the nose as it articulates with the two pairs of the nasal bones and the frontal processes of the maxillae.

The Frontal Processes of the Maxillae

Both processes provide a stout base for the bony pyramid as they are made of thick strong bones which are natural continuation of even stronger bodies of the maxillary bones.

The frontal processes provide the largest contribution to the bony pyramid.

The Nasal Bones

They make a nice round caping to the already strengthened base.

The Bony Septum

The bony septum provides a midline support for the bony pyramid. It acts as a strut that connects the apex or the dorsum of the bony pyramid to the bony nasal floor.

The nasal bony pyramid therefore stands on two side walls and a central septal support. All three-walls are strongly held superiorly by the nasal process of the frontal bone.

The size and shape of the bony pyramid is variable in different according to age, ethnic group and in different individuals.

In children the nasal bony pyramid is always small in relation to the rest of the nose which makes it less liable to traumatic fractures than adults.

2.2.1.6 Bilateral Maxillary Asymmetry

The human face is not symmetrical. The two sides of the face are always different in **size** and **shape** in **all individuals**.

Minimal asymmetry is usually overlooked and hardly noticeable. Asymmetry is only noticeable when the difference in size and shape between the two sides is wide.

The two unequal sides is the result of unequal facial bones including the **two maxillae** and the **two nasal bones**.

The frontal processes of the maxillae have the largest contribution to the nasal bony pyramid. Noses of these individuals have **unequal sides** of their bony pyramids, and their noses are therefore **oblique** and **deviated** towards the smaller side.

Facial and nasal asymmetry can be seen both **clinically** and **photographically**, especially in the frontal, the basal and the backwards tilting views (Fig. 2.3).

Consequences of Bilateral Maxillary Asymmetry

A noticeable maxillary asymmetry is associated with the following changes:

Unequal Wide Base of Bony Pyramid

The larger side of the nasal bony pyramid is **lateralized farther** from the midline than the smaller side.

Nasal Hump

An osteocartilagenous hump is almost always associated with the bony pyramidal asymmetry.

Oblique Bony Pyramid

The bony pyramid is oblique **off the midcoronal plane** towards the **smaller side**.

Deviated Bony Pyramid

The bony pyramid is deviated **off the midsagital plane** towards the **smaller side**, away from the midline.

In conclusion, severe bilateral maxillary asymmetry has a consequent aesthetic effects on the nasal bony pyramid so that it becomes both **oblique** and **deviated**. There is almost always an elevation caused by the larger maxilla to produce an **osteocartilagenous hump**.

Differential Diagnosis of Maxillary Asymmetry

The asymmetrical obliquely deviated nasal bony pyramid is to be differentiated from the post-traumatic bony pyramid. In traumatic cases, only the bony pyramid is driven and deviated to one side while the distal cartilaginous part of the nose remains in the midline. The outcome is a **crooked** rather than a deviated and oblique nose. One or both sides of the bony pyramid may show the **irregularities** of the broken bones.

If the traumatic event took place earlier in life, i.e., at the growing age between 8 and 15 years, then **growth** of the traumatized side may become

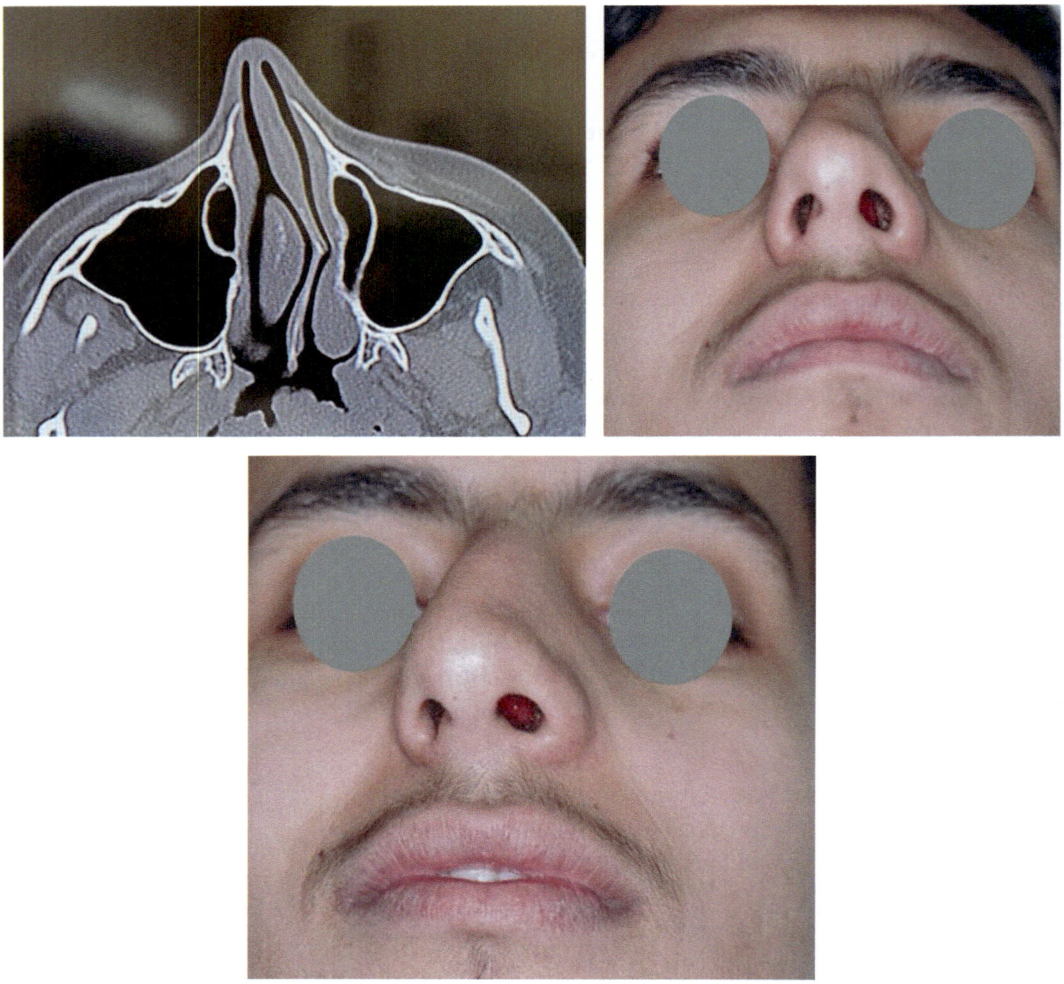

Fig. 2.3 Bilateral Maxillary Asymmetry, the right cheek is wide and low and the left cheek is high and narrow (According to the angle of Radiology and photography)

affected. Growth retardation may also affect the same side of the **upper lateral cartilage**.

The traumatized side therefore may have **less** bony or cartilaginous tissue and looks **depressed** both **clinically** and **photographically** over the area of the nasal bone and occasionally the upper lateral cartilage.

On performing aesthetic rhinoplasty to these post-traumatic cases an additional **augmentation graft** may be necessary over the affected bony or upper cartilaginous side.

This is unlike case of an asymmetrical oblique and deviated nasal bony pyramid which never needs any additional grafts as there are no defective areas (Fig. 2.4).

2.2.2 Anatomy of the Upper Lateral Cartilage the MidVault

The upper lateral cartilage is triangular in shape and has an anteriorly convex body. It constitutes the midvault of the nasal dorsum, as it **extends** from the nasal bones of the **bony pyramid** superiorly to the **lateral crurae** of the lower lateral cartilages inferiorly.

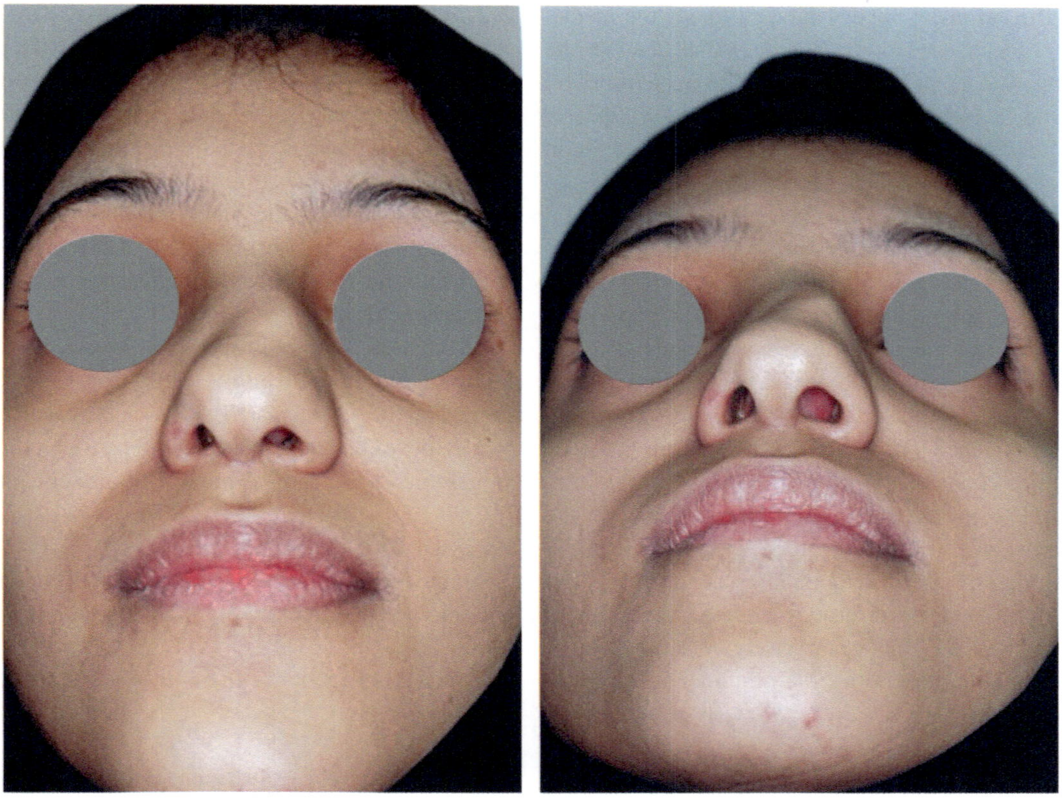

Fig. 2.4 The left deviation of the bony pyramid is secondary to old trauma of the nose. Maxillary asymmetry is minimal

2.2.2.1 Boundaries of the Upper Lateral Cartilage

Superiorly: The upper lateral cartilage is overlapped by the nasal bones on both sides to variable degrees. The cartilages are firmly attached to the nasal bones by fibrous tissues (Key stone area).

Laterally: There is a sheet of dense fibrous tissue that connects the **posterior margins** of the upper lateral cartilage to the bony margins of the nasal aperture i.e., frontal processes of maxillae.

Inferiorly: The **two inferior divisions** of the upper lateral cartilage are overlaped by the right and left **lateral crurae**.

This overlap takes many different anatomical shapes. This is further detailed by Eugene Tardy as shown in his diagrams.

2.2.2.2 Anatomy of the Upper Lateral Cartilage

The **upper lateral** and the **septal cartilages** are therefore considered anatomically to be **one unit**. The **quadrilateral cartilage** of the nasal septum is completely **intergrated** with the **upper lateral cartilage** at the midline summit of its curve posteriorly. One body is thus made by these two components.

At the junction between the three-walled, upper two-thirds of the nose, with the four walled lower third, the body of the upper lateral cartilage bifurcates into two divisions, right and left. They disunite from their intergrated bond with the anterior border of the cartilaginous septum. The latter is now released and becomes the free caudal cartilaginous septum. Despite **inferior**

bifurcation of upper lateral cartilage, the medial border of each division remains attached to the anterior septal border by a **medial perichondrial fold** or **web** that varies in length and width.

Bifurcation of the upper lateral cartilage is an important anatomical necessity for the creation of the weak triangle. The latter marks the junction between the upper three-walled with the lower four walled parts of the nose.

Internally the junction between the upper two-thirds and the lower third corresponds with the junction between the nasal cavities proper lined by the respiratory mucosa, with the vestibular cavity lined with the vestibular skin i.e., the muco-cutaneous junction.

The lower end of the each division of the upper lateral cartilage proceeds under the upper border of the corresponding lateral crus. The inferior margin protrudes into the nasal cavity pushing its lining precisely at the **muco-cutaneous junction**. This prominence is clearly seen inside the nasal cavity and is known as the **limen nasi**.

The **medial perichondrial fold** (web) on each side is similarly covered by a muco-cutaneous fold. This fold bridges the gap between the **limen nasi** and the **septum**. The medial fold meets the septum at an angle of 10–15°. This angle is known as the **anterior angle of the internal valve**. The latter plays an important role in nasal physiology (Refer to physiology of nasal respiration).

The free anterior border of the cartilaginous septum **continues** inferiorly **beyond the muco-cutaneous junction** to end at the supratip area as the **anterior septal angle**. The anterior septal angle supports the floor of the weak triangle and is bisecting it. Together with the rest of the caudal part of the septum they make the superior part of the medial vestibular wall which is covered by **vestibular skin**. This part of the caudal septum is called the **vestibular septum** (see Histology Section).

2.2.3 Anatomy of the Nasal Septum

The nasal septum is a midline structure that divides the nasal cavity into two completely separate aerodynamic systems that regulate the entry and exit of the respiratory air. **The nasal septum is one of the four major areas of Rhinoplasty**. As well as its structural **supportive** and **aesthetic roles** it has an equally important **physiological** role.

The nasal septum is made of **bony, cartilaginous and membranous** parts. The latter is present at the distal part of the septum and is mostly devoid of internal bony and cartilaginous support hence the name is **membranous septum**.

2.2.3.1 The Bony Septum

The bony septum is mainly made of the **vomer** and the **perpendicular plate of the ethmoid bone**.

Other contributions from the surrounding facial bones are:

- The **nasal crest** and the **nasal spine** antero-superiorly from the **nasal** and **frontal bones**.
- The **rostrum** and the **sphenoid crest** postero-superiorly.
- The **incisor crest** with its **anterior nasal spine**. This is a contribution from the palatine process of the maxillary bone. Despite their small sizes, the incisor crest and anterior nasal spine are of special aesthetic importance because of their location at the **naso-labial angle**.

i. <u>The Vomer</u>

The vomer is **the only purely septal bony structure**. It forms the postero-inferior part of the septum. It is almost **trapezoid** in shaped. It extends all the way from the **sphenoid sinus** postero-superiorly to the **incisor crest** of the maxilla antero-inferiorly.

Along this long distance the upper margin of the vomer is attached to the **ethmoid plate** and then the inferior margin of the **septal cartilage**.

ii. **The perpendicular plate of the ethmoid**
It is a thin quadrilateral bone. It comes down from the **cribriform plate superiorly** to be attached to the **vomer** and **septal cartilage postero-inferiorly**. Otherwise it is attached to the surrounding nasal and frontal bones as well as the **sphenoid sinuses**. The weakest part is at the cribriform plate superiorly while the thickest is its inferior articulating border with the septal cartilage.

Surgical Significance:

A **high deviation** in the ethmoid plate may not be seen clinically, or interfere with the nasal airway, but it may **obstruct the midline adjustment of the bony pyramid** after osteotomies.

2.2.3.2 The Cartilaginous Septum

The septal cartilage is surgically the most important part of the whole of the nasal septum, both functionally and aesthetically.

It has an almost **quadrilateral** shape. The four borders are:

i. The **caudal border:** The inferior caudal border is totally subcutaneous and is **part of the membranous septum.** It has an **anterior septal angle** that bisects and supports the weak triangle, and a **posterior septal angle** which is attached to the incisor crest of the maxilla. The posterior angle is the only fixed point of the caudal border.

ii. The **superior border** is almost parallel to the caudal border and is attached to the perpendicular plate of the ethmoid.

iii. The **anterior border** is attached to the internasal suture between the two nasal bones. The anterior border then merges and completely **fuses with the upper lateral cartilage** providing it with support and keeping it straight.
The septum finally leaves the upper lateral cartilage and becomes free in its last one fifth. This distal end is attached to the medial margins of the two division of bifurcated upper lateral cartilage by a right and left **perichondrial web** (see Anatomy of the Weak Triangle).

iv. The **inferior border** is **the thickest** of all borders. The cartilage is thickened at this border in order to **articulate** with the **vomer** and the **incisor crest** successively. This border is **an excellent source of graft material** especially for alar margin augmentation.
The thick inferior border is accommodated in special grooves of the vomer and the incisor crest, where it is attached by firm connective tissue fibers (Gray's anatomy).
If displaced out of these grooves the whole of the caudal cartilaginous septum will be directed to the same side thereby narrowing the anterior valve angle of the **internal valve**. In severe cases it pushes the nasal sill band laterally thus narrowing the **external valve** as well.
The cartilaginous septum is covered on each side by a tough mucoperichondrial layer which in turn is lined by **respiratory mucosa**. The only exception is the **caudal septum** which is covered by a layer of **vestibular skin** on top of the perichondrial layer (see histology).
At the junction between the caudal and proximal parts of the septum the cartilage is thickened to make the **tuberculum of Zukerkandle**. It is located at the junction between the vestibular skin and the respiratory mucosa i.e., at the area of the internal nasal valve. The internal valve is important for the physiology of nasal respiration.

2.2.3.3 The Membranous Septum "The Weak Area of the Nose"

The membranous septum is a midline structure that joins the **fixed** caudal cartilaginous septum to the relatively **mobile** medial crurae of the lower lateral cartilages i.e., the columella.

This part of the septum is devoid of supporting osteocartilagenous structures, hence the name membranous septum.

The caudal cartilaginous septum is covered by vestibular skin (see histology section). It is **the only firm structure** in the membranous septum.

The membranous septum is made of two layers of **loose vestibular skin** which are separated by an abundantly **loose connective tissue layer**. The length of the membranous septum can be increased by pulling it down from the medial crural end.

Contents of the Membranous Septum

The two skin layers of the membranous septum have important structures between them:

i. A pair of Depressor Septi muscles:

   They are also called the alae muscles. They **originate** from the incisive fossae in the **anterior surface of the maxillae** just lateral to the nasal spine. The muscles then run between the two layers of the membranous septum to be **inserted** into the **caudal margin of the cartilaginous septum** as well as the **caudal margins of both medial crurae** of the lower lateral cartilages.

   The main job of this pair of muscles is **fixing** the lower third of the nose during forced respiration. They also have a role in **facial movements** and **expressions**.

The Mobile Tip and The Sliding Tip

Mobile tip is a condition where the nose moves down on smiling. It is also called **animation** if there is more movement of the nose during talking and eating (Fig. 2.5).

While the mobile tip is caused by overactive Depressor Septi muscles, the **sliding tip** is caused by loose membranous septum as well as the overactive Depressor Septi muscles. The lower lateral cartilages and the nasal tip are at a

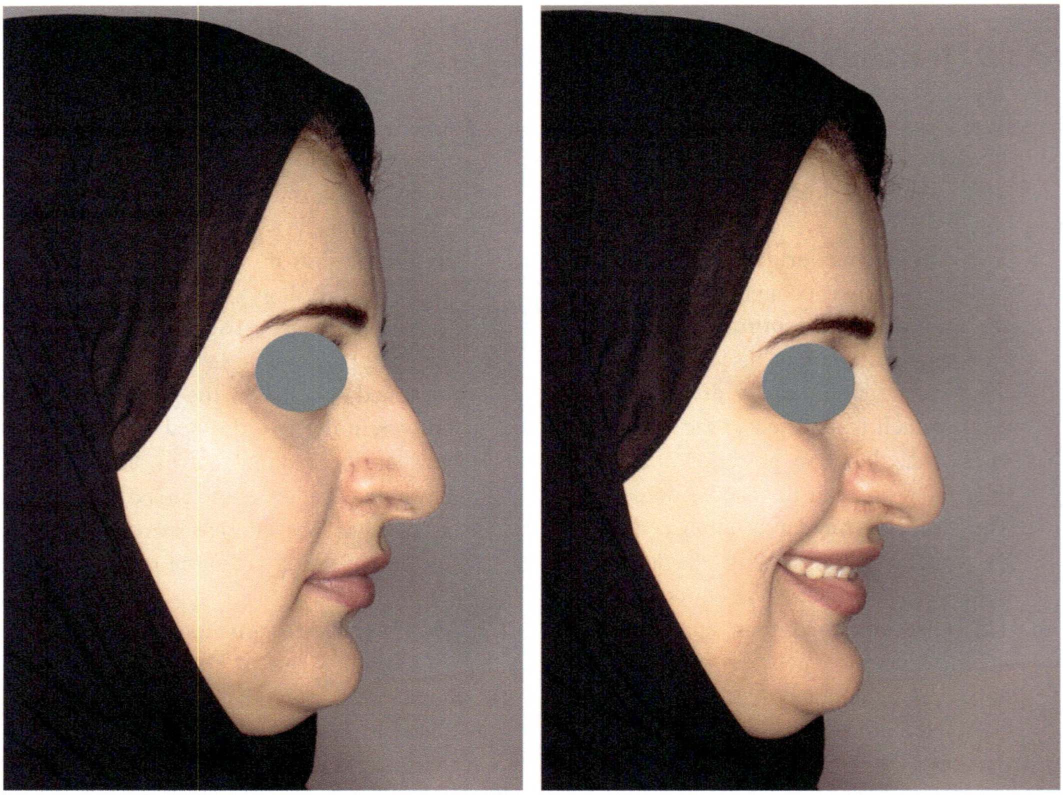

Fig. 2.5 Mobile Tip, nasal tip moves downwards on smiling (inferiorly)

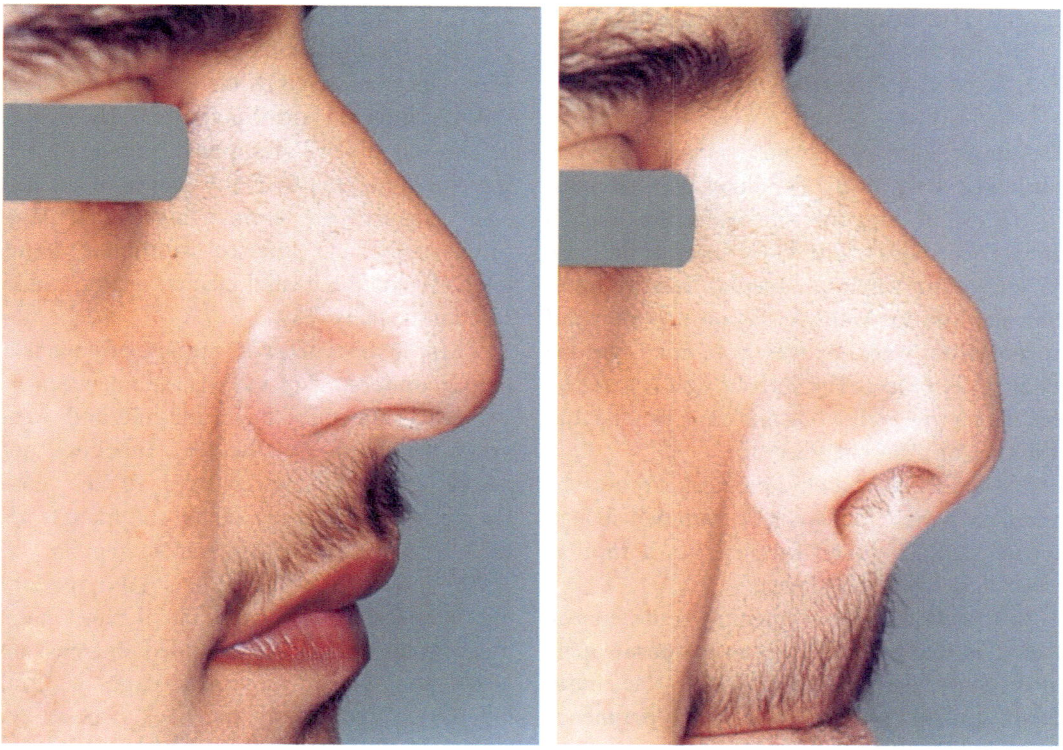

Fig. 2.6 Sliding Tip, nasal tip moves backwards (posteriorly)

lower level than the nasal dorsum. The nasal tip can be pushed up back to its place by the tip of the finger (Fig. 2.6).

ii. A pair of upwards and forwards extensions of the **nasal sill bands** (see History section).

iii. The caudal cartilaginous septum.
The vestibular skin of the membranous septum continues for a few millimeters over the caudal cartilaginous septum i.e., the adherent respiratory mucosa **does not** start strictly at the caudal margin of the septum (see histology).

The caudal cartilaginous septum is considered to be a **vestibular septum** as it is covered by a layer of loose vestibular skin with underlying loose connective tissue (see histology section).

The Weak Area of the Nose

The membranous septum is an **internal weak area of the nose**. The nose lacks support in the area between the caudal vestibular septum superiorly and the columella inferiorly. The membranous septum is the counter part of the weak triangle externally. This weak areas is the transitional area between the solid three-walled upper two-thirds with the relatively mobile four walled lower third of the nose.

2.3 Anatomy of the Lower Third of the Nose

The principle of the four walled structure of the lower third of the nose must be clearly understood before studying the detailed anatomy of each wall. Anatomy of the lower third of the nose includes two main sections:

1. **The Four Walled Structure of the lower third of the Nose.**
2. **Anatomy of the Four Walls.**

2.3.1 The Four Walled Structure of the Lower Third of the Nose

The lower third of the nose is made of **two conjoined rooms**. By definition a room must have six walls, viz., four side walls, a roof and a floor. Each room of the lower third of the nose has only **four walls** i.e., **medial, lateral, anterior** and **inferior walls**. It has **no superior and no posterior walls**, as they both open into the nasal cavity proper. The anterior wall is made by the thin narrow body of the middle crus. The four walls are of **different sizes**.

For aesthetical and physiological purposes the meetings of these four walls are **rounded** and not angulated. Each room therefore has a **tubular** rather than a box appearance.

Inferiorly there is an **opening** in the floor in each side that makes the **external nasal aperture**. **Superiorly** and **posteriorly** the **nasal cavity proper** begins at the **muco-cutaneous junction** (Fig. 2.7).

It is imperative to understand the four walled structure of the lower third of the nose so that the three-dimensional course of the lower lateral cartilages can be clearly understood as they run from one wall to the other. The physiology of nasal respiration is better understood.

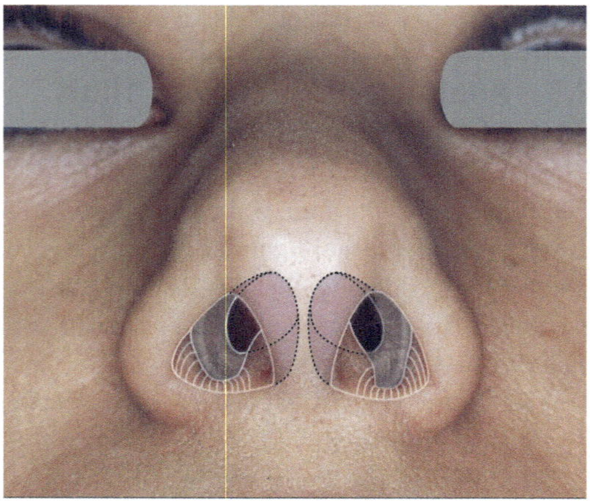

Fig. 2.7 The two nasal aperture tubes

2.3.1.1 The Lower Third is not a Solid-Walled Tube

The walls are covered by the **external** nasal skin and the **internal vestibular** skin. In between these two layers of skin **support is made by firm structures** i.e., the fibrofatty tissues of the **alae nasi** laterally, the **lower lateral cartilages** antrolaterally, the **inferior vestibular bands** inferiorly and the **medial crurae** and the **caudal septum** medially.

These firm structures support only parts of the circumference of the walls. In between the supportive structures there are **soft and weak areas** that allow **for the best functions and aesthetics** of the lower third of the nose. Examples of these areas are the soft triangle, the weak triangle and the membranous septum.

The lower third of the nose is **not** in the form of a **static** and **solid tube**, but it rather has a **pleasant looking kinetic rounded alae nasi** and nicely **curved lower lateral cartilages** that form the medial and lateral crurae as well as **the domes**. Both domes are incorporated in the formation of the utmost beauty of the nasal contours i.e., **the nasal tip**.

The **semi-separation** of the lower lateral cartilages and **the almost full separation** of the alae nasi give them **increasingly more freedom to move** and fulfill their physiological role in nasal respiration and facial expressions.

2.3.1.2 The Physiological Role of the Lower Third

The skin lined aperture tube is known internally as the **nasal vestibule**. Physiologically it is known as the **external valve**. The main role of this valve is to act as a **reservoir** that is capable of expansion to allow for the **maximum amount of air** to come into the nose before it passes through the narrow cleft of the internal valve.

In order to become as **wide** as possible, **internally,** the walls of the aperture tube i.e., the nasal vestibule, has to be as **mobile** as possible. At the same time it maintains an aesthetically **attractive** shape **externally**.

The nasal aperture tube possesses the two most attractive rounded features of the external nose, viz., the nasal tip and the alae nasi.

Internally all of the four walls of the aperture tube are both **concave** and **expandable** to give more room for the inspired air.

The vestibular walls are quite versatile, having great potentials for both **expansion** and **movement.** This is shown in each wall individually and coordinately as they harmoniously move with each other.

Because of the versatility, the strechability and the width of the vestibular walls the surgeon is capable of introducing a nasal speculum, opens it up to expand the vestibule and then moves it around with the vestibular walls to inspect the various parts of the nasal cavity.

It is equally possible for a person to use the tip of his finger to scratch, decrust or remove any loose body inside the nasal vestibule as it moves freely within the expandable mobile vestibular walls.

2.3.1.3 The Shape of the Nasal Aperture Tubes

Each aperture tube is pear shaped with wide, rounded stretchable walls inferiorly made of the ala nasi, nasal sill and columella. Superiorly the walls are narrower, less mobile and rigid walls. These walls are made of the upper lateral cartilage and the caudal cartilagenous septum respectively. Each tube is sliced superomedially and infrolaterally, producing the superior and inferior openings of the nasal aperture tube (Fig. 2.8).

Each pear shape tube is slightly **tilted backwards** as well as **laterally**. The **backwards tilt** is 40–60° to the coronal plane according to the natural angulation of the nose. The backwards tilting of the nasal aperture tube places the vestibular floor in an inferior plane so that the nasal sill is located anteriorly and the vestibular margin posteriorly.

2.3.1.4 The Openings of the Nasal Aperture Tubes

Each aperture tube has a superior and an inferior opening. The **inferior opening** has the free external aperture margins, while the **superior opening** has margins that can only be seen internally.

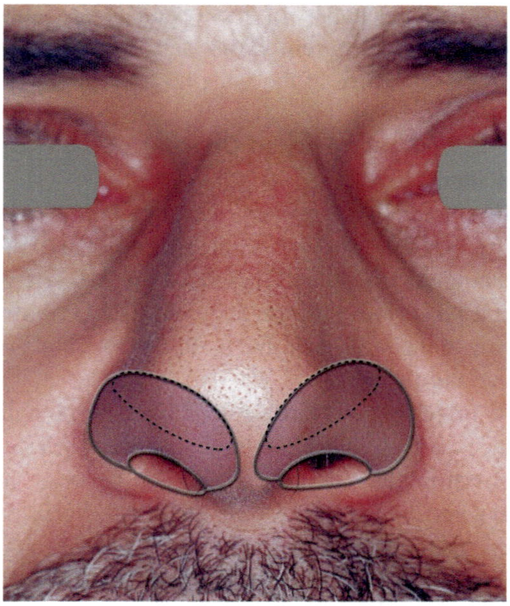

Fig. 2.8 The superior aperture openings are looking towards each other while the inferior openings are looking away from each other. The pear-shaped aperture tubes sliced by the upper and lower openings

The **two inferior** openings, right and left, are mainly facing an **inferior** direction with slight **lateral** and **forwards** inclinations. This is due to the effect of the alar muscles on the alae nasi that place them in the **alar flare** position.

Both inferior openings are therefore looking away from each other i.e., downwards, forwards and laterally.

The two **superior openings** on the other hand are mainly facing a superior direction with more **medial** and **posterior inclination**. This is due to the narrow upper end and the strictly vertical medial wall of the aperture tube i.e., the nasal septum.

The two superior openings of the aperture tube are therefore **looking towards each other** i.e., **upwards, backwards** and **medially**. It must be realized that both the superior and inferior openings have the **same direction of angulation towards the midline or the sagital plane**.

The superior openings have more acute angles of rotation towards the midline than the inferior openings.

The angulations of the openings are quite **variable** in **different noses** and in **each individual aperture** of the same nose.

The Triangular Shaped Opening of the Four Walled Tube

Despite of its **four walls**, the superior and inferior openings of the nasal aperture tubes are **triangular in shape.** They have **medial, lateral** and **posterior** margins. They do not have **anterior margins**. This is due to the **narrow body** of the **middle crus**.

Inferiorly the cartilaginous body of the middle crus is **short of reaching the inferior aperture margin**. Instead the gap between the **ala nasi**, in the lateral wall, and **medial crus**, in the medial wall, is bridged by the skin fold of the **flat (soft) triangle**, covering and bypassing the anterior wall.

Superiorly the cartilaginous body of the middle crus is short of reaching **the superior aperture margin**, instead the gap between the lateral crus and the nasal septum is bridged by the protruding margin of the **limen nasi**.

The dome is the **narrowest** and **thinest** part of the lower lateral cartilage. The **flat (soft) triangle** below each dome and the **weak triangle** above both domes are created.

A **triangular external aperture** is **aesthetically** more atractive than a quadrangular one. On the other hand a **triangular internal aperture** is **physiologically** important to enhance the speed of inspired air.

The Inferior Margins of the Nasal Aperture Tube

The aperture tube ends inferiorly by the free margins of its walls i.e., the **alar rim** laterally, the **nasal sill** posteriorly and the **lateral columellar margin** medially (Fig. 2.9).

The transition between the **ala nasi** and the **nasal sill** is made of a soft fold of unsupported skin i.e., the **rim-sill fold**.

Likewise the transition between the **lateral columellar margin** and the **alar rim** is made by the soft skin of the **flat triangle (soft)**.

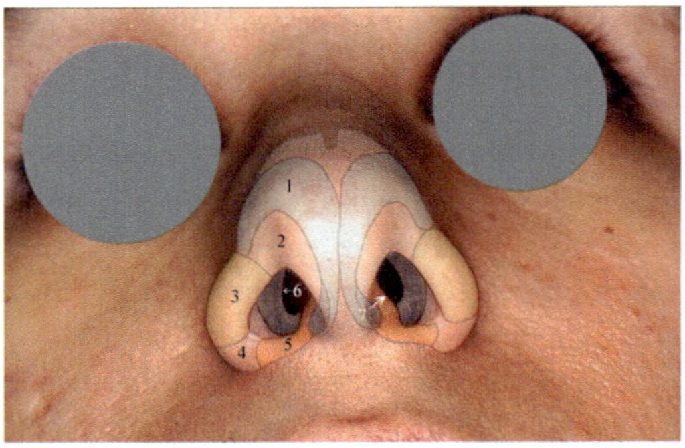

Fig. 2.9 The two nasal aperture tubes: showing the inferior margins (No. 3, 4, 5 and 7) and the posterior vestibular margin as part of the superior margin (No. 6) Lower Lateral Cartlidge (No. 1). Flat Triangle (No. 2). Inferior Alar Margin (No. 3). Rim-Sill Fold (No. 4). Inferior Vestibular Band (No. 5). Posterior Vestibular Margin (No. 6). Lateral Columellar Margin (No. 7)

Although the inferior margins of the nasal aperture form a complete circle, yet the **true supportive structures only share in parts of this circle**.

These supportive structures are the **alar rim,** laterally, the **nasal sill band** posteriorly and the inferior margin of the **medial crus** medially.

Soft areas of skin complete the circle of the aperture margin i.e., the **flat (soft) triangle** anteriorly, the **rim-sill fold** postro-laterally and the **soft posterior columellar fold** medially (Fig. 2.9).

The Superior Margins of the Nasal Aperture Tube

The aperture tube is limited superiorly by the **muco-cutaneous junction** i.e., between the vestibular skin and respiratory mucosa at the **septum medially**, the **limen nasi anteriorly**, just **anterior** to the **inferior turbinate head laterally** and the **posterior vestibular fold inferiorly**.

The limen nasi, as described by Zukerkandel in 1892, lies at the **inferior border of the upper lateral cartilage** exactly at the **muco-cutaneous junction** (Fig. 2.10).

The superior opening thus has two **prominent margins** antro-laterally and posteriorly, and two **flat** areas at the nasal septum **medially** and just

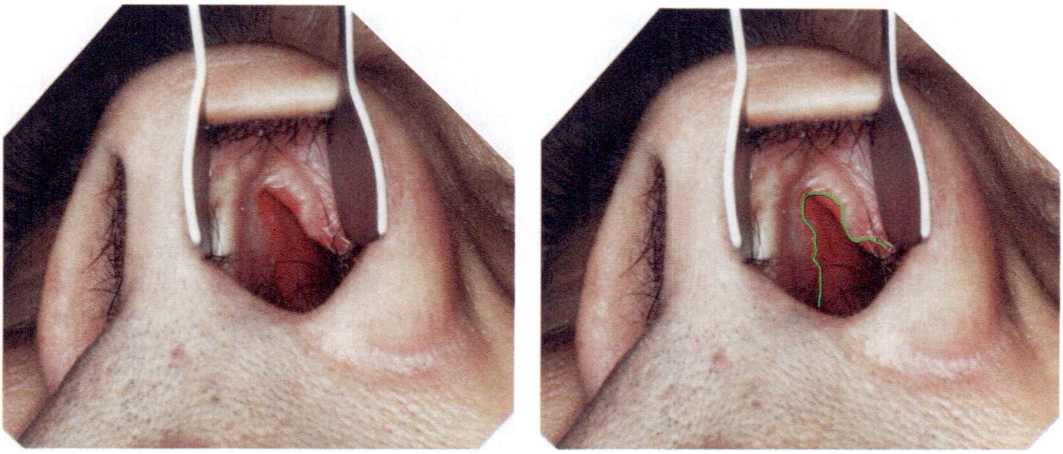

Fig. 2.10 The left limen nasi and the caudal septum meet at the muco-cutaneous junction anteriorly. The muco-cutenous junction is seen at the limen nasi and on the septum as an irregular line

anterior to the inferior turbinate head **laterally** in between the two prominent margines of the limen nasi and the posterior vestibular fold.

Surface Anatomy of the Superior Internal Aperture

The superior opening is represented **externally** at the line that starts from the **midpoint of the weak triangle** just below the anterior septal angle, to the **scroll area** at the junction between the upper and lower lateral cartilages, then finally to the **posterior half of the superior alar groove**.

The Four Walls of the Nasal Aperture Tube

Each aperture tube is formed by four walls, medial, lateral, anterior and inferior wall. There are **no posterior or superior walls** to allow for the passage of air. The **anterior** wall is made by the **dome** of the middle crus. There is a **common medial wall** made by the **columella** and the membranous septum. The **lateral wall** is made by the **ala nasi** and the **lateral crus**, while the **inferior wall** is made by the **vestibular floor** and the inner surface of the **flat triangle**.

The anterior and the lateral walls are seen both externally and internally, while the inferior and medial walls are mostly seen inside the nasal vestibule. The external surfaces of the flat triangle and the columella are the only parts that are seen externaly from the floor and the medial walls successively.

The morphological description of the aperture walls is better done **from within the cavity** of the aperture tube in order to have better correlation with their functions.

The Anterior Wall

The anterior wall is made by the concave cartilage of the **dome of the middle crus.** The maximum curvature of the lower lateral cartilage takes place at the dome.

The anterior wall therefore has a **deeply concave surface**. The **depth** of the concavity of the anterior wall is **increased further** by the posteriorly protruding skin fold of the **flat (soft) triangle inferiorly** and the protrusion of the **limen nasi superiorly**. The curved anterior vestibular wall therefore has two prominent margins, the limen nasi **superiorly** and the flat triangle **inferiorly**.

The main characteristic of the anterior wall is that it is **the deepest** of all of the four walls.

The muco-cutaneous fold of the limen nasi is short and has a more acute angle with the vestibular wall, while the skin fold of the flat triangle is longer, and looks like a lower shelf that gives the anterior wall a reversed, curved L-shaped appearance.

In order to shave the vestibular hair (vibrecae) of the anterior wall during surgery, the surgeon must **evert** the inner wall of the flat triangle by a sharply pronged alar retractor and counter-push it externally by his ring or middle finger.

The Lateral Wall

The lateral wall is made by the body of the **lateral crus** and the **curved inner surface of the ala nasi.** The body of the ala nasi is **free** from any crippling attachments. It has a long **free inferior margin**. The **superior margin** lies against the soft area of the muscular triangle, while the **posterior margin** is partially attached to the orbicularis oris through its upper half. The ala nasi is therefore **attached to the nose only by muscle fibers** and **skin tissues**. The alae nasi are **the most mobile** of all of the **aperture walls** and the rest of the nasal structures in general. They expand upwards, backwards and laterally. The degree and force of expansion depends on the amount and speed of air needed in conditions of quite and forced respiration (Refer to the chapter of the Physiology of Nasal Respiration).

From the free alar margin inferiorly the curved lateral alar wall extends **backwards** to the **muco-cotaneous** line, just in front of the anterior end of the inferior turbinate at the bony nasal margin. This is the location of the entrance to the posterior wider part of the **internal valve**.

Superiorly the lateral alar wall is followed by the lateral crus before reaching the muco-cutaneuos junction at the limen nasi.

The Inferior Wall

The inferior wall is made by the **vestibular floor posteriorly** and the inner surface of the **flat triangle** as it folds backward, **anteriorly**. In fact, the external nasal opening is no more than a **hole in the anterior part of the vestibular aperture floor**.

The **flat triangular surface** runs horizontally from before backwards till it ends up in its free posterior margin. The detailed anatomy of the flat triangle is explained in a separate chapter.

The vestibular floor is lined by a very loose hair bearing skin and essentially takes a **horizontal plane**. It is limited by two distinctive elevated margins, the **nasal sill** anteriorly and the **posterior vestibular margin posteriorly**.

The **nasal sill band** lies horizontally at the anterior end of the vestibular floor. It is firmly attached to the superfacial layer of the **orbicularis oris** muscle **inferiorly**. Its external **anterior surface** is covered by a firmly adherent, thin, smooth non-hair-bearing **skin layer**.

From the prominent ridge of the nasal sill, the loose vestibular skin slopes **posteriorly down** to make the horizontal vestibular floor which again curves **upwards** and **backwards** to make the second palpable prominent ridge i.e., the **posterior vestibular fold**. This fold is seen curving in a **semi-lunar fashion** from medial to lateral **at the level of the bony nasal margin**. It is **not** attached to this margin, but rather separated from it by a loose connective tissue layer. The posterior vestibular margin is the exact location of the **muco-cotaneous junction**.

The **posterior vestibular margin** therefore has double relations to the **nasal sill band**. It lies **posterior** to the nasal sill and at a **higher level** i.e., **more prominently elevated**. This is due to the fact that the **nasal bony margin** is more posterior and higher than the **orbicularis oris muscle**. The vestibular floor on the other hand remains in the horizontal level as an inferior wall.

The **high elevation** of both the nasal sill and the posterior vestibular margin **moves them out of the horizontal plane** so that the **nasal sill** becomes the **posterior margin** of the **inferior opening** of the nasal aperture tube, while the **vestibular** margin becomes the **inferior margin** of the **superior opening** of the nasal aperture tube.

The Medial Wall

Both nasal aperture tubes share a **common medial** wall which at the same time separates them from each other. It is made by the **columella**, the **medial crurae** of the lower lateral cartilages and the **membranous septum**. The medial aperture wall is the **least concave** of all four aperture walls.

The **medial crurae** have their lateral concave surfaces facing the vestibular cavity inferiorly, while the **membranous** septum is almost straight in the midline. The **lower half** of the membranous septum is made by a segment of abuntantly loose connective tissue layer which is sandwiched by two layers of equally loose skin, while its **upper half** is made by the most inferior skin covered caudal cartilagenous septum i.e., the vistibular septum.

2.3.2 Anatomy of the Four Walls

I. Anatomy of the **Medial Wall**
The medial wall separates the two chambers of the lower third of the nose. This wall is made of the following structures:

A. The **columella**
B. **The medial crurae** of the lower lateral cartilages
C. **The membranous septum** (see nasal septum).

II. Anatomy of the **Lateral Walls**

A. The **lateral crurae** of the lower lateral cartilages
B. The **alae nasi**

III. Anatomy of the **Anterior Wall**
The anterior wall is made by the **two conjoined middle crurae**

IV. Anatomy of the **Inferior Wall**
The inferior wall of the nose is made of two sides, right and left. On each side the inferior wall is made of

A. The **Vestibular Floor**
B. The **Flat Triangle**
The **Nasal Opening**: Each nasal opening is no more than a gap in the nasal floor that separates the vestibular floor from the flat triangle.

2.3.2.1 Anatomy of the Medial Wall

The Columella

Columella in latin means little or small column. The columella is a unique anatomical structure that contains cartilages, bands and muscles i.e., the medial crurae, the Inferior Vestibular Bands (I.V.B.) and the Depressor Septi muscles. The columella is attached to the Orbicularis Oris via the Inferior Vestibular Bands.

Anatomy of the Columella

The columella is covered by the **external nasal skin**. It begins **posteriorly** from the upper lip at the filtrum and ends **anteriorly** at an imaginary transverse line that joins the **posterior angles of both flat** (soft) **triangles**.

Shortly after its commencement, the inner surface of the external columellar skin becomes adherent to the inferior borders and the lateral surfaces of both medial crurae. The columella is therefore subdivided into two components:

(a) **The Firm Anterior Segment:**

This is the main segment of the external columella. It **starts** from the beginning of the posterior borders of the two medial crurae and **ends** at the transverse line that joins the posterior angles of the two flat triangle.

Compared with the posterior soft fold this segment of the columella is **longer**, **wider** and is **firmly supported** by the curved most inferior parts of the **bodies** and the **inferior margins** of the medial crurae (Fig. 2.11).

As the lower borders of the medial crurae curve laterally, they push the external columellar skin laterally to make the **lateral columellar margins**.

The outer convex surfaces of the inferior parts of the bodies of the medial crurae are exposed inferiorly to become attached to the external columellar skin. They can be seen externally as clear subcutaneous structures.

Bifid columella is an easily diagnosed surface anatomical condition.

(a) **The Soft Posterior Fold:**

This is a short segment of the columella that **starts** from the firltrum of the upper lip and **ends** at the posterior ends of the **inferior borders** of the medial crurae. It is made of **soft unsupported skin** that has a **rounded** external surface and is **narrower** than the anterior firm segment.

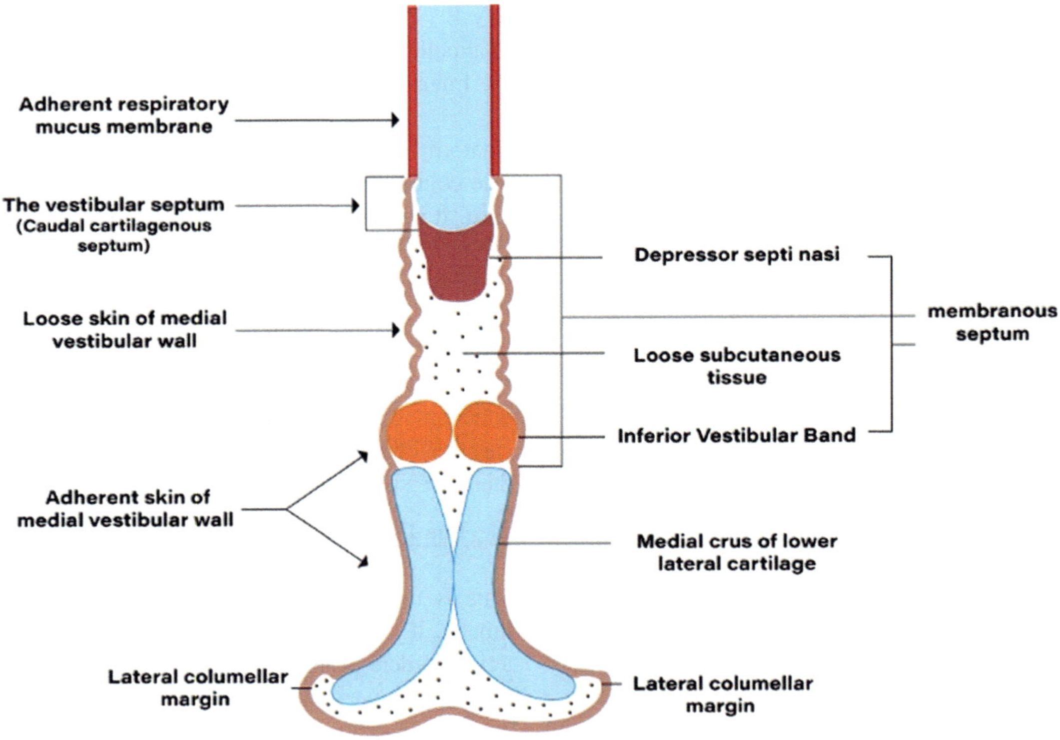

Fig. 2.11 Coronal section in the columella and the membranous septum

The posterior soft fold covers the gap between **medial crurae** anteriorly and the **Orbicularis Oris muscle** posteriorly.

Surgical significance

i. The presence of important anatomical structures.

Despite the lack of support to the walls of the soft segment, yet it contains two important structures:

- The Depressor Septi Muscles.
- The anterior nasal spine which provides deep support to the soft fold.
- The naso-labial angle.

Any changes in the anatomy or physiology of the content of the soft fold will directly affect the aesthetics of the nasofrontal angle.

- Long caudal septum will lead to a protruding columella with a wide naso-labial angle. The nasal opening of the affected side is distorted and narrowed.

  A small nasal spine may lead to a rectracted columella and an acute naso-labial angle.
- Strongly active Depressor Septi muscles will lead to unpleasant animation of the nose.
- Skin of the lateral columellar margin.

Exactly at the lateral columellar margin the thin adherent hairy vestibular skin is immediately followed by the thick less adherent hairless external skin.

This junction is the exact location for the incision to explore the medial crus of the lower lateral cartilage in the process of delivery of the lower lateral cartilages.

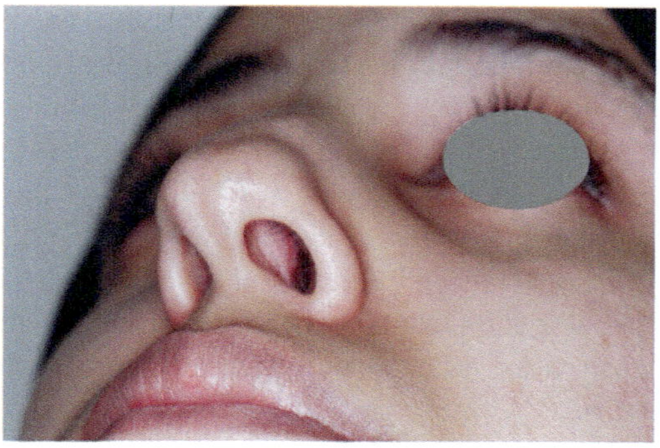

Fig. 2.12 Bifid Columella

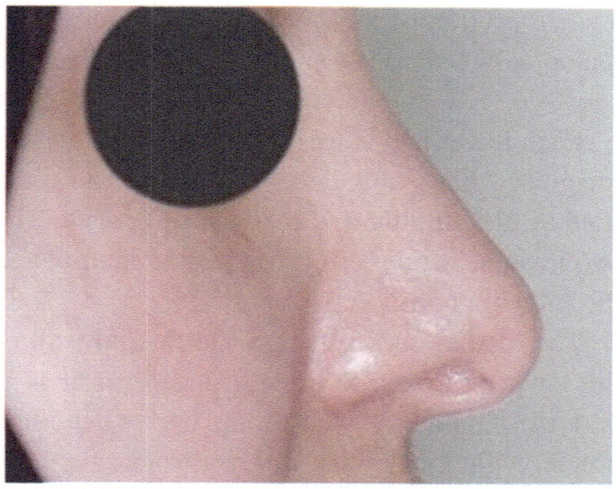

Fig. 2.13 Protracted Columella

Aesthetic Conditions of the Columella

(a) **Grooved or Bifid Columella**
The inferior margins and bodies of the medial crurae are semidetached from each other producing an unpleasant bifidity of the columella (Fig. 2.12).

(b) **Protracted columella**
This is a condition where the columella is at a lower level than the alar margins. A large nasal spine and/or long caudal cartilaginous septum may lead to **elongation of part or all of the columella** below the level of the alar margins on both sides. The medial vestibular wall is unpleasantly exposed (Fig. 2.13).

(c) **Hanging Columella**
This is a condition where there is downwards curved projection of the columella **at the level of the medial crurae**, just anterior to the posterior columellar fold. Much of the lateral surfaces of the crural bodies are exposed below the level of the alar margins. The medial crurae look like the handle of a ladies bag, hence the name "hanging" columella. Although the caudal septum may have a contribution to this deformity, yet many cases may require direct reduction of the medial crural size. This condition is to be differentiated from the protracted columella. Combination of the two conditions may present in the same nose (Fig. 2.14).

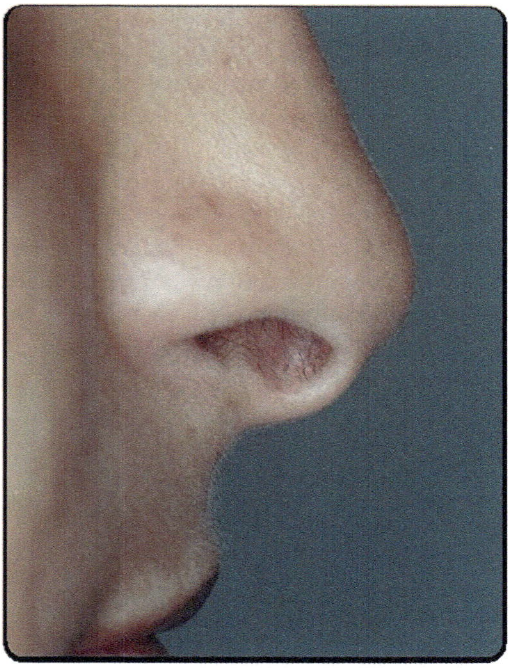

Fig. 2.14 Hanging Columella

The Medial Curae

The two medial of the lower lateral cartilages are conjoined in the midline to be part of the medial wall of the lower third of the nose. The lower lateral cartilages, right and left, are also known as the **major alar cartilages**. The author finds the term lower lateral cartilage is more appropriate as the cartilage's only contribution to the ala nasi is a small portion of its lateral crus i.e., there is no major contribution to the ala nasi by this cartilage.

Each lower lateral cartilage is divided, by two imaginary lines into three components i.e., the **medial**, the **middle** and the **lateral crurae**. The two imaginary lines are known as the **medial** and the **lateral genua**.

The **medial crus** is part of the **medial wall** of the lower third of the nose. The **lateral crus** is part of the **lateral wall** while the two middle crurae, alone, make the **anterior wall**.

Location of the Medial Crus

The medial crus is a **rectangular** structure that lies essentially in the **sagital plain** with its long axis antro-posteriorly, parallel to the lower border of the columella. It is the **thickest** of all three crurae of the major alar cartilage. It is called medial crus mainly because it is **located in the medial wall** of the nasal aperture tube. It also lies medial to the lateral crus.

Both medial crurae are juxtra adherent to each other at their convex surfaces to make a united though midline structures that share in the formation of the columella.

The medial crurae are sandwiches by the vestibular skin. Their inferior border can always be **palpated** and sometimes clearly **seen** on the external skin throughout their course. They are felt as rigid margins when pushed against a midline caudal septum.

Anatomical Course of the Medial Crus

The medial crurae **begin** posteriorly, just anterior to the vertical part of the **inferior vestibular bands** (Refer to histology).

They continue to run forwards with **their inferior parts abutting the inner surface of the external comullar skin** and their **medial surfaces facing each other**. The body of each medial crus is curved like a saucer that has a deep gutter between the **lateral columellar margin** inferiorly and the **inferior vestibular band** superiorly (Refer to Histology).

The **posterior** and **superior** margins are **in close contact with the inferior vestibular band**. The latter curves upwards (inwards) from its transverse course on the aperture margin to run **on the medial vestibular wall along the posterior** then **superior** margins of the medial crus.

The two medial crurae **end** anteriorly at the **medial genua** as they begin to separate and depart from each other to become the **middle crurae**.

The medial crus is **the only crus that is closely related to the nasal aperture margin.** It is directly involved in the making of the medial aperture margin.

The location of the medial crurae with their characteristic courses are a **fixed anatomical finding**. The medial crurae are **the most predictably stable** in their anatomical **locations** and **courses** of three crurae.

Anatomical variations may affect their **length**, **width, thickness**, **curvature** and the **distance from each other** but **rarely** their **location** and **course**. Even if they protrude inferiorly, as in cases of hanging or protruding columella, they continue to be in the **most inferior** part of the medial vestibular wall.

Vertically the medial crus extends from the skin margin **inferiorly** to a variable distance inside the medial vestibular wall superiorly.

Curves of the Medial Crus

The bodies of the medial crurae are **curved** both vertically in the **sagital plane** and antro-posteriorly in the **axial plane** along their long axes. These two planes of curving produce two concave vestibular surfaces covered with hair-bearing vestibular skin. These are equally two juxta-opposed convex surface that are attached to each other by tough connective tissues. In other words the medial crural bodies are **curved in all their axes** especially near to their margins.

The degree of curving in the **axial** plain i.e., antro-posteriorly determines the extent of the **medial crural prominence** posteriorly, while the degree of the vertical curving in the **sagital** plane decides the **width** of the columella inferiorly i.e., the distance between the two **lateral columellar margins**. This is because the vertical curving affects the lower borders of the medial crurae which tend to project **laterally** rather than inferiorly. This helps in making of the lateral columellar margins.

The convex surfaces of the extreme lower parts of the bodies of both crurae are facing directly downwards. This is clearly seen externally. The increase in the convexity and in the distance between the two crura will lead to a wider columella. This may appear externally as a midline grove i.e., bifid columella.

The degree of curving in the body of the **right** medial crus is usually different from that of the **left** one. This fact is clearly shown in the **different** medial crural prominences, as well as in the columella externally.

The Lateral Columella Margin

The **inferior margin** of the medial crus protrudes laterally, rather than inferiorly, due to the curved body of the medial crus (Fig. 2.15).

The lateral columellar margin is therefore made by the inferior margin of the medial crus.

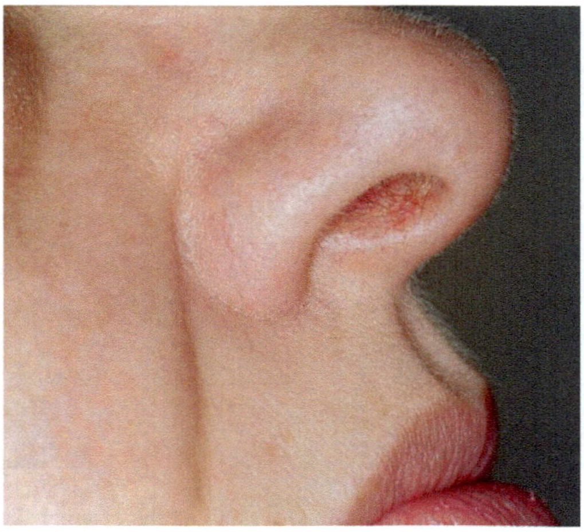

Fig. 2.15 Lateral Columellar margin caused by lateral crural prominence. Note the light reflex

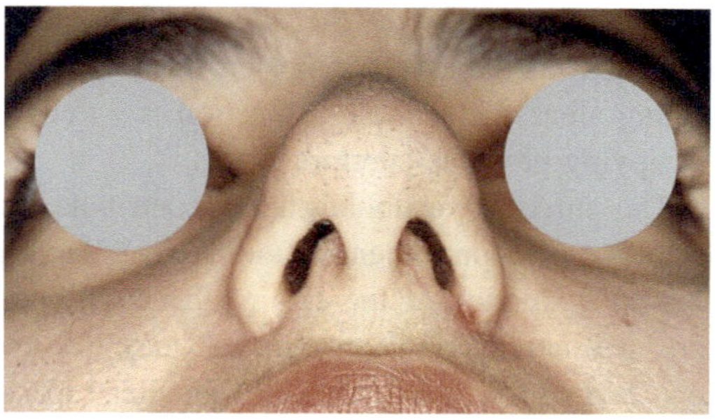

Fig. 2.16 Right and left lateral crural prominences caused by the posterior margins of the medial crurae

The Lateral Crural Prominence

The lateral crural prominence is made of the **posterior margin** of the medial crus as it protrudes inwards inside the nasal cavity.

The size and degree of curving in the body of the medial crus determined the extent of encroachment on the size of the nasal aperture.

A dislocated caudal septum may push the medial crus further inside the nasal cavity (Fig. 2.16).

The Skin Cover of the Medial Crurae

The lateral concave surfaces of the medial crurae are covered with hair bearing thin adherent vestibular skin. The inferior margins and the exposed lower parts of their convex bodies are covered by smooth less adherent hairless external skin.

The thin adherent hair bearing vestibular skin on the lateral concave surface of the medial crus is therefore, immediately and suddenly followed by the smooth less adherent hairless external skin over the inferior margin of the medial convex surface of the lower part.

Surgical Significance

The medial crural prominence may have an effect on the **shape** and **size** of the nasal aperture as follows:

The posterior margins of the medial crurae may overproject into the nasal aperture wall.

Encroachment upon the **shape** of the nasal aperture wall takes place postero-medially producing unaesthetic wall projection as well as occupying precious aperture space.

The inferior vestibular band contributes to further crural prominence (vid supra). During surgical reduction of the size of the nasal aperture, **a normal** crural prominence may become **too large** for the available smaller space. Reduction of the medial crural prominence becomes then necessary.

Exploration of the Medial Crus

For surgical exploration incision is made **exactly at the lower margin of the medial crus** i.e., at the junction between the thin adherent hairly **vestibular skin** and the thick less adherent hairless **external skin**.

The medial crus is tucked **immediately under the lateral columellar margin**. The surgeon gently places the **edge** of the knife at the **junction** between the external skin and the vestibular skin. Using the **side** of the knife the thick hairless loose external skin is pushed medially in order to place the knife **edge** exactly on the inferior border of the medial crus (Fig. 2.17).

A Transcolumellar Stitch is Sometimes Used to Reduce the Medial Crural Prominence (Refer to Surgical Section)

2.3.2.2 Anatomy of the Lateral Wall

Each of the two lateral walls of the nasal aperture tube is made by the two main structures:

(a) **The lateral cruae of the lower lateral cartilages**.
(b) **The ala nasi**.

The Lateral Crus

The lateral crus is the **largest** and **widest** of the three crurae of the lower lateral cartilage. It is called the lateral crus as it is **lateral to the medial crus**, and most importantly because it is located in the **lateral wall** of the nasal aperture tube. It is variable in size, shape, position, thickness and consistency according to age, sex and ethnicity.

Each lateral crus has **inner** and **outer** surfaces which are completely covered by the **vestibular** and the **external skin** successively i.e., the **lateral crurae are entirely subcutaneous** both internally and externally.

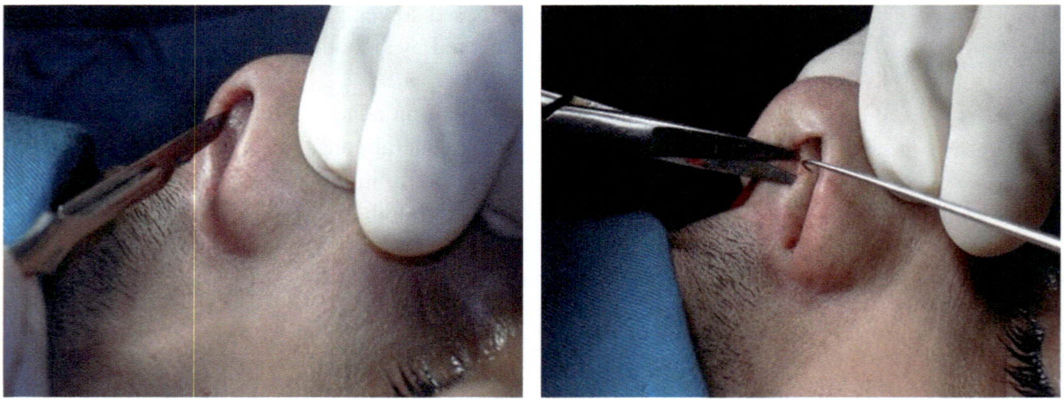

Fig. 2.17 Exploration of the medial crus incision is at the junction between the vestibular skin and the external skin

The size final look of each lateral nasal wall is determined by the size, shape and the three-dimentional location of each lateral crus and ala nasi.

Anatomical Course of the Lateral Crus

The lateral crus **begins** at the **lateral genu** (see anatomy of the middle crus). It is partly responsible for the formation and shaping of the lateral wall of the lower third of the nose.

The lateral crus has **superior, inferior** and **posterior** borders. The **inferior** and **superior** borders of the lateral crus have **similar courses**: upwards, backwards and laterally, yet they have **different relations**.

The **inferior border** starts from the **inferior end** of the **lateral genu**. It runs upwards, backwards and laterally abutting the ascending curve of the superior margin of the ala nasi, to share in the formation of the anterior third of the **superior alar groove**. It then departs gradually **away** from the ala nasi. It **ends** by curving upwards to make the posterior border of the lateral crus.

The **superior border** starts from the **superior end** of the **lateral genu**. From this point it runs upwards, backwards and laterally, **overlapping the lower border of the upper lateral cartilage all along its course**, before it finally **ends** by curving downwards to make of the posterior border.

The superior border of the lateral crus varies in its course from one person or one side to the other so that it may **curve suddenly, rapidly** or **smoothly upwards** to give the body of the lateral crus its characteristic large size. It is this part of the lateral crus that is surgically excised in cephalic trimming of the lateral crus if indicated.

The **inferior borders** of **all three crurae**, medial, middle and lateral, continue with each other as **one smooth uninterrupted arc**. This can always be observed during surgery while performing a rim incision.

The **posterior border** of the lateral crus marks the anterior border of the muscular triangle of the nose. It is connected to the frontal process of the maxilla by a **tough fibrous membrane.** There are 3-4 sessamoid cartilages usually present within this membrane.

The lower margin of this membrane can be palpated by the tip of the little finger when introduced into the nose. It is felt as a clearly distinguished margin high up on the lateral nasal wall above the nasal vestibule.

In some individuals there is a **cephalic extension** or **tail**, to the lateral crus, with the sessamoid cartilages.

This helps as an additional supporting factor, known as the hinge effect. It plays very little role in the nasal aesthetics and is better avoided during surgery.

Curves of the Body of the Lateral Crus

The **body** of the lateral crus is usually **convex laterally** i.e., externally. The relative degree of its convexity in conjunction with the convexity of the dome has an important effect on nasal aesthetics.

The **less** the convexity of the **body** of the lateral crus the more prominent is the **domal** convexity and the nasal **tip** projection and vice versa.

If the body of the lateral crus is less convex or even concave, it will show externally as a smooth slope or depression that is followed by a nicely prominent convex dome and nasal tip.

Conversely, should the convexity of the lateral crus be higher than the dome, the tip appears low and less projected.

The degree of convexity of the body of the lateral crus not only varies from one nose to the other but also from one side of the same nose to the other.

As well as the curving of its body, the lateral crus has **two other curves** along its **posterior** and **superior borders**.

(a) **The posterior border**:

This border tends to fold inwards and protrudes sometimes as a **prominence** inside the lateral vestibular wall. This can clearly be seen clinically in some individuals.

(b) **The superior border**:

The superior border of the lateral crus overlaps the lower border of the upper lateral cartilage.

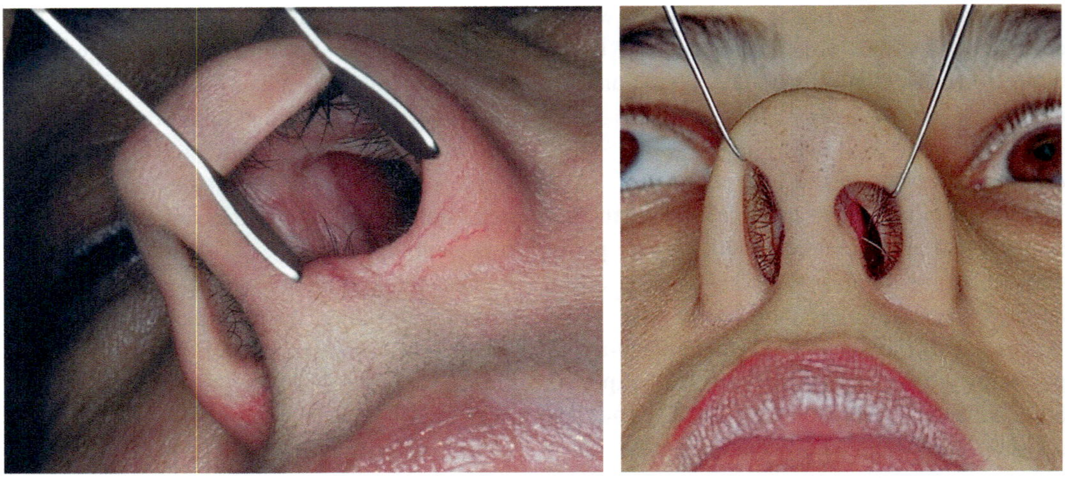

Fig. 2.18 The left limen nasi at the muco-cutaneous junction

The details of this overlap are of particular clinical interest and importance.

The lateral crus overlaps the lower margin of the upper lateral cartilage by a **fold** of cartilage rather than a simple marginal overlap.

The superior margin of the lateral crus is **rolled in** so that in fact this margin is looking **downwards**, rather than upwards. Together with the **lower border** of the **upper lateral** cartilage, they both protrude into the nasal cavity to form the prominence of the **limen nasi**. This is the site of the **muco-cutaneous junction** i.e., the nasal valve and the upper limit of the aperture tube (Fig. 2.18).

The **outcurving** of the upper lateral cartilage and **incurving** of the lateral crus is called the **"Scroll"**.

At this junction the two cartilages are well supported by strong connective tissue fibers that firmly hold them together. The scroll area may be the site of a bulky nose.

Surgical Significance

- The curve of the superior margin of the lateral crus lies at the roof of the **intercartilaginous fold** which is the site for the **intercartilaginous incision** for rhinoplasty. The intercartilaginous fold is covered by a vestibular skin, and it is **not** the site of the muco-cutaneous junction.
- **Aging** affects the connective tissue that holds the upper and lower cartilages. It becomes thinner and weaker, and there is gradual unfolding of the upper margin of the lateral crus.

  The relations between the two cartilages changes into various other forms, and the lower third of the nose gradually droops **caudally**.
- The scroll area of overlap may be the site of a bulky nose that may need surgical reduction.

The Skin Cover of the Lateral Crus

The lateral crus is covered by skin both externally and internally. The nature of skin on both sides is quite different from each other.

The internal vestibular skin cover of the lateral crus has special characteristics that makes it uniquely different from the rest of the vestibular skin.

These characteristics are almost the same in all individuals. They do not change with age, sex or race. They are summarized in being delicately **thin**, tightly **adherent and** smoothly **hairless**.

The internal skin cover of the lateral crus is **the most delicate** of the whole of the vestibular skin, as it is tightly **adherent** directly to the perichondrium.

It is **the only skin** in the nasal vestibule that is **devoid of hair** (vibrecae). The hair line is a rough guide to the lower margin of the lateral crus if it is to be surgically explored.

The **external skin** on the other hand is the **thickest** and **greasiest** of all of the external nasal skin. Unlike the internal skin, the external skin thickness **varies with the age and race** for each individual.

Immediately under the **epidermal** layer, and adherent to it, there is a smooth, thick and tough **fibrous tissue layer**of the **dermis**. This is followed by the **subdermal** layer. The latter acts as a plane of cleavage that separates the external two layers from the **middle** and the **lateral crurae**. This plane is bridged by **bands of fibrous tissue** and contains variable amounts of **fat**.

The subdermal **fibrofatty tissue layer** makes it easier for the surgeon to dissect the lateral and the middle crurae off the external skin using a pair of scissors to cut these bands i.e., the external skin is **less adherent** to the middle and lateral crurae than the vestibular skin.

Removing the fibrofatty layer, after full delivery of the lower lateral cartilages i.e., **defattening**, helps greatly in reducing the **size** and the **bulk** of the lower third of the nose.

The Alae Nasi

The alae nasi are also known as the **external naris**. They are the two outwards protrusions on the sidewalls of the lower third of the nose. As the name linguistically implies, they are two **winglike** structures that form the major part of the lateral wall of the nasal aperture tube.

The alae nasi are major contributors to nasal aesthetics. They give the side wall of the lower third of the nose its characteristic appearance. Their beautiful **round bodies** must not be hidden by a large bulky nasal front, nor they should be too large, thick and bulky. The **alar margin** should be at an acceptable aesthetic level.

As well as their **aesthetic** effect, they play a major role in the **physiology** of nasal respiration and in various facial expressions. The **size**, **shape** and **position** of the alae nasi are important not only to the nasal aesthetics but also to allow **sufficient** amount of air to enter towards the **right direction inside the nasal cavity.**

It is important for the bodies of the alae nasi to be solidly firm in order to withstand the force of the inspired air stream. The bodies are made of **tough fibrofatty tissues** which give **natural** and **strong attachments** for the small muscles of the nose.

The Size and Shape of the Ala Nasi

The ala nasi has a **firm** and **fixed** curved shape. It is usually **wider posteriorly** than anteriorly i.e., winglike especially in long noses. It takes the shape of a quarter of the wall of an egg with its wider part posteriorly placed. In Asian and African noses it may take a more rounded shape.

The size, shape and position of the alae nasi affect the overall size and shape of the nose i.e., the aesthetics of the lower third of the nose.

Position of the Ala Nasi "The Alar Flare"

The ala nasi tends to have very characteristic **stable position** which is maintained by the tone of the facial muscles. It becomes dynamically active during respiration and in various facial expressions.

The body of the ala nasi tends to be **tilted backwards** and **rotated outwards** i.e., **everted**. At the same time it is maintained in a highly **elevated** position. The **tilted**, **everted** and **elevated** position of the alae nasi is known clinicaly and aesthetically as the **alar flare** (Fig. 2.19).

This graceful position is maintained and dynamically moved by the **direct** and **indirect** actions of the facial muscles.

The firm bodies of the alae nasi are acted upon **directly** by **special alar muscles** that move them **inwards** and **outwards** as well as **upwards** and **downwards**. These are the compressors, the

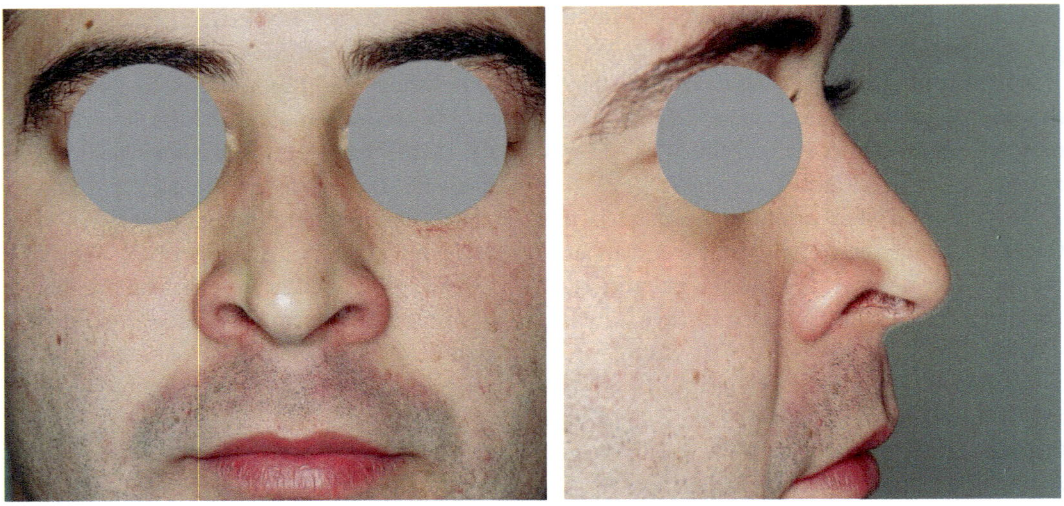

Fig. 2.19 The alar flare, alae nasi are tilted backwards and rotated outwards (Everted). Note that superior and posterior alar grooves

dilators, the elevators as well as the orbicularis oris.

The **levator labii alaeque nasi** and the **alar part of the nasalis** are attached to the **outer surfaces** and **lower borders** of the alae nasi. They are the main contributors to the **alar position and flare**. Their contraction will lead to further elevation, eversion and tilting of the alae.

The **orbicularis oris** is attached to the **posterior margin** of each ala nasi i.e., the alar base. Laughing and whistling may widen and narrow the nasal aperture.

The alar flare is very important for the nasal physiology. This position of the alae turns the external opening i.e., the **external valves** so that they look **forwards** and **laterally** which is the same direction of the **internal valves** that look **backwards** and **medially**. The inspired air thus has a direct path from the external to the internal valves (Fig. 2.19).

Indirectly the alae nasi are acted upon by other facial muscles e.g., the levator and depressor labii muscles as well as the zygomaticus major and minor muscles.

The level of the **alar margin** in relation to the **columella** and the **nasal sill band** is of significant **physiological** and **aesthetical** values. The alar margins should be **slightly higher** than the lateral columellar margin without exposing the internal vestibular skin over the medial crus.

Not only the **size** and **shape** of the ala nasi but also its degree of **backwards tilting**, **eversion** and **elevation** that decide the final level of the alar margin.

The Alar Grooves

They are also known as **alar creases**. This is a very important feature of the nose anatomically, physiologically and aesthetically. Starting from these grooves the lateral nasal wall bulges out to make the external naris. The extent of bulging and grooving is affected by the size of the ala nasi, the thickness of the skin and the general shape of the nose and face. They are variable according to age, race and from one nostril to the other.

It is of great surgical and aesthetic importance to differentiate anatomically between the two components of the alar grooves:

The Superior Alar Groove

The superior alar groove is an **Alar-Nasal** groove i.e., between the **superior margin of the ala nasi** and the **lateral wall of the nose** which includes, from before backwards, the **flat triangle**, the **lateral crus** of the lower lateral cartilage and finally the **muscular triangle**. It **starts** from the **alar margin** at the **lateral angle of the flat triangle** (soft) anteriorly, curves smoothly **upwards** and **backwards**, then **downwards** and **backwards till** it reaches **the upper lip** posteriorly.

The Posterior Alar Groove

The posterior alar groove is an **Alar-Lip groove** i.e., a groove between the **posterior margin of the ala nasi** and the **upper lip**.

It **starts** superiorly at the **posterior end of the superior alar groove** where it curves **sharply downwards** in an almost right angle, and **ends** inferiorly **at the inferior aperture margin** where the rim-sill fold begins.

It has a **shorter** and **less curved** course than the superior alar groove.

The superior alar groove is the result of the **medial inclination** of the **superior border** of the firm body of the ala nasi abutting the inferior margin of the **lateral crus** and then the soft area of the **muscular triangle**.

By the same token, the **backwards tilting** and **elevation of** the **posterior border** of the ala nasi abutting the relatively soft **orbicularis oris** muscle results in the **posterior alar groove**.

The more the **eversion** of the ala nasi the deeper is the **superior** alar groove and vice versa, while the more the **elevation** and **backwards tilting** the deeper is the **posterior** alar groove.

Skin Cover of the Alae Nasi

The external surface and lower margin of each ala nasi is covered with **smooth hairless** and **glistening** skin. The skin is rich in sebaceous glands and is usually **thick** and **tightly adherent**.

Internally the ala nasi is covered by **thin adherent hair-bearing** vestibular skin.

Relations of the Alae Nasi

The body of the ala nasi is bounded by the **superior** and **posterior grooves** superiorly and posteriorly, while inferiorly it has the rounded and firm free **alar margin**. The alar margin extents from **lateral angle of the flat (soft) triangle** anteriorly to the **lateral end of the rim-sill fold** posteriorly (see chapter of nasal gaps).

The Bodies of the Alae Nasi

The **external surface** convexly curves antro-posteriorly with maximum curvature just before reaching the posterior groove.

The most **anterior margin** of the ala nasi delineates the lateral margin of the flat triangle.

The **superior curved margin** forms the characteristic **superior alar groove,** which is related in its anterior third to the inferior border of the **lateral crus**, while the posterior two-thirds marks the **inferior border of the muscular triangle.**

The superior two-thirds of the **posterior margin** is firmly attached to the **orbicularis oris**, while the lower third is separated from the upper lip by a wedge of soft tissue extension of the **rim-sill fold** (see chapter of Soft and weak areas).

The Physiological Role of the Alae Nasi

The alae nasi constitute the active, kinetic lateral walls of the external nasal valves. The **widely placed** and **firm consistency** of the alae nasi as well as their relative **free mobility** are the important factors that enable them to perform their valuable physiological role.

It is important for the external naris to **remain widely** open at all times to allow for the maximum air entry during normal and forced respiration, both in the conscious and subconscious states e.g., during sleep or coma.

This goal is only achieved by having a well-supported firm alar walls that do not collapse by the force of air entering during inspiration, thus maintaining the patency of the external valves.

The alae nasi are the most mobile parts of the external nose. Their mobility are very important for nasal respiration and various facial expressions e.g., smiling, snarling, sarcasm, anger and discontent.

The small alar muscles are **directly** responsible for their movements. Other facial muscles may have an **indirect** contribution to their activities. The free **lateral** mobility of the alae nasi, as in smiling, is allowed by the **stretchable rim-sill folds** and the **loose skin of the vestibular floor**.

On the other hand, freedom for **eversion**, **elevation** and **backwards tilting** is allowed because of the **free margins** of the alae against the **soft areas** of the **muscular triangles** superiorly and the **rim-sill folds** and the **orbicularis oris muscle** posteriorly.

The role of the external valve i.e., alae nasi in the physiology of nasal respiration is explained in details in the physiology of nasal respiration.

Factors Affecting the Alar Flare

The stable position of the alae nasi i.e., the alar flare, may be influenced by many factors. The **firm** and **fixed rounded shaped bodies** of the alae nasi are the **first** major contribution to the appearance and stability of their flare. The size and shape of the alae nasi as well as the size and shape of their closely related **lateral crurae** of the lower cartilage also play a role.

Nevertheless by definition, the **second** most important factor that is responsible for the **positioning** of the alae nasi is the **tone and actions of the facial muscles**. They are by far the most major contributing factor not only for maintaining the **alar flare** but also for enabling the alae to perform their physiological role.

This fact is better appreciated and clearly demonstrated in the case of a long-standing **unilateral facial palsy**. In these case there is loss of the **direct** and **indirect** muscular support to the ala nasi on the affected side (Fig. 2.20).

The alae nasi therefore **loses its elevated**, **backwards tilted** and **everted** position. Consequently it droops **downwards**, **forwards** and is **inverted medially** i.e., the alar flare is lost and is almost reversed.

The **alar margin** is at a **lower level** and is **turned medially** (inwards). The **nasal aperture** consequently becomes **smaller** and looks **downwards**, **backwards** and **medially** instead of upwards, forwards and laterally (Fig. 2.20).

The **superior alar groove** is at a **lower level**, more **forwards** and **shallower**, while the **posterior alar groove** is more **medial**, **forwards** and **flatter**. The cheek skin fold with the lip and nose i.e., the **naso-labial fold is lost** (Fig. 2.20), while the level of the nasal sill is minimally affected.

The **physiology** of nasal respiration is devastated. The **amount** and **speed** of air entry is reduced both at rest and in forced respiration. Both the **external** and **internal valves are reduced in size, paralyzed and malaligned** i.e., their position to each other is changed. The **active widening** of the alae nasi i.e., the external valves, as well as the **active counter-action** to the natural collapse of the internal valves is therefore lost during normal and forced respiration e.g., in moderate efforts, physical exercise or in the circumstances of respiratory distress.

The air column from the external valve is no longer at the same direction to that of the internal valve, even during comfortable respiration.

2.3.2.3 Anatomy of the Anterior Nasal Wall the Middle Crurae

The anterior nasal wall is **only present in the lower third of the nose**. The lower third is the only part of the nose that has **four walls**. The upper two-thirds of the nose has three-walls.The whole of the nose i.e., the upper two-thirds and the lower third, is divided into two similar, but not identical, halves by the nasal septum.

The anterior wall has **aesthetic** and **functional** roles:

(b) **Aesthetically** the main feature of the anterior wall is the creation of the gracefully projecting **nasal tip**, which is the most beautiful part of the nose.

(b) **Functionally**: The anteriorly convex middle crurae are part of the external valve of the nose.Together with the large sized alae nasi, they widely expand the size of the vestibular cavity during inspiration (Refer to the physiology of nasal respiration).

The Middle Crurae

The anterior wall of the lower third of the nose is made solely by the two convex bodies of the **middle crurae**.

The middle crus is the intermediate cartilaginous segment of the lower lateral cartilage that

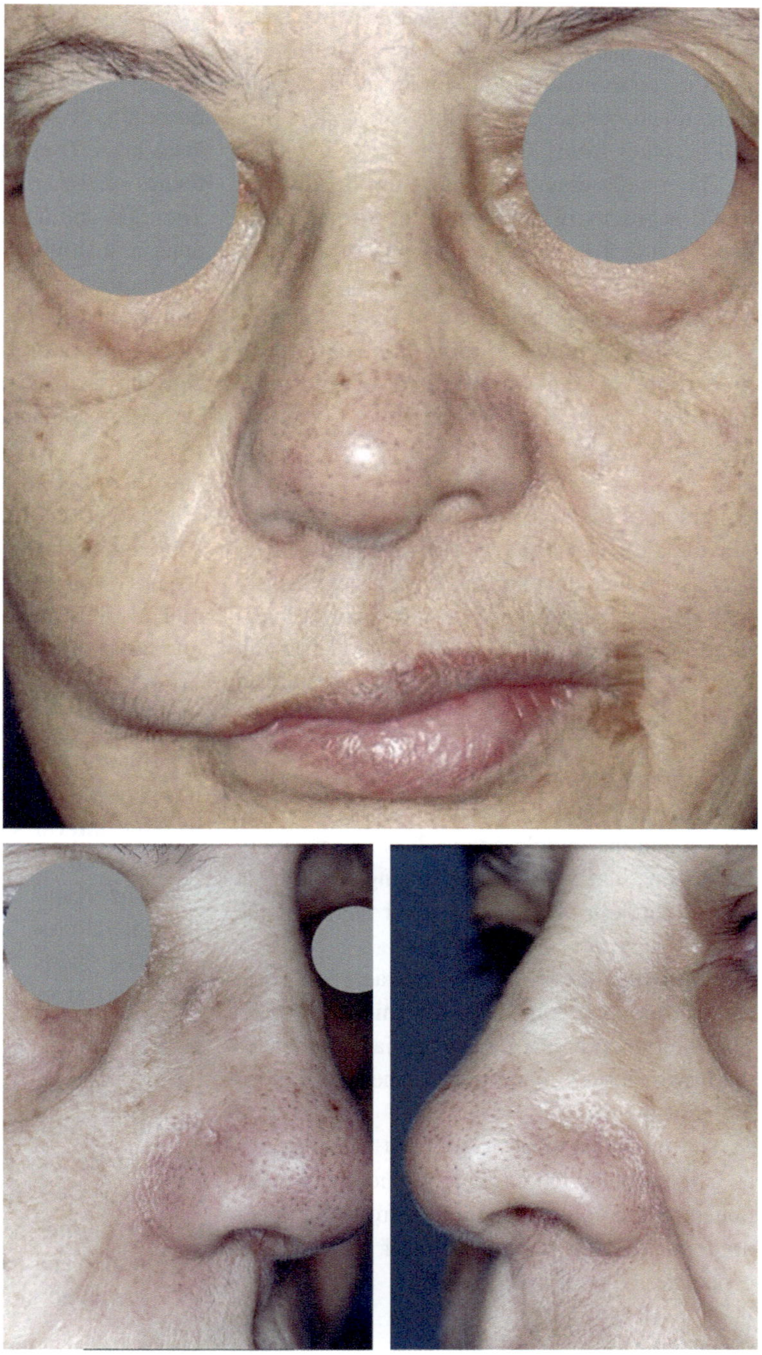

Fig. 2.20 Right facial palsy: the right alar flare is lost with flattening of the superior and posterior alar grooves

communicates the medial crus in the medial nasal wall to the lateral crus in the lateral nasal wall.

In its course the middle crus loses its attachment to all of the surrounding fixed structures and becomes **totaly free.**

The middle crus is **the most important aesthetic segment of the whole of the external nose** as it is the skeletal foundation of the nasal tip.

Understanding the anatomy of the middle crus is **the key for understanding the anatomy of the whole of the lower third of the nose** including the surrounding gaps (Refer to the Soft and Weak Areas of the nose).

Definition of the Middle Crus

The middle crus is **the free segment** of the lower lateral cartilage that makes the **anterior nasal wall** i.e., the **dome**. It is the **intermediate segment** between the medial and the lateral crurae.It begins at the **medial genu** and ends at the **lateral genu (Fig. 2.22)**.

Definition of the Medial Genu

The Medial Genu is the junction between the medial and the middle crurae. It is an imaginary curved line that joins the medial angle of the flat (soft) triangle to the apex (inferior angle) of the weak triangle.

At this line the two medial crurae **evert from each other** to become the **free middle crurae**. The inferior margin of each medial crus leaves the nasal aperture margin at the medial angle of the flat triangle.

The **medial angles** of both flat triangles can be both **seen** and **felt** externally. Sliding an index finger on the columella, starting from the upper lip forwards, the point of medial crural divergence can be easily palpated (Fig. 2.22).

Definition of the Lateral Genu

The lateral genu is the junction between the **middle** and the **lateral** crurae. It is **an imaginary curved line** that joins the **lateral angle of the weak triangle** to the piont of meeting between the **inferior border of the middle crus** with the **upper border of the ala nasi**. At this line the eversion process of the middle crus is completed (Fig. 2.22).

P.S. The medial and lateral genua are two **immaginary lines**. There are **no angulations** at these lines. They follow the curved surface of the bodies of the crurae i.e., they are **curved lines**. The right and left **medial genua** meet with each other at a **single point** of contact in the midline. This point is located at the maximal convexities of the curved bodies at the ends of the two medial crurae. This marks the last contact between the two **crurae**, after which they are completely separated from each other.

The Three-Dimensional Movements in the Body of the Middle Crus

Although both **the medial** and **the lateral** crurae are in **two almost parallel sagital planes** in the **medial** and **lateral nasal walls**, yet they have **four anatomical differences**:

(1) As the name implies the **medial** crus is present in a sagital plane which is **medial** to that of the lateral crus.
(2) The **medial surface** of the medial crus is the **lateral surface** of the lateral crus i.e., **everted**.
(3) The medial crus is at a **lower** level than the lateral crus.
(4) The lateral crus slightly **medially rotated** i.e., towards the midline.

The **middle crus** therefore is not in the form of a simple fold. Its body undergoes an upwards **helical** (spiral) movement. **Three concurrent movements** take place in free space in order to transform the **medial, inverted**, **lower** and **strictly sagital** medial crus to the **lateral, everted**, **higher** and **rotated** lateral crus.

These three movements are:

(1) **Lateral curving**: The middle crural body curves laterally in order to **cross over** from the **medial wall** in the paramedian plain, to the **lateral wall** in a more lateral plane. Not only does the middle crus **curve laterally** but it also **folds** upon itself, at the dome, to come **backwards** as the lateral crus. While

curving laterally and folding backwards the body of the middle crus gradually **everts**. The **medial surface** of the **medial** crus therefore becomes the **outer surface** of the **middle crus** and the **lateral surface** of the **lateral crus**.

(2) **Cephalic Elevation**: to reach from the **lower** medial crus to the **higher** lateral crus, the body of the middle crus makes an upwards helical movement.

(3) **Medial Twisting:** The body of the middle crus twists medially so that the superior border of the lateral crus is more medial to the inferior border.

Details of the Three-Dimensional Movements

Detailed knowledge of the curves and twist **in the body** of the middle crus is essential for the understanding of the surgical anatomy of the nasal tip and the two anatomical gaps around it i.e., the weak and the flat (soft) triangles.

It is important to realize that **the three movements of the lateral curving, the cephalic elevation** and **twisting**, take place **simultaneously**, from the beginning of the middle crus at the **medial genu** and continue throughout its body until it finally **ends** at the **lateral genu.**

Lateral Curving of the Middle Crus:

Lateral curving is the most **significant** and **important** of the three movements due to its magnitude.

In order to reach from the medial to the lateral crus, the middle crus has to curve laterally, then folds upon itself backwards making the dome.

This process of external backwards folding leads to the **eversion** of the **medial surface** of medial crus to become the **external surface** of the **middle** and the **lateral** crurae.

The **medial crus** is in a **sagital plane**, while the **dome** is in a **coronal plane**. The **lateral crus** is **halfway** between the **sagital** and the **coronal** planes.

The Angle of Anterior Folding:

The angle of anterior folding measure the extent of forwards then backwards rotation of the lateral crus from the location of the medial crus. Maximum folding takes place at **the dome** of the middle crus.

The degree of folding varies from one ethnic nose to another e.g., 150° in African and Asian noses as compared to 170° in Caucausian nose (Fig. 2.21).

Cephalic Elevation of the Middle Crus

Cephalic elevation is the upwards movement of the middle crus in its helical journey from the **inferiorly** placed medial crus to the **superiorly** placed lateral crus. As this movement takes place in the **sagital plane,** it is best appreciated when observed from a **lateral view**.

The upwards helical movement in the body of middle crus causes an upwards tilting of the body of the lateral crus which is the **angle of elevation.**

The Angle of Elevation:

As elevation starts from the **medial genu** and ends at the **lateral genu**, the angle of elevation is therefore measured between these two lines.

In a direct **lateral view**, the **first line** for the elevation angle is drawn along the **long axis of the medial crus** and passes by the **mid point of the medial genu.** This called the **medial crural line**. The **second line** is drawn along the long axes of the lateral crus and passes by the **mid-point of the lateral genu.** This is called **lateral crural line.** The **anterior angle** between these two lines demonstrates the exact degree of upwards movement of the lateral crus as it elevates from its original location at the medial crus i.e., **the angle of elevation** (Fig. 2.21).

The angle of elevation ranges between 45 and 75°. It varies according to the nasal height, age and ethnicity. It may vary from one side of the nose to the other.

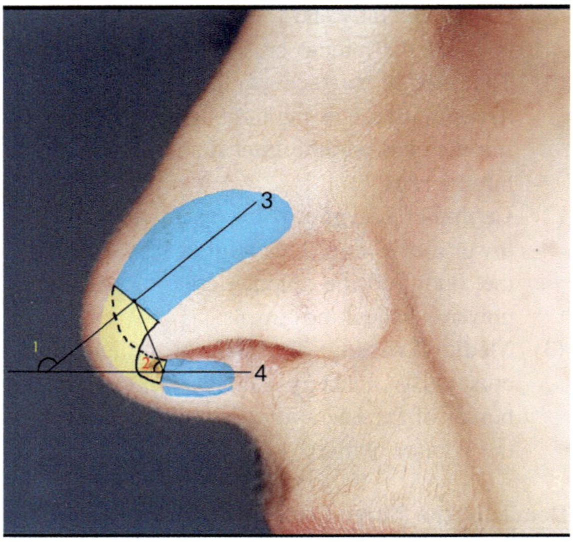

Fig. 2.21 1. The angle of anterior folding 2. The angle of elevation 3. Lateral Crural Line 4. Medial Crural Line

Young children, Africans and Asians, have wider angles, while long Caucasian noses have narrow angles.

Twisting of the Middle Crus

The body of the middle crus twists **medially**. This leads to the **medial rotation of the lateral crus** so that its **superior border** becomes **medial** to the **inferior border**.

The Angle of Rotation:

Twisting of the middle crus causes **rotation** of the lateral crus.The degree of medial displacement of the superior border of the lateral crus as compared to the inferior border decides the angle of rotation.

For direct comparison, it helps to look simultaneously at the vertically placed **medial crus** in which the location of its superior border is in the same vertical line as the inferior border. There is **no horizontal displacement**. In contradistinction, the location of the **superior border** of the lateral crus is medial to that of the **inferior border**.

The angle of rotation is best appreciated in the **backwards tilting views**.

The **Angle of rotation** is measured by the **angle between** the **body of the lateral crus** and **the sagital plane**. A central nasal septum is usually a good guide to this plane. The angle of rotation ranges between 20 and 45°.

The African or Asian noses have **more twist** in their middle crurae and therefore flatter lateral crurae. Their **angles of rotation are wider** than the Caucasian noses.

The Course of the Middle Crus

The two middle crurae **start** at the **anterior ends of the medial crurae** i.e., at the **medial genua**, where the two medial surfaces begin to separate from each other by the process of gradual **eversion**. The two medial surfaces are gradually exposed **from below upwards** like a **blossoming flower** (Fig. 2.22).

All three moves of the middle crurae i.e., lateral curvings, cephalic elevation and medial twisting proceed **from below upwards**. Eversion of the **inferior border** of the middle crus **begins before** the **superior border**, as it takes a **longer** journey for it to reach to the lateral nasal wall.

The **inferior border** therefore has a **different course** from that of the **superior border.**

The Course of the Inferior Border of the Middle Crus:

The **inferior border** of the middle crus **begins** exactly at the **medial angle of the flat (soft) triangle**. This point can be both **seen** and **palpated** externally by the tip of an index finger. It is the anterior end point of the medial crus and external skin part of the columella.

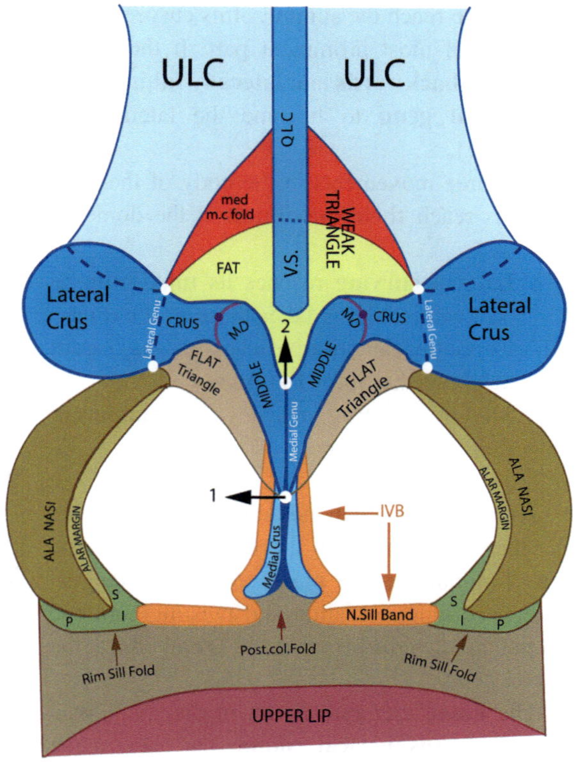

Fig. 2.22 The lower two-thirds of the nose. ULC: Upper Lateral Cartledge. QLC: Quadrilateral Cartledge of Nasal Septum. VS: Vestibular Septum (Caudal). Med M.C Fold: Medial Muco cutaneous fold. MD:Mid-Domal Line and Mid-Domal Point. IVB: Inferior Vestibular Band. Rim-Sill Fold S: Superior Segment. Rim-Sill Fold I: Inferior Segment. Rim-Sill Fold P: Posterior Segment. 1: The starting point of the middle crural body eversion (inferior margins). 2: The end point of the middle crural body eversion (superior margins)

From this point of the medial genu, the **inferior border** curves **upwards, forwards** and **laterally,** marking the medial border of the flat (soft) triangle. As it folds to make **the dome,** it forms the **anterior angle** of the flat triangle and then the **posterior border** of the **flat triangle**. It finally reaches the **superior border of the ala nasi**. The inferior border of the middle crus **ends** at this point to become the **inferior border of the lateral crus.** The latter briefly abuts the superior border of the ala nasi before curving upwards away from it (Fig. 2.22).

The Course of the Superior Border of the Middle Crus:

The **superior border** of the middle crus **begins** exactly at the **apex (inferior angle) of the weak triangle**. This point can be both **seen** and **palpated** by the tip of an index finger, just inferior to the anterior angle of the nasal septum.

At this point the two superior borders of the **medial crurae** end by departing from each other to become the **middle crurae**.

Each superior border continues its course **upwards, forwards** and **laterally** till it reaches the **highest point** of the middle crus, i.e., **the dome.** It then moves **upwards, backwards** and **laterally** making the sidewall of the weak triangle, before it finally **ends** at the **lateral angle** of the weak triangle. At this point the superior border of the middle crus becomes the superior border of the lateral crus.

The Nasal Tip

The nasal tip is the most graceful and beautiful midline structure. It is made harmoneously by the **two domes** as they are held together by the interdomal fibrous bands and the covering skin.

The Dome

The dome is defined as the **highest**, **most prominent**, **exposed**, **free** and **unattached** fold of the lower lateral cartilage.

Each dome begins with the formation of the middle crus from the medial genu. The body of each dome curves **upwards**, **forwards** and

laterally to reach the summit of its curve i.e., the highest and most prominent part. It then turns **upwards**, **backwards** and **laterally** till it ends at the **lateral genu** to become the lateral crus (Fig. 2.22).

All three movements in the body of the middle crus reach **their maximum** at the dome so that

i. **Lateral curving** reaches its **maximum** as backwards folding takes place **at the dome**.
ii. **Cephalic elevation** reaches its **maximum** height at the tip of **the dome**.
iii. **Medial twisting** reaches its **maximum** shape **at the dome**.

After the maximal movements at the dome, the three movements in the body of the middle crus continue to take place, to a lesser degree. Lateral curving, elevation and twisting continue till the middle crus becomes the lateral crus at the lateral genu.

The **dome** therefore is **not** in the shape of a typical **hemispherical dome** as the name implies, it rather a **fold of cartilage** that has a **twist** in its body.

The **tip of the nose** looks like a hemispherical dome as it is made of the **two domes of the middle crurae** and their **covering skin** including the two flat triangles. The simple external shape of the dome gives no indication of the complex internal anatomical structures.

The term **dome** is more applicable to the surface anatomy of the **nasal tip** rather than anatomy of middle crus.

Skin Cover of the Middle Crus

The **inner surfaces** of the middle crurae are covered by **thin adherent** hair-bearing **vestibular skin**, while the **outer surfaces** as they become gradually exposed are covered by the much **thicker** and **less adherent external nasal skin.** There is a thin **fatty layer** that separates the smooth dermal layer of the external skin from the perichondrium of the middle crurae. This layer may be removed in defatting of the lower lateral cartilages.

Tip Projection and Tip Definition

Tip projection and tip definition are two gold standards in nasal aesthetics (refer to Guide for Atlas in clinical cases of Rhinoplasty for further details).

For better nasal aesthetics the tip should project as the highest point at the caudal end of the nasal dorsum.

The antroinferior end of the tip should not be amorphously rounded but rather have a more distinctive shape i.e., well defined.

The domes of the two middle crurae are the skeletal foundation of the nasal tip.

For better clinical assessment and management the nasal tip is defined anatomically as follows:

The MidDomal Lines and Points

There are two lines of **maximum projection**: the **right** and the **left mid-domal lines**. They represent the **highest levels of the domes and the nose**. Each line begins from the **apex** (anterior angle) of the **flat triangle** and goes upwards and medially to reach the superior border of the middle crus **halfway** between the **apex** and the **lateral angle** of the **weak triangle** (Fig. 1a). This line is **convexly curved forward**. The top of this curve represents the **point of maximum projection**. Ideally the two points should be at the same horizontal level and of equal distance from the midline (Fig. 2.22).

Photographically these points reflect the light in the frontal view photographs. The two points may vary in their location from one side to the other.

It is not uncommon or unusual to find the **two domes**, on each side of the nose, are **different** in their **sizes**, **curves** and **positions**. In these cases the lines and points of maximum projections are **different on each side** with a somewhat irregular nasal tip. This is not necessarily unaesthetic. On the contrary, the nose may continue to be quite attractive. In that context it is similar to the beauty of an apple that has quite different contours in every direction.

The Angle of Divergence of the Domes

This angle measures the extent of lateral curving of the middle crurae. The angle of divergence

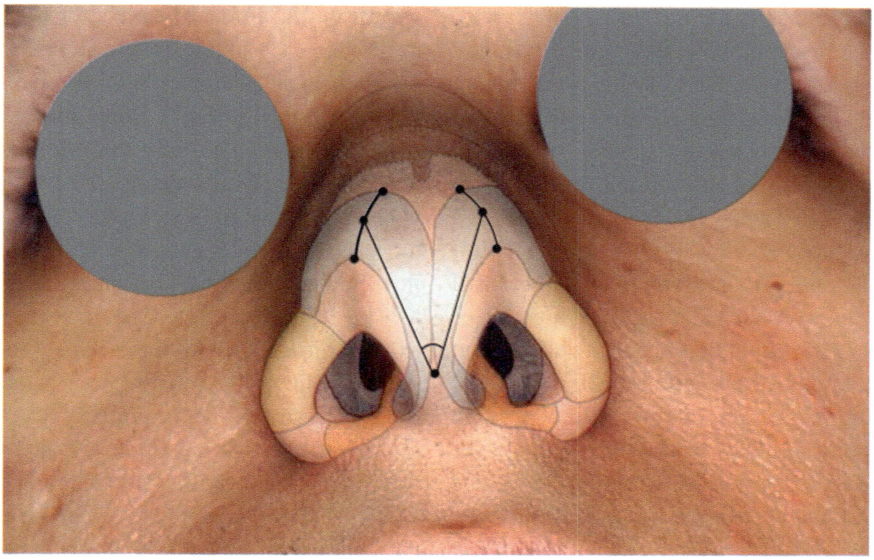

Fig. 2.23 The angle of divergence of the Domes

is best seen from a backwards tilting view. Anatomically it is defined as the angle between the **inferior end point of the medial genu and**, in the midline, to the middle of the **lateral genu** on each side.

From the practical point of view the angle of divergence is best measured from the **inferior end point of the medial genu** to the **mid domal point on each side**. The **angle between the apecies of the two domes** is of clinical and aesthetic significances.

The aesthetically acceptable angle of divergence is between 30 and 60°. The wider the angle of divergence the broader is the nasal tip and vice versa. Caucasian noses have narrower tips than African, Asian and Middle Eastern noses (Fig. 2.23).

Aesthetic Effects of the Middle Crus

The aesthetics of the **frontolateral** walls of the nose, i.e., the nasal tip is **directly** and **indirectly** affected by the degree of **twist** and **curves in** the bodies of the middle crurae.

Direct Effects on the Nasal Tip

The direct effects are mainly due to the anatomical changes in **the domes**. The two domes are approximated to each other by **interdomal bands** and by **the covering external skin** in order to reduce the gap between them. The **lines and points of maximum projection** including the apecies of the two flat triangles are brought **as close as possible to each other** nearer to the midline. A unified midline prominent structure is now formed, viz., the **nasal tip**.

The **prominence** of the nasal tip is directly affected by the following factors:

The Degree of Maximal Domal Twisting and Elevation

The more the **twisting** and **elevation** the **more prominent** is the nasal tip.

Lateral Curving

The degree of lateral folding at the dome affects the **width** of the nasal tip. Acute folding produces **narrow** tip and vice versa wide folding produce **broad** nasal tip.

The Length of Middle Crurae

The **longer** the body of the middle crus the more the direct effect it has on the nasal tip. The Caucasian nose has **longer** middle crurae resulting in a more **prominent** nose than African and Asian noses.

Indirect Effects on the Lateral Nasal Walls

The indirect effects of the middle crural twist and curves are mainly due to the consequent anatomical changes that take place on **the lateral crurae**.

In contradistinction to the almost fixed location of the medial crus, **the lateral crus** shows wide range of variation in its final **position** (medial and lateral)**, level** (high and low) and **plane** (sagital, coronal and axial). The location of the **lateral crus** is greatly influenced and decided by the variations of the **anatomical twist and curves that take place in the body of middle crus**. These movements of **the twist** and **curves** in the body of the **middle crus** may have the following indirect effects on the lateral crus.

The Degree of Lateral Folding

Depending on the degrees of lateral folding, the lateral crus may be placed **medially** or **laterally** producing narrow or broad sidewalls. This consequently affects the anesthetics of the nasal tip.

The relative differences in the convexities of the middle and lateral crurae have an indirect effect on tip projection.

If the lateral crus is **concave** or **less convex** than the dome, the supratip area will show a smooth slope that gives the nasal tip better projection and vice versa. If the convexity of the lateral crus is more, it will negatively affect the tip projection.

Elevation

The more the elevation movement in the body of the middle crus the higher is the lateral crus and vice versa. **Lower placed lateral crurae** may produce a **prominent nasal tip**.

Twisting

The **more the medial twisting**, in the body of the middle crus, the more the lateral crus goes to settle in a more transverse (coronal) plane and vice versa **the less twisting** the less the lateral crus moves away from the vertical sagital plane.

2.3.2.4 Anatomy of the Inferior Nasal Wall

For the normal physiological flow in the nose during respiration, the air needs to have a **free way** from the **inferiorly** placed nasal apertures, to the lateral nasal clefts **superiorly**, then to the nasal choanae **posteriorly**. Naturally, therefore, the nasal aperture tubes has **no superior** or **posterior walls**.The only **roof** for the nose is located at the skull base including the cribriform plate i.e., at a much higher level than the aperture tube. **Posteriorly** the first wall that hits the air flow is the posterior pharyngeal wall.

The **inferior wall** of the lower third of the external nose is mostly replaced by the external nasal opening. The inferior nasal aperture is no more than an opening within the nasal floor that separates its two components i.e., the **vestibular floor** posteriorly and the **flat triangle** anteriorly.

The flat triangle is the backwards deflexion of the long excess soft skin from the anterior nasal wall. It is discussed in details in the chapter of the weak and soft areas of the nose.

The inferior wall of the lower third of the external nose is therefore made of:

(a) The Two Vestibular Floors
(b) The Two Nasal Apertures
(c) The Two Flat Triangle.

The Vestibular Floor

The vestibular floor, as the name indicates, lies **inferiorly** to make the **floor** of the nasal aperture tube. It is lined by a very **loose** and **thin** layer of the hair bearing skin, which in turn overlies a **thick** layer of abundantly **loose connective tissue**. The latter rests on the orbicularis oris muscles.

The vestibular floor lies just in front of the inferior bony margin of the nasal aperture.

The Shape and Position of the Vestibular Floor

The vestibular floor is curved down like a saucer between two elevated margins i.e., the **nasal sill band anteriorly** and the **posterior vestibular margin posteriorly** at the muco-cutaneous junction. **Medially** it is limited by the membranous septum, the medial crus and the anterior nasal spine, while **laterally** there is the firm wall of the ala nasi.

The **posterior vestibular margin** is at a **higher** level than the **nasal sill** band in order to take the inspired air in a mostly **superior** direction.

The vestibular floor is therefore **tilted slightly forwards**. The vestibular floor is continuous with the rest of the nasal floor proper lined by respiratory mucosa over the hard palate.

The vestibular floor is part of the **external valve area.** Its contribution to the physiology of the external valve is provided via its main unique feature of the **loose skin** with its abundantly loose **subcutaneous** tissue as follows:

- The vestibular floor allows the **free movement** of the mobile lateral **alar wall.** The lack of bony attachment and the presence of the abundantly loose skin and subcutaneous tissues allows for the rigid lateral alar wall to move freely.
  In addition, contribution is also made to the ala nasi by the **stretchable non-wrinkable** soft skin of the **rim-sill fold**.
- The vestibular floor **expands** during inspiration with the widening ala nasi transforming the vestibular cavity into a **large receptacle** that takes in the maximum amount of the inspired air.

The Inferior Vestibular Band (IVB)

The Inferior Vestibular Band (IVB) is a **subcutaneous firm fibroelastic band** that is present in the **inferior part** of the **medial** and **inferior** walls of the nasal vestibule (see histology chapter).

Course of the IVB

The Inferior Vestibular Band starts laterally from a variable point near the inferior alar margin i.e., the alar rim. It runs a **transverse course** medially at the **junction between the vestibular floor and the upper** lip. It is covered by a tightly adherent hairless thin skin. This part of the IVB is known as the **nasal sill.**

The band then leaves the **inferior vestibular wall** and moves to the **columellar wall**, by sharply turning **upwards** then **forwards**, passing **behind** then **above** the **medial crus** of the lower lateral cartilage. It continues **forwards** along the superior border of the medial crus (Figs. 2.24 and 2.25).

The medial crus thus lies in a **deep gutter** that is bounded by the lateral columellar margin inferiorly and the IVB both posteriorly and superiorly.

The vertical part of both bands **can be felt** by rolling them between an index finger and the thumb if placed inside the two nostrils.

Movements of the upper lip are associated with movement of the inferior vestibular bands together with the whole of the lower third of the nose.

All along its course, the inferior vestibular band is covered externally by **adherent**, **thin** and **hairless skin.**

Both bands are attached to each other by connective tissue fibers along their course in the columellar wall. Along their course on the lip they are firmly adherent to the underlying Orbicularis Oris muscle (see Histology section).

The Supportive Role of the IVB

The inferior vestibular band is made of firm fibrous tissues intermingled with elastic tissues (see histology). This makes it a truly supportive structure to both the inferior and the medial nasal aperture walls.

Both bands help in **holding the inferior vestibular floors to the columellar wall**. They prevent the **medial crurae** from springing inwards and encroaching upon the nasal openings.

This prominent band is the junctional margin that **separates the nasal cavity from the upper lip**. It helps in keeping the nasal discharge inside the nasal cavity and prevents it from spontenous dripping.

Caucasian noses usually have **thin skin** and **firm lower lateral** cartilages including the medial crurae. These are associated with thick and more prominent bands, while African, Asian and Middle Eastern noses have thick skin and softer cartilages with thinner and less prominent bands.

The Nasal Sill

The nasal sill is **the anterior boundary of the vestibular floor**. It extends from the **beginning**

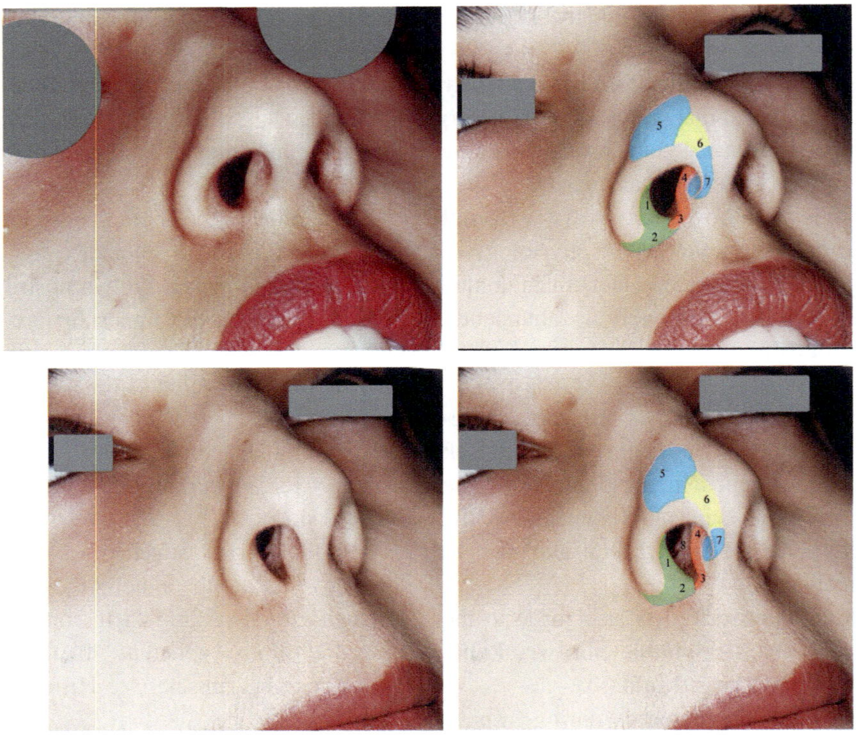

Fig. 2.24 The inferior vestibular band moves from the nasal sill then upwards and forwards posterior and then superior to the medial crus. 1—Superior segment of the Rim-Sill Fold 2—Inferior and posterior segments of the Rim-Sill Fold 3 and 4—Inferior Vestibular Band (IVB) 5—Lateral Crus of the lower lateral cartilage 6—Middle Crus of the lower lateral cartilage 7—Medial Crus of the lower lateral cartilage 8—Caudal Margin of the Cartilaginous Septum

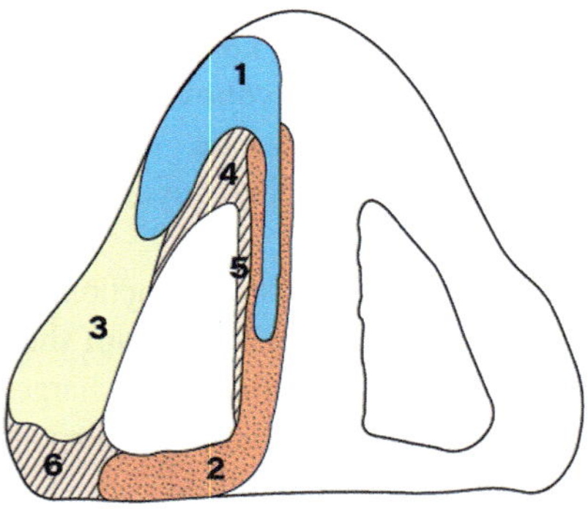

Fig. 2.25 Anatomic look into a right aperture view. 1—The right lower lateral cartilage 2—Inferior Vestibular bans 3—Right Ala Nasi 4—The Right Flat Triangle (soft) 5—The Lateral Columellar Margin 6—The Right Rim—Sill Fold

of the IVB laterally, till its sharp **upwards turn medially**. The nasal sill is therefore **only part of the IVB**. Clinically the nasal sill is a **ridge of skin** that is both **seen** and **felt** at the anterior margin of the vestibular floor. It is made of a rolled fibrous band that is covered by a closely adherent skin anteriorly, superiorly and inferiorly (see histology).

There are soft folds of skin that continue the circle of the aperture margin both medially and laterally. They join the nasal sill with the alar rim laterally and the columellar margin medially.

At a variable point away from the center of the nasal sill, an **upwards** and **forwards branching** takes place on the **lateral** end to make the upper lateral soft folds of the skin.

The Upper Lateral Fold of the Nasal Sill

The **lower** margin of the nasal sill is continuous with the **lower** margin of the alar rim. The **upper** margin of the nasal sill diverges **upwards** (inwards) and **forwards** on the inner surface of the ala nasi making a prominent fold of soft skin that fades away gradually anteriorly (Fig. 2.24).

It is an **unsupported** soft fold of skin. Anatomically it is part of the natural extension of the **rim-sill fold**. Its prominence and length are variable in the different individuals, the two nostrils of the same individual and with age and race.

Sometimes it is so prominent and long that it almost makes a second alar rim. In some noses it may not be so clear and cannot be seen except by moving the alar rim in various directions. It may be absent all together.

This fold is very little for any surgical or physiological significance.

Surgical Significances

a. The columellar incision in **septoplasty** should be placed strictly at the **caudal margin of the nasal septum**, i.e., above the IVB. This avoids cutting through the band which will make dissection more difficult, painful post-operatively and may affect the anatomical transverse position of the nasal sill. On the other hand it keeps the surgeon away from the naso-palatine nerves as they pass down to the incisive canal.
b. The incision in **rhinoplasty** should be a transfixing one i.e., the wound is exactly at the same position on both sides. This provides the best possible chance for surgically symmetrical apertures. It can be helped by using **Cottle's columellar forceps** to retract and **stretch the loose skin of the membranous septum** until the caudal part of septum becomes prominently clear. Incision is then made strictly on the cartilaginous margin going through the other side i.e., a transfixing incision antro-posteriorly.
c. The insertion of an intercrural columellar graft i.e., a columellar strut: Attempts at placing a graft from above via a superior columellar incision are a difficult and cumbersome procedure. Having to go through the tough tissues of the IVB in a reverse direction from above downwards makes it almost an impossible task.

   A much easier and more direct way is to go through an inferior incision at the lower margin of the medial crus of the lower lateral cartilage.
d. Reducing the **medial crural prominence** only needs to approximate these two bands by a transfixing stitch.

The Nasal Base

The **nasal base** is not the same as the **alar base**. Although the **alar base** is the widely used expression, yet the **nasal base** is the more anatomically accurate term. Anatomically, the alar base is the part of the nasal base.

Definition:

The nasal base is defined as **the location where the lower third of the nose is attached to the upper lip**. This is a **junctional area** which has a **nasal side** and a **facial side**.

(1) The nasal side:

   a. The **vestibular floors** including the posterior vestibular margins.
   b. The posterior margins of the alae nasi i.e., the **alar base**.
   c. The **nasal sill bands** (Parts of the inferior vestibular bands).

(2) The facial side:
   The upper lip that includes the **lip skin** and the underlying **Orbicularis Oris muscle**.

Each of the structures from the nasal side is attached to either of the two components of the upper lip, i.e., skin and muscle, in its own unique way to adapt for its physiological role.

It is better to deal with the **nasal base as a whole** including the floor and the boundaries, as each of its components has its own anatomical, aesthetic and surgical characteristics and significance.

The **vestibular floor** is separated from the Orbicularis Oris muscle by a **thick loose connective tissue layer**. The alar base is thus **fully mobile**. The loose areolar tissue is an excellent **sliding platform** for the whole of the lower third of the nose, providing it with the freedom to move and perform its various physiological and expressional tasks.

Movements of the **lower third** of the nose including the alar base are the tasks of the **small muscles of the nose** as well as the **Orbicularis Oris**.

The **nasal base** is mainly moved by the **Orbicularis Oris muscle** via its intimate and direct attachments of its fibers into two important lines:

(a) **The nasal sill band**:

This is the **anterior attachment line** of the nasal base to the upper lip. The nasal sill band is **directly** and **intimately attached** to the muscle fibers of the **orbicularis oris muscle** inferiorly and posteriorly (see the histology section).

Additionally, the nasal sill band is **closely adherent** to the overlying **skin of the naso-labial junction** both anteriorly and superiorly.

In this area the **skin** over the nasal sill band **suddenly** and **abruptly** becomes **thin, glistening, hairless** and tightly **adherent** to the underlying band fibers (see histology section). Hair grows again **on both sides** of the nasal sill, viz., as a mustache in the skin of the upper lip and as vibrecae in the vestibular skin inside the nose.

(b) **The alae nasi**:

This is the **lateral attachment line** of the nasal base to the upper lip. The **upper half** of the posterior alar margin is attached to the **skin** and the underlying **Orbicularis Oris muscle**, while the **lower half is only** attached to the **upper lip skin** via the rim-sill fold.

The posterior alar margins of the alae nasi delineate the lateral limits i.e., the width of the nasal base.

The alar base can move with the lip **sideways** across the midline, **backwards** and **forwards** as well as **upwards** and **downwards**. Each side may move independently.

The skin cover of the nasal aperture tube:

The **alae nasi**, the **middle** and the **lateral crura** are all covered by **external skin**. This skin is relatively thick and full of sebaceous glands, sweat glands and occasional hairs. The skin cover of the alae nasi is directly attached to them, while the skin cover of the middle and lateral crura is separated from them by a layer of fibro-fatty tissue.

All walls of the nasal aperture are covered **internally** by the **vestibular skin**. The vestibular skin contains sebaceous glands, sweat glands and hair (vibrissae). The skin is tightly adherent to the inner surface of the lateral alar wall as well as all three crurae of the lower lateral cartilage.

On the **floor** of the nose the vestibular skin is quit loose with abundant subcutaneous tissue.

The skin is soft both internally and externally in the areas of the **flat triangle**, **rim-sill folds** and the **posterior columellar folds**.

The **marginal** skin is tightly **adherent** to the nasal sill band posteriorly and the alar rim laterally, while it becomes **soft** and unsupported over the areas of the flat triangle, the rim-sill fold, the lateral columellar margin and the posterior columellar fold.

The Flat Triangle

The flat triangle is also known as the soft triangle. It is a triangular fold of soft skin that **covers a gap in the anterior nasal wall**. This gap is located between the **medial crus** in the medial wall and the **ala nasi** in the lateral wall of each side of the lower third of the nose.

The gap is created where the **medial crus** is transformed into the **middle crus** as it moves **upwards, forwards** and **laterally** away from the nasal aperture margin. The **middle crus** has a narrow body that is too high and too short to reach the aperture margin.

A double layered fold of soft skin covers the gap in the anterior wall between the two firm structures of the medial and the lateral walls. Due to the **lack of support,** this skin fold is stretched like a web as an **inferior flat sheet**. It cannot maintain the firm external rounded contour of the anterior cartilaginous wall of the middle crus.

The flat tringle is not strictly triangular in shape as its lateral angle is made by the rounded body of the ala nasi.

The **inner surface** of the skin fold is made of hair bearing **vestibular skin**. It makes **the anterior part of the vestibular floor**, which is separated from the vestibular floor proper at the nasal base by the external nasal opening.

The **flat triangle** and the **nasal sill band** are the **only parts of the vestibular floor that have externally exposed surface skin**.

Aesthetic Effect of the Flat Triangle on the Aperture

Margins:

The skin fold of the flat triangle crosses directly from the **medial crus** to the **ala nasi** i.e., from the **medial wall** to the **lateral walls** of the lower third of the nose.

The flat triangle thus covers the inferior margin of the dome of the middle crus so that it is not a high unaesthetic forth aperture margin to the external opening of the nose.

This arrangement is responsible for the **transformation** of the **external nasal opening into a triangular shape** rather than a quadrangular one.

The posterior free margin of the flat triangle becomes the **anterior margin of the nasal aperture**, which is continuous with the **inferior free alar margin** laterally and the **lateral columellar margin** medially.

Why the Term Flat Triangle and not Soft Triangle

The flat triangle is a **more accurate descriptive anatomical term** than the soft triangle. Flattening **is the most important and significant event** that takes place in this triangular skin fold at this critical part of the nasal aperture wall.

Flattening results in important anatomical changes:

(a) The vestibular Floor: this fold of skin is part of the vestibular floor. It therefore takes more of a horizontal plane that is in the same level of the posterior part of the vestibular floor.
(b) The flat triangle covers the inferior margin of the dome of the middle crus i.e., the anterior wall of the lower third of the nose. This is responsible for transforming the nasal opening into a triangular rather than a rectangular shape.
(c) This triangular fold appears as a flat area at the inferior aspect of the nose that has a posterior margin.

Flat triangle is therefore a true descriptive term to the **surface anatomical appearance** of the fold.

Anatomy of the Flat Triangle

The skin fold of the flat triangle is made of **two layers of skin** that are separated from each other by a thin layer of **loose connective tissue**. Each of these layers is significantly important because they are dealt with as **three separate layers** i.e., **external skin**, **connective tissue** and **vestibular skin**.

Anatomically the flat triangle has, by definition, an **external surface,** an **internal surface, three borders** and **three angles**.

The External Surface

The external surface of the flat triangle is made by **smooth hairless** external nasal skin (Figs. 2.26, 2.27 and 2.28).

Each triangle is located at the **most inferior**, **medial** and **anterior** part of the nasal aperture tube with its external surface looking **infro-laterally**. This represents an acute deflection from the anteriorly curved surface of the dome (Fig. 2.27).

The infro-lateral inclination of the external surface is caused by the lower level of the medial margin of the flat triangle as compared with its higher lateral margin.

The Internal Surface

The internal surface is made by the **hair-bearing vestibular skin**. The skin fold of the flat triangle creates **shelf-like floor** to the anterior vestibular wall.

The concavity of the anterior vestibular wall, made by the inner surface of the dome, which is further deepened by the acutely angled fold of the triangle.

To see and shave the internal skin surface of the flat triangle, in preparation for Rhinoplasty,

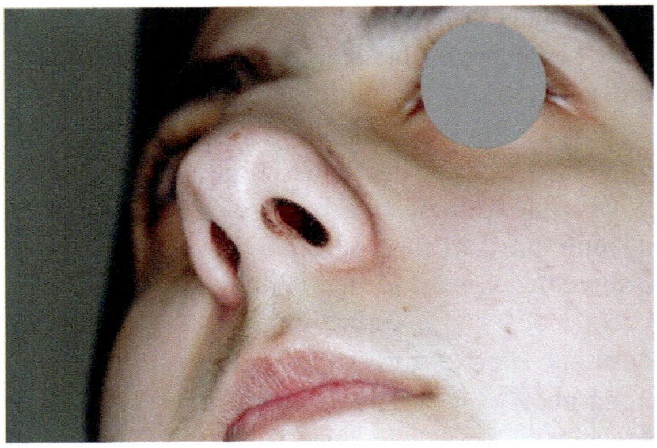

Fig. 2.26 The left flat triangle crossing between the lateral and medial crurae

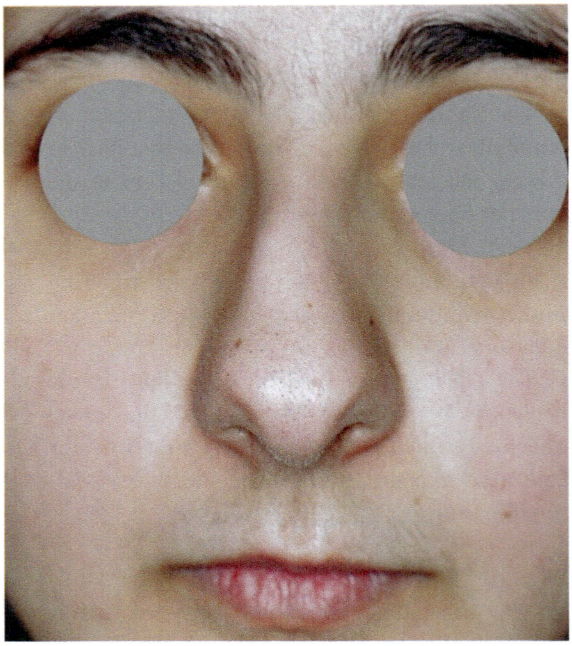

Fig. 2.27 The two flat triangles deflecting posteriorly at the lower margins of the middle crurae. The outer surfaces are looking downwards and laterally

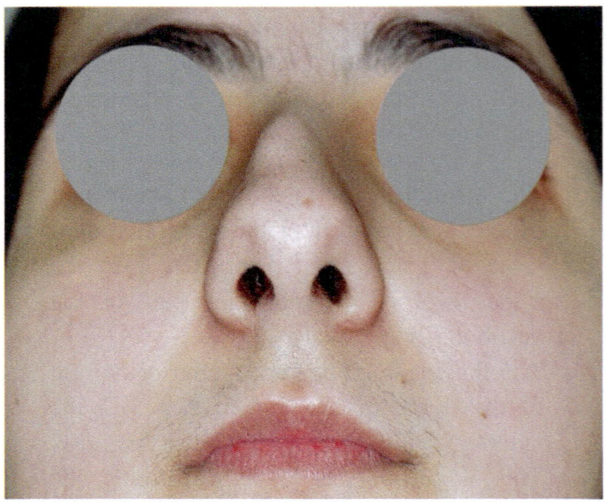

Fig. 2.28 The two flat triangles transforming the nasal opening from quadrangular into triangular shape

we have to **evert** it using a sharp pronged alar retractor with the help of an external finger pressure.

Borders of the Flat Triangle:

The **medial border** of the flat triangle is made by the upwards and forwards going **inferior border of the middle crus**. It ends at the apex of the flat triangle anteriorly i.e., the dome of the middle crus.

The **lateral border** is made by two structures, viz., anteriorly by the backwards and upwards going **inferior border of the middle crus**, while posteriorly it is made by the curving **anterior border of the ala nasi**.

The **posterior border** is made by the **free skin margin** of the flat triangle. This border is usually a curved one and makes the anterior free margin of the inferior opening of the nasal aperture tube.

Angles of the Flat Triangle:

The **anterior angle** is the **apex** of the flat triangle. It is made by the **inferior border of the middle crus** as it bends backwards in the process of the dome formation.

The medial angle is made between the ascending inferior border of the middle crus and the free posterior skin margin of the flat triangle.

The **lateral angle** is made between the curving anterior border of the ala nasi and the free posterior skin border of the flat triangle (Fig. 2.29).

The Surgical Significances

The surgical importance of the flat triangle stems from its important physiological role, anatomical location and histological structure.

The anterior gap, between the medial and the lateral aperture walls, is closed by the **inferiorly** placed skin fold of the flat triangle. It transforms the **four walled nasal aperture** into a **three marginal nasal opening**. The **anteriorly looking** gap is closed now by an **inferiorly looking** skin fold in order **to adapt for the proper nasal function.**

This is an **important task**, both aesthetically and physiologically, which is achieved by this **small** delicate fold of skin.

In order to maintain its role, the skin fold of the flat triangle is uniquely balanced by **accurately structured** anatomical factors, viz.:

(a) The skin fold is stretched between the firm medial and lateral walls with certain degree of **tension** that keeps its external flat appearance in an exact infro-lateral location so that its free skin margin is directed **posteriorly** at the **same level** with the alar and columellar margins.
(b) It is made of **two layers of skin** separated by **connective tissue** layer. Each of the three layers has its own unique

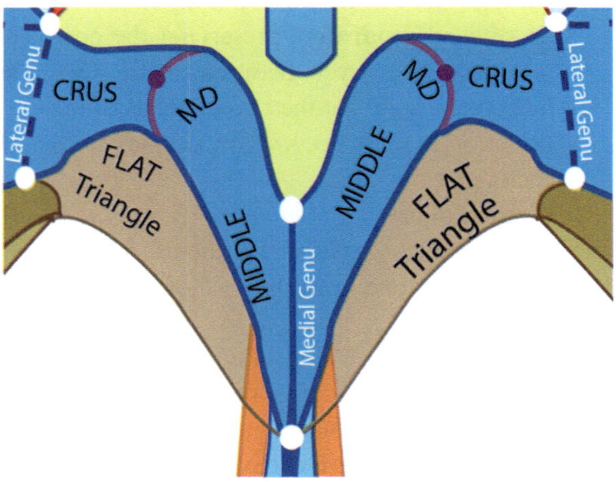

Fig. 2.29 Anatomy of the two flat triangles. MD: Mid-Domal Lines and Mid-Domal Points

characteristic that gives this fold its overall **soft, pliable** and yet **tight consistency**.

(c) The **external** skin is quite **different** from the **internal** skin. The **external** being thick smooth, hairless with sebaceous glands, while the **internal** is thin and hair bearing. Both layers meet each other at the posterior smooth free margin.

(d) The two skin layers are **completely separated** from each other by the loose layer of connective tissue.

Aesthetics of the Flat Triangle

From the **aesthetic** point of view there are **no positive constructive work** that is required in the area of the flat triangle as it has **no skeletal** structure that requires reformation or modification.

The most important attitude nevertheless is the careful **preservation** of this delicately balanced triangular fold with its three layers.

Loss or **injury** to one or more of its layers may have major aesthetic consequences that are difficult to regain.

Management of Injury of the Flat Triangle

(1) Acute injury:

If the flat fold is **inadvertently** cut during surgery or injured as part of nasal trauma, it has to be re-stitched meticulously and immediately at the time of surgery or trauma using thin six zero nylon or vicryl stitches. Each of the **two skin layers** has to be stitched **separately** preserving the connective tissue layer between them. One must make sure that the two cut ends of the posterior margin become continuous with each other.

(2) Chronic injury:

Chronic injury or damage of the flat triangle results in one of the following two situations:

(a) **Chronic scarring** of either one or the two layers of the skin. More commonly the damage may only affect **the loose connective tissue layer** of the flat triangle which is lost and become replaced by a **contracting fibrous tissue layer**.

The triangular fold loses its flat smooth appearance. The skin is contracted into a deep irregular **ugly looking notch** with or without external scarring of the skin.

(b) **Total loss** of the whole of the skin fold of the flat triangle including all of its three layers.

The gap in the anterior nasal wall, which was originally covered by the flat triangle, is now disclosed. It appears as a notch in the anterior nasal wall between the anterior end of the **medial crus** and of the **alar body**.

Although the **flat triangle** is located **infro-laterally** i.e., at an **inferior location** yet its absence or deformity is unsightly gap or disfigurement that appears **anteriorly**.

Chronic scarring or loss of the whole of the flat triangle may happen in the following conditions:

i. Maltreated or neglected acute traumatic injury or surgical cuts to this fold.
ii. Long standing pressure on the flat skin fold:

All types of **plastic nasal tubes** e.g., nasogastric tubes, anesthetic tube, nasal stents or the tubes inside merocel nasal packings. All of these tubes tend to **slide forwards** and rub against the area of the flat triangle causing chronic irritation, inflammation, scarring or even **loss of the whole of the flat triangle** with **notching** of the nose anteriorly.

Chronic scarring or loss of **one** or the **two skin layers** is very difficult to **repair, replace, reproduce** or **camouflage**. Considerations of the **thickness, colour** and **pliability** of each layer to **adapt and fit exactly at the same level** on the external surface and **in line** with the alar and columellar margins is not an easy task.

The **loose connective tissue** layer is particularly hard to reproduce or replace if injured, scarred or lost.

3 The Weak Areas and Soft Folds in the Nasal Walls

Abstract

The walls of the lower third of the nose are different from the walls of the upper two-thirds. The lower third of the nose has **kinetic** walls that contribute to the physiology of nasal respiration and facial expressions while the upper two-thirds have **static** walls.

Keywords

The muscular triangles · The weak triangle · Two vestibular floors · Two flat triangles

The walls of the lower third of the nose are different from the walls of the upper two-thirds. The lower third of the nose has **kinetic** walls that contribute to the physiology of nasal respiration and facial expressions while the upper two-thirds have **static** walls.

The small muscles of the nose act on the four firm structures in the walls of the lower third, i.e., the **lower lateral cartilages**, **alae nasi**, **the caudal vestibular septum** and the **inferior vestibular bands.** The walls of the lower third of the nose are not in the form of a solid-walled tube. In order for them to move, these four structures have gaps in specific locations between them and at their **superior** and **inferior junctional areas**. These gaps are covered by weak areas and soft folds of skin.

These gaps **are created during the developmental process of the nose** in the areas of meeting between the **fronto-nasal process** and the **maxillary processes.**

a. **Gaps of the superior junctional area**

Gaps are present at the junction between the solid immobile three-walled **upper two-thirds** of the nose with the soft mobile four-walled **lower third** of the nose, i.e., between the bony pyramid and the cartilaginous midvault superiorly and the lower lateral cartilages and alae nasi inferiorly.

b. **Gaps of the inferior junctional area**

Gaps are present at the junction between the **firm structures** in the walls of the lower third of the nose and the upper lip including **Orbicularis Oris muscle,** i.e., between the lower lateral cartilages and the nasal sill bands and alae nasi anteriorly and the Orbicularis Oris posteroinferiorly

Imagine if the nose is denuded of the skin and subdermal tissues. The following will be found:

i. **The upper two-thirds**: There are no gaps in the bony pyramid and the midvault of the upper lateral cartilage.
ii. The **lower third**: The lower lateral cartilages, the alae nasi, the caudal vestibular septum and the inferior vestibular bands are **separated by gaps** that are variable in sizes and shapes.

These gaps are bridged and covered by **weak areas** and **folds of soft skin** that are present both

M. H. A. Shafy, *Innovations in Rhinoplasty*,
https://doi.org/10.1007/978-3-030-94573-2_3

externally and intranasally. A layer of **loose connective tissue**, **fat** and/or **muscles** separates the two skin layers.

3.1 Significance of the Weak Areas and Soft Folds

The weak areas and soft folds are **necessary for the physiology and the aesthetics of the firm structures** in the walls of the lower third of the nose.

The **weak areas and soft folds** give the firm structures their relative **freedom to move**, while at the same time they are the site of nice-looking areas, folds or creases, i.e., **they contribute to nasal aesthetics**.

The firm structures in the lower third of the nose are not meant to completely fill the walls of the nasal aperture tubes. They **only support parts of these walls.** They serve as **functional** as well as **aesthetic structures**.

If the firm cartilaginous and fibrofatty structures were to completely fill the four walls, the lower third of the nose would end up having totally **rigid** and **motionless** nasal walls. These walls would be **incapable** of performing their physiological role in nasal respiration and facial expressions. They may look attractive but lifeless and motionless like a statue.

3.2 Locations of the Gaps

A total of **thirteen gaps** are present within the walls of the nasal aperture tubes. These gaps are accurately arranged **between and around the firm structures** of the walls of the lower third of the nose. Eleven of these gaps are closed by weak areas and soft folds. The two nasal openings are the remaining two unclosed gaps.

There are **three single** midline gaps and **five paired** gaps in the walls of both aperture tubes.

3.2.1 Gaps in the Medial Nasal wall: "Midline Gaps"

Two single gaps are present in the common medial wall between the two nasal aperture tubes.

3.2.1.1 The Membranous Septum, the Weak Area of the Nose

The membranous septum fills the gap that is present between the **caudal septal margin superiorly** and the **medial crurae** including the **columella inferiorly**. It is a weak transitional area between the upper two-thirds and the columella.

The membranous septum is devoid of firm structures. It is an internal weak area of the nose and the counterpart of the weak triangle externally.

3.2.1.2 The Posterior Columellar Fold

There is a fold of soft skin that fills the gap between the two **medial crurae** anteriorly and the **orbicularis oris muscle** posteriorly.

3.2.2 Gaps in the Lateral Nasal Walls

3.2.2.1 The Rim-Sill Folds

These are two gaps, right and left, that are present between the lower ends of the **alar bodies** and the lateral ends of the **nasal sill bands**. Both structures are firmly attached to the orbicularis oris, leaving two gaps between them. These gaps are filled with **folds of soft skin**.

3.2.2.2 The Muscular Triangles

These are a pair of gaps that are bounded by

- The **alae nasi,**
- **The lateral crurae,**
- The **upper lateral cartilage** and
- The **inferior margins** of the nasal **bony pyramids.**

The muscular triangles are the only gaps that contain **muscle fibers**, Panniculus Carnosus, as well as areolar connective tissue between their covering two layers.

3.2.3 Anterior Wall Gap "The Weak Triangle"

The weak triangle is a gap that **appears** as a result of the evolution of the anterior wall in the lower third of the nose, i.e., the middle crurae. The gap is located between the upper lateral cartilage superiorly and the two middle crurae inferiorly.

This gap is a single midline gap that is known as the weak triangle.

3.2.4 Gaps in the Inferior Nasal Walls

3.2.4.1 Two Vestibular Floors

The **right** and the **left vestibular floors** fill a pair of gaps that are present in the **inferior nasal walls** between each **nasal sill** anteriorly and the **posterior vestibular margin** posteriorly. The two gaps are separated from each other by the nasal septum.

3.2.4.2 Two Flat Triangles

They are two flat soft folds of skin that fill the gaps between the medial crurae and the alae nasi. The medial crurae are part of the medial wall while the alae nasi are part of the lateral walls of the lower third of the nose.

3.2.4.3 The Two Nasal Openings

The two nasal openings are gaps in the floor of the nose. Each nasal opening separated the vestibular floor posteriorly from the flat triangle anteriorly.

A detailed anatomy of each gap with its corresponding weak area or soft fold is discussed in a special individual chapter.

3.3 The Posterior Columellar Fold

The posterior columellar fold is a small **midline fold of soft skin** that is present at the most posterior part of the columella, as it meets the upper lip. It covers the **gap** between the **two medial crurae** anteriorly and the **orbicularis oris** muscle posteriorly. The soft columellar skin fold lacks support for a short distance till it joins the upper lip with its underlying Orbicularis Oris muscle.

This gap is created during development, in the midline, at the meeting between the median process of the fronto-nasal process and the two maxillary processes.

3.3.1 Boundaries

Anteriorly: The posterior margins of the **two medial crurae.**

Posteriorly: The **upper lip** with its underlying **Orbicularis Oris**.

Superiorly: The inferior end of the **anterior nasal spine**.

Laterally: The medial ends of the transverse parts of the **inferior vestibular bands.**

3.3.2 Skin Cover

The posterior soft columellar fold is covered externally, i.e., inferiorly by hairless external skin. The sides of the folds are covered by the hair-bearing vestibular skin.

3.3.3 Contents

The posterior columellar fold is a soft fold of skin that contains **loose connective tissue** and **muscle fibers**. The muscle fibers of **both Depressor Septi muscles** pass through this fold, as they originate just lateral to the nasal spine, underneath the orbicularis oris muscle, to be inserted into the caudal septum and the medial crurae anteriorly.

The posterior columellar fold is of great surgical importance due to its crucial anatomical location at the naso-labial angle. This will be discussed in detail in the surgical section.

3.4 The Rim-Sill Folds

The right and left **rim-sill gaps** are two of the thirteen gaps present in the lower third of the nose. Each rim-sill gap lies between the lower end of the ala nasi, the nasal sill band and the Orbicularis oris muscle. The gap is filled by a soft fold of skin, i.e., the Rim-Sill fold.

From the surface anatomical point of view, this fold lies between the two prominences of the inferior **alar rim** and the lateral end of the **nasal sill band**, hence the name **Rim-Sill fold** (see anatomy and histology of the Inferior Vestibular Band).

The rim-sill fold is a **transitional area between the two firm** structures of the **lateral** and the **inferior** nasal aperture walls, i.e., the **free anteriorly** directed ala nasi and the less freely **attached horizontally directed nasal sill band** in the floor of the nose. Both structures are attached to the Orbicular Oris muscle. The softness of the rim-sill folds allows for the physiological roles of the surrounding firm structures.

The Rim-Sill fold has an inferior and a posterior segment that play significant aesthetic as well as surgical roles in alar base surgery.

3.4.1 Boundaries

The mechanism of anatomical appearance of **the gap** between the **three structures** of the **ala nasi**, the **nasal sill band** and **Orbicularis Oris** must be clearly understood in order to know the exact extensions of the rim-sill fold.

This gap is created during the development of the nose, between the **median** and the **lateral fronto-nasal processes.** As the **lateral process** fully develops, it produces the lateral aperture wall including the alae nasi, while the **median process** produces the **columella** and both nasal sill bands as parts of the premaxilla. The **upper lip** and the **floor of the nose** are developed from the two **maxillary processes**.

The firm fibrofatty wing of an ala nasi has a characteristic **alar flare,** i.e., **elevated**, **everted** and **backward tilted**. Each of these movements has its anatomical effect on the **rim-sill gap** and hence the **size and shape of the rim-sill fold**.

3.4.1.1 Elevation

Under normal anatomical conditions, the ala nasi and the alar margin are elevated and at a slightly higher level than the lateral columellar margin. The columellar margin can just be seen below the alar margin in an oblique view photograph. The rim-sill fold, therefore, takes a **slightly oblique course upwards and laterally** from the nasal sill band to the alar margin**.** If the alar margin is **high** or **low**, in certain anatomical variations, the obliquity of the rim-sill fold varies accordingly (see anatomical variation Vol. I Chap. 8).

3.4.1.2 Evertion

The degree of the **lateral alar rotation** from the midline affects the **location** of the inferior alar margin in relation to the nasal sill band. An **increased alar eversion** will **widen** the rim-sill **gap** and increase **the length** of the **inferior segment** of the rim-sill fold.

3.4.1.3 Backward Tilting

This is the most important and constant move that affects the rim-sill gap. Backward tilting creates a **wedge-like gap** between the inferior part of the posterior margin of the ala nasi and the Orbicularis Oris. This gap is filled by the **posterior segment** of the rim-sill fold.

3.4.2 Anatomy and Histology of the Rim-Sill Fold

According to the anatomical nature of the gap, the rim-sill fold has two main components.

3.4.2.1 The Posterior Segment

The rim-sill fold starts laterally as a **wedge-shaped** piece of soft skin which fills the gap **behind the lower third of the posterior margin of the ala nasi**. It shares in the formation of the posterior alar groove with the upper lip (Fig. 3.1).

3.4.2.2 The Inferior Segment

As the posterior segment continues medially, it takes the shape of a **rounded fold** and runs obliquely downwards from the inferior alar margin to the **nasal sill band** in the nasal floor (Fig. 3.1).

This segment of the rim-sill fold has an outer (anterior) rounded contour which usually, but not always, takes the same shape and contour of the nasal sill band and the alar margin, so they are **one continuous** margin.

A **large posterior segment** is a major contributor to the **bulk** of the skin of the alar base. A **long inferior segment** is a major contributor to the **width** of the nasal base. **Both segments** contribute to the overall **size** of the nasal aperture.

Histology of the Rim-Sill Fold.

Histologically, Rim-sill fold is made of skin that has a hypodermis which is rich in connective tissues. No specialized tissues were found.

3.4.3 Aesthetics of the Rim-Sill Fold

A large **posterior segment** of the rim-sill fold has **excess soft skin** that usually rests on the upper lip like a flat tire of a car, with an unpleasant acute angle. This gives the nose a heavy and thick-looking appearance. A well propped up ala nasi is like a well-inflated tire, i.e., **less acute angle** with the upper lip which aesthetically is more pleasing.

An **inferior segment** with a uniformly thin fold that has the **same shape and thickness** as the **alar rim** and the **nasal sill** gives the nose a

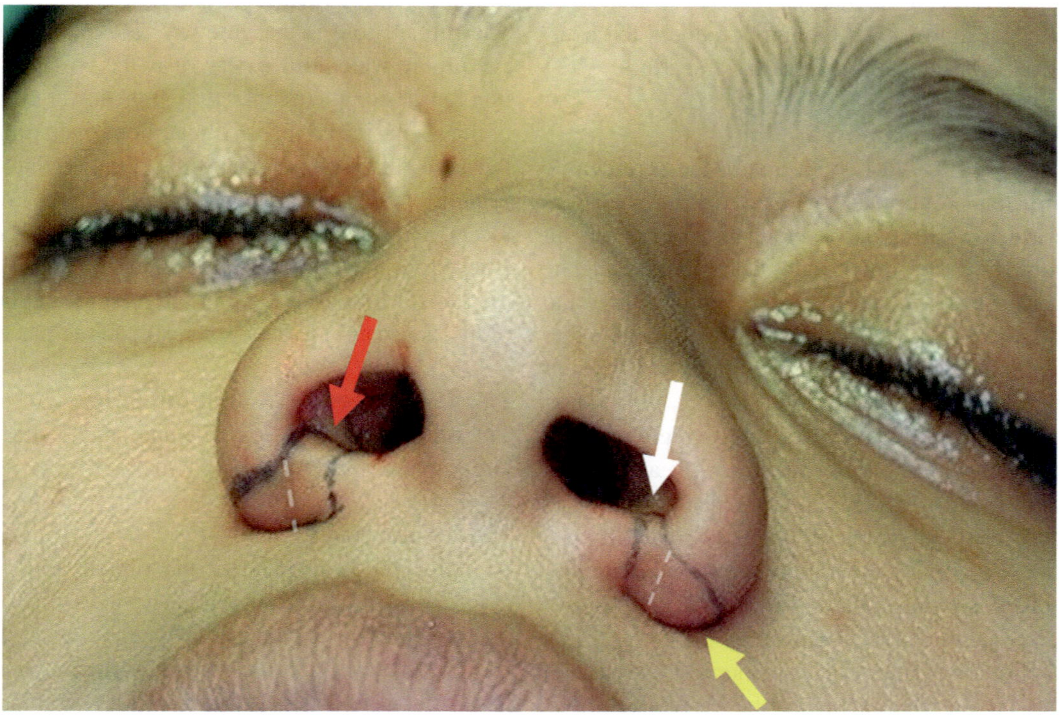

Fig. 3.1 The inferior segment of the left Rim-Sill fold is shown by the white arrow. The posterior segment is shown by the yellow arrow. The demarcation between the posterior and inferior segments is made by the dotted line on the right and left sides. Note that the right inferior segment is longer than the left segment (red arrow)

good aesthetic appearance. A thinner or thicker inferior segment results in an unaesthetic appearance.

3.4.4 Surgical Significances

The rim-sill fold is an important structure that plays a key role in alar base surgery:

3.4.4.1 Effects on the Size and Bulk of Nasal Aperture

The **inferior segment** of the rim-sill fold mainly affects and contributes to the **width** of the nasal aperture, while the **posterior segment** contributes to the **bulk** of the alar base.

These facts are of great importance while considering aesthetic surgery of the **alar base.**

- Excision of the **inferior segment** reduces the **width** of the alar base and the embarrassing wide smile.
- Excision of the **posterior segment** reduces the **bulk** of the alar base.
- Excision of **both segments** reduces the overall **size** and **bulk** of the nasal aperture.

3.4.4.2 Effects on Smiling

The rim-sill fold is both a **soft** and **stretchable** structure. A normal-sized nasal aperture becomes **wide on smiling** due to elongation of the rim-sill fold. It is **the only** anatomical structure in the nasal aperture that expands on smiling and therefore responsible for its widening. After smiling, it goes back to its original size **without wrinkling**.

On smiling, the contracting **orbicularis oris** muscle pulls the **alae nasi** laterally away from the **nasal sill bands**. The rim-sill folds elongate and the nasal apertures increase in **width** and **size**. Excision of the inferior segments of the rim-sill folds reduces the embarrassing widening of nasal apertures on smiling (Fig. 3.2).

Note: Smiling will also increase the size of nasal vestibules including the vestibular floors. The increase in their sizes follows the stretch of the rim-sill folds and is governed by them. Excision of the folds abolishes the expansion of the nasal vestibules. There is no need to excise the loose vestibular skin in the vast majority of cases.

3.4.4.3 Surgical Incisions

The rim-sill fold is the only location for alar base surgical incisions for the following reasons:

The Posterior Segment

The location of the incision is **at** the **naturally hidden and well camouflaged, posterior alar groove**. No scar is seen.

The Inferior Segment

This is the only excisable soft skin segment in the alar base. The cut edges are on the margins of the nasal sill band and the alar rim. Both have similar rounded margins that can be stitched together with a natural continuation. The wound heals nicely with minimal if any apparent scar.

3.4.4.4 Exploration of Nasal Vestibule

The rim-sill fold is the **gateway to explore the vestibular walls and cavity**. It is the best location for the complete separation of the lower third of the ala nasi from the vestibular floor, including the nasal sill. Surgery in the walls of the vestibule becomes more accessible, e.g., for the removal of ulcers and tumors. The **alar margin** may be stitched to the **nasal sill band** after resection of the rim-sill fold, if needed, or after the relocation of the alar margin to an aesthetically better place.

3.4.4.5 Unaesthetic Rim-Sill Fold

The rim-sill fold may itself be unaesthetic and a target for surgery.

The Inferior Segment

A **long** inferior segment of the rim-sill fold is associated with a **wide** nasal aperture.

The inferior segment may be **thicker** or **thinner** than its surrounding alar margin and nasal sill band. This gives the aperture margin an unaesthetic appearance.

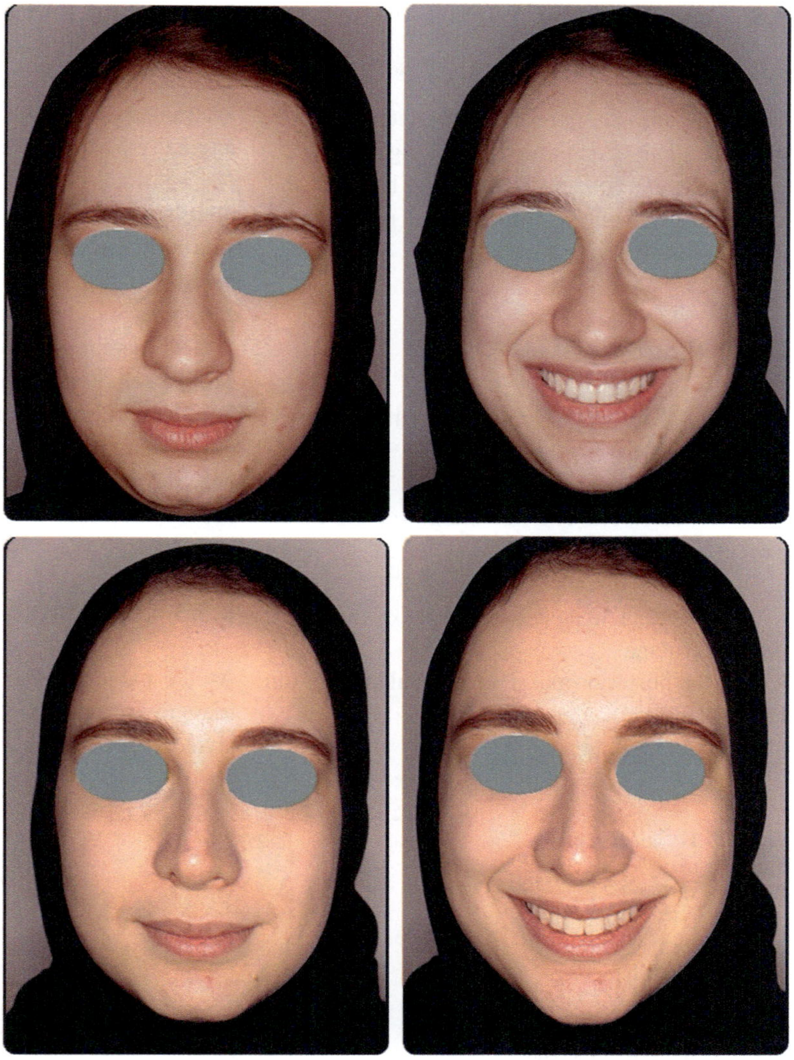

Fig. 3.2 Excision of the Rim-Sill folds has overcome the wide flare of nasal apertures on smiling

Partial or total excision of a **long** or **oblique** rim-sill fold will

- Reduce the aperture **size** by reducing the gap between the ala nasi and nasal sill band.
- **Lower** and **invert a** high or everted ala nasi.

Total excision of a **thin** or **thick** segment improves the aesthetics of the aperture margin. The overall outcome is a **narrower** aperture with **lower** and **inverted** alar margin. The **triple relation** between the **alar margin**, **nasal sill** and **columella** is, therefore, greatly improved.

The Posterior Segment

A thick posterior segment produces a **bulky alar base** that lies flatly and acutely on the face. Its excision is part of reducing the nasal **bulk**.

3.4.4.6 The Light Reflex

The anterior margin of the **rim-sill fold** is a direct continuation with that of the **nasal sill** medially and the inferior border of the **ala nasi** laterally. Together they all produce **one continuous line of light reflex** (see photography section). This line is the site for **marking lines** used as a guide in surgery of the alar base (vid supra).

3.5 The Muscular Triangle “The Hinge Area”

This is a gap that is present in the lateral wall of the nose. This gap is created during the development of the nose at the junction between the lateral process of the **fronto-nasal** process and the **maxillary process** on each side (Fig. 3.3.).

3.5.1 Boundaries

Inferiorly: The upper margin of the posterior two-thirds of the

ala nasi.

Posteriorly: The anterior margin of the **nasal process of the**

maxilla.

Anteriorly: The posterior margin of the upper lateral cartilage

and the posterior margin of **lateral crus** of the **lower**

lateral cartilage.

3.5.2 Roof and Floor

The **roof** of the muscular triangle is made of the external nasal skin, while the **floor** is made internally by the respiratory nasal mucosa.

The floor is supported by a **tough fibrous membrane** in which are found three to four **sesamoid cartilages**. This membrane is attached mainly to the lateral crus of the lower lateral cartilages and the nasal process of maxilla.

The membrane has a **free lower margin** that can be **palpated** by the tip of a little finger when introduced inside the nose. It is felt as a distinct tough margin that can be traced from its origin near the lateral crus till the root of the anterior nasal spine.

3.5.3 Contents

As the name implies, the main contents of this triangle are parts of the muscular bodies of the levators and dilators of the alae nasi, viz., the two

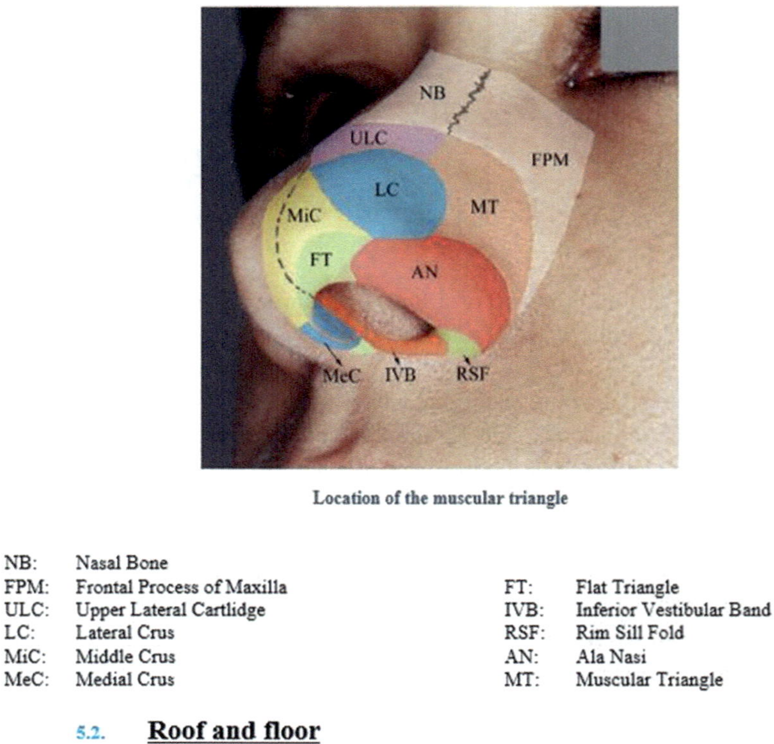

Fig. 3.3 Location of the muscular triangle. NB: Nasal Bone. FPM: Frontal Process of Maxilla. FT: Flat Triangle. ULC: Upper Lateral Cartlidge. IVB: Inferior Vestibular Band. LC: Lateral Crus. RSF: Rim-Sill Fold. MiC: Middle Crus. AN: Ala Nasi. MeC: Medial Crus. MT: Muscular Triangle

parts of the **nasalis** and **the levator labii superioris alaeque nasi**.

The muscles triangle can be **palpated** externally by placing the tip of a finger just anterior to the nasal process of the maxillary bone. Contraction and relaxation of the muscular contents can be easily felt on moving the alar nasi, nasal tip and the upper lip.

3.5.4 Surgical Significances

The muscular triangle is a soft gap that is filled only with muscle tissues and is strongly supported by a tough membranous floor.

It has two **kinetic structures along** its margins, the **ala nasi** and the **lower lateral cartilage**. The muscular triangle gives them a **free** area for their active movements during respiration and facial expressions hence the name the **hinge area**.

The area of the muscular triangle, including its tough membranous floor, moves inwards after lateral osteotomies.

The muscular triangle has no direct aesthetic effect. Its exploration is of no surgical value both functionally or aesthetically. It is an area that did not stimulate the interest of the surgeons along the whole history of the surgical rhinology.

3.6 The Weak Triangle

The weak triangle is a **midline gap** that appears between the **lower border of the upper lateral cartilage** superiorly and the **upper borders of the two middle crurae** inferiorly.

It is the transitional area between the **three-walled upper two-thirds** and the **four-walled lower third** of the nose.

The gap is initiated **superiorly** by the **bifurcation of the body of the upper lateral cartilage** into two branches, to embrace the four-walled lower third of the nose. Each branch is tucked under the lateral crus of each side of the nose. **Inferiorly,** the gap is initiated by **the divergence of the two bodies of the middle crurae,** i.e., the anterior nasal wall. A gap is,

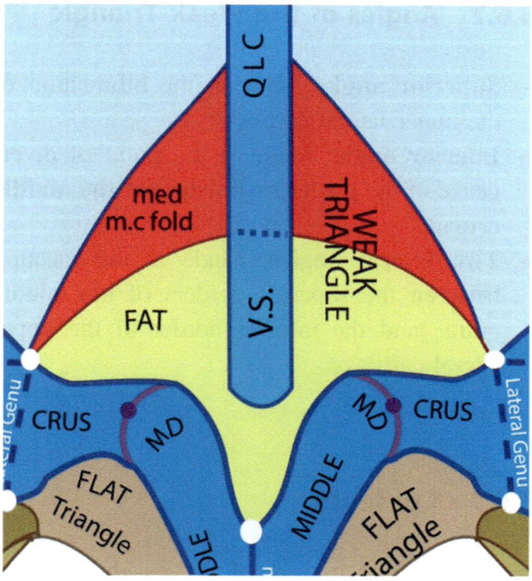

Fig. 3.4 The weak triangle. Med M.C Fold: Medial Muco-cutaneous Fold. MD: Mid-Domal Line and Mid-Domal Point. QLC: Quadrilateral Cartlidge of Nasal Septum. V.S: Vestibular Septum

thus, created between the upper lateral cartilage and the middle crurae (Fig. 3.4).

The weak triangle is strictly not triangular in shape. It is in fact a **quadrilateral space,** i.e., bounded by four borders. It lacks support in its roof, while the floor is only partially supported by the anterior angle of the caudal septum. Hence, the name is the **weak triangle**.

3.6.1 Boundaries of the Weak Triangle

As a quadrilateral space, it is bounded by two superior borders and two inferior borders. It has four angles, superior, inferior and two lateral angles.

- The **superior borders**: They are made by the **inferior borders** of the two branches of the **upper lateral cartilage**. They are separated by an angle that varies from 20–30 degrees depending on the width of the nose.
- The **two inferior borders**: They are made by the two **superior borders of the middle crurae.**

3.6.2 Angles of the Weak Triangle

- **Superior angle**: Made at the bifurcation of the upper lateral cartilage.
- **Inferior angle**: Made at the point of divergence of the **posterior borders of the middle crurae**.
- **Two lateral angles**: Made at the meeting between the superior borders of the middle crurae and the inferior border of the upper lateral cartilage.

3.6.3 Contents

- The anterior margin of the **caudal septum** with its **anterior angle** bisects the weak triangle. The septal angle represents the end-point of the dorsum of the nose.

This part of the cartilaginous septum is totally **subcutaneous**. It can be felt by palpating the supratip region. It may also be seen in some noses as a prominent protrusion. **It fills up the weak triangle** so that if it is inadvertently over-reduced, this will lead to a supratip depression.

Histologically, **all** of the skin-covered **vestibular septum** as well as **part** of the mucosally covered septum are present in the weak triangle, i.e., the junctional area (Fig. 3.4).

- On both sides of the cartilaginous septum, the weak triangle is filled with **loose connective tissue** and **copious amounts of fat** (Daniel & Palhase anatomical and clinical Atlas). This layer of fat may extend over the upper lateral cartilage to a variable degree.

3.6.4 Support:

The **walls** and **contents** of the weak triangle are held together by stabilizing fibrous tissues and bands. The **two middle crurae** are held together at the domes by the inter-crural connective tissue band. The two crurae are attached to the **septal angle** with fibrous bands which act as a **suspensory ligament** for the tip of the nose (never proved histology).

Ideally, the nasal tip is held at a slightly higher level than the septal angle in order to have a pleasing tip projection.

In the **lower margin of the upper lateral cartilage**, even though it is separated from the caudal septum, yet there remains a **perichondrial web attachment** at the angle of their meeting.

3.6.5 Roof and Floor

The **roof** of the weak triangle is made by the **skin cover** of the external nose, while the **floor** is made on each side of the nasal septum by the **medial muco-cutaneous folds**. These are the most medial unsupported folds of the limen nasi (see histology). They differ from the rest of the limen nasi as they have no **underlying cartilage** due to abscent continuation between the lower margin of the upper lateral cartilage and the caudal septum on both sides. They are only made of a muco-cutaneous lining with underlying loose connective tissue.

Although it is **a very short fold**, it has **a potential length** that is needed during active respiration **to open the anterior nasal valve angle** (see physiology of the nasal respiration). Because of this fold, the anterior valve angle is not a rigidly fixed one but rather more versatile and changes by the effect of the active small nasal muscles of respiration.

3.6.6 Surgical Importance of the Weak Triangle

The area of the weak triangle needs special attention and care from the surgeon both internally and externally. **Internally,** its location at the transitional muco-cutaneous nasal valve angle makes it very special during internal surgical handling.

Externally, the weak triangle represents the transitional area between the three-walled solid fixed pyramidal upper two-thirds of the nose and the four-walled lower third. The lower third is the more significantly important **physiologically** and **aesthetically**.

At this junction, **the nasal tip** is held tightly against the **nasal dorsum** to complete the nose into one unit.

The **slightest** surgical or traumatic change in this area **internally**, at the anterior angle of the **nasal valve**, or **externally**, including the **septum**, crurae, bands and ligaments or the covering skin, may have a **profound** effect on the **function**, the **aesthetics** of the nose or both.

There are two anatomical areas of surgical importance in the weak triangle, these are as follows:

3.6.6.1 The Medial Muco-Cutaneous Fold

The medial muco-cutaneous fold is at a much **higher** level than the anterior septal angle. The intercartilaginous incision, when communicated with a transfixing columellar incision, should, therefore, be made **inferior** to the valvular angle. A carefully planned incision should not disturb the anterior angle of the nasal valve. This is a point of great surgical significance (Fig. 3.5).

The medial muco-cutaneous fold has a significant value in the physiology of the nasal respiration.

It must not be disturbed by inadvertent injury or a wrongly placed surgical incision.

3.6.6.2 The Vestibular Septum

The caudal cartilaginous septum is lined by the vestibular skin and is called the vestibular septum (see Histology section).

The vestibular septum fills the weak triangle and is **a totally subcutaneous structure**. Therefore, it has a direct effect on the aesthetics of the supratip region.

There are **anatomical specifications** for the vestibular septum which have to be **precisely accurate** in order to fulfill its aesthetic role. These specifications are as follows:

(i) **The central course**

The vestibular septum has to have a **strictly central course**. **Deviation** or crookedness of the dorsal course of the vestibular septum may lead to a **tip** or **supratip crookedness or deviation**.

(ii) **The length**

The vestibular septum has to **have the exact length that fills the weak triangular area**. A **short septum** may either be associated with **supratip depression** or it may pull on the nasal tip upwards, thus unduly exposing the nasal apertures, i.e., **pig snout deformity**.

A **long vestibular septum** stretches the supratip region and pushes the domes down with a consequent **elongation of the nose and nasal tip.**

(iii) **The height**

The vestibular septum is the inferior end part of the nasal dorsum. It continues to have the same height as the dorsum.

As it fills the weak triangle, the vestibular septum should be at a slightly lower level than the nasal tip for a better aesthetic appearance.

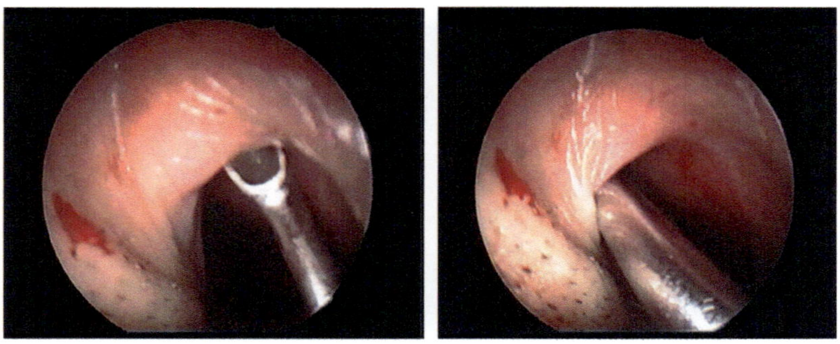

Fig. 3.5 The left medial muco-cutaneous fold

Traumatic or surgical **reduction of the height** of the vestibular septum will lead to a **supratip depression**.

On the contrary, if the vestibular septum is **higher** than the nasal tip, this leads to either of the following two deformities:

(a) **Parrot beak** deformity.
(b) **Sliding tip** if the middle crurae are loosely attached to the vestibular septum.

Combinations of all the above changes may take place in the septum so that.

- A **short** and **deviated** septum will not reach the tip. The nasal tip is still in the midline. The result is a **short deviated or crooked** supratip of the nose. This may be disclosed and clearly seen by smiling.
- A **long, deviated** septum drives the tip to one side leading to a **long deviated tip**.
- In both cases, the septum may be **high** or **low** leading to a **long**, **deviated parrot beak** or a **short, deviated** and **depressed** supratip deformities successively.

Significance of Nasal Base Attachment to the Orbicularis Oris

4

Abstract

The lower third of the nose is the most significant functionally, aesthetically and hence clinically. Anatomically and physiologically, it is different from the upper two-thirds. The nasal base attachment to the Orbicularis Oris is of significant surgical importance.

Keywords

The Oro-Nasal act of smiling · Smile Asymmetry

The lower third of the nose is the most significant functionally, aesthetically and hence clinically. Anatomically and physiologically, it is different from the upper two-thirds.

While kinetically and vitally active, the three-dimensional structure and position of the lower third of the nose are maintained at all times.

The Superior and Inferior Junctional Areas

The lower third of the nose joins the immobile upper two-thirds and the extremely mobile upper lip, with its inclusive Orbicularis Oris muscle, in the **superior** and **inferior junctional areas**. These two junctional areas have very important distinctive anatomy. The lower third is **semidetached from upper two-thirds** by areas of overlap, weak areas and soft folds, while **intimately attached** to the Orbicularis Oris in definite attachment areas.

The lower third of the nose is, therefore, **firmly held** and supported by the solid immobile walls of the upper two-thirds **superiorly** with limited movement. **Inferiorly** as well as the effects of the small muscles of the nose, the lower third follows the wide range of movements of the upper lip with its inclusive Orbicularis Oris.

The three-dimensional **shape** and **position** of the lower third are maintained at all times by the firm bodies of the lower lateral cartilages and the alae nasi.

Surgeons must understand the intimate relationship of the lower third of the nose with the **skin** of the upper lip and the **Orbicularis Oris** in order to perform accurate, aesthetically pleasing and successful alar and nasal base surgeries. It also helps in understanding the nasal involvement with the upper lip in other important physiological roles, e.g., facial expressions, eating, drinking and pursing.

The **upper lip** is an important **base** for the **lower third of the nose**. The **orbicularis oris** muscle is the main founder of the lips. It provides **direct attachments** to the **vestibular floor**, the **nasal sills,** the **alae nasi** and the **caudal septum**. **Indirectly,** it affects **the medial crurae** and consequently the rest of the lower third of the nose.

Of all parts of the lower third, the orbicularis oris has more powerful effects on the alae nasi. From this unique **firm, stable** and **actively mobile base**, the **alae nasi** are capable of both

M. H. A. Shafy, *Innovations in Rhinoplasty*,
https://doi.org/10.1007/978-3-030-94573-2_4

standing gracefully, producing their characteristic **aesthetic contribution** and at the same time **actively moving** to share in the **physiology** of nasal respiration and facial expressions. For successful nasal base surgery, it is essential to clarify the anatomy of this important junctional area.

4.1 Surgical Anatomy of the Orbicularis Oris

The orbicularis oris was known as the sphincter of the mouth. It is now recognized that its muscle fibers do not make a complete circular sphincter. It is clear that the orbicularis oris is made of **four independent groups of muscles** (right, left, upper and lower). Each group is made of **larger superficial** and **smaller deep groups,** i.e., the orbicularis oris is made of eight smaller subgroups of muscles.

4.1.1 Pars Peripheralis

This makes the **main bulk** of the orbicularis oris muscle. It is made of **fan-shaped cylindrical muscle fibers** that originate from the **modiolus** on each side. **The modiolus** is a **mobile fibromuscular mass** 12 mm. lateral to the buccal angle, **opposite to the second upper premolar tooth**.

It has no clear histological boundaries and varies with age, sex and ethnic group. It can be palpated by the opposite thumb and index finger.

The **highest fibers** of the pars peripheralis run through, and some are attached to, the **naso-labial sulcus**, then pass to the **nasal ala** and **septum**. The **lowest fibers reach** and are attached to the **mento labial sulcus** (Fig. 4.1).

4.1.2 Pars Marginalis

In each quadrant, the pars marginalis is made of a **single band of muscle fiber** that goes within the vermillion zone of each lip. Laterally, they are attached to the **deepest part** of the **modiolus**.

Most of the stem fibers are originated from the **modiolus. Reinforcement** comes from **other muscles** like the **buccinator, levator anguli oris** and the superficial part of the **zygomaticus major** in the **upper lip** and from the **buccinator** and **depressor anguli oris** in the **lower lip**.

The **upper most** and **lower most** fibers from the **buccinator pass directly** to corresponding upper and lower lips, while the **middle fibers decussate** at the modiolus to the **opposite lip**.

All parts of the orbicularis oris can be **palpated intraorally** and bimanually, starting from the modiolus laterally to naso-labial and mento-labial folds to the superior and inferior vestibular sulci.

4.1.3 Direct Labial Tractors

These are muscles that **pass directly to the upper and lower lips** at a right angle to the oral fissure. They do not come via the modiolus (Fig. 4.1).

They elevate, depress and evert the whole or part of the corresponding upper or lower lip.

The tractors of the upper lip, from medial to lateral, are as follows:

- The labial part of the levator labii superioris alaequae nasi.
- The levator labii superioris.
- The zygomaticus minor

Tractors of the lower lip are as follows:

- The depressor labii inferioris.
- Pars labii of the platysma.

The tractor muscles blend into a **continuous sheet** that divides into a **series of coronal sheets** which run between the bundles of the pars peripheralis and marginalis until they reach and are **inserted into the dermis of the kin** of the **lip** and **vermilion zone**.

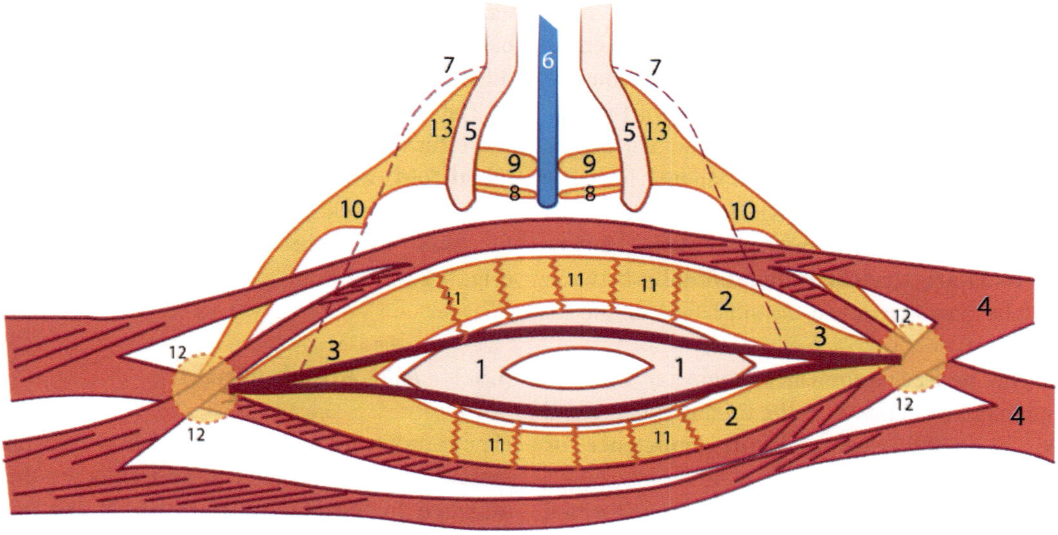

1. Lip Vermelion Skin
2. Pars Peripheralis
3. Pars Marginalis
4. Buccinator
5. Alae Nasi
6. Caudal Cartilagenous Septum
7. Naso Labial Fold
8. Septal Attachment of Pars Peripheralis
9. Vesticular Floor Attachment of Pars Peripheralis
10. Naso Labial Attachment of Pars Peripheralis
11. Direct Labial Tractors
12. Modiolus
13. Alar Attachment of Pars Peripheralis

Fig. 4.1 Anatomy of the Orbicularis Oris

4.2 Effects of the Orbicularis Oris on Nasal Base

The Orbicularis Oris has very important and unique anatomy that suits its variable and complicated tasks.

The main role of this muscle is the making of the structural **anatomy** and **physiology** of **both lips**. It also plays a key role in the **anatomy** and **physiology** of the **lower third of the nose**.

Unlike the Orbicularis Oculi, the Orbicularis Oris is **not** just a simple sphincter. An ultrasound study found that although the Orbicularis Oris muscle may be regarded as a single muscle anatomically, it appears functionally to consist of different parts acting independently or together with other facial muscles (Joe Iwanaga, et al. September 2017).

The Orbicularis Oris muscle works on both the lips and the nose in order to perform its various functions that include **speech** and articulation, the **facial expressions** of sadness, happiness, doubt, discontent, disdain, the canine snarl, **eating**, **drinking** and the original **sphincteric job of pursing** as in blowing, sucking, whistling and kissing.

Contraction of the marginalis muscle produces the **labial cord** in the vermilion border of the lips, by changing its cross-sectional profile. These cords are responsible for the fine vibrating movements of the lips.

In all of these jobs, the lips are required to **move in almost all directions**.

They are capable of moving, either **separately** or **together**, upwards and downwards, forwards and backwards against the teeth, from side to side, eversion and inversion as well as the pursing action. The **lower third of the nose follows the upper lip in all of its movements.**

Pursing has a **very powerful effect on the alae nasi**. During pursing, the bases of the alae nase are pulled downwards, and the alar bodies are rotated forwards and flared slightly laterally. The alae nasi are **strongly held** and **fixed** in this position which **secures good air entry**. The **rim-sill folds are stretched longitudinally** between the alae nasi above and the sill bands on the lip below.

This perfect performance requires a complete command and control of the lip musculature and skin in order to have **total oral competence for air, fluids and solids.**

Muscle fibers have, therefore, to be **inserted directly** into the **skin** and the **mucous membrane** without any loose tissues underneath.

The **smooth, thin** and **delicate vermilion skin** is quite suitable and specially suited for the fine and accurate control of the oral fissure. **Speaking** needs a very smooth **lip to lip and lip to teeth** relationship. **Drinking** and **eating** also need equally smooth and sensitive touch and seal at this important inlet of the mouth.

All of these acts of the lips are **very basic functions**, which **must not be disturbed** or **lost during lifetime**.

The **anatomical structure** and the **physiological performance** of both **lips** and consequently the **nose**, therefore, remain **stable** and **competent without affection by aging or any generalized bodily changes and illnesses**, e.g., body weight, hormonal and metabolic disorders. Only neurological, traumatic or direct pathological diseases may affect their functions.

4.3 Nasal Base Attachments of the Orbicularis Oris

There are definite nasal extensions of the Orbicularis Oris muscle to the base of the lower third of the nose. All three components of the nasal base, i.e., the alae nasi, the two vestibular floors and the caudal septum are attached to the Orbicularis Oris muscle. Each part of the nasal base is attached to the muscle in a completely different way.

The uppermost fasciculus of the pars peripheralis runs through and is attached to the **naso-labial fold**, which is the site of folding of the fat-bearing cheek skin over the firmly adherent lip skin over the orbicularis oris muscle (Fig. 4.1).

4.3.1 Alar Attachments

Having gone through the naso-labial fold, the muscle fibers of the **pars peripheralis** are then **attached to the upper two-thirds of the posterior margin of the ala nasi on each side** (Fig. 4.1), i.e., the **alar base** of the nose is attached to the face at this **firm meeting between the alae nasi and the orbicularis oris.**

The **nasal fasciculus** of the **pars peripheralis** can be **palpated intraorally** between the modiolus laterally and the superior vestibular fold medially. The muscle act on the alae nasi by **moving them laterally and medially,** thus, **widening** and **narrowing the alar base** of the nose as in smiling and whistling.

4.3.2 Vestibular Floor Attachments

The nasal fascicular fibers of the pars peripheralis run into the vestibular floor where the nasal **sill bands** take **direct and firm** attachments, while the **loose vestibular skins** are **separated** from the muscle by an **abundant connective tissue layer** (Fig. 4.1).

4.3.3 Caudal Cartilaginous Septal Attachment

The muscle fibers are finally attached to the caudal nasal septum. They may interlace with fibers from the opposite side over the midline (Fig. 4.1).

4.4 Effect of Upper Lip Skin on Nasal Stability

Unlike the rest of the facial skin, the **lip skin neither wrinkles nor droops down** with age, as it is directly attached to the underlying muscle layer. It may have **firm surface furrows** rather than loose redundant skin wrinkles.

Likewise, **the increase in cheek fat never affects the lips**. This explains the deepening in the naso-labial grooves in conditions of aging and increased facial fat.

These facts are important so that

(a) The basic physiological work of the mouth and lips is maintained, i.e., **oral competence** for air and fluid and solids. These are basic needs of life, i.e., breathing, eating and drinking.
(b) **Nasal stability,** i.e., the nose does not move forwards or backwards with the change in body weight, neither do the alae droop down with the atrophied skin of an aging person.

4.5 The Oro-Nasal Act of Smiling

Although **the act of smiling** is primarily linked with the **mouth**, the **lower third of the nose is inseparably involved in the procedure**.

Smiling is an **active process** that involves the **lips**, the **alae nasi**, the **medial crurae** and the **caudal cartilaginous septum**.

The facial, oral and nasal muscles are all involved so that

4.5.1 The Lips

The **orbicularis oris** is **acted upon** on each side by two groups of muscles, viz.,

i. The **buccinators**:

They pull on the **modiolus** on each side of the muscle **directly laterally.**

ii. The **levators**, labii and anguli, and the **zygomaticus**, major and minor. They pull on the modiolus **upwards** and **laterally**.

4.5.2 The Alae Nasi

The **alae nasi** are **acted upon** by two groups of muscles:

i. The **alar extensions** of the **orbicularis**:

They pull on the posterior margins of both alae **widening the alar base** and hence the nasal apertures.

ii. The **dilator** and **levator alae,** i.e., the alar parts of the nasalis and the **levator labii alaeque nasi** successively:

As they are attached to their outer surfaces, both alae are **elevated, everted** and **dilated.**

4.5.3 The Nasal Septum and Medial Crurae

The **depressor septi** muscles tend to **fix the caudal septum** and the **medial crurae** by pulling them down. An act which, **if exaggerated, may lead to animation**, i.e., **mobile tip**.

The outcomse of these three active processes are as follows:

(a) **Wider oral fissure** due to elongation of the lips. **The angles of the mouth are elevated** producing the happy curved appearance.
(b) **Wider nasal apertures with elongation of the rim-sill folds** between **the two fixed ends** of the **alae nasi** and nasal **sill bands**. The two **vestibular floors** with their loose skin and subcutaneous tissue are equally stretched, widening the size of both nasal apertures.

Further widening of the aperture is added by the **elevation** and **eversion** of the **alae nasi.**

(c) The position of the **caudal septum, medial crurae** and consequently the lower lateral cartilages is strongly maintained and stabilized in a **lower position**.

In the case of the **stronger act of laughing**, more muscles are involved in the **face, neck** and **body**.

4.6 Smile Asymmetry

Normal individuals may have an asymmetrical smile so that the lateralization of one side of the face is different from the other side. The angle of the mouth, the naso-labial fold and ala nasi is wider and higher on one side than the other. The ball of the cheek is bigger on the side of the larger maxillary bone.

This must be noted especially in patients who had alar base surgery. They maintain the same asymmetry of their smile post-operatively.

The asymmetrical smile does not change a patient's surgical management. Some patients may only notice their smile asymmetry for the first time after they have their surgery. This is especially true if they underwent alar base reduction.

Pre-operative non-smiling and smiling photographs are quite essential in helping patients to understand this normal and natural fact.

The Seven Types of Nasal Skin Anatomy and Surgical Significance

5

Abstract

Before studying the skin of the nose, it is essential to understand the basic structure of the skin in general. This will shed the light on how the nasal skin is suitably adapted to its **functions** and **aesthetics**.

Keywords

The seven types of nasal skin · The hypodermal two fatty layers (Panniculus Adiposus)

Before studying the skin of the nose, it is essential to understand the basic structure of the skin in general. This will shed the light on how the nasal skin is suitably adapted to its **functions** and **aesthetics**.

The skin invests the external surface of the whole body. It provides cover and protection to the various parts of the external surface of the body from head to toe.

It has to adapt for function according to the stresses and exposures of the various areas of the external surface of the body. Examples of these are the palms and soles, the areas of flexion and extension, the scalp and face, etc.

5.1 Basic Anatomy of Skin

The following information is mainly derived from Gray's Anatomy (chapter).

The main layer of the skin is the **dermis (corium)**. It is made of **strong fibrous tissue** that is **rich in blood vessels**, **nerves** and **lymphatics**. The manufacturing of leather depends on the drying and dying of this layer.

The dermis is covered and protected by the layer of **the epidermis**. Loss of the epidermis will lead to ulceration, infection and the consequent loss of the underlying dermal layer.

The skin is attached to the body via the **subcutaneous tissue layer** or **the hypodermis**. This layer is made of **areolar connective tissue** and is rich in **fat**.

The thickness of the skin mainly depends on the thickness of the **dermis** and the **horny layer** of the epidermis.

The body is invested and wrapped deeply by a **deep fascial layer**. From the surface inwards the **skin layers,** therefore, are:

(a) The Epidermis.
(b) The Dermis.
(c) The Hypodermis, i.e., The Subcutaneous tissue layer.
(d) The Deep Fascial Layer.

Each of these layers is subjected to wide **variations** in the different parts of the body.

M. H. A. Shafy, *Innovations in Rhinoplasty*,
https://doi.org/10.1007/978-3-030-94573-2_5

5.1.1 The Epidermis

The epidermis is made of five layers starting from the deepest layer to the surface:

(1) **The Geminal layer "Stratum Germinativum"**.

This is the basal columnar cell layer that undergoes continuous mitosis.

(2) **The Prickle cell layer "Malpighian layer"**.

These are made of many daughter cell layers that gradually flatten toward the surface.

(3) **The Granular cell layer "Stratum granulosum"**.

Granules of the pre-keratin appear inside the cells.

(4) **The clear cell layer "Stratum lucidum"**.

This is a thin clear layer.

(5) **The Keratine layer "Stratum corneum"**.

This layer is made of varying thicknesses of the horny layer.

5.1.2 The Dermis

This is **the most important layer** of all the skin layers for the following reasons:

(1) It is a **tough fibrous layer** that provides a good cover and protection to the underlying structures.
(2) It is rich in **blood vessels** and **nerves**.
(3) **The adnexa** are mostly present in this layer:
  i. The **sweat glands**: They are present under the surface of the dermis. The ducts are spiral in the dermis and dilate in the epidermis.
  ii. The **sebaceous glands**: They are grape-like and only present and open into the hair follicles.

Both of these glands help in **wetting** and **greasing** the skin.

  iii. The **hair:** It is present in variable amounts in the different areas of the nose.
(4) **Langer's lines**: The collagen fibers in the dermis lie in parallel bundles. The directions of Langer's lines are of great surgical importance to have a wound that heals with minimal scar. The surgical incision should be parallel to Langer's line.
(5) **The yellow elastic fibers**: They are essential for **the vital look** of the skin. They progressively **atrophy with age**.

5.1.3 The Hypodermis

This is also known as the **subcutaneous tissue layer**.

It is the intermediate layer that connects and attaches the skin to the underlying parts of the body, i.e., deep fascia, bone or cartilage.

It is made of varying degrees of **areolar connective tissue** and **fat "Panniculus adiposus".**

Through this layer, the vessels, nerves and lymphatics pass to and from the skin.

The fibrofatty tissue under the skin is divided by **fibrous bands** that connect the **skin** to the **deep fascia**. These bands are especially significant in the skin area that covers the nasal tip and the lateral crura.

These fibrous bands fix the external skin to the crurae so that it does not slide over them (see the anatomy of Lower Lateral cartilages).

In certain areas, within the **hypodermis,** there are sheets of flat muscles **"Panniculus carnosus"** that connect the **skin** to the **deep fascia** or **bone,** e.g., the platysma, the occipitofrontalis and in other areas of the body as in the nipple and scrotum. In the nose, it can be seen in the **procerous** and many other **small muscles of the nose (SMAS).**

5.1.4 The Deep Fascial Layer

This is a deep investing **fibrous tissue layer** that usually wraps the deep tissues and muscles of the body, i.e., the scalp, neck abdomen, back and limbs.

This layer is **totally absent in the face**. Over the **bones** and **cartilages,** it is replaced by the **periosteal** and the **perichondrial layers**. Examples of these are the skin over the tibia and over the **ears** and nasal **cartilages**.

The **perichondrium** of the nasal cartilages gives attachment to the **fibrous bands** that connect it **to the dermal skin layer**.

5.2 The Seven Types of Nasal Skin

The skin of the nose is a perfect example of the adaptation of tissues for function. As a three-dimensional structure, the nose has a **physiologic** role as well as **aesthetic effects**. In order to achieve these functions, the skeletal components of the nose, i.e., the bones, the cartilages and the fibrofatty tissues are linked to each other in unique and very specialized transitional areas.

These transitional areas are in the form of **sutures, overlaps** and **gaps**. The **bones** are attached to each other by **sutures**, while the **upper lateral cartilage** is linked to the nasal bones and lower lateral cartilages via specialized **overlapping areas**. Other parts are separated by gaps that are filled with weak areas and soft folds of the skin.

All these skeletal structures and the transitional areas are covered by skin which varies **widely in these limited and small parts of the nose** in order to meet the **physiological** and **aesthetic** functions.

Although all **the layers** of the nasal skin are important, the **dermis** and the **hypodermis** are the two most important layers.

The **dermal layer** is more concerned with the nasal **functions** while the **hypodermal layer** is more concerned with the nasal **aesthetic**.

These two components of the skin are quite variable in the different areas of the nose according to their aesthetic and physiologic roles.

The skin of the external nose is divided into **seven areas** (Fig. 5.1). Each area has a **histologically different skin** in order to adapt for **function** and **aesthetics**. These areas are as follows:

(1) The bony pyramid.
(2) The upper lateral cartilage.
(3) The lower lateral cartilage.
(4) The alae nasi.
(5) The nasal vestibules.
(6) The weak areas and soft folds.
(7) The junctional areas.

5.2.1 The Skin Cover of the Bony Pyramid

The skin covering the bony pyramid is **very thin** and the **most mobile** of all the nasal skin areas. This is as a result of the loose areolar connective **tissue** in the hypodermis (Fig. 5.1).

The **mobile** skin over the **fixed bones protects both structures** from the effect of trauma. In cases of direct trauma, **the skin slides** as it takes away the direct force off the underlying bone. In the meantime, the skin itself is less injured or damaged.

5.2.2 The Skin Cover of the Upper Lateral Cartilage

The **skin** covering the upper lateral cartilage is **less mobile** than that of the nasal bones.

The **hypodermis** has less areolar connective tissue and **more fibrofatty** and **muscle tissues,** i.e., panniculus adiposus and panniculus carnosusu. Fibrofatty tissues spread within the loose connective tissue layer, e.g., SMAS.

5.2.3 The Skin Cover of the Lower Lateral Cartilages

The external skin of the lower lateral cartilages only covers the **middle** and **lateral crurae,** i.e., the **frontolateral walls** of the lower third of the nose (Fig. 5.1).

This is the **most important skin** of all the nasal skin areas. Not only does it cover the most aesthetically significant frontolateral walls,

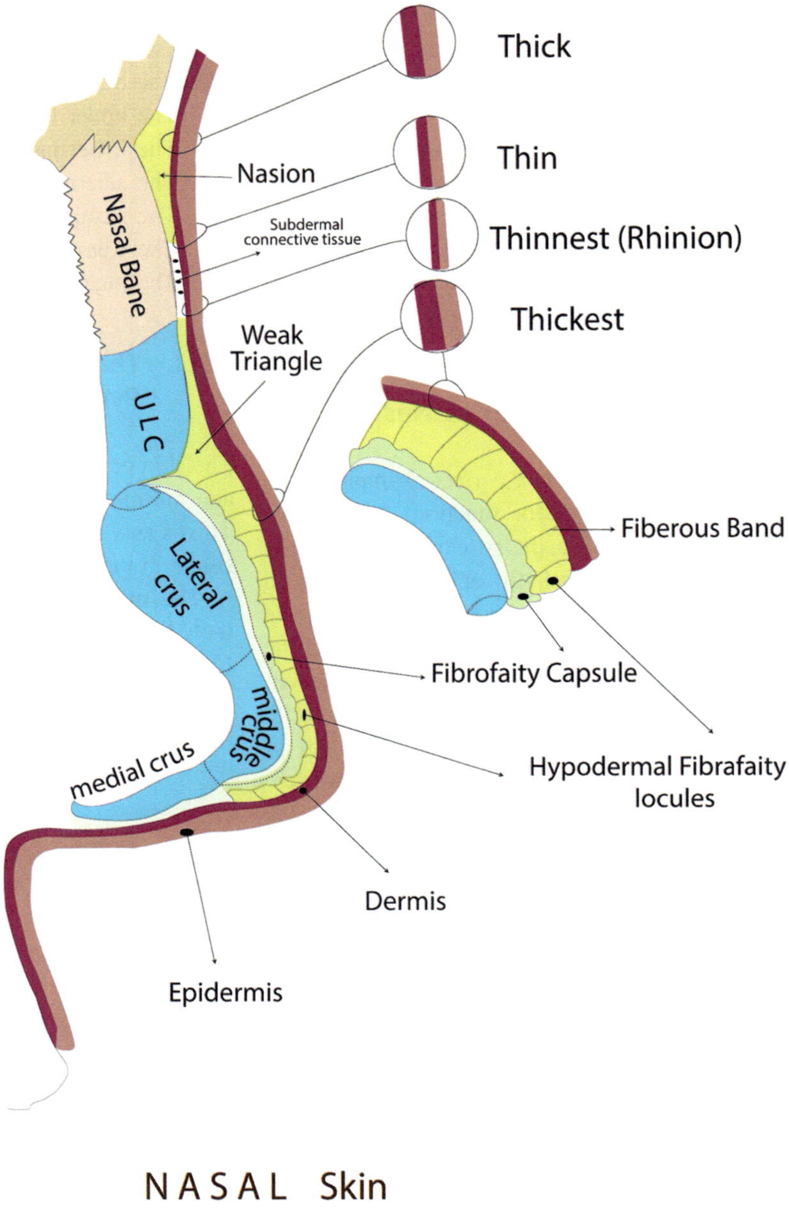

Fig. 5.1 Nasal skin. ULC—Upper Lateral Cartilage

including the nasal tip, but it also has unique characteristics that make it **share in the structuring of these walls.**

It is the **thickest** and **greasiest** of all of the nasal skin and is **totally immobile** as it is fixed to the relatively mobile middle and lateral crurae.

The **Middle Eastern** and **Hispanic noses** are generally characterized by the **thick frontolateral skin of the middle and lateral crurae**, while the **African** and **Asian noses** have **thick alae nasi skin**. Clinically, the bulky Middle Eastern and Hispanic noses are mainly due to the bulky frontolateral walls while bulky Asian and African noses are mainly due to bulky alae nasi.

The **dermis** and the **hypodermis** of the skin over the middle and lateral crurae have unique characteristics that make them very special for this important location of the nose.

5.2.3.1 The Dermis

The dermal layer over the middle and lateral crurae is **the thickest** and **the toughest** of all nasal skin areas. It acts as a protective cover and protects this important front of the nose.

The dermal thickness and toughness vary from one side of the same nose to the other. It is also variable in the different sex, age and ethnicity, being **thicker** in **males**, **adults** and **Middle Eastern** noses than **females**, **children** and **other ethnic groups**.

5.2.3.2 The Hypodermal Two Fatty Layers (Panniculus Adiposus)

This layer is also known as the **hypodermis** or the superficial fascia. It is this layer that gives the lower lateral skin its unique important characteristics of shape and thickness.

Both, the **dermal skin surface** and the **crural cartilages,** are covered by **two separate layers of fat** (Fig. 5.1).

(a) **The hypodermal fibrofatty locules**

The **hypodermal layer** is made of fibrofatty tissue that spreads under, and is quite adherent to, the dermal layer. As **this layer is unique to the lower lateral cartilaginous skin**, it ends abruptly at its junction with the upper lateral cartilaginous skin by a distinctly **prominent fibrofatty ridge.**

There are many **bands** (Fig. 5.1) which are close to each other that connect the dermis with the fibrofatty crural capsules. These bands pass through the hypodermal fatty layers. The bands are **normal anatomical findings of the skin** all over the body. In this area, the nose bands are much more **numerous, closer** to each other and **tougher**. The hypodermal fat is, thus, enclosed into small locules of fat.

(b) **The crural fibrofatty capsules:**

The outer surfaces of the middle and lateral crurae are covered with fibrous capsules that are studded with variable amounts of fat (Fig. 5.1).

The outcome is the presence of **two layers of fibrofatty tissues** that are neatly and firmly loculated in **closed chambers**. These chambers are made by the hypodermal **fibrous bands** that bind with the fibrofatty **capsular layers** of the cartilaginous crurae. They all are integrated in the formation of **one complex unit** that finally forms the frontolateral wall of the nose, including the nasal tip.

The two-step Enlargement of the Middle and Lateral Crurae

The fibrofatty capsules that fit the outer surfaces of the middle and lateral crurae **take their exact shapes** but **at a larger scale**. The fatty capsules are then attached to the external skin by the hypodermal fibrous bands. The bands pull the external skin tightly toward the crurae. The external skin of the **frontolateral walls,** thus, takes the **exact same shapes** of the middle and lateral crurae at a further larger scale **for the second time**. The middle and lateral crurae, therefore, are enlarged twice in two steps.

The **external look** and the **shape** of the frontolateral wall of the nose are determined not only by the shape of the lower lateral cartilages, but also by the thickness and the distribution of the two layers of fibrofatty tissues that cover them.

The **thickness** of each of the two fibrofatty layers is **variable** from one person to another and from one side of the same nose to the other. These layers help in smoothing the surfaces and the margins of the bodies of the lower lateral cartilages.

A nose with a thick frontolateral wall always has thick fibrofatty layers and vice versa.

Surgical significances

The hypodermal double fibrofatty layers play an essential part in the **stability** and **aesthetics** of the frontolateral wall of the nose.

i. **Stability of the frontolateral wall**

The fibrofatty layers fix and immobilize the skin over the middle and lateral crurae.

If the fibrofatty layers were loosely mobile, the external skin would slide over the mobile crurae and the nasal front would be floppy and lose its fixed projection.

ii .**Aesthetics of the Nasal tip**

In noses with large, boxy, bulbous or clown-looking tips, **the fibrofatty tissues are in excess** and so thick that they are much larger and **overshadow the real sizes and shapes of the crural cartilages**.

Removal of the fibrofatty layers clears the way for the cartilaginous shapes to be shown under the thinner skin which enhances the natural nasal aesthetics.

Skin over the junction between the upper and lower lateral cartilages.

The two subdermal fibrofatty layers over the lateral crurae end abruptly at their junction with the upper lateral cartilage. There is a prominent margin of hypodermal fibrofatty tissue.

The sudden end of these two layers of fat means the **sudden reduction in the thickness of skin** between the two areas. This is shown **externally** by the **sudden drop in the height** of the skin level from the lateral crurae to the upper lateral cartilages. This junction might be marked by a **crease**, **step** or a **slope** on the external skin.

As well as with the difference in the level of the skin, there is a sudden change in the **nature** of the skin, from the **thick, immobile, greasy** type over the lower lateral cartilages to the **thin, mobile, non-greasy** type over the upper lateral cartilage.

5.2.4 The Skin Cover of the Alae Nasi

The skin cover of the alae nasi has **no hypodermal tissue layer,** i.e., it is directly adherent to the underlying fibrofatty layer of the alae nasi.

The alae nasi are covered by **external** and **internal** skin. Internally, it is covered by **hairy vestibular skin**. The external skin has an epidermal layer that is similar to that of the middle and lateral crurae, i.e., is **thick, immobile, greasy** and **hairless**.

5.2.5 The Vestibular Skin

The vestibular skin is generally thin and hairy (vibrissae) and greasy. It contains some sebaceous and sweat glands. Each vestibule, right and left, has medial, lateral, inferior and anterior walls. The skin of each of the vestibular walls has its own characteristics as well as its own relations to the underlying structures.

5.2.5.1 The Lateral Vestibular Wall

The lateral vestibular wall has two components, the **ala nasi** and the **lateral crus**. Each has a vestibular skin cover of different characteristics.

i. The skin cover of the **alar nasi** is a natural continuation of the external skin. It continues to be directly **adherent** to the underlying fibrofatty layer all around the alar margin and the internal vestibular wall.

Similar to the rest of the vestibular skin, it is **thin, greasy** and has extensively **dense vibrissae**.

ii .The lateral crural vestibular skin becomes **suddenly devoid of vibrissae**. It is a useful surgical anatomical guide to the lower margin of the lateral crus. The skin is paper-thin and incisions are made extremely lightly.

5.2.5.2 The Anterior Vestibular Wall

The vestibular skin cover of the middle crus is thin, greasy and has dense vibrissae despite its direct continuity with the lateral crural skin.

5.2.5.3 The Inferior Vestibular Wall

The inferior wall skin is abundantly loose with an equally abundantly loose hypodermal connective tissue layer. The skin is thin, hairy and greasy.

5.2.5.4 The Medial Vestibular Wall

The skin is **adherent** to the **vestibular** septum and the **medial crus**. In between these two structures is the **membranous septum** and the two skin layers are extensively loose with abundant hypodermal connective tissue layer. Only the medial crural vestibular skin has dense vibrissae, and the membranous septal skin is devoid of hair.

5.2.6 Skin Cover of the Weak Areas and Soft Folds

The flat, **the weak** and **the muscular triangles** are covered extremely with the same greasy skin that covers the lower lateral cartilages and alae nasi. **Internally,** they are covered by the vestibular skin and respiratory mucosa successively.

The skin cover of the **muscular triangle** has **no hypodermis** as the small muscles of the nose are directly attached to the skin (panniculus carnosus).

The **rim-sill** and **posterior columellar folds** are covered by soft hairless skin.

The **vestibular floor** is covered by thin, hairy and greasy skin, while the **membranous septum** is devoid of hair.

Over-reduction of a nasal hump is to be observed in this area. Allowance is made for the **thin bone, skin** and **hypodermis**. Slightly **less reduction** is needed here.

5.2.7 Skin Cover of Transitional Areas

The nasal dorsum covers two main transitional areas:

The Rhinion, i.e., the junction between the nasal bones and the upper lateral cartilage. The skin cover in this area is the thinnest of all nasal skins (Fig. 5.1). Care must be taken during undermining the dorsal skin and while rasping or excising osteocartilaginous hump. The skin may easily be pierced or injured.

The scroll area, i.e., the junction between the upper and lower lateral cartilages. The skin is thick, hairless and greasy. It is less thick than the skin cover of the middle and lateral crurae.

5.3 Incisions and Scars of Nasal Skin

Clean surgical wounds generally almost always leave minimal or no visible scar if made in the right location and neatly stitched at the appropriate time with the appropriate stitches in the appropriate layers. This is especially true on making external incisions on the nasal skin.

5.3.1 Location of Incision

The location and type of skin where incisions are made play a major role in the aesthetic outcome of the final scar.

The best location for a planned external nasal incision is at the soft folds of skin located at the posterior alar grooves, i.e., the rim-sill folds. They almost always leave no visible scars if stitched in layers and the skin margins are appropriately approximated.

- Any inadvertent cut in the external skin of the nose, e.g., in the frontolateral wall or nasal dorsum leaves no visible scar if stitched immediately at the time of surgery.
- An inadvertent cut in the flat triangle (soft) is dealt with by immediate separate stitching of the two skin layers, external and internal. The skin will take a few weeks before it finally heals with no visible scarring.
- The thin skin over the nasal bones is more likely to leave visible scarring.

5.3.2 Time of Stitching

Immediate stitching of clean wounds has the best chance of better aesthetic results. The longer the delay, the less chance of better results especially after the first 24 hours.

5.3.3 Types of Stitch

Nylon (Proline) stitches for the external skin and Vycril for the subdermal tissues are the best for these layers. The thinner the type of the stitch, the better, i.e., 5-0 or 6-0, depending on the location, the results produced. The margins of skin edges must match on the same level on both sides.

5.3.4 Layers of Stitch

All the cut layers of the skin must be stitched separately so that

- Alar wounds after alar resection are stitched in two layers, viz., skin and the hypodermal tissue layer.
- An inadvertent cut of the flat triangle and the two layers of its skin are stitched separately, viz., external and vestibular. The same applies for all other nasal skin areas.

6 Histological Studies of New Anatomical Structures

Abstract

Two new anatomical structures are studied histologically for the first time. Both are firm structures that are present in the dynamically important lower third of the nose.

1. The Inferior Vestibular Band
2. The Vestibular Septum

Keywords

The Inferior Vestibular Band · The Vestibular Septum #Caudal Cartilagenous Septum

6.1 The Inferior Vestibular Band

The floor of the nose has clear anatomical and physiological significances. It is part of the external valve of the nose. The nasal sill was studied histologically in several methods. The tissues of the nasal sill band lose their structure quickly after death because of their delicate consistency. It was found that the **nasal sill band is not just a small free band at the anterior end of the vestibular floor,** but the tissues of the band **extend to the medial vestibular wall**. It was important to have extensive study to find out the exact nature and extensions of this band in the inferior vestibular area of the nose.

6.1.1 Material and Methods

Tissues were taken from fresh cadavers within the first five hours of death, to avoid disintegration of the elastic tissues.

Histological studies were made on sagittal cuts across the **floor of the nose (nasal sill)** and coronal cuts along the **columella**.

Two staining techniques were used to reveal the nature of tissues, viz., **hoematoxellin** and **eosin** and **Verhoeff Van Gieson** stains.

Twenty cases were studied in various age groups, i.e., between the ages of 20 and 70 years. Originally, tissues were taken from more than sixty fresh cadavers. Only twenty of them were valid for the study. This was due to various factors including the trial of making cuts in more distant places in the nose and the use of other methods of preparations and staining.

6.1.2 Histological Findings

Tissues made of condensed **yellow elastic** fibers interdigitating with bundles of **collagen fibers** were found to be running along the anterior margin of the nasal floor making the nasal sill (Fig. 6.1). They then sweep around the **posterior** and the **superior** margins of the **medial crus** of the lower lateral cartilage (Figs. 6.2, 6.3, 6.4 and 6.5).

M. H. A. Shafy, *Innovations in Rhinoplasty*,
https://doi.org/10.1007/978-3-030-94573-2_6

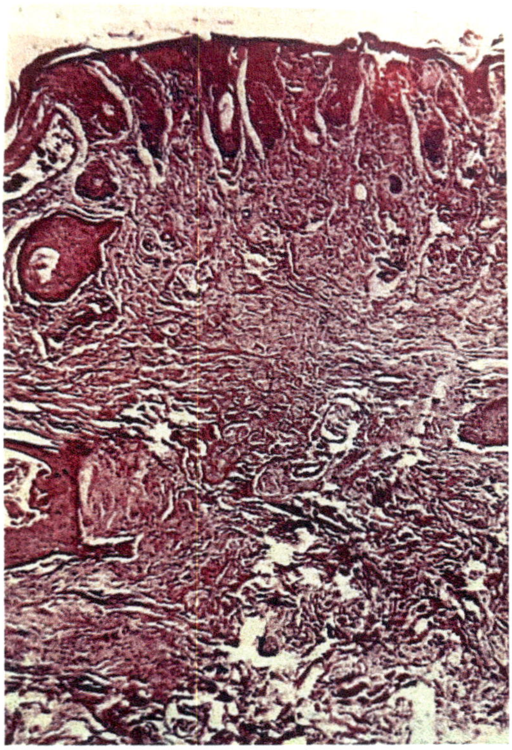

Fig. 6.1 Section across the nasal floor (nasal sill): Thick fibro-collagen reaching directly to the skin surface and deeply to Orbicularis oris muscle. (H. and E. stain) Red: collagen fibers., Black: elastic fibers.Yellow: muscle fibers

Collagen and **elastic fibers** were found to be **reaching the skin directly** without intervening subcutaneous tissues both in the **columellar** and the **nasal sill** cuts. The skin over these fibers was devoid of hair at the nasal floor cuts, while in the columellar cuts vestibular hairs (vibrissae) were found (Fig. 6.6).

Muscle fibers were found to be **directly attached to the deeper side** of the fibro-collagenous fibers at the nasal floor cuts. These are fibers of the Orbicularis oris muscle.

Muscle tissues were found in loose connective tissue higher in the columellar cuts (Fig. 6.1).

6.1.3 Conclusion

There is a constant finding of a **free band** formed of **yellow elastic** and **white collage fibers** which runs transversely in the anterior margin of the vestibular floor at its junction with the upper lip. These fibers pass **superiorly behind** than **above** the **posterior** and the **superior margins** of the medial crus (Fig. 6.7). The two bands can be felt rolling between the thumb and the fingers if introduced in both nostrils. The bands constantly raise an adherent layer of thin skin along their course. It helps in the formation and support of the nasal floor and the medial columellar wall.

6.2 The Vestibular Septum

The caudal cartilaginous septum has an important anatomical and aesthetic significance. Microscopic studies have proven that it has a different histological structure than the rest of the nasal septum.

6.2.1 Material and Methods

Intraoperative specimens were obtained. The membranous septum was fully stretched by Cottle's columellar forceps. **Stripes of the cartilaginous septum with their lining on one side** were obtained. The specimen site was halfway between the anterior and posterior septal angles. Cuts were made, **starting from the caudal end of the septum going cephalically for two cen-**

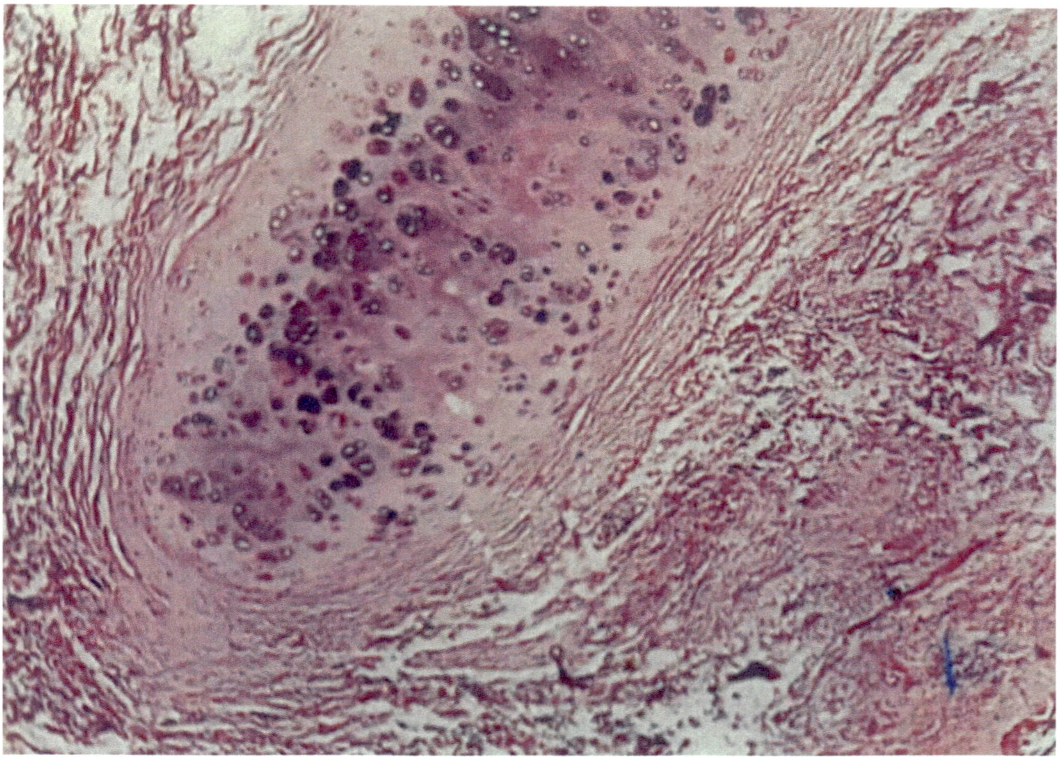

Fig. 6.2 Columellar cut: The medial crus surrounded by sweeping fibro-collagen fibers that reach the skin (H. and E. stain)

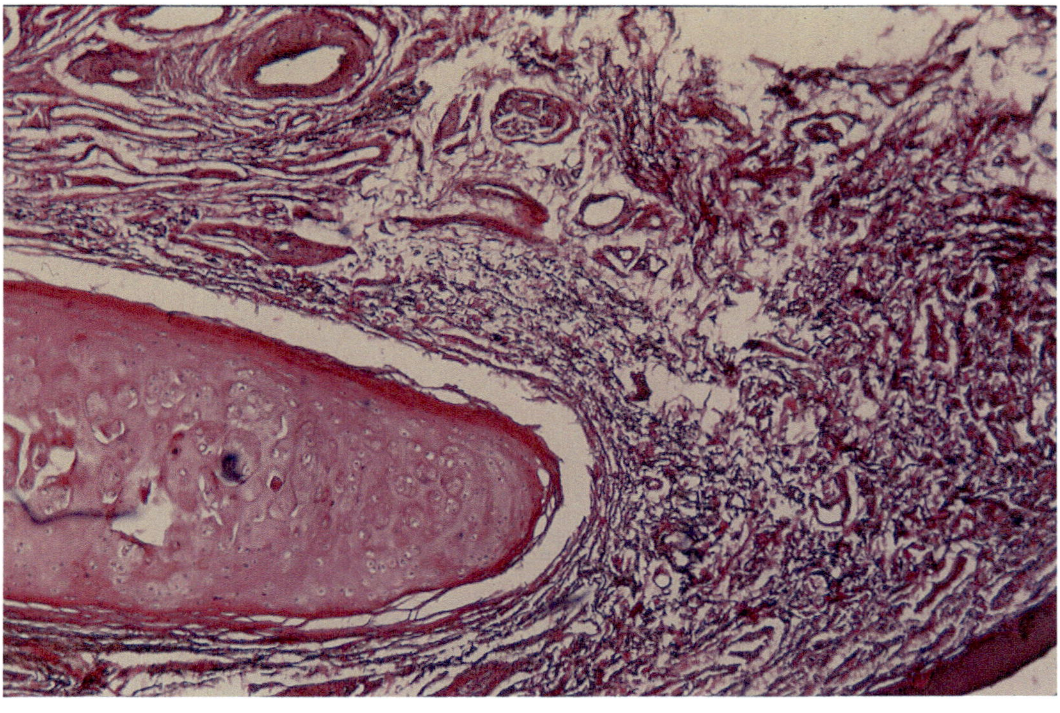

Fig. 6.3 Sweeping fibro-collagen fibers around medial crus reaching the skin. (Verhoeff Van Gieson stain)

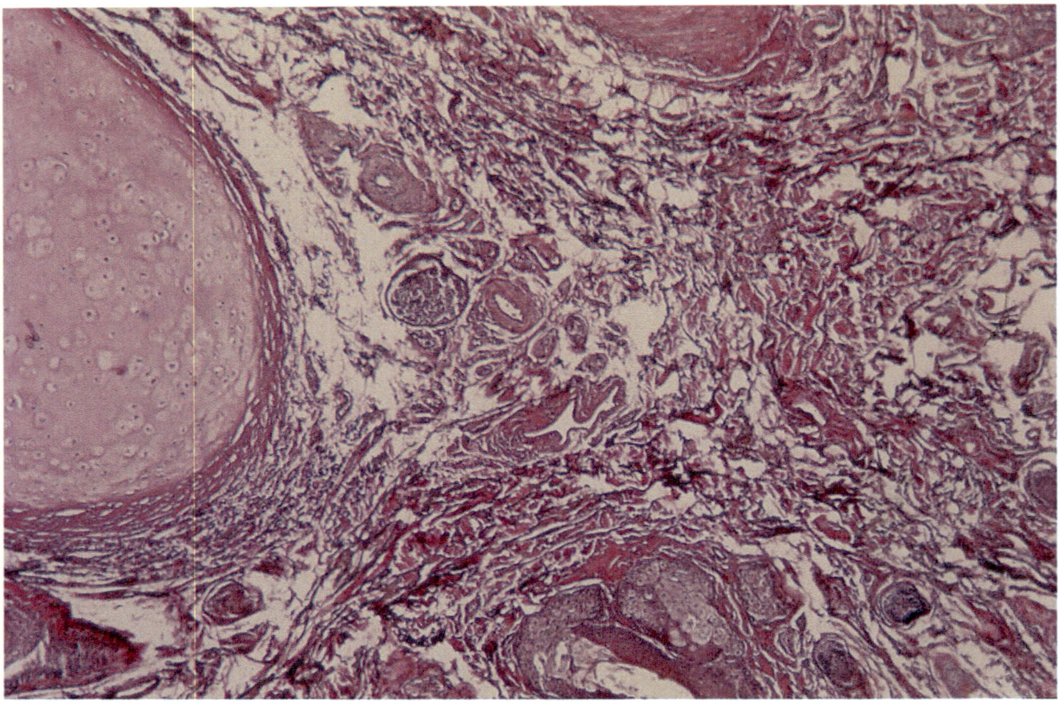

Fig. 6.4 The medial crus and fibro-collagen fibers (high power) V.V.G stain

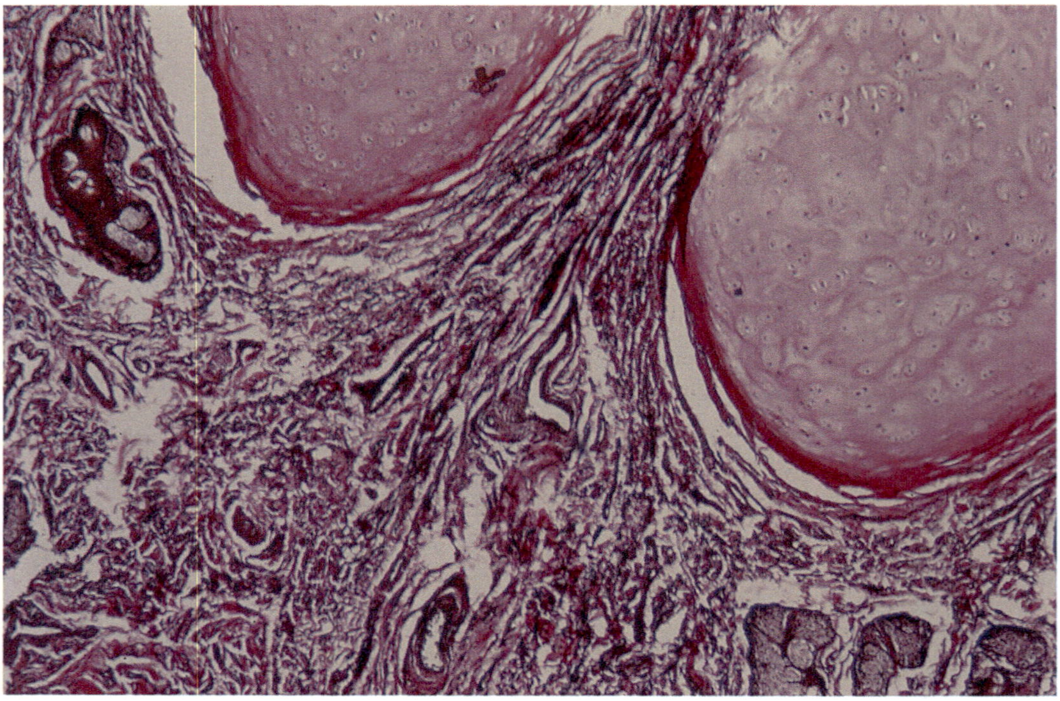

Fig. 6.5 High midline columellar cut: The upper ends of the two medial crura with the sweeping fibers still present (V.V.G stain)

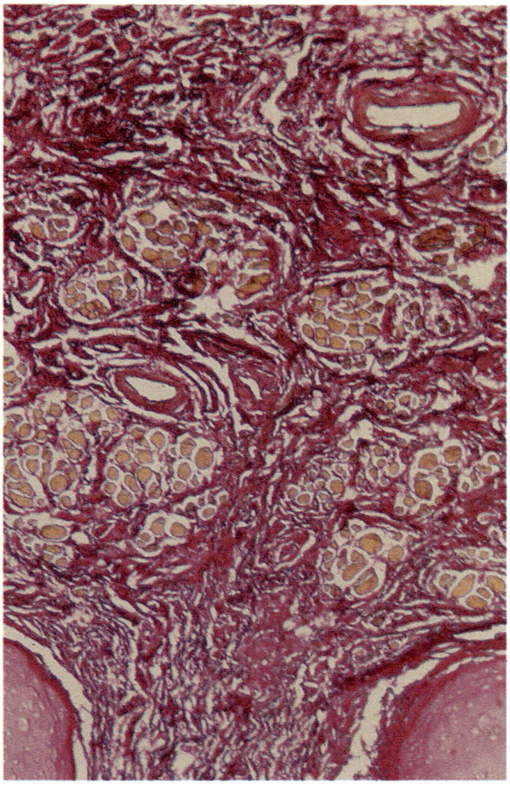

Fig. 6.6 High cut in the membranous septum: Muscle fibers are in excess (depressor septi) V.V.G stain

timeters. The specimens were mainly from adult patients between the ages of 20 and 30 years.

6.2.2 Histological Findings

Coronal sections were histologically studied. Starting from the caudal end of the septum upwards, **three types of histological areas** were seen.

6.2.2.1 Area of Keratinized Stratified Squamous Epithelium

This area is characterized by **moderate keratinization**. There is gradual maturation of the squamous epithelium with the preservation of all cell layers, i.e., the **basal**, the **prickle**, the **granular** and the **cornified** cell layers (Fig. 6.8).

The **granular cell layer** is composed of two to three layers of flattened cells containing keratohyalin granules. These are coarse, intensely basophilic granules which are rich in histidine. They are the precursors of the protein filaggrin, which is responsible for the aggregation of keratin filaments.

Underneath the epithelial layer, there is a wide **subcutaneous layer of loose connective tissue** before reaching the perichondrium of the cartilaginous septum. This is part of the membranous septum.There are **no adnexal tissues** in the subcutaneous layer, i.e., no hair follicles, sebaceous or sweat glands (Fig. 6.9).

6.2.2.2 Transitional Area

There is a **gradual change** in the epithelial lining from the **skin** to **respiratory** type. The **keratinized** stratified squamous epithelium becomes **less keratinized** with one or two granular cell layers, then **non-keratinized** stratified epithelium devoid of granular cell layer with a **flattened** (squamous) top layer. This top layer becomes **cuboidal** just before the transformation into pseudo-stratified columnar epithelium (Figs. 6.8 and 6.10).

6.2.2.3 Area of Pseudo-Stratified Columnar Epithelium With Goblet Cells

Only with the appearance of the respiratory type epithelium that the lamina propria of fibroelastic tissue and the layer of seromucinous glands appear.

The subcutaneous **loose connective tissue layer continues** throughout the skin and the **transitional areas** that cover the caudal part of the septum. It stops **abruptly** when the respiratory mucosa appears. The latter comes in direct contact, i.e., adherent to the perichondrium of the cartilaginous septum (Fig. 6.11).

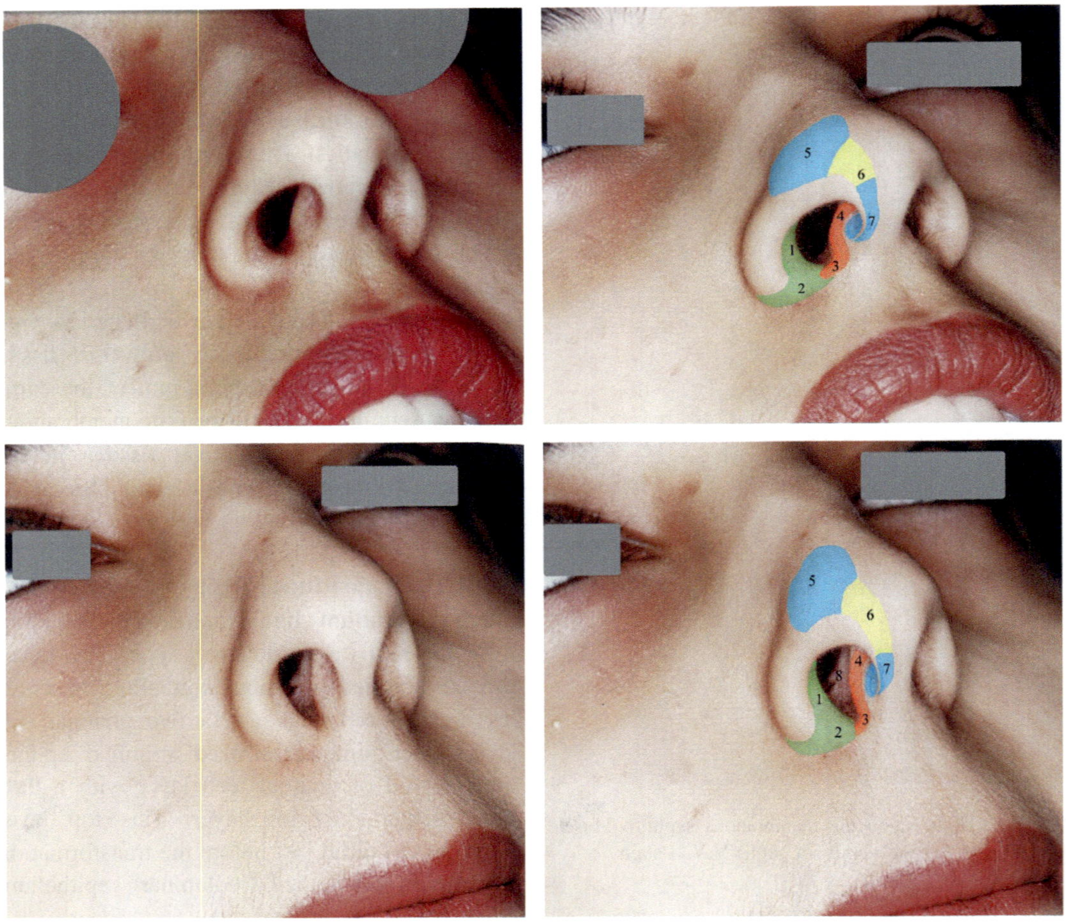

Fig. 6.7 The inferior vestibular band moves from the nasal sill then upwards and forwards posterior and then superior to the medial crus. 1—Superior segment of the Rim-Sill Fold, 2—Inferior and posterior segments of the Rim-Sill Fold, 3/4—Inferior Vestibular Band (IVB), 5—Lateral Crus, 6—Middle Crus, 7—Medial Crus, 8—Caudal Margin of the Cartilaginous Septum

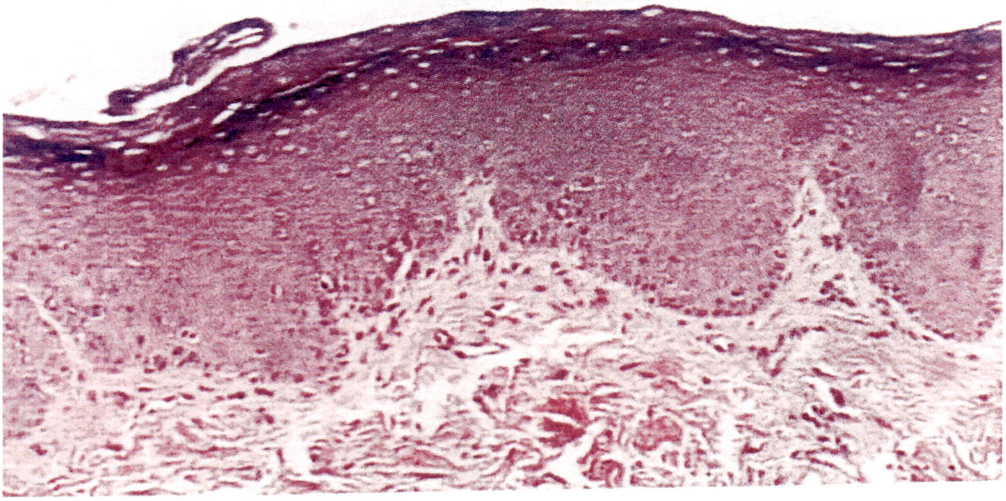

Fig. 6.8 Keratinized stratified squamous epithelium is well-preserved granular cell layer and moderately thick keratin. Wide area of loose subdermal connective tissue (H. and E. original magnification X250)

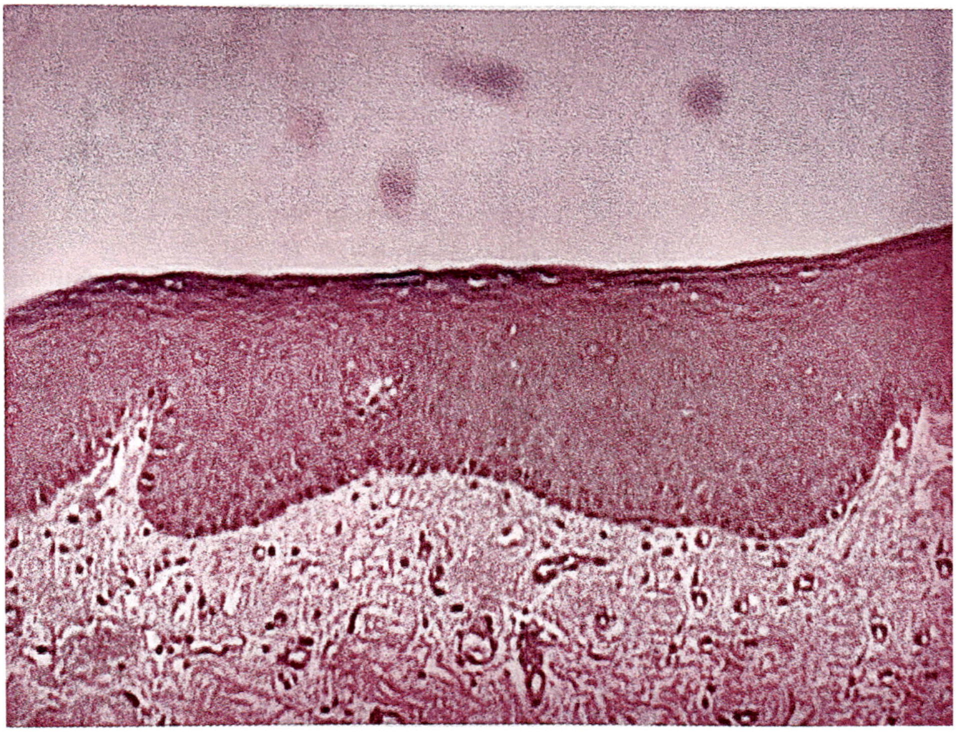

Fig. 6.9 The granular cell layer gradually decreases with the keratin from left to right (H. and E. original magnification X100)

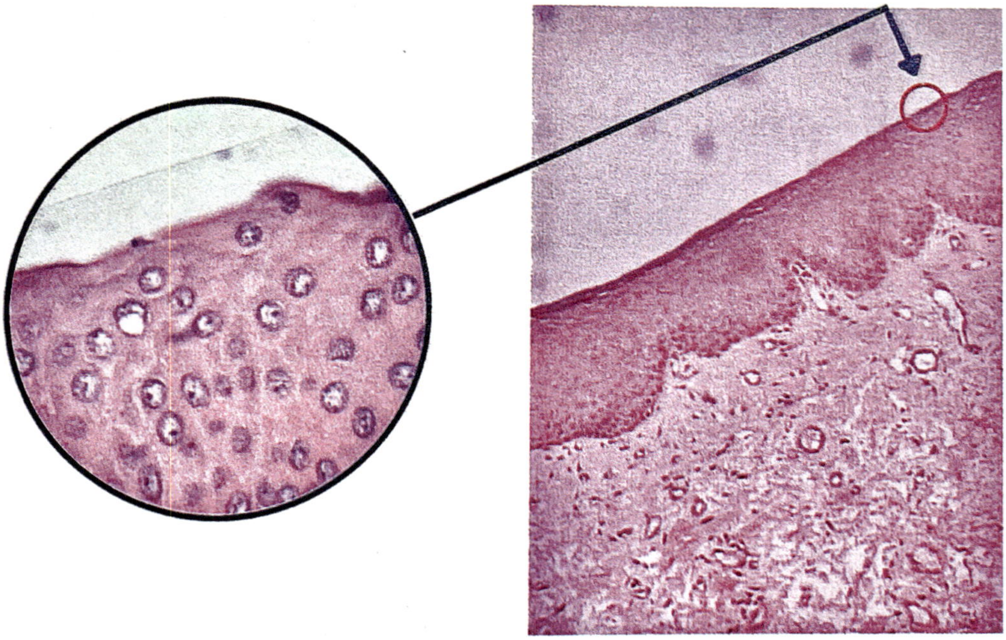

Fig. 6.10 Gradual disappearance of granular cell layer and keratin. Note that cuboidal top layer (arrow) with rounded nuclei (H. and E. original magnification X100)

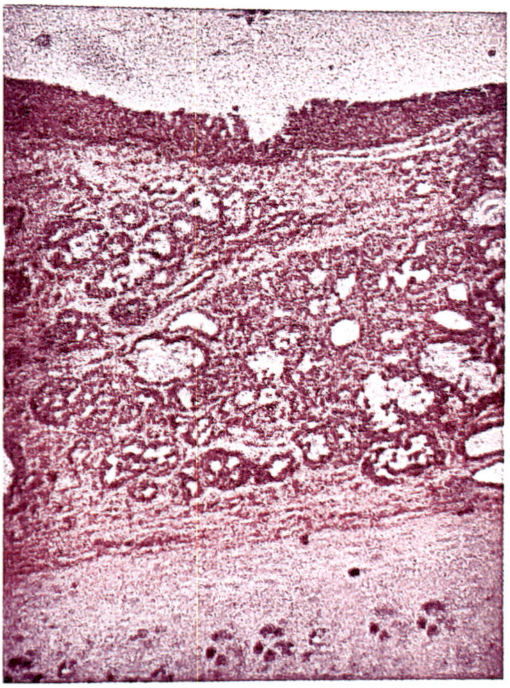

Fig. 6.11 Respiratory pseudo-stratified columnar epithelium. Note the appearance of seromucinous glands in the submucosa and disappearance of the wide loose subcutaneous layer. (H and E original magnification X100)

6.3 Conclusion

The caudal cartilaginous septum is different histologically from the other septal parts. It is a free subcutaneous structure that has a different lining. It is defined as the vestibular septum.

The **vestibular septum** is defined histologically as that part of the caudal cartilaginous septum that is **covered by loose vestibular skin overlying the loose subcutaneous connective tissue layer**. It **starts** from the **caudal margin** and **ends** with the **appearance of the respiratory epithelium.**

7 The Anatomy and Physiology of Nasal Respiration

Abstract

Rhinoplasty is not only concerned with an aesthetically pleasing outcome. It is imperative that the surgeon maintains good nasal respiration. The nasal valve is responsible for the physiology of nasal respiration.

Keywords

The nasal valve · The physiology of nasal respiration

Rhinoplasty is not only concerned with an aesthetically pleasing outcome. It is imperative that the surgeon maintains good nasal respiration. The nasal valve is responsible for the physiology of nasal respiration.

As Rhinoplasty takes place in the exact location of the nasal valve, surgeons must be aware of the anatomy and physiology of the valve to avoid compromising the nasal airway.

Patients may have a successful aesthetic result yet be miserable because of a compromised airway.

7.1 The Nasal Valve

The nasal valve has gained a great deal of care and attention because of its delicate and valuable anatomy and physiology. The term nasal valve was first introduced by Mink in 1903. It is **not a true valve** that allows the air to move in one direction only. It is, rather, a kinetic bottleneck that physiologically regulates nasal respiration.

It is important to have clear and accurate anatomical and physiological definitions of the nasal valves. **Anatomically**, it is necessary to know the exact **location** and the **structures** that share in the formation of the valve. **Physiologically**, it is important to recognize the role of the valve in nasal respiration.

The nasal valve is further subdivided into two complementary valves, the **external** and the **internal** valves. The **external value** is lined by **vestibular skin** and has **four walls**, while the **internal valve** is lined by **respiratory mucosa** and has **three walls**. The external valve is part of the four-walled lower third, while the internal valve is part of the three-walled upper two-thirds of the nose.

The nasal valve is the **only** structure in the external nose that has **mobile lateral** walls which **actively move with** the help of **the small muscles of the nose**, the **orbicularis oris** muscle and the **aerodynamic forces**.

The nasal valve is therefore **defined anatomically** as the **segments of the nasal airway passage that lies underneath its mobile lateral walls.** These mobile walls are the **alae nasi** in the case of the external valve and the **lower free margin** of the **upper lateral cartilage** in the case of the **internal** valve.

The **main task** of the nasal valve is the delicate **coordination of its two parts,** external and

M. H. A. Shafy, *Innovations in Rhinoplasty*,
https://doi.org/10.1007/978-3-030-94573-2_7

internal, in regulating the nasal air entry, i.e., the **physiology of nasal respiration**.

The nasal valve is **defined physiologically** as the segment of **kinetic widening and narrowing** of the anatomical components of the **external** and **internal** valves successively **in order** to **physiologically regulate the inspired air**.

The mobile parts of the lateral walls play an important role in these mechanisms. The dynamics of air entry to the nasal cavity proper, i.e., lined by respiratory mucosa, is greatly influenced by the effects of the **small nasal muscles** on the **external** and **internal valves**. It is therefore important that we should be familiar with each and every one of these muscles.

7.1.1 Anatomy of the Nasal Valve

7.1.1.1 The External Valve

Definition:

The external valve is defined anatomically as the segment **of the nasal airway that lies underneath the freely mobile ala nasi**.

The Inferior and Superior Ends of the External Valve:

The external valve is the nasal aperture tube that **begins** inferiorly at the **aperture margins** and **ends** superiorly at the **muco-cutaneous junction**.

Walls of the External Valve

The external valve is located in the **four-walled lower third of the nose.** It therefore has four walls:

- The **lateral wall** is the dynamic part of the valve that is made of the freely mobile **ala nasi**.
- The **medial wall** is made by the medial crus of the lower lateral cartilage and the membranous septum, i.e., the vestibular part of the columella.
- The **anterior wall** is made by the inner surface of the middle crurae.
- The **inferior wall** is made by the loose skin of the floor of the nasal vestibule as well as the vestibular surface of the flat triangle.

The external valve is covered by the surface skin **externally** while **internally** it is covered by the vestibular skin.

The main physiological task of the external valve is to act as a large receptacle that expands widely in order to receive the **largest amount** of external air before it passes into the narrowest area of the internal valve.

It is important to have an external valve before the internal valve. It helps in collecting, channeling and directing the external air toward the internal valve. This two-stage procedure increases the efficiency of the internal valve.

7.1.1.2 The Internal Valve

Definition:

The **internal valve** is defined anatomically as **the segment** of the nasal airway that lies **underneath the lower one-fifth to one–fourth of the freely unattached and relatively mobile margin of the upper lateral cartilage**. The internal valve segment represents the **beginning of the nasal cavity proper**, i.e., lined by respiratory mucosa. The internal valve has a more significant and sophisticated anatomy and physiology than the external valve.

The Inferior and the Superior ends of the Internal Valve

The internal valve begins at the superior opening of the aperture tube, i.e., at the **muco-cutaneous junction.** Anatomically, it is made of the **limen nasi** and the **vestibular crest** laterally, the **posterior vestibular fold** posteriorly and the **superior end of the vestibular septum** medially.

Superiorly, the valve segment extends inside the nasal cavity for a distance that corresponds to **the length of the free mobile lower one-fifth to one-fourth of the upper lateral cartilage**.

The inlet of the internal valve therefore has **two prominent margins** anteriorly and posteriorly, i.e., the limen nasi and the posterior vestibular margin. It also has **two flat areas**, medially at the septum and laterally just in front of the turbinate head. The prominent margins of the **limen nasi** and the **posterior vestibular fold** occupy almost two-thirds, or more, of the circumference of the nasal valve inlet.

The prominent margin of the limen nasi constricts and reduces the size of the valve. **The inlet of the internal valve** consequently **is the narrowest area of the whole of the nasal airway passage**.

The opening of the internal valve is **pear-shaped** being narrow anteriorly and wide posteriorly.

The right and left openings of the internal valves are looking toward each other **upwards**, **backwards** and **medially**.

Externally the surface anatomy of the **valve inlet** is marked by the line that starts at the **apex of the weak triangle** then passes to the **scroll area**, at the junction between the **upper and lower lateral cartilages**, and finally goes down to the **superior alar groove**.

The superior end of the internal valve is marked **externally** by the transverse line that passes a few millimeters **above the base of the weak triangle,** i.e., the lower margin of the upper lateral cartilage.

The inlet of the internal valve **anatomically** represents the entrance or the gateway to the internal nose. **Physiologically,** it represents the **transitional** phase between the **external** air and the **inspired** intranasal **air**.

The Medial Soft Fold of the Limen Nasi

The lower one-fifth to one-fourth of the upper lateral cartilage is not continuous with the dorsal cartilaginous septum. It is only attached to it by a thin layer of perichondrium.

The **extreme medial part** of the prominent margin of the **limen nasi,** i.e., at its meeting with the nasal septum, is therefore made **only of a mucocutaneous perichondrial fold.** Unlike the rest of this margin, it is **devoid of underlying cartilage.** This is called the **medial soft fold** of the limen nasi. This fold is supported internally by the **perichondrial layer** that joins the dorsal cartilaginous septum to the lower margin of the upper lateral cartilage. The medial soft fold is therefore made of a layer of perichondrium that is covered by a mucosal layer superiorly and vestibular skin layer inferiorly, i.e., mucocutaneous perichondrial fold.

This **soft mobile fold** meets with the **solid immobile septum** at the point of the **anterior angle of the valve**. As the upper lateral cartilage moves with respiration, the **soft fold** becomes suitably **adaptable** and **versatile** against the **rigid septum** which may be irregular, deviated or thick.

The soft medial folds of the two internal valves are part of the **floor of the weak triangle** on both sides of the septum. The health of these folds is very important **for the** relatively **free movement of the lower margins of the upper lateral cartilage**. The loss or scarring of these folds will lead to restriction of movements of the lateral walls. Should scarring proceed, it will cause **vestibular stenosis** of varying degrees and the physiology of the internal valve will be greatly hindered.

7.1.1.3 The Walls of the Internal Valve

The internal valve is located in the three-walled upper two-thirds of the nose. Therefore, it has three walls: a **lateral**, **medial** and an **inferior wall**. All walls of the internal valve are lined by respiratory mucosa in a **segment** that begins from the muco-cutaneous junction inferiorly and extends to the level of the lower one-fifth to one-fourth of the upper lateral cartilage.

The Medial wall:

The medial wall is made by the rigidly fixed cartilaginous septum anteriorly and part of the vomerine bone posteriorly.

The Lateral wall:

The lateral wall is made up of two parts:

(a) The **anterior dynamic** part of the lateral wall is made by the relatively mobile lower one-fifth to one-fourth of the **upper lateral cartilage**.
(b) The **posterior fixed** part of the lateral wall is made by the nasal surface of the body of the **maxillary bone**. At this location, there is an upwards and backwards oblique ridge,

termed the **conchal crest** for articulation with the inferior nasal concha. The **conchal crest** is covered directly by **respiratory nasal mucosa,** while the **inferior concha** is covered by the erectile tissue of the **inferior turbinate**.

The **head of the inferior turbinate** therefore is part of the **lateral wall** and **the contents** of the internal valve segment.

The **conchal crest, inferior concha** and their covering of mucosa and erectile tissues contribute to the **reduction in the size** of the internal valve segment.

The size of the inferior turbinate head has considerable importance because of its anatomical location within the valve segment.

The Inferior wall:

The inferior wall is made by the nasal surface of the **palatine process of the maxillary bone**. It is lined by respiratory mucosa.

N.B. The vestibular floor is not part of the internal valve.

7.1.1.4 The Anterior Angle of the Internal Valve

It is the angle between the **limen nasi** and the **caudal septum,** i.e., between the lower margin of the **upper lateral cartilage** and the **soft medial fold** of the limen nasi on one side and the **caudal cartilaginous septum** on the other side, **at the level of the muco-cutaneous junction**.

This is not a rigidly fixed angle, but it is rather a **versatile** one as it changes with the active nasal respiratory movements because of its mobile lateral wall.

It is the **most physiologically important** part of the internal valve for two reasons:

(a) **Most of the inspired air** is directed toward the anterior valve angle.

(b) It is **the only actively kinetic** part of the internal valve.

Movement is only possible at the free lower margin of the upper lateral cartilage. It moves under the effects of both the **aerodynamic forces** of the respiratory air and the active contractions of the **small muscles** of the nose.

The small muscles of the nose act upon the upper lateral cartilage moving its lower margin medially and laterally **with** and **within** the loose muco-cutaneous folds of the limen nasi.

The upper lateral cartilage is acted upon **directly** by the nasalis muscle (the transverse part) and **indirectly** by the alar muscles and the procerus. **Each small nasal muscle** has to be reintroduced to us **as an important well-known muscle for a specific action** in the physiology of nasal respiration, rather than collectively as one group of the small muscles of the nose.

For comfortable nasal respiration, the **valve angle must not be less than ten degrees**. This **clinically** means that the sides of the angle are **not touching each other**, and a **slit** is seen between the caudal septum and the lower margin of the upper lateral cartilage.

There are definite ethnic differences in the degree of this angle, being narrower in Caucasians and wider in Africans and Asians.

The final **functional outcome** of the anterior angle of the valve is affected by **its width**, the **strength of the small nasal muscles** and the **health** and **anatomy** of the **structures that make the valve**.

7.2 The Physiology of Nasal Respiration

The physiology of nasal respiration is a mechanism which describes how the nose **actively** transports the **external air** across the nasal valve transforming it into the **inspired air** that has acquired completely new dynamic properties and a specific direction. The wide alae nasi together with the negative inspiratory pressure invite the largest amount of air inside the nasal vestibule, i.e., the external valve chamber. The air then suddenly passes through the dynamically narrowed inlet of the internal valve.

7.2.1 Physiological Definitions

The **external valve** is defined physiologically as the **area of maximal dynamic expansion** in the nasal airway passage.

The **internal valve** is defined as the **area of** maximal **dynamic narrowing** in the nasal airway passage.

The physiological outcome is the introduction of the **maximum amount of air** to the **external valve** and the gain of **maximum speed** in the **internal valve** (Fig. 7.2).

7.2.2 Inspiration

The fast inspired air moves mainly from the **anterior angle of the internal valve** to the direction of **the middle meatal cleft**.

The nasal valve is mainly concerned physiologically with changing the **speed** and the **direction** of the inspired air.

7.2.2.1 Changing the Speed of the Inspired Air

i. <u>The Kinetic Part of the Valve</u>

The external valve and the anterior half of the internal valve are the kinetic parts of the nasal valve.

1. During normal **inspiration,** as the speed of the inspired air increases, there is an **active dilatation** and **elevation** of the alae nasi by the dilator naris posterior (the alar part of the nasalis) and the levator labii superioris alaeque nasi. The size and consequently the capacity of the external valve chamber thus increase (Figs. 7.1 and 7.2).
   Simultaneously, there is a tendency toward **passive** inwards **collapse** of the limen nasi. This paradoxical narrowing of the internal valve inlet is greatly resisted and **counteracted** by the effect of the dilator naris anterior (the transverse part of the nasalis).
   This dynamic **action** and **counteraction** on the internal valve create some **resistance** to the entry of air.
   The final outcome of these two forces is a **slight narrowing** of the internal valve.
2. In **forced inspiration**, there is an increased speed of the inspired air. This leads to reduced air pressure inside the valve that tends to **close both** the external and the **internal** valves.
   The **dilator** and **elevator** muscles will come into more powerful action in order to **counteract** the passive collapsing effect of air (Fig. 7.2).
3. In **extremely forced inspiration,** more muscles will come into action so that the procerus muscle (pyramidalis nasi), through its action on the superficial muscular aponeurotic system (SMAS) in conjunction with the nasalis, and sometimes the frontal part of the occipitofrontalis, will all contract forcibly to share in this powerful act (Fig. 7.1).
   Fixation and stabilization of both alae nasi, the caudal septum and the upper lateral cartilages are achieved by the depressor and the compressor muscles. The depressor septi muscles (also called the depressor alae nasi) act on the caudal septum and both medial crurae, while the nasalis act both as an elevator (alar part) and dilator (transverse part) in forced respiration.

ii. <u>The Static Part of the Valve</u>

The posterior half of the nasal valve has less complicated physiology. At this part of the valve, the air has to pass from the **widest area** of the external valve to the much narrower fixed walled posterior segment of the internal valve. The head

Fig. 7.1 Small Muscles of the Nose and Related Facial Muscles

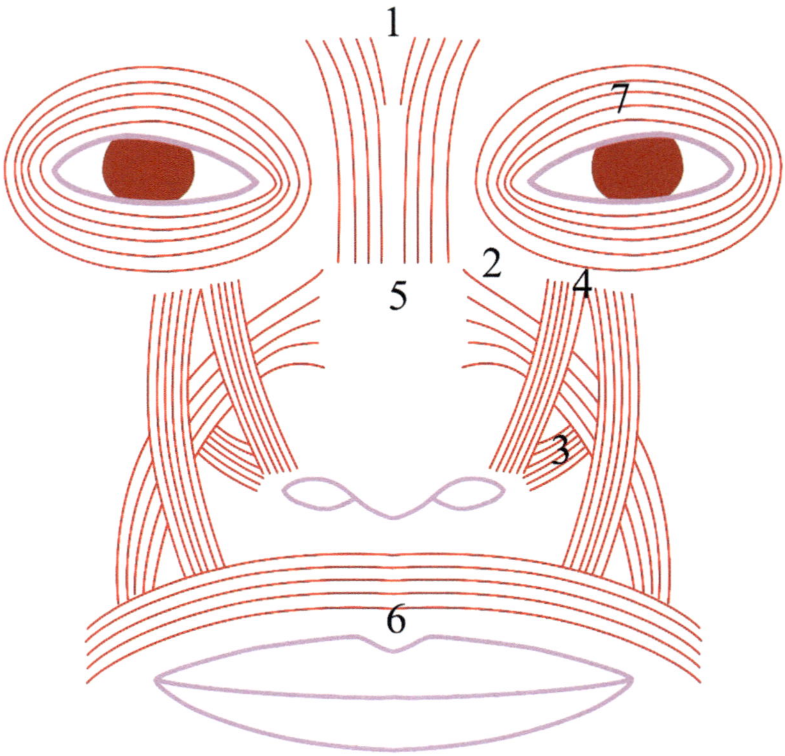

1. Procerus (Pyramidalis Nasi)
2. Dilator Naris Anterior (Transverse part of nasalis)
3. Dilator Naris Posterior (Alar part of nasalis)
4. Levator Labii alique nasi
5. Superfacial muscular aponeurotic system (SMAS)
6. Orbicularis Oris
7. Orbicularis Occuli

of the inferior turbinate and the conchal crest are the main contributors to this narrowing.

This mechanism greatly enhances the **amount** and the **speed** of air entry to the respiratory lined nasal cavity.

7.2.2.2 Changing the Direction of the Inspired Air

Both parts of the nasal valve, external and internal, coordinate in moving the inspired air column into the desired physiological path, i.e., upwards and backwards from the nasal valve to the middle meatal cleft.

The **position** of the alae nasi, i.e., the alar flare, turns the **external** opening together with the whole of the **nasal aperture tube**, in an **upwards, forwards** and **lateral** directions which is the same direction as the internal valve that looks **upwards, backwards** and **medially**.

The **column of air** is thus directed from the external to the internal valve in an **upwards, backwards** and **medial** directions.

The static posterior half of the **internal valve** also plays an important role in directing the column of the nasal air. The anterior end or **the head of the inferior turbinate** carries the stream of the inspired air in an **upwards** and **backwards** direction toward the middle meatal cleft.

The **conchal crest** is an oblique bony elevation at the entrance of the internal valve just

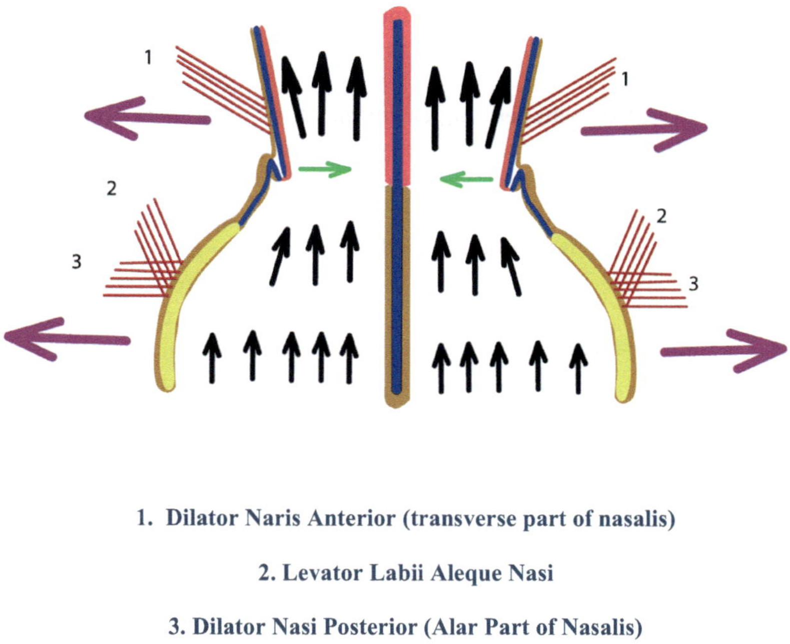

Fig. 7.2 Inspiration

anterior to the turbinate head. It helps the natural physiological role of this part of the valve, **even after total turbinectomy**.

Fortunately, it is rather difficult to completely excise the turbinate head during total surgical turbinectomy, as the intimate location of the **prominent conchal crest** produces a **solid obstacle** and a **difficult angle** for the cutting scissors of the surgeon.

7.2.2.3 The Middle Meatal Cleft

After passing through the narrowed **anterior valve angle** at a high speed, the inspired air is directed **upwards** and **backwards** toward the angle and the cleft between the anterior margin of the **middle turbinate** and the **lateral nasal wall**. It is in the form of an inverted v-shape. Obliteration of this cleft produces a strong sensation of nasal obstruction. On the other hand, securing an

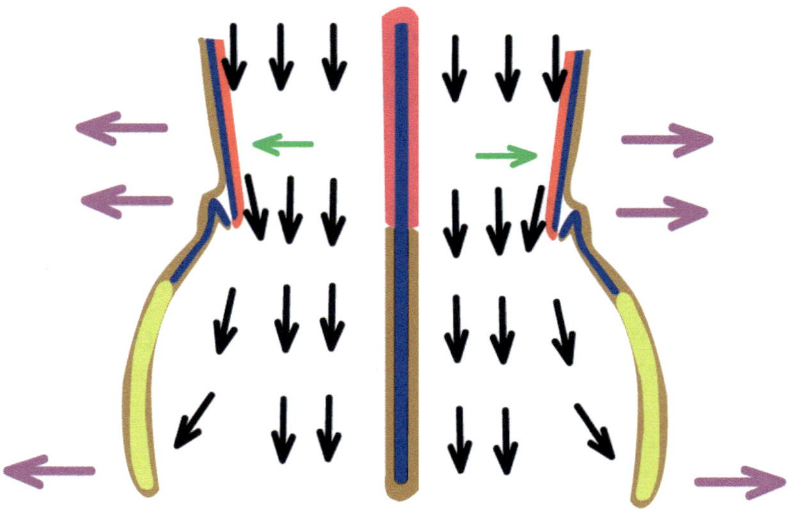

Fig. 7.3 Expiration

open middle meatal cleft and an intact middle turbinate physiologically enhances an open nasal airway.

Two inverted v-shaped angles are therefore important to secure a physiologically open and comfortable nasal airway, viz., **the anterior valve angle** and the **angle between the middle turbinate and the lateral nasal wall.**

7.2.3 Expiration

Expiration is a totally **passive** procedure where the **positive pressure** of the expired air simply pushes its way out expanding both the internal and external valves.

It is of interest that the **internal valve** is **wider** during **expiration** than inspiration, while the **external valve** is **wider** during **inspiration** than **expiration**.

7.3 Surgical Significance of the Nasal Valve

The surgical importance of the nasal valve stems from its significant role in the physiology of nasal respiration.

Although the opening of the internal nasal valve is **small**, controlled by the small nasal muscles and is made by delicately small anatomical structures, **all the inspired and expired air** passes through this valve segment.

Even the **slightest** disturbance in any of the valve's structural components may have a **profound** effect on the physiology of air entry with a strong sensation of **nasal blockage**.

Incisions in rhinoplasty and septorhinoplasty always involve the nasal valve area, i.e., the limen nasi, nasal septum and the alae nasi.

Care must be taken to avoid injury to the **anterior valve angle** which is at a **higher** level than the level of the incision (Fig. 7.4).

7.4 Factors Affecting the Nasal Valve

Any **deformity**, **damage**, **scarring** or **paralysis** of the structures that make the nasal valve may affect its function in the form of varying degrees of reduced nasal air entry.

Lesions in **nearby structures** may have an indirect effect on the valve with similar consequences on the air entry.

Functionally, the **internal valve** is divided into a **narrow kinetic anterior angle** and a **wide static posterior half**. Despite being smaller and narrower, the **anterior half is more dynamic and physiologically active**. It only takes a **small** lesion, scar or deformity to produce a **profound** effect on the valve and the nasal air entry in general.

The **external valve** on the other hand combines being **static and kinetic** at the same time. The firm bodies of the alae nasi have to maintain the external naris open at all times, while their kinetic free mobility controls the amount, speed and direction of air entry.

7.4.1 Factors Affecting the Anterior Kinetic Parts of the Valve

(a) The alae nasi:
   i. Congenital Deformities:
      Congenital deformities are seen in cases of small or absent lateral crus, hare-lip or a unilateral change in size, shape, position or depth of the alar groove.
   ii. Injury and scarring:
      This may be accidental or surgical trauma during alar base surgery.
      A **high** posterior alar wound may cause injury to the muscular attachments to the ala nasi.
      Overzealous excision of the thin **adherent vestibular** skin over the ala nasi

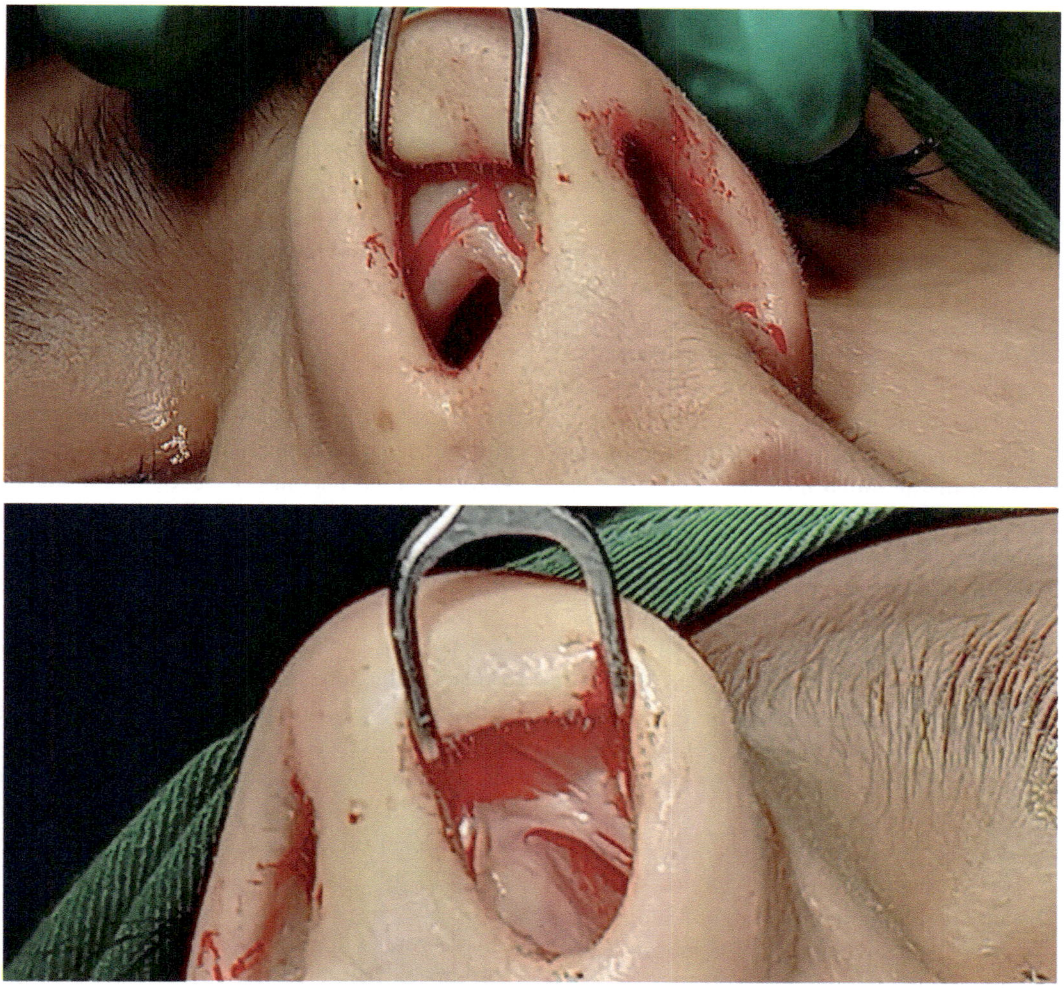

Fig. 7.4 Location of the Intercartilaginous Incision

leads to a **crippling scar** and **ugly angulation** at the area of alar attachment. Surgical **malalignment** of the rim-sill margins may lead to unsightly deformity and abnormal restricted movement of the ala nasi.

iii. Paralysis:

In cases of partial or complete **facial paralysis**, the alae nasi lose their **postural tone**, i.e., the alar flare, as well as their ability to move. This will have a devastating effect on the physiology of nasal respiration.

(b) The anterior angle of the internal valve:

The importance of the anterior angle stems from the fact that it is anatomically very **small,** yet the only **kinetic** part of the internal valve and allows entry of a **large volume of the inspired air**. It only takes a **small lesion** and equally **small surgery** in order to have a **major effect** on nasal air entry.

i. Deformities:
Crookedness or thickening of the **cartilaginous septum** or the lower margin of the upper lateral cartilage.
Deformities may affect the **medial soft fold of the limen nasi**.
The most obstructing deviation or thickening of the cartilaginous septum is **at**, or **just superior** to the anterior angle of the internal valve.

ii. Injury and scarring **"vestibular stenosis"**:
This is the most vulnerable area for iatrogenic injury and scarring.
The **length** and **health** of the **medial soft fold of the limen nasi** are of great surgical importance. Damaged and shortened by injury and scarring will lead to obliteration and blunting of the anterior valve angle which is the earliest form of vestibular stenosis.
If damage proceeds further to affect the **lower margin of the upper lateral cartilage**, scarring will progress from before backwards leading to increasing degrees of vestibular stenosis.
Vestibular stenosis not only reduces the **size** of the anterior angle that reduces the nasal airway, but more importantly it reduces and cripples the dynamics of the **mobile lateral wall** of the internal valve.
Direct injury to the **superficial muscular aponeurotic system (SMAS)** may take place as a result of rough manipulations, incision in the wrong plane or aggressive removal of the lower border of the upper lateral cartilage.

iii. Paralysis:
Facial palsy affects both the external and internal valves with consequent major effects on the physiology of nasal respiration.

7.4.2 Factors Affecting the Static Posterior Parts of the Nasal Valve

Usually, there are less problems encountered in this posterior wide part of the nasal valve. Nevertheless, it is not uncommon to have narrowing in this area after alar base reduction rhinoplasty or functional surgery for chronic sinus disease. Structures that may be affected are

i. The heads of inferior turbinates:

Hypertrophy of the anterior end of the inferior turbinate not only reduces the size of the **internal valve area** but may also intrude into the narrow **inlet** of the valve at the muco-cutaneous junction, leading to its further considerable narrowing.

ii. The caudal septum:

A dislocated or thickened posterior half of the caudal cartilaginous septum reduces the size of both valve areas, **internal** and **external** on the affected side, i.e., reduces the size of the whole of the aperture tube as it pushes the **medial crus** inwards and the nasal **sill band** inferiorly leading to additional **unaesthetic** consequences.

iii. The posterior vestibular fold:

This is the widest part of the internal valve posteriorly. It is hardly encountered in any surgical procedure and is rarely the cause of any valvular affection.

iv. Alar base:

Surgical, traumatic injury or paralysis to the alae nasi affect the valve mechanisms (vid supra).

7.4.3 Extra-Valvular Factors

Adhesions, swellings and granulomas that take place near the area of the nasal valve may have the same obstructive effect on air entry.

7.5 The Physiological Role of the Nasal Septum

Having a nasal septum secures **two separate aerodynamic systems** which in turn **avoids undue turbulence**. This helps the air to gain the right **speed** and **direction**. This separation helps in better **mucociliary circulation** on the nasal walls. If the air does not gain enough speed at the valve angle, it will not have enough force to go through the middle cleft.

The job of the nasal septum is severely disturbed and well appreciated in cases of septal defects of varying sizes and locations. Patients usually suffer from dryness and crustations due to disturbed mucociliary circulation. An unpleasant loud sound or whistling may take place due to turbulent airflow. Patients suffer from breathing discomfort and halitosis.

The nasal septum may look apparently deviated, but it is clinically and radiologically in the middle between the two unequal sides. For better physiological performance, the nasal septum is situated between **the two unequal structures** on the lateral nasal walls to allow for almost equal and suitable shares of air flow on each side.

Nasal septal deviation, per se, is not a disease. It is found in more than 70% of normal individuals (Gray's Anatomy). Septal deviations of varying degrees may have very little if any symptoms. Careful history, clinical and C-T scan studies must be considered before contemplating any form of septal surgery.

Despite the ambiguity of nasal septal physiology, there are certain key areas that have considerable effects on nasal respiration. These areas are

(a) The nasal valve areas:
   i. The valve angle: A localized area of septal deviation is one of the causes of obliteration of the nasal valve angle. Deviation may be developmental or secondary to surgical or accidental trauma. The latter may also produce localized adhesions of varying degrees.
   ii. The external valve: caudal septal dislocation drives the posterior septal angle laterally, thus narrowing the external valve area which may cause varying degrees of nasal obstruction.

(b) Severe Septal Deviations:
Severe nasal septal deviations that affect the nasal airway take place at the caudal, osteo-cartilaginous junctions or at the junction between the vomer and ethmoid plate. These deviations may be natural or post-traumatic.

7.6 Clinical Picture of Nasal Valve Disorders

Lesions of the nasal valve strongly affect the physiology of nasal respiration. Depending on the extent of the lesion, patients may suffer from progressive degrees of **reduced air entry** rather than internal nasal obstruction, i.e., the patient can have the joy of inspired air if it bypasses the initial obstruction. The patient discovers the trick of laterally pulling his cheek to improve the airway. He sometimes uses a pillow or his hand to do this job during his sleep. The patient is usually distressed, frustrated and angry, as he feels deprived of natural comfortable respiration.

Clinical assessment should be **patiently** and **orderly** performed in order to reach the exact cause and location of the lesion as follows.

7.6.1 Inspection

1. The patient is asked to **breathe normally and quietly**. Observe if his mouth is closed or open and if the lips are dry and cracked. He is then asked to take a **deep breath** through his nose with his mouth closed. The degree of nasal obstruction is observed. **Alar collapse** is clearly seen in an **external** valve lesion or severe weakness of the nasal muscles (Fig. 7.5).
   In **milder forms**, collapse of the **internal valve alone** is seen externally as the lateral wall of the nose is **sucked in** just **above the superior alar groove.** This is due to the

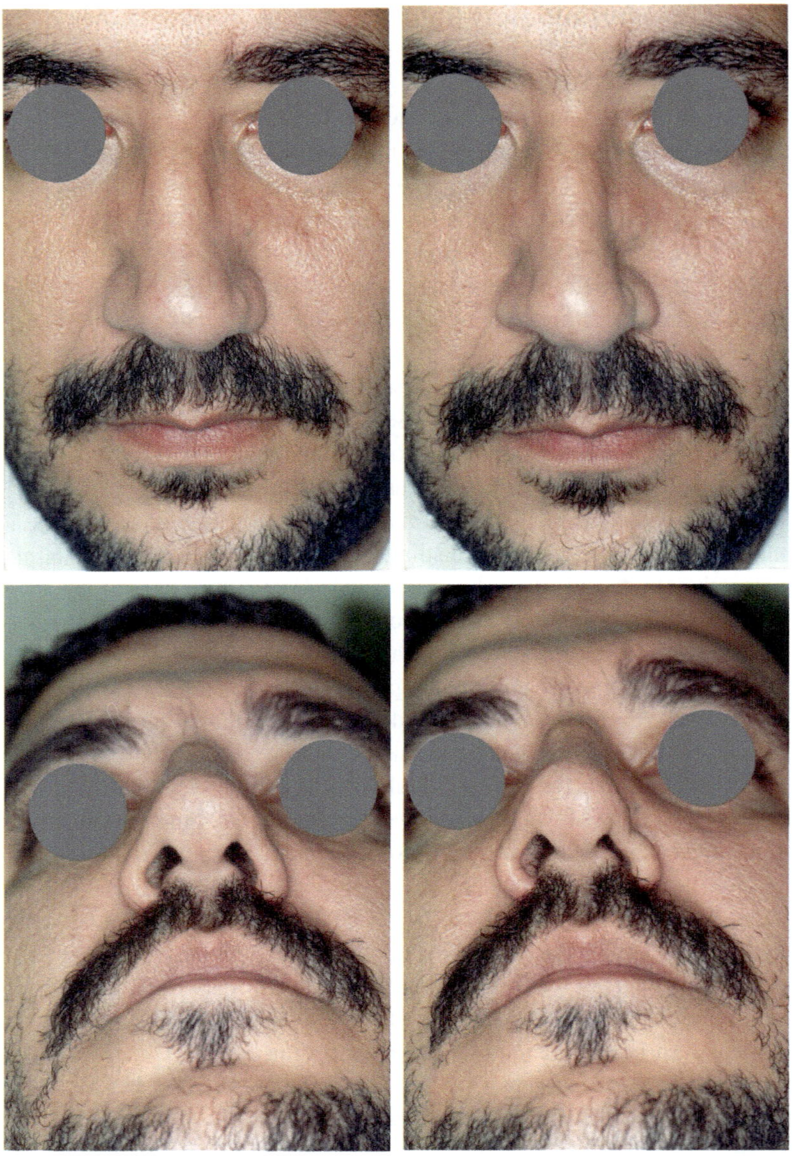

Fig. 7.5 Nasal Valve Disorder- Collapse of the Left Ala Nasi on Forced Inspiration

inwards collapse of the lower margin of the upper lateral cartilage.

2. The nasal aperture is observed for signs of **caudal septal deviation** either **anteriorly** at the anterior valve angle or **posteriorly** where there is medial crus displacement and lowering of the nasal sill.
3. The **position of the ala nasi** and the **depth of alar grooving** are observed. In chronic cases of muscle weakness, the ala nasi of the affected side is totally flaccid with **flattening of the alar groove** and **narrowing of the nasal opening**. A clear example of this is seen in **unilateral facial palsy**.

7.6.2 Examination

1. **Cottle's test**:

The examining physician or the patient himself is asked to pull the cheek next to the ala nasi

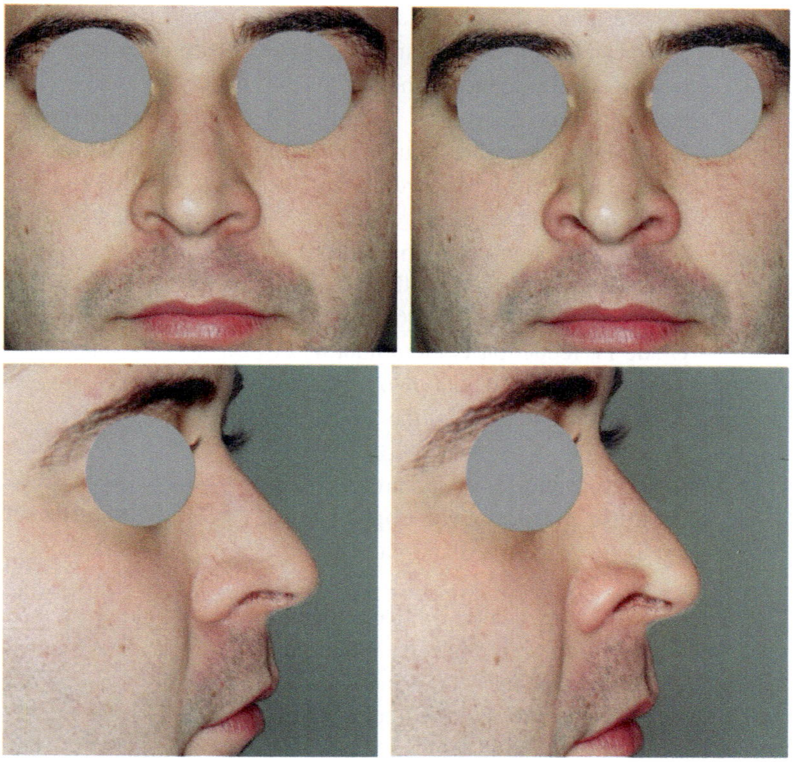

Fig. 7.6 Increased Alar Flare on Forced Inspiration

laterally while breathing in. The air entry improves in cases of nasal valve collapse and caudal septal deviation. This test is negative in cases of vestibular stenosis.

Cottle's test may be directly enhanced by using a blunt probe to elevate the limen nasi laterally at the anterior angle while asking the patient to breathe in.

2. **Examination of the nasal vestibules**:

Rushing directly into vestibular examination is the commonest cause of missing the diagnosis of a nasal valve disorder. It should be the **last step** in the clinical assessment.

The nasal vestibule is examined in three steps, the **first** is by simply elevating the nasal tip, **then** using the nasal speculum and **finally** by using the optical telescope.

Close observation and then gentle **palpation** of both normal and diseased structures are to be carefully assessed as follows:

(a) **The Anterior valve angle**:

i. The anterior valve angle is too far anteriorly placed, as it is hidden and obscured **above the inwards skin fold angulation of the flat triangle.** It is best examined while **the patient's head is** tilted backwards so that the angle is directly facing the examining physician.

The two walls of the angle should be separated from each other by a **slit,** i.e., the angle is 10 degrees or greater. The **effect of deep inspiration** on the angle is tested.

ii. The length and health of the **medial soft fold** of the limen nasi are observed. **Gentle palpation by** a **probe** to feel its consistency and free mobility.

Early vestibular stenosis appears as a **blunt obliteration** of the angle and **stiffness** of the soft fold.

As vestibular stenosis advances, it continues to proceed from this angle postro-laterally reducing the size of the nasal vestibule.

Jack Sheen describes four grades of vestibular stenosis according to the reduction in the vestibular volume:

Grade I reduction up to 15%.

Grade II reduction is 15–40%.

Grade III reduction is 40–65%.

Grade IV reduction is more than 65%.

iii. **The septum**: any deviation or thickness is observed especially at the area of the valve angle.

iv. Any deformities or undue protrusion of the **lower margin of the upper lateral cartilage** is observed and palpated.

Obliteration of the anterior valve angle is **much more common** than clinically found during routine examination using the nasal speculum. Even with the use of the optical telescope, it is not very easy to see the angle properly and assess its mobility. The thick vestibular hair, vibrecae and the difficult location of the angle make it almost impossible for some noses to examine the angle properly.

Many cases, where the nasal septum is clinically diagnosed as being straight and not the least deviated, are found **intraoperatively** to have **severe localized obliteration of the anterior valve angle**, which can be a major source of nasal obstruction.

The lower margin of the upper lateral cartilage, i.e., the limen nasi is found to be in **direct contact** and almost **pushed** laterally by the anterior septum.

Most cases are diagnosed under favorable conditions during surgery. The patient is **lying down** with the head elevated **under general anesthesia** and the **vestibular hair is closely shaved**. The anterior valve angle can now be easily inspected by the naked eye and fully assessed by the **optical telescope**.

Endoscopic examination of the anterior valve angle should be a mandatory routine in any surgical procedure on the nose in order to avoid a disappointing post-operative nasal obstruction after the great efforts of all types of fancy surgical procedures.

(b) **The wide posterior half**:

i. The **head of the inferior turbinate** is observed for its **size** and **location** in relation to the internal valve size and inlet.

ii. Posterior septal dislocation and prominent **anterior nasal spine** are additional factors which may affect the external valve area.

7.7 Management of Nasal Valve Lesions

(a) Prophylactic measures:

i. The intercartilaginous and septal incisions for Rhinoplasty are anatomically **inferior** to the location of the valve angle. These wounds must be accurately stitched back at the end of the operation especially if tissue structures are unstable after the surgery.

ii. The dissection level in the subcutaneous tissue must be **deeper than the muscular layer**, i.e., as close as possible to the cartilaginous surface of the upper lateral cartilage.

iii. Trimming of a medial triangular sector of the upper lateral cartilage is a wise prophylactic routine after osteotomies to keep the valvular angle open.

(b) Surgical treatment:

i. **Mild forms** of valve disorders are either asymptomatic or the patients may suffer very slight nasal obstruction. They may not require treatment, e.g., slight muscle weakness, first grade vestibular stenosis or minimal septal deviation. Patients are encouraged to **exercise the nasal muscles** and are advised **to avoid heavy eyeglasses** which may slide down over the valve areas compressing them from outside.

ii. **Symptomatic cases** which need surgical interference:

The main objectives of the treatment plans are

1. To open the valve angle.
2. To restore the free mobility of the upper lateral cartilage and alae nasi.
3. To remove any anatomical structures that obstruct the opening of the valve.

Once an accurate diagnosis is made to locate the exact cause of valvular disorder or obstruction, treatment is then planned:

(1) Nasal septum:

An abnormal nasal septum is the **commonest cause** of localized obliteration and narrowing of the anterior valve angle.

The wide use of endoscopes in nasal surgery has disclosed more cases of anterior valve angle obliterations than clinically found in outpatient clinics.

Common examples of these are

(a) **Localized acute curving or bulge of septum**: This is dealt with by localized correction or limited excision of the curved part of septum with or without excising the overlying septal mucoperichondrium. A soft nasal splint may be needed for 2 weeks.

(b) **Unilateral anterior angle obliteration** due to **one-sided inferior veering or deviation of the septum**: These cases are dealt with by proceeding to a routine **formal septoplasty,** i.e., anatomically freeing the quadrilateral cartilage from its bony attachments from the vomer inferiorly and the perpendicular plate of the ethmoid, superiorly with the exception of the key area, i.e., near to the nasal dorsum.

The **angle usually opens up** at the end of this procedure alone, as the whole quadrilateral cartilage shifts to become almost centralized.

Finally, a very small localized part of the cartilaginous septum at the **area of the valve angle** may have to be excised inclusive or exclusive of the overlying mucoperichondrium.

A successful outcome of surgery results in a clearly seen slit at the anterior valve angle. Bilateral nasal splints are placed for 2 weeks.

(2) Vestibular Stenosis:

The main purpose of treatment is to restore and secure the presence of an **angle** and the **mobility** of its lateral wall, i.e., **mobile angle**. Treatment of vestibular stenosis therefore means the release of the lower margin of the upper lateral cartilage, i.e., the lateral wall of the internal valve, from the crippling effect of the scar tissues. Not only does the size of the nasal cavity and the airway become wider but also the dynamic movement of the valve is restored.

According to the degree of stenosis, surgery is planned so that the following may be done:

- Simple division and the insertion of silastic stent that remains for 2 weeks.
- Local Z-plasty or M-plasty.
- Free skin graft.
- Composite skin and cartilage graft.

(3) Inferior turbinate:

If the **anterior end of the inferior turbinate** enlarges and intrudes into the opening of the nasal valve, then **localized trimming of the turbinate head** or **submucosal diathermy** will clear the way for air entry.

(4) The upper lateral cartilage:

i. Excision of a **triangular segment** from its lower margin (Gray) with proximal flap removal (Lopez-Infante flap) opens the angle of the valve.
ii. **Spreader cartilage** graft is useful in certain cases of acute valve angles.
iii. **Collapse of the upper lateral cartilage**, usually secondary to overzealous dorsal resection. There is a bilateral **collapse of the anterior valve angles**. The middle third of the nose looks extremely thin.

Total **conchal graft**, when used to support the upper lateral cartilage over the cartilaginous septum, **opens up the valve angle bilaterally**, and impressively improves the nasal air entry on both sides. There is an equally impressive improvement in the **external appearance**.

(5) The lower lateral cartilage:

Fibrosis, malposition or total absence of the **lateral crus** of the lower lateral cartilage may happen primarily or secondary to surgical over-resection. This will lead to a collapse of the **external valve,** i.e., the expanding air reservoir before entering through to the internal valve. There is a strong sensation of reduced air entry on the affected side.

A **cartilage graft** expands the external valve and acts both **functionally** improving the air entry and **aesthetically** elevating the collapse on the affected side. An **ear conchal** or a **cartilaginous septal graft** is usually suitable for this defect.

(6) The ala nasi:

Overzealous alar base resection, extensive manipulations in the aponeurotic muscle layer or paralytic lesions may all reduce cripple or totally abolish movement at one or both of the alae nasi, i.e., the only mobile wall in the **external valve**. This has major consequences on the physiology of nasal respiration as well as the aesthetic effects.

The management of each of the conditions is dealt with separately in the surgical section.

(7) Other conditions:

Relatively large anterior nasal spine or caudally dislocated septum in a narrow nose markedly reduces the size of the external valve.

Cysts, adhesions, tumors or granulomas may take place in either the external or internal valve areas.

Anatomical Variations of the Nose 8

Abstract

This chapter studies the range of diversities of the different anatomical parts of the nose.

Keywords

Anatomical variations of the nose · Nasal skin variations

This chapter studies the range of diversities of the different anatomical parts of the nose.

Variations may all be **acceptable** within the range of the **normal anatomy**, but may **not be totally acceptable aesthetically**. Different parts of the nose may vary in **size**, **shape** and **position**.

It is important to realize that noses are like fingerprints, i.e., they are different and variable from one person to another and from one side, of the same nose, to the other. No two noses or even two halves of one nose are the same.

Anatomical variations of the nose are mainly **developmental**, but some changes may be acquired.

Embryologically, the **nasofrontal process** is the main contributor to nasal structures. In a developing nose, the median and the two lateral processes may not be completely **descended** (lowered), **rotated** or **approximated** to each other (medialized). This in turn will affect the **size**, **shape** and **position** of each component of the nasal walls and consequently the overall aesthetics of the nose.

Acquired variations may be **accidental**, **surgical trauma** or **pathological**, e.g., infection, neoplastic or burn.

Anatomical variations are classified into

(I) Variations in the **three-walled upper two-thirds** of the nose.
(II) Variations in the **four-walled lower third of the nose.**
(III) Variations in the **weak areas and soft folds.**
(IV) **Ethnographic** Variations.
(V) **Bilateral** Variations.
(VI) Age Variations.

8.1 Variations in the Three-Walled Upper Two-Thirds of the Nose

Variations in the three-walled upper two-thirds of the nose include two areas:

(A) The Bony pyramid.
(B) The Upper lateral cartilage, i.e., Midvault.

8.1.1 The Bony Pyramid

The bony pyramid is variant in its **size**, **deviation** from the axial plane and **obliquity** from the sagittal plane.

M. H. A. Shafy, *Innovations in Rhinoplasty*,
https://doi.org/10.1007/978-3-030-94573-2_8

Deviations and obliquities of the pyramid are associated with bilateral maxillary asymmetry. It is discussed in further detail in the surgical section.

8.1.2 The Upper Lateral Cartilage

(a) The **upper lateral cartilage** makes **one unit** with the **cartilaginous septum.** Most of the variations in this united structure are associated with its **size** and **position.**
The size of the midvault is large in cases of a nasal hump, which usually include the bony and cartilaginous parts of the septum and the lateral walls.

(b) A smaller side of the upper lateral cartilage may be seen in forgotten early childhood injuries and in maxillary asymmetry. Clinically, it appears as a one-sided area of defect or depression as compared to the other side.

8.2 Variations in the Four-Walled Lower Third of the Nose

The lower third of the nose is the **highest**, **widest** and the most contributing to the **aesthetics** and **dynamics** of the external nose.

Any of the components of the four walls may show anatomical variations as follows.

8.2.1 The Lateral Wall

The ala nasi including the alar body, the alar margin and the alar groove, with its two components, the superior and posterior grooves.

The **lateral crurae** of the lower lateral cartilage.

8.2.2 The Medial Wall

- The columella.
- The medial crurae.
- The membranous septum.

Loose membranous septum leads to the condition of a sliding tip (see Surgical section).

8.2.3 The Inferior Wall

The Nasal Sill Bands
The soft vestibular floors and posterior vestibular margins are versatile and do have any variations.
The **Flat Triangle**

8.2.4 The Anterior Wall

The **middle crus** of the lower cartilage on each half of the nose is the only component of the anterior wall.

8.2.5 The Weak Areas and Soft Folds

(a) The rim-sill folds.
(b) The weak triangle.
(c) The flat triangle (discussed with the inferior wall).

8.2.6 The Lateral Wall

8.2.6.1 The Ala Nasi

The **body** of the ala nasi may vary in **size, shape, thickness** and **position**. These variations not only have a **direct** effect on the overall aesthetics of the nose, but they also have **indirect** effects on the important surrounding structures, viz., the **alar groove**, the **flat triangle,** the muscular triangle and the **rim-sill fold.**

The Size of the Ala Nasi

Small Ala Nasi
The ala nasi may be **genuinely or relatively small** as compared to the overall size of the nose. As the **major contributor to the lateral nasal wall**, the small alae nasi may have a considerable effect on **nasal aesthetics** (Fig. 8.1).

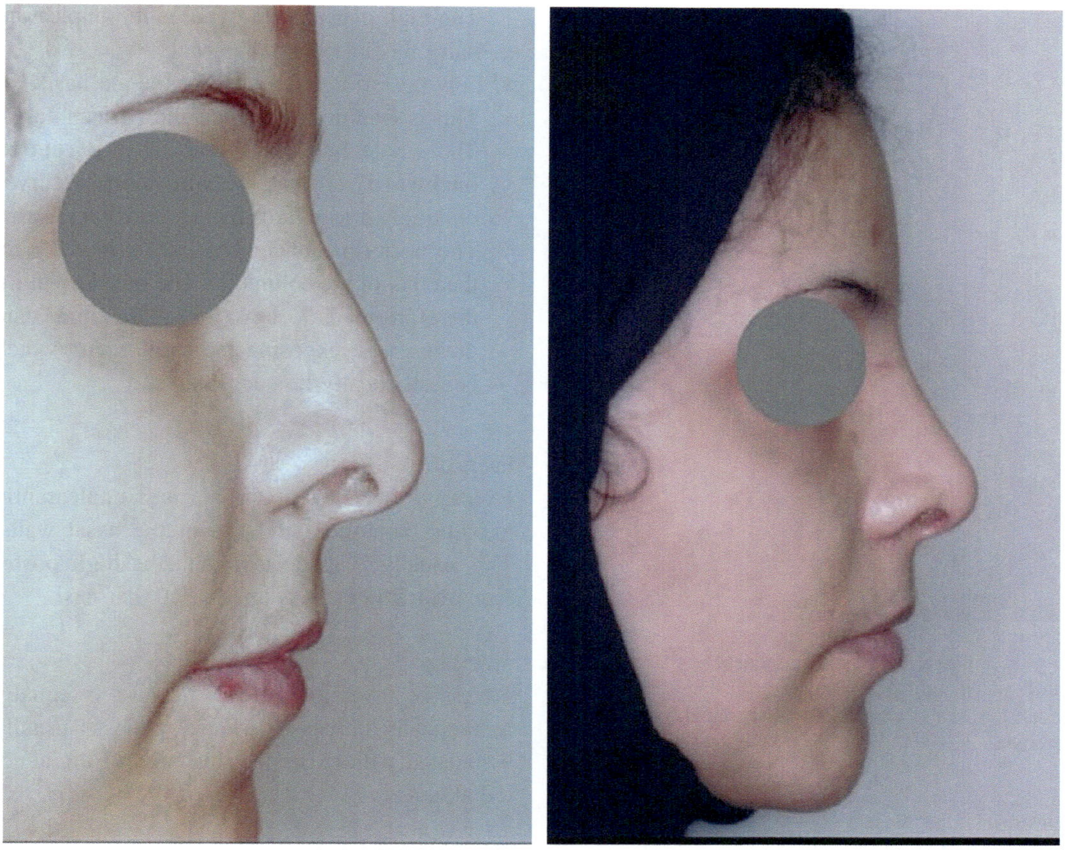

Fig. 8.1 Small Ala Nasi Consequences of small right ala nasi: large flat triangle, wide muscular triangle, columella is exposed and short superior alar groove. Improved aesthetics post-operatively

The nasal **functions** are **not** usually affected by the size of the body of the ala nasi. The consequent aesthetic effects may be:

- **High arched alar margin** exposing the medial columellar wall.
- **Short alar margin** which leads to a **large flat triangle**. An unpleasant notch may replace the flat triangle if its skin fold is too small.
- **Short superior and posterior alar grooves**. The short **posterior** alar groove means **short attachment** of the ala nasi to the **upper lip**, while the short superior alar groove means a **wide** area of the **muscular triangle** and vice versa.

Large Ala Nasi

This is commonly seen in the **Asian** and **African noses** (Fig. 8.2). It has exactly the opposite effects of the small ala nasi on the surrounding areas:

- The **alar margin** may be **lower** than the lateral columellar margin.
- The **flat triangle** is **small**.
- The **muscular triangle** is exceedingly **small**.
- The superior and posterior **alar grooves** are **long**, i.e., longer length of attachment to the upper lip.

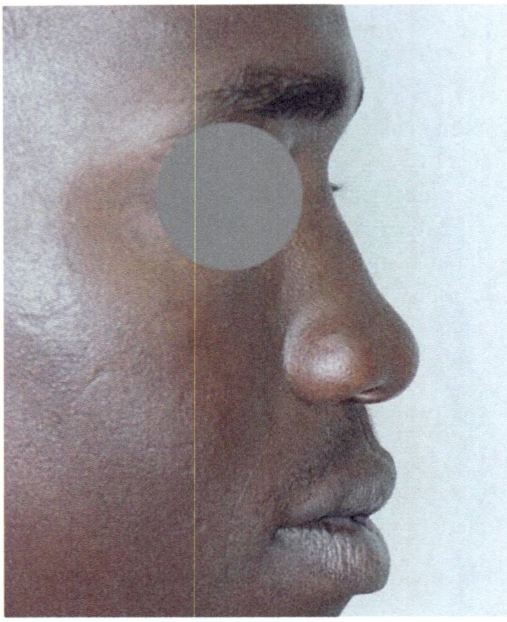

Fig. 8.2 Large Ala Nasi: Consequence of large right ala nasi: alar margin is at a lower level than the columella, small flat triangle, small muscular triangle and long alar grooves

Unequal Alae Nasi

Unequal alae nasi on both sides may lead to an unbalanced shape of the lower third of the nose.

The Shape of the Ala Nasi

The usual **oval** shape of the ala nasi may change in some individuals to become more **circular**. This is usually seen in African and Asian noses. Both **alar grooves** become **equal** in length. The ala nasi tends to be **larger** in size.

The Position of the Ala Nasi

High or Low Alar Margin

The height of the alar marginal arch may be related to the **position** of the body of the alar nasi **rather than its size**.

- High posterior attachment of the ala nasi: This leads to an **oblique rim-sill fold** as it has to cross the gap between the higher alar margin to the lower nasal sill band. The high alar margin exposes the unpleasant hairy medial columellar wall.
- Low posterior attachment of the ala nasi: This is seen in some Asian and African noses. The whole body of the ala nasi is **rotated backwards** so that the **alar margin** curves obliquely downwards from before backwards. The posterior attachment is at a lower level than that of the columella. The **nasal opening** therefore tends to look **forwards** rather than downwards, exposing the nasal cavity which is aesthetically less acceptable.

Eversion

Excessive eversion of the ala nasi unpleasantly exposes the **inner surfaces** of the nasal walls. This usually is associated with the **high posterior attachment** of a small-sized alar nasi.

Inversion

Excessive inversion of the ala nasi is equally aesthetically unpleasant. Facial palsy is usually associated with excessive inversion of the affected ala nasi.

Lateral Attachment of the Posterior Alar Margin

This consequently leads to a wide alar base. The **rim-sill** fold and/or the **nasal sill band** are elongated. The end result is a wide nasal aperture and an overall large lower third of the nose.

The Indirect Effects of Alar variations

The anatomical variations of the alae nasi indirectly affect the neighboring anatomical structures, i.e., the alar grooves, the rim-sill fold, the flat triangle and finally the muscular triangle.

The Alar Grooves

The Superior Alar Groove

The **length**, **depth** and **curvature** of this groove are related to the **size**, **position** and **shape** of the ala nasi successively, as well as the size and shape of the lateral crus of the lower lateral cartilage. The latter shares in the formation of the anterior third of the superior alar groove.

- Deep superior groove:
  This makes the ala nasi look as if it is semidetached from the nose. The aperture tube is compressed antero-posteriorly and the nasal opening takes a transversely long axis. The asymmetrical appearance of nasal openings may result from a unilateral deep superior alar groove (Fig. 8.3).
- Shallow superior alar groove:
  In these cases, the lateral nasal wall is flattened and looks like a solid tube. The affected nostril takes a more rounded shape (Fig. 8.4).

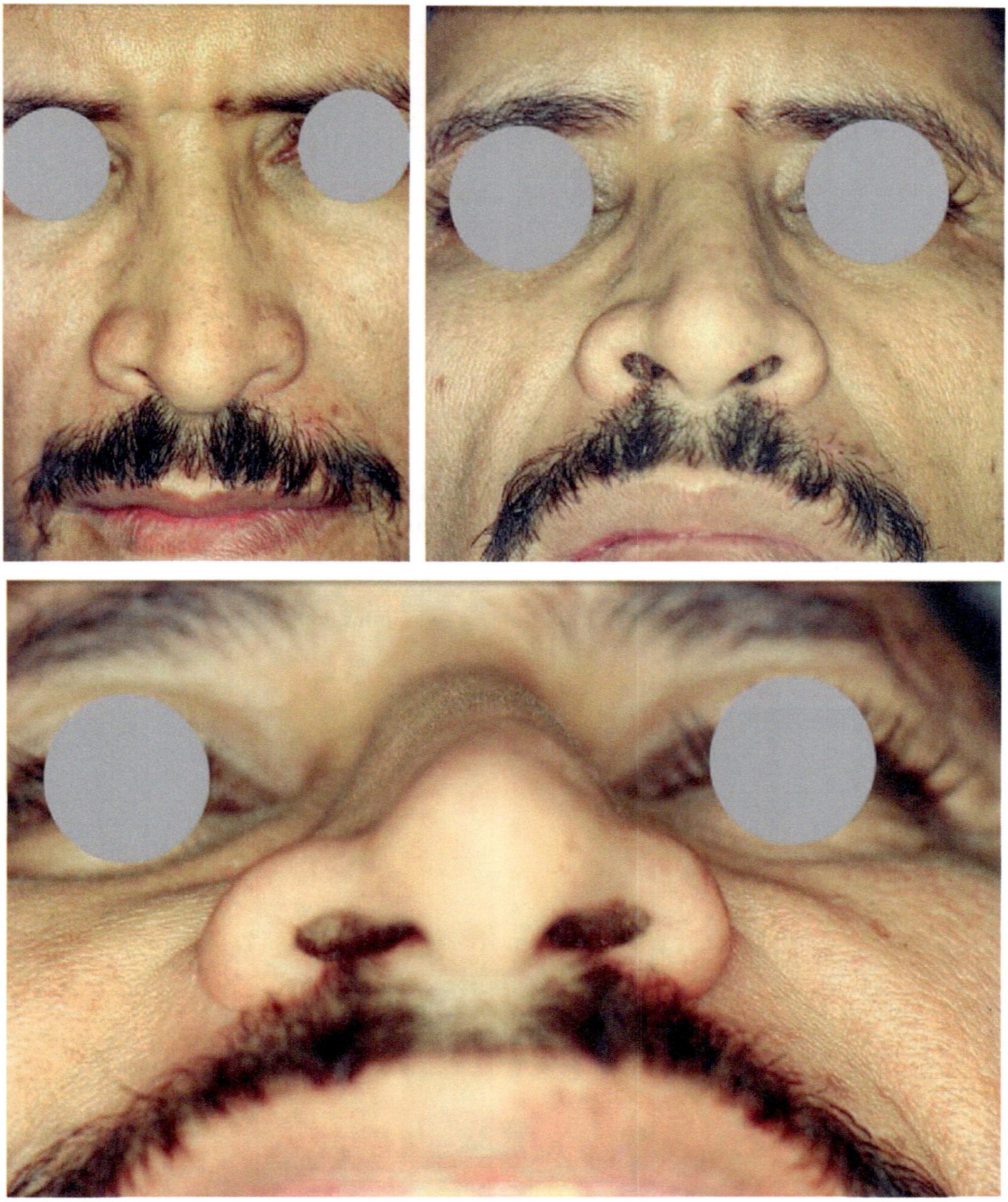

Fig. 8.3 Naturally Deep Right Superior Alar Groove

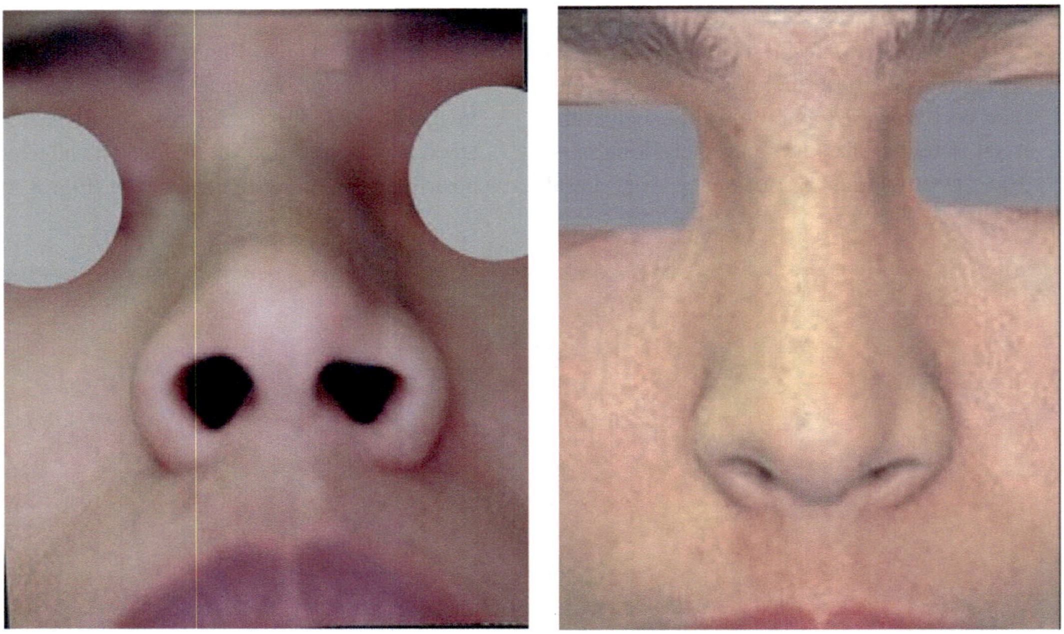

Fig. 8.4 Naturally Shallow Right Superior Alar Groove

The Posterior Alar Groove

- Deep posterior alar groove:
  Deep groove is seen in cases of **thick-skinned** nasal apertures. Thickness is caused by the posterior segment of the rim-sill folds. The folds lay down, over the upper lip, like a **flat tire** of a car, creating a very deep alar groove. The **angle** between the ala nasi and the upper lip is quite **acute**. Their junction can only be seen after elevating the ala nasi away from the lip (Fig. 8.5).

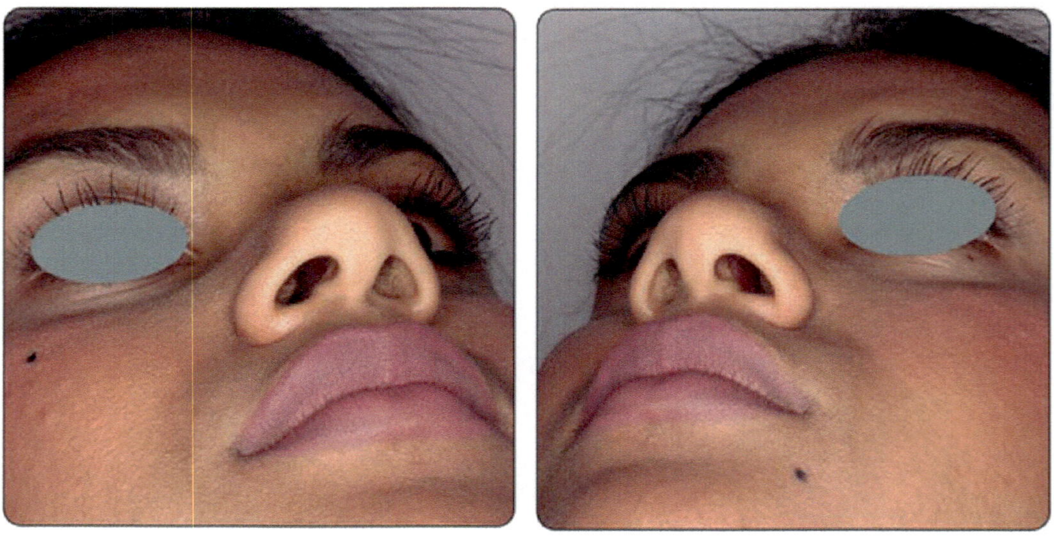

Fig. 8.5 Deep Posterior Alar Groove

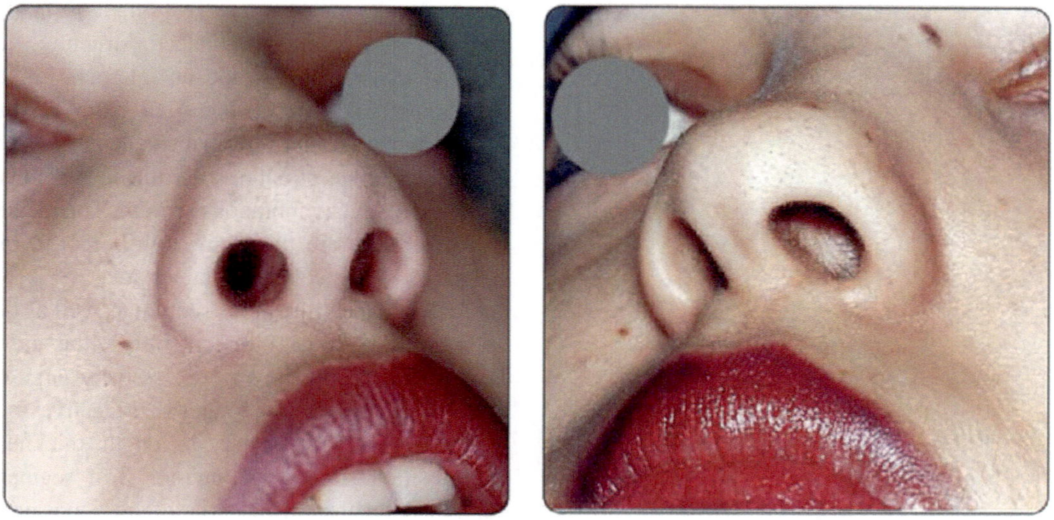

Fig. 8.6 Shallow Posterior Alar Groove

- Shallow posterior alar groove:
  This is commonly seen in the Asian and some African noses which have more spherical apertures. The **angle** between the ala nasi and the upper lip is very **wide** more than 90 degrees. Their junction is therefore clearly exposed and seen (Fig. 8.6).

8.2.6.2 The Lateral Crus

Variations in the lateral crus may affect its **size**, **shape** and **position**.

Size

The increase or decrease in the size of the lateral crus directly affects the overall size of the lower third of the nose and inversely affects the size of the muscular triangle.

Shape

The lateral crus may vary in its shape from being **oblong** to widely circular. The body of the lateral crus may continue to be as **convex** as the dome of the middle crus, less convex or the curvature of its body may reverse its shape to become **concave** (Fig. 8.7).

The combination of a **large size** and **increased convexity** of a lateral crus produces a **large boxed** type nose (Fig. 8.8).

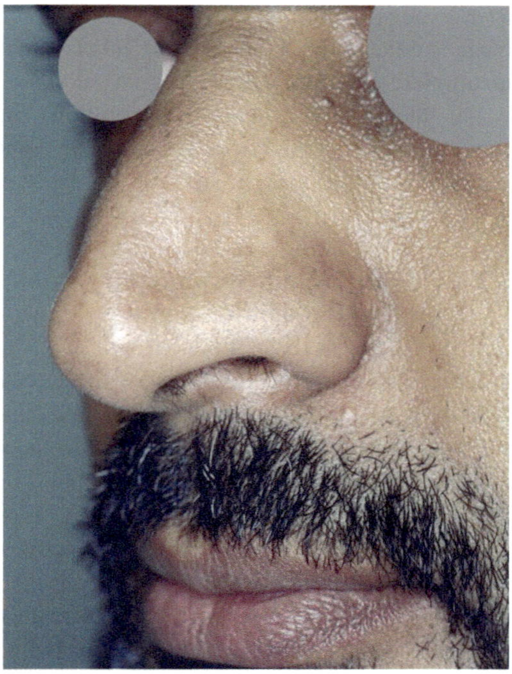

Fig. 8.7 Concave Left Lateral Crus

Position

The position of the lateral crus may vary according to the degree of **cephalic rotation**, **twisting** and **lateral curving**.

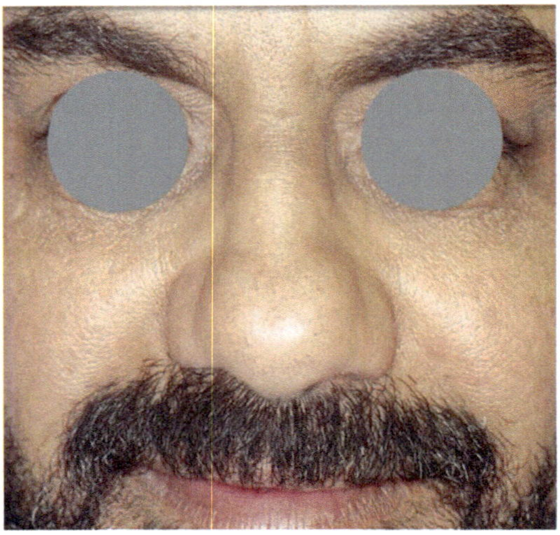

Fig. 8.8 Large Boxy, Lateral Crurae

The lateral crus may not reach its place in the lateral wall leaving a soft area between the cartilage and the body of the ala nasi. This is due to **incomplete rotation** and **curving** laterally.

On the contrary, **excessive rotation** and **curving** may take the lateral crus and the dome nearer to the nasal margin and over the body of the ala nasi.

8.2.6.3 The Prominent Superior Overlap of the Lateral Crus

Overlapping of the upper border of the **lateral crus** over the lower border of the **upper lateral cartilage** (scroll area) may become **unaesthetically prominent**. Not only that but it may also contribute to the bulk of a large nose (Fig. 8.9).

Bulky folding of the upper marginal cartilage of the lateral crus is the site of this prominence. Direct surgical reduction of this fold via the intercartilaginous incision reduces this prominence without affecting the nasal function.

8.2.7 The Medial Wall

8.2.7.1 The Columella and the Medial Crurae

The columella constitutes the common medial wall between the two nasal aperture tubes. As mentioned in the anatomy section, it is in the form of an inverted T-shaped structure, an external transverse part and an internal vertical membranous septum. The medial crura are the only structures that are subcutaneously seen externally. Other structures are all hidden internally within the membranous septum. The medial crura therefore are the main contributors to the aesthetics of the columello-labial area.

The caudal cartilaginous septum as well as the anterior nasal spine indirectly affect the naso-labial aesthetics, if they are excessively large or extensively retracted or reduced surgically.

The columella may vary in length, thickness and position. It has an anterior firm segment supported by the medial crurae and a posterior unsupported soft segment. The caudal cartilaginous septum and nasal segment. The caudal cartilaginous septum and nasal spine indirectly affect the aesthetics of the columella.

Length

i. Short columella: this is seen in cases where the medial crura are short, e.g., cases of hare lip.
ii. Long columella: this is seen in cases where the medial crura are long, e.g., in long Caucasian noses.

Thickness

The thickness of an aesthetically acceptable columella is closely comparable to the thickness of the inferior margins of the alae nasi. The external inferior surface is usually smoothly round. Unaesthetic columella tends to be **wider** than normal. Both parts of the external columella may be affected as follows:

i. Bifid columella: The inferior part of the columella is grooved and wide. This may be caused by the increased **coronal** curvature in the bodies of the medial crura which leads to the wide lateralization of their inferior borders.
   The distance between the two medial crura is wide in some other cases.
ii. Wide posterior columellar fold: It is usually associated with the **overprojection of the posterior margins of the medial crura**.

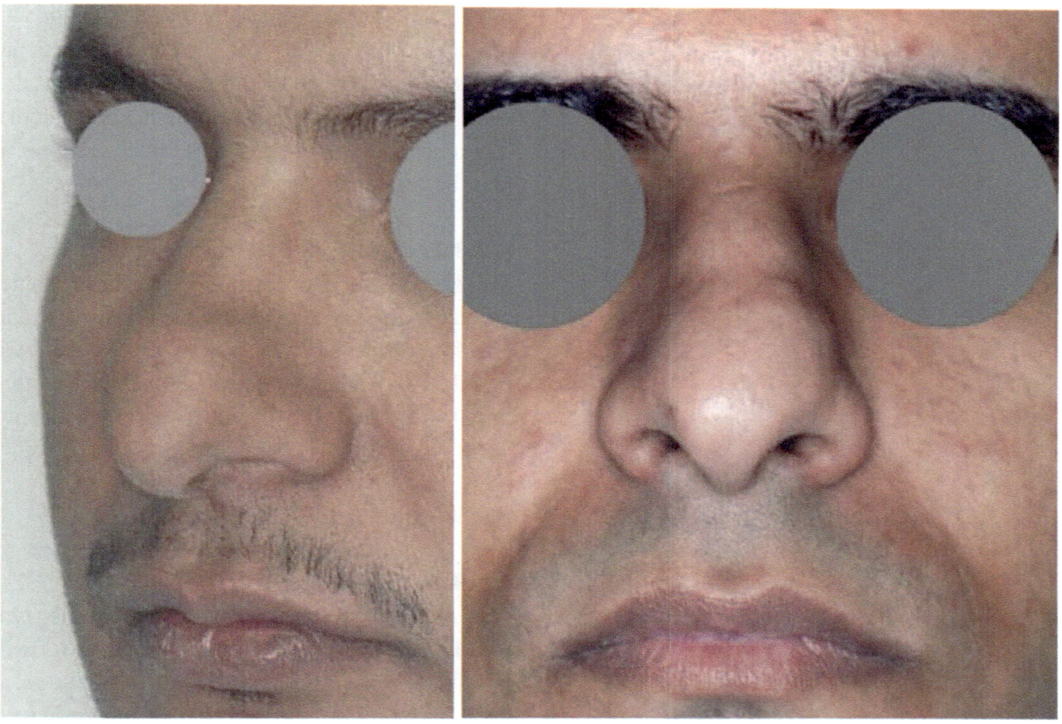

Fig. 8.9 Prominent, Bulky Overlap of the Lateral Crus

This is due to the increased axial curvature in the bodies of the medial crura.
The increased **medial crural prominence** usually affects the aesthetics and the width of the nasal aperture by encroaching upon its wall and the aperture space.

Position

i. Retracted columella: In these cases, the **posterior columellar fold loses its bony support by the anterior nasal spine**. This is either post-traumatic or iatrogenic after surgical over-reduction of the spine.
ii. Protracted columella: This is caused by the overprojection of the posterior columellar fold either by a misplaced caudal cartilaginous septum or a large anterior nasal spine.
iii. Hanging columella: This is a case of protruding large-sized medial crura anteriorly, exposing their hairy medial surfaces. A long caudal septum may contribute to the crural hanging.
iv. Oblique columella: This is caused either by an obliquely dislocated caudal cartilaginous nasal septum or rarely by an oblique alar base.

8.2.8 The Inferior Aperture Wall

The only two structures that may have aesthetic variation in the inferior aperture wall are the **nasal sill** band and the **flat triangle**. They are **the only externally appearing structures** in the nasal floor. The vestibular floor on the other hand is an internal unsupported loose structure.

8.2.8.1 Variations in the Nasal Sill Band

Length

A very **long** nasal sill produces a **wide** alar base and hence a wide nasal aperture. A **short** nasal sill, on the other hand, produces a **narrow** alar base and narrow nasal aperture.

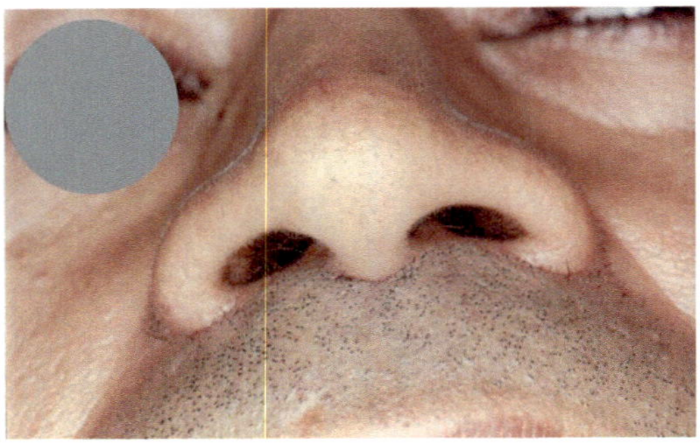

Fig. 8.10 Flat Nasal Sill Bands

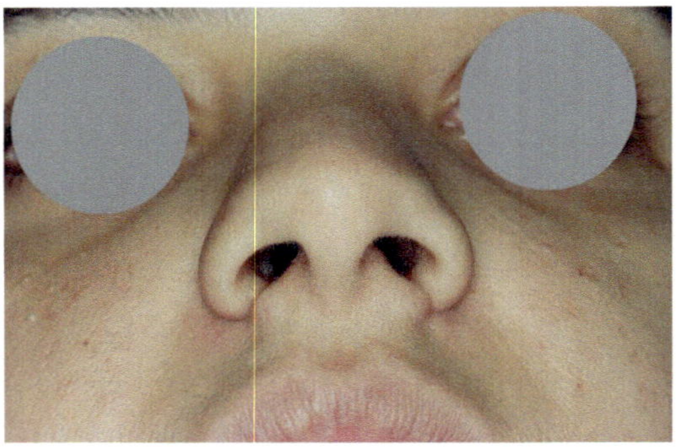

Fig. 8.11 Prominent Nasal Sill Bands

Thickness and Prominence

Middle Easterners and Africans, in general, have highly **prominent** and thick nasal sills (Fig. 8.11), while Asians tend to have **flat** sills (Fig. 8.10). In all cases, the sill band can be easily and distinctly palpated as a definite margin.

Position

The nasal sill should be just seen off the alar margin in the oblique and lateral views.

A very high nasal sill produces an unaesthetic appearance to the nose.

The nasal sill may be pushed **down** by a dislocated and long **caudal septum** or displaced **upwards** by an excessively reduced anterior **nasal spine** or in cases of **unilateral facial palsy**.

The upper lateral fold of nasal sill

This soft fold of skin only exists if the ala nasi is externally rotated so that the alar margin is not in line with the nasal sill. It varies in length and prominence in a way that affects the external aesthetic appearance of the nose.

It may be so prominent that it almost looks like a second alar rim. On the other extreme, it may be too small or absent.

8.2.8.2 The Flat Triangle

The size, shape and position of the flat triangle, i.e., all indirectly affected by the size, shape and position of its surrounding structures, i.e., the middle crus and the alar nasi. Other factors that might affect the degree of flatness is skin thickness.

8.2.9 The Anterior Wall

8.2.9.1 The Middle Crurae

The anterior wall is **only made** by the **two middle crurae** of the two halves of the lower third of the nose, clinically known as the nasal tip. Variations in this important structure have a direct influential effect on the external appearance.

The middle crurae may vary in **size**, **shape** and **position**. The interdomal relations may also be variable.

Size

A large or small middle crus reflects itself on the size of the nasal tip.

Shape

The dome is always convex. The degree of convexity either produces a narrow pointed or broad wide tip (Fig. 8.12).

Position

The dome may be **elevated** exposing the nasal opening causing a "**pig snout**" deformity or **depression** in cases of a **plunging tip**. The most aesthetic nose is when the dome is in a truly anterior position giving the nose its ideal projection. Both domes are attached to each other producing one unit, the nasal tip.

The separation of the domes from each other may produce a **bifid** tip or a **boxed** tip if both have large quadrangular domes.

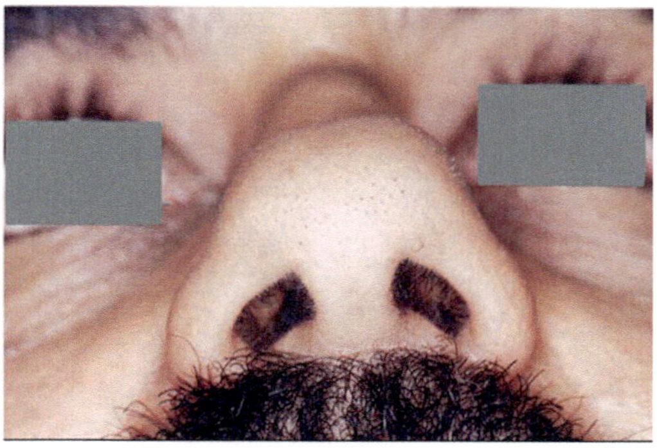

Fig. 8.12 Large, Boxy, Unequal Middle Crurae

8.2.10 The Weak Areas and Soft Folds

8.2.10.1 The Weak Triangle

The weak triangle is the gap between the upper three-walled two-thirds and the two lower four-walled one-third of the nose.

The weak triangle varies in its **size**, **shape** and **position** according to the effects of its surrounding boundaries.

(a) The **size of the middle crurae** and the degree of their divergence. A large widely divergent middle crura will lead to wide-angled weak triangle and vice versa.

(b) The **anterior septal angle**:
A long caudal septum will lead to a long weak triangle and vice versa.
A high anterior angle will lead to parrot beak deformity, while a low angle leads to supratip depression.

(c) The **pad of fat** that fills the weak triangle affects the supratip aesthetics. Unwise removal of the weak triangular fat may lead to supratip depression. Decision to remove the weak triangular fat may be part of a reduction of a bony cartilaginous hump in a large nose.

8.2.10.2 The Rim-Sill Fold

Variations in the rim-sill fold may take place during the embryological development of the nose. They result in two main situations:

i. **Incomplete descent**, **medialization** and **inversion** of the lateral process of the fronto-nasal process that mainly develops into the **ala nasi** in the lateral nasal wall.
The affected ala nasi becomes **higher**, **laterally placed** and **everted**. It is usually **small** in size as it is less developed.
The **alar margin** therefore is not only farther **away** from the **nasal sill**, but it is at a **higher** level and **everted**.
The natural smooth **circular continuation** between the alar margin and the nasal sill is **lost**.
The **rim-sill fold** of soft skin has to **cross** this wide gap between the two structures. The **second fold of soft skin** is elevated from the inner surface of the everted ala nasi that becomes continuous with the nasal sill margin. The rim-sill fold therefore becomes **long**, **oblique** and **bifid**.

ii. **Excessive descent, medialization** and **inversion**:
This is usually seen in large ala nasi and in facial palsy. The rim-sill fold becomes short and compressed.

The rim-sill fold therefore may vary in its **length**, **thickness** and **position**:

Length

i. Long rim-sill fold results in a wide aperture. This is more common in rounded nasal apertures (Fig. 8.13).
ii. Short rim-sill fold is seen in oval nasal apertures and in cases of the long nasal sill. It may be reduced to become just a fissure between the alar rim and nasal sill (Fig. 8.14).

Thickness

i. Rim-sill fold may take **the same shape**, **thickness** and **prominence** of both **alar rim** and **nasal sill** so that these three structures are joined uniformly in **one smooth continuous fold**. This is common in noses with rounded apertures.

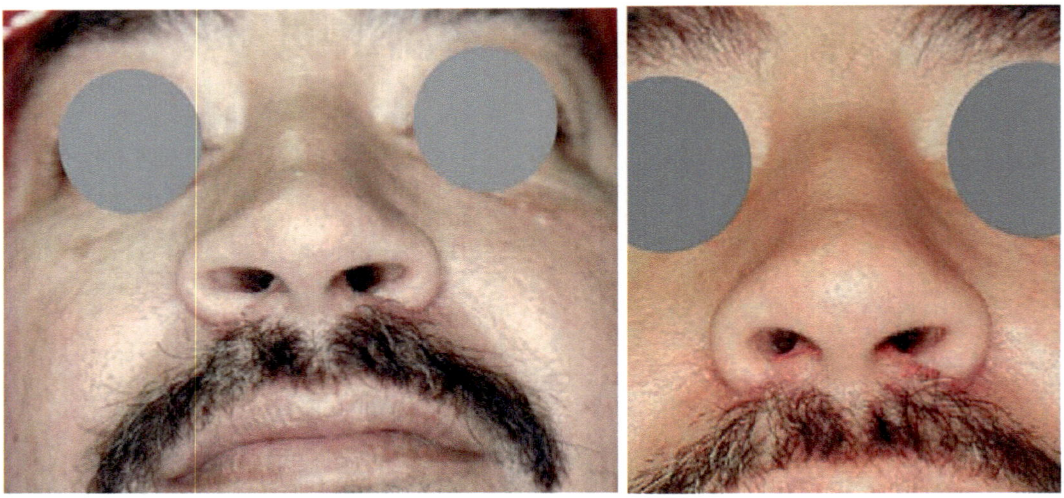

Fig. 8.13 Long Inferior Segments of Rim-Sill Folds. Post-operative reduction of long inferior segments of the rim-sill folds (Right Image)

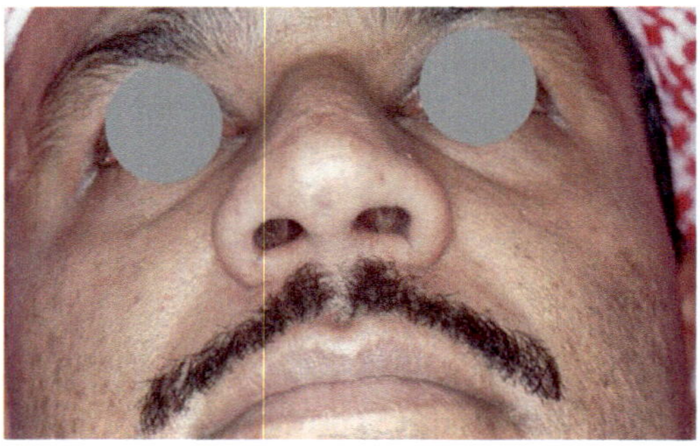

Fig. 8.14 Absent Rim-Sill Folds. Rim-Sill Folds are replaced by skin crease

ii. Partial or complete **absence** of the rim-sill fold, i.e., loss of natural continuity between the nasal sill and the alar rim. This is more common in noses with oval or long apertures where there is a sharp change of direction between the alar rim and the nasal sill from antero-posterior to transverse.

The communicating fold of skin loses its prominent shape in part or all of its length. Thus, a **flat area** may separate the alar rim from the nasal sill.

This area varies from being a **simple fissure** or crease to a much **wider space**. Flatness happens more commonly on the medial side, nearer to the nasal sill, making the lateral end point of the nasal sill appear as a clear prominence. The soft skin fold that remains in continuity with the alar rim is variable in length.

The postero-lateral end point of the alar rim therefore does not correspond to the apparently seen one. Gentle medial displacement of the alar rim using a blunt angle probe (rim-sill test) will show clearly the real margin of the alar rim.

iii. **Localized thickening** of the rim-sill fold is unaesthetic.

iv. **Thinner** rim-sill fold gives unnatural communication between the alar rim and nasal sill.

Position

i. The rim-sill fold may take a **transverse** or **oblique** course according to the level of the ala nasi in relation to the nasal sill.

ii. It may take a long-angled course making a **fourth aperture wall**, i.e., rectangular nasal aperture.

iii. If the alar rim is much higher than the nasal sill, i.e., high alar postero-lateral attachment, the rim-sill fold may take an **oblique**, or almost a vertical direction (Fig. 8.15). Lowering of this unduly high alar rim is achieved by simply excising the rim-sill fold (8.16).

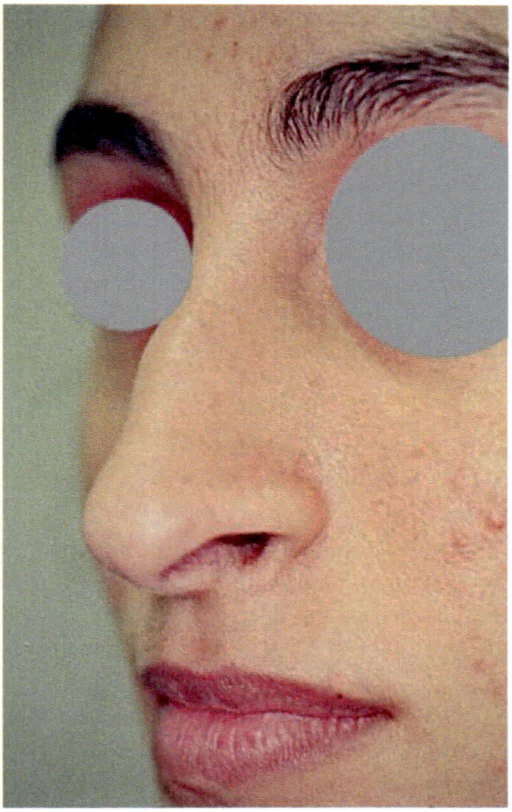

Fig. 8.15 Oblique Left Rim-Sill Fold

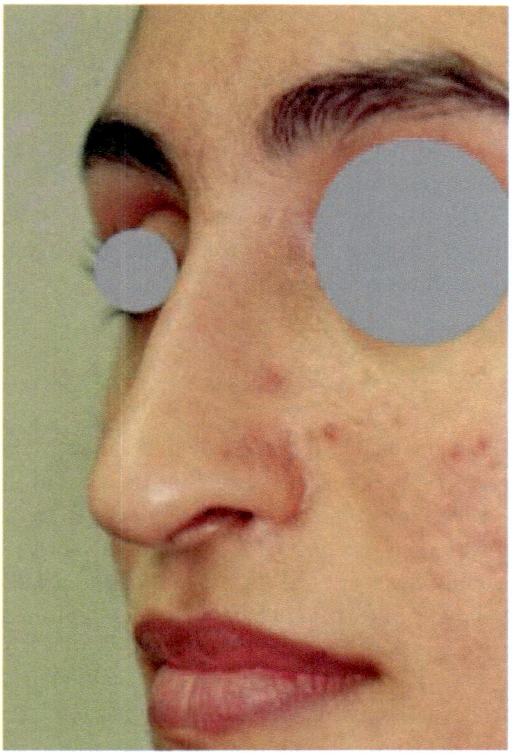

Fig. 8.16 Oblique Rim-Sill Fold - Excised

8.3 Nasal Skin Variations

The nasal skin is mainly variant over the **lower third** of the nose, i.e., that covers the frontolateral walls of the middle and lateral crurae as well as the alae nasi.

Skin cover of the upper two-thirds, i.e., the bony pyramid and the upper cartilage are usually more consistently thin with less fat underneath.

Skin variations in the lower third are mostly related to geographic ethnicity. African, Middle Eastern and Hispanic and Asians generally have thicker skin over the lower third than Caucasian noses.

8.4 Ethnographic Variations

Clinically, there are four main groups of noses that are seen in different parts of the world:

(1) The **Caucasian** noses: They include Europeans and white Americans.
(2) The **African** noses.
(3) The **Asian** Noses.
(4) The **Middle Eastern** Noses: These include **Hispanic, Arabs** and **Iranian, Indian** and **Pakistani** noses.

The noses of each of these groups have their own characteristics in the general shape, bulk and size. They are affected by the shapes, bulks and sizes of the **frontolateral walls**, the **bony bridges** and their covering **skin**.

8.4.1 The Caucasian Noses

The Caucasian noses are characterized by having a high nasal bridge, firm cartilaginous framework and oval nasal openings that have an oblique antero-posterior axis.

The covering skin is generally thin over the firm cartilaginous framework of the middle and lower thirds of the nose.

8.4.2 The African Noses

The main characteristics of the African noses are that they are **generally large**, **bulky** and **flat all over the bony** and **cartilaginous parts**. Both the dorsum and the lower third look as if there are forcibly flattened, i.e., dish face. The **main bulk** is in the **alae nasi** which has thick fibrofatty tissues as well as the thick covering skin.

The **nasal tip** is **small** and **low positioned** in between the two more projecting sizable alae nasi. In taking the **oblique view photographs**, the nasal tip cannot be seen as the highest projecting point. The **alae nasi are more projecting forwards**. The **lower lateral cartilages** are **small and weak**. They are not surgically capable of reshaping the covering thick skin. The **nasal openings** are **rounded**, **wide** and have a **transverse long axis**. The covering **skin** of the frontolateral walls is generally **the thickest** of all the Ethnographic groups. The bony pyramid is wide and low.

8.4.3 The Asian Nose

The Asian noses are generally **small in size as compared to the size of the face**. The typical Far Eastern face has very wide and large cheekbones (Zygomatic bones) with a comparatively small nose. Sometimes, the nose is too small to project against the wide cheek margin in the oblique view photographs.

Asian noses are generally **flat** and **bulky** but in a different way than African noses. They are less bulky. The **alae nasi** may be less bulky but comparatively have a **larger size**. They are relatively large compared to other structures of the nose. The alar margin may be lower than the columellar level. The **alae nasi** are **tilted more posteriorly downwards**, affecting the final alar flare. The **nasal opening** therefore tends to be **looking forwards** rather than downwards.

The **lower lateral** cartilages are comparatively **larger** and slightly **stronger** than in the African noses. The tip therefore is not as low and flat. The **bony bridge** is **shorter**, **thinner** and is equally **flat** as compared to the African noses.

8.4.4 The Middle Eastern and Hispanic Noses

These noses have **high** and strong **bony bridges**.

The **skin** of the frontolateral walls tends to be to a thicker side but not as thick as the African noses. The lower third of the nose tends to be bulky.

Although the **nasal tip** has a proportionately good size, it is generally rounded and **lacks a clear definition and projection**.

The **lower lateral cartilages** are of **good size**, generally **firm** and reliable in reshaping the nasal tip especially after thinning the skin by defatening procedure.

There are tendencies for **wide nasal apertures** that may need alar resections.

8.5 Bilateral Nasal Variations

The differences between the two sides of the body are quite natural and normal findings, e.g., the right eye, ear, hand or foot is naturally different from the left one. They differ both in shape and size.

The nose is no exception. **The two halves of the nose are not exactly mirror images**. They vary from each other in almost every nose.

The natural variations between the two sides of the body are mostly accepted aesthetically as long as they are not extremely different, as the **two organs are wide apart** and no direct comparison between the two sides.

The visual effect is quite different in the nose, being a single midline organ where a **direct comparison between the two sides is more clear to the eye**. In addition, there is a form of a balanced situation between the two sides which might be disturbed in cases of wide variations in the shape or size.

The unbalanced nose may look **crooked, deviated** or **defective** in one area. All areas of the nose may be affected, but the commonest are the nasal bones, the rim-sill folds and the lateral cartilages, upper and lower.

8.5.1 Bony Pyramid

Large nasal bone on one side is usually associated with larger zygoma on the same side, i.e., bilateral facial asymmetry. The **whole pyramid of the nose is deviated toward the smaller side**.

The nasal bone alone may be smaller in size. The affected side will have a localized depression or defect.

8.5.2 The Upper Lateral Cartilage

The right side may be smaller than the left side giving the impression of a **localized defect on** the affected side of the nose.

8.5.3 The Lower Lateral Cartilages

Both domes and lateral crura may be different in size, shape and position.

One lateral crus may be concave while the other is convex. The medial crural projections are variable from one side to the other.

8.5.4 Alae Nasi

Bilateral variations in shapes and sizes of the alae nasi are not uncommon (Fig. 8.17).

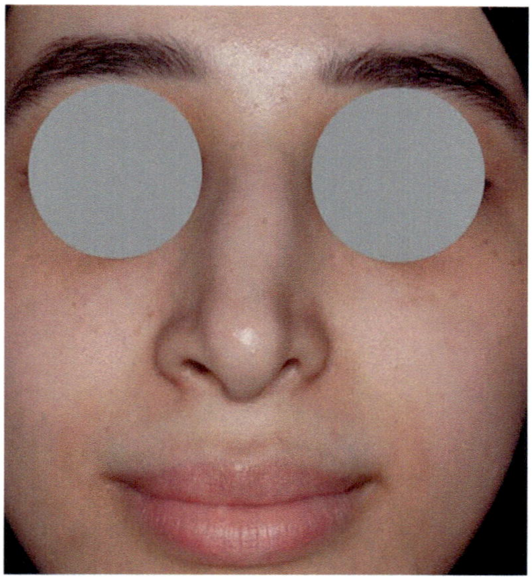

Fig. 8.17 Unequal Alae Nasi. The right ala nasi is naturally larger than the left

8.5.5 Unequal Nasal Openings

Both nasal openings may be **different** in **size** and/or **shape**. This is due to the difference in the shape and length of the **nasal sill bands**, **rim-sill folds** as well as **medial crural prominences**.

These three factors are to be addressed in the surgery to equalize both sides.

8.5.6 The Natural Unilateral Nasal Defects

In a normal unoperated nose, there may be **one or more areas of natural defects**. These are areas where one or more structures on one side of the nose are different in **size** and/or **shape** from the equivalent other side.

The commonest areas of these natural defects are the **nasal bone**, **one side of the upper lateral cartilage, the lateral crus** and finally the **rim-sill fold**.

The nose continues to be unbalanced until the **defected** sides are **compensated** by **suitable grafts** or the **larger** sides are **reduced** by the **suitable surgical reduction**.

Part II
Rhinoplasty Photography of Surgeons

Rhinoplasty Photography of Surgeons

9

Abstract

Photography is discussed here from the surgeon's point of view. Details of the technical aspects of photography are avoided as this is not meant to be a text in the science of photography, which is rather highly technical and vast. Equipments, setup and techniques are made simple and inexpensive so that high standard photography is achieved by the surgeon or any trained personnel in a surprisingly small area in the office practice.

Keywords

Patient consent for photography · The necessity of photography · Photographic equipment · The lighting system · The set up for photography · Preparing the patient for photography

Photography is discussed here from the surgeon's point of view. Details of the technical aspects of photography are avoided as this is not meant to be a text in the science of photography, which is rather highly technical and vast.

Photographic techniques described in the text are aimed to be as simple as possible without compromising the basic clinical photographic rules.

Although professional photographic advice is always needed and sought, **professional photographers** are **not always** available in many practices and clinical situations.

Many surgeons have the idea that photography is a complicated procedure that needs a qualified photographer and expensive equipments.

With the simple setup described below, any surgeon, or his well-trained assistant, will be able to take good quality photographs for his own patients in his practice. Surgeons must make every effort to take their own patient's photographs or else work closely with their professional photographers in every single case.

It is usually the surgeon's eyes that decide the area of clinical interest for the best photographs. A photographer's guidance is necessary every now and again in practices where the photographic department is not available.

With the growing knowledge and interest in the surgical anatomy of the nose, as well as the science and art of photography, there is a need for the development and evaluation of the science of **photographic anatomy**.

The medical photographers and **the surgeons** must come together and **share their knowledge** to give each photograph its meaningful **surgical anatomical description**.

M. H. A. Shafy, *Innovations in Rhinoplasty*,
https://doi.org/10.1007/978-3-030-94573-2_9

9.1 Patient Consent for Photography

A well-informed written consent must always be obtained before photography is undertaken. It is accepted, however, that in some circumstances patient is unable to give consent, for instance under anesthesia. Retrospective informed consent must be obtained or otherwise photographs are destroyed (Institute of Medical Illustration IMI National Guidelines). Each patient must understand the important need for photography and documentation. The clinician must spare good time to answer all the questions and concerns of the patients.

A **well-informed written consent** has three levels:

1. Consent for use medically
2. Consent for use in teaching healthcare staff
3. Consent for publication. This should be for specific single use only or for general release in the journal, book electronic media, etc. Patients should be warned that once published the consent cannot be withdrawn. This is especially important for internet publication.

9.2 The Necessity of Photography

Photographs in rhinoplasty are necessary for the following two important reasons:

9.2.1 Medicolegal Documentation

9.2.2 Photographic Anatomy

A method designed to enhance diagnosis and improve surgical planning.

The photographs highlight certain **anatomical areas** in the nose and the face that are missed and could not be seen by the surgeon's eyes at the time of the clinical examination in the first interview with the patient. Not all information could be seen live. The surgeon needs to have time to study and absorb more facts in the photographs.

In a way this is similar to the **forensic investigators** who take photographs of the scene of an incident or a crime to critically and carefully study them later. They discover many details that were overlooked at the time of their first inspection of the place. Both sides could be seen at the same time, e.g., two lateral, two oblique views, basal and overhead view.

9.3 Photographic Equipment

There are three basic prerequisites in order to have good quality photographs:

9.3.1 The Camera Body

A good quality DSLR (Digital Single-Lens Reflex) camera is necessary to have a photograph with high resolution.

A digital camera with a sensor of 16 megapixels or higher is more than sufficient. A memory card of 16 Gb or larger is needed. The author uses Canon EOS Rebel T7/EOS 2000 camera. An equivalent camera is Nikon D3400. These are not expensive cameras but efficiently suitable (Fig. 9.1).

9.3.2 The Lens

Close-up photographs with satisfactory **magnification** are important to see the different **anatomical details** of the nose and the face. The rim-sill test and light reflexes are also better seen in the magnified pictures.A 55 mm/60 mm f/2.8 or f/2 macro lens on a DX format camera is suitable for this purpose. This will allow close-up magnified images. The author used Tamron SP 60 mm f/2 D11 1:1 macro lens. For Nikon Camera Micro-NIKKOR 55 mm f/2.8 macro lens is suitable (Fig. 9.2).

9.3.2.1 Depth of Field

Depth of field is the amount of a subject that appears **sharp** in front of, and behind, the point of focus. The smaller the lens aperture, the greater the depth of field. This is particularly critical in the close-up work of the nose.

Aperture size is denoted on a lens by **f-numbers**. The **higher the number,** the **smaller**

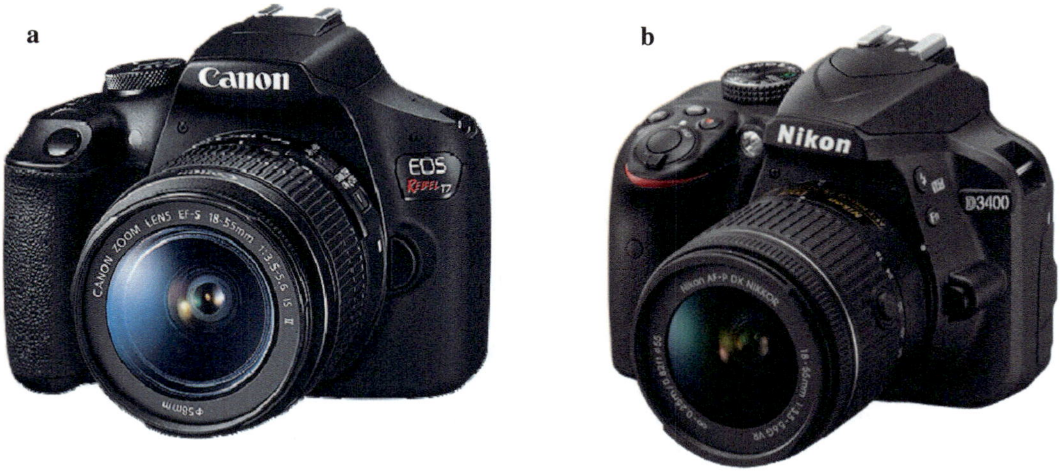

Fig. 9.1 **a** Canon EOS Rebel T7/EOS 2000 **b** Nikon D3400

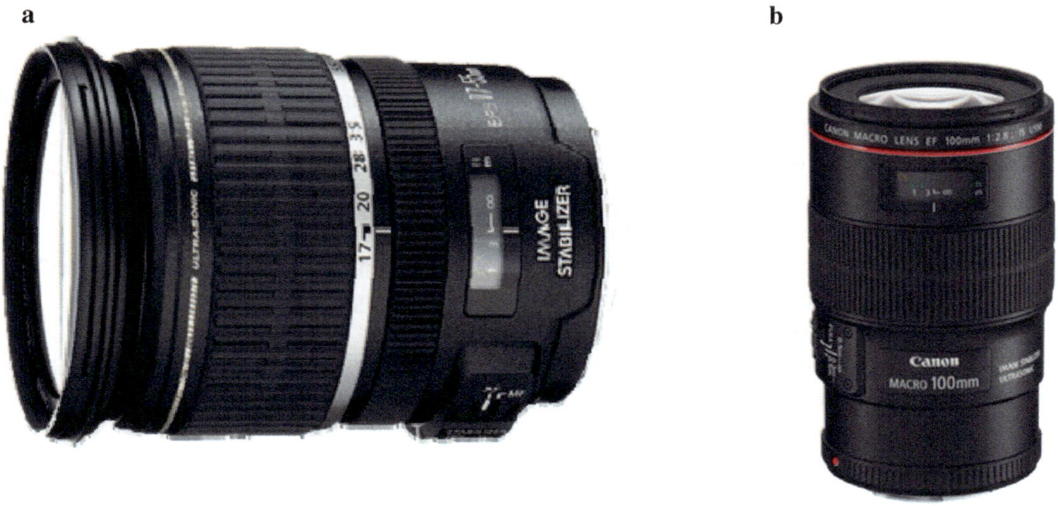

Fig. 9.2 **a** Micro-NIKKOR 55 mm f/2.8 **b** Tamron SP 60 mm f/2 D11

the amount of **light** that passes through the lens but the **greater the depth** of field.

On photographing the nose we need the **maximum depth of field**. The flash should be **bright** enough to allow for the use of the **smallest possible aperture** (Naylar JR). The **f-stop** is, therefore, an indication of the **size of** the **aperture** and consequently the **depth of field**.

f-stop in the Omicron System (Depth of Field)

(a) Full face photographs, i.e., at a distance of 60 cm (for the anther's system)
f/8–f/13 for white and brown skins
f/7–f/10 for the dark African skins

(b) Close-up photograph to the middle-third of the face from eyebrows to the lips at a distance of 40 cm
f/16–f/20 for white and brown skins
f/14–f/16 for dark African skins

f-stop in Alien Bees Flash System

Almost the same as the Omicron System with minor differences.

In all cases, ISO is 400 and shutter speed is 1/125th of a second.

9.3.3 The Lighting System

A good lighting system is critically important in order to have the following outcome:

i. Shadowless photographs
ii. Even illumination
iii. Sufficiently strong for a clear depth of field.

All folds and creases of the nose and cheeks must be shadowless and well illuminated so that the different anatomical parts can be clearly seen. The rim-sill folds and the light reflexes are well demonstrated.

The best and simplest lightning system for this purpose is the direct and the indirect **ring flash systems**.

9.3.3.1 Direct Ring Flash

The suitable ring flash must have a **wide-circled ring** so that **the diameter of the ring flash must be as wide or wider than the human face**.

The direct light of the ring flash is **uneven**, being brighter in front of the area of the ring light and less bright in front of the central area. This results in a **ring area of overexposure in the peripheral parts of the face** and an area of underexposure in the center of the face.

To correct this problem the light of the ring flash must be defused by a **light diffuser**. This is usually provided with the ring flash. The diffuser is a plastic sheet that has a **frosted** or **prominent crisscross grating surface**.

Two systems of direct ring flashes are used:

Metz Ring Flash

The Mecablitz 15Ms—1 digital Ring Macro Flash is the simplest ring flash that has a **wide ring** and is as wide as the normal human face (17.5 cm in diameter). It has **two small lights** at the sides of the ring. The bounce diffuser is in the form of a crisscross grated plastic cover over the two light sources. The light from this unit is almost shadowless (Figs. 9.3 and 9.4).

The camera's own flash system is **switched on** to allow the impulses through, but the **camera's flash** itself is **covered with a plastic infrared clamp** (provided with the Metz flash) to prevent its light from causing shadows. No further adjustments are required for the flash.

Omicron System

Quantum Omicron OM3 TTL Flash is another direct ring flash, which has a ring that **is as wide as the normal human face** (Fig. 9.4). There is a **ring tube** of **light** that is covered by a **frosted plastic sheet** all around. The Omicron flash system is **stronger** than the Metz system and has an evenly distributed light (Fig. 9.5).

9.3.3.2 Combined Direct and Indirect Ring Flash

The Alien Bees System ABR 800

This is a combined, direct and indirect ring flash system. It has a higher light output than the two previous flash units (Fig. 9.6).

It is made of a central tube of light that is mostly reflected backward and sideways on a wide metal dish. Some of the light directly goes forward, after being diffused by a frosted plastic cover diffuser. The size of the dish is the same or slightly larger than the human face.

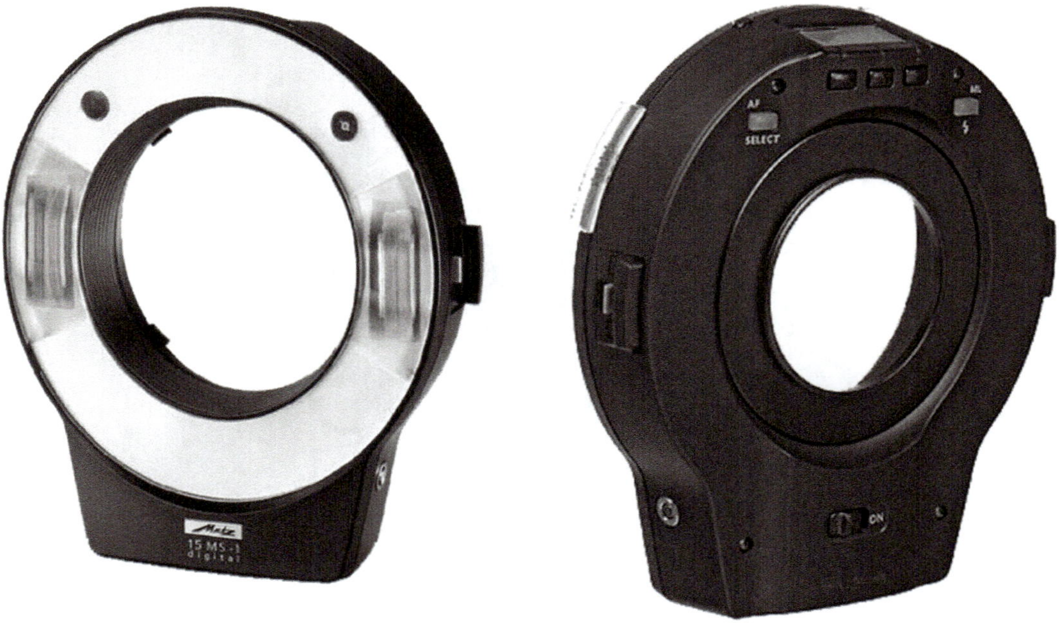

Fig. 9.3 Mitz Mecablitz 15Ms ring flash

Fig. 9.4 Camera's flash is covered with a plastic infrared clamp

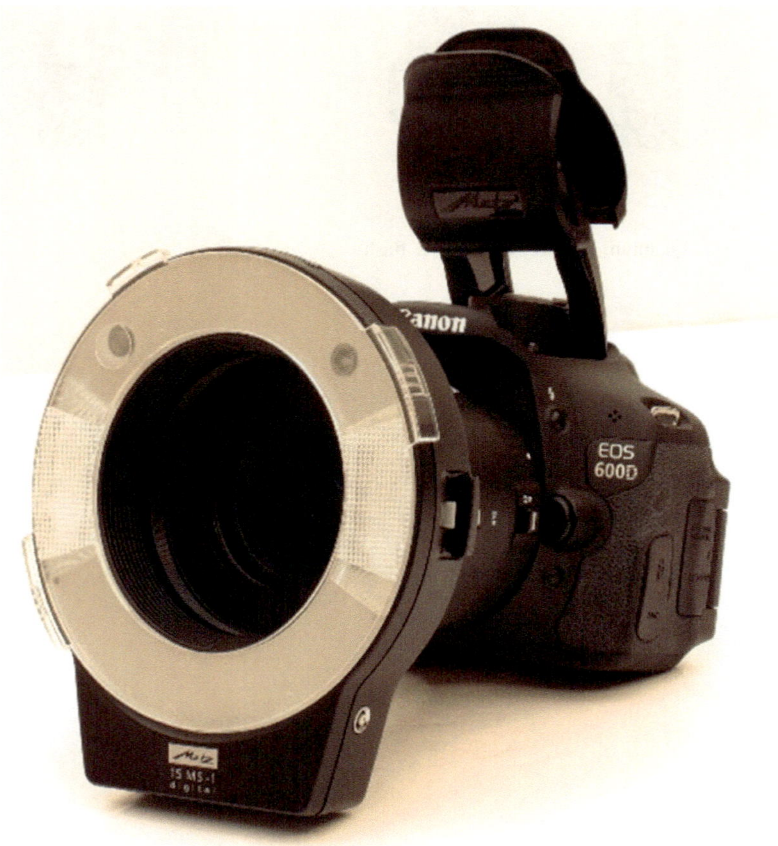

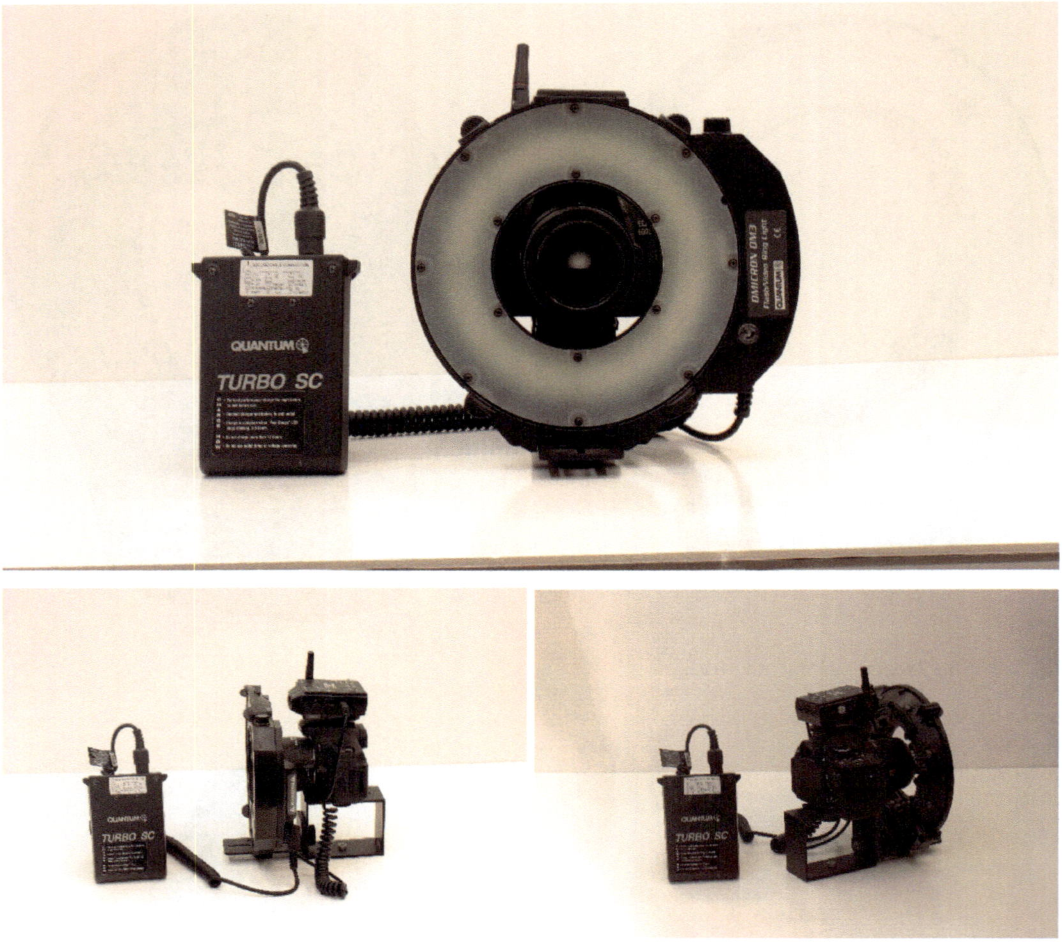

Fig. 9.5 Quantum Omicron OM3 TTL flash

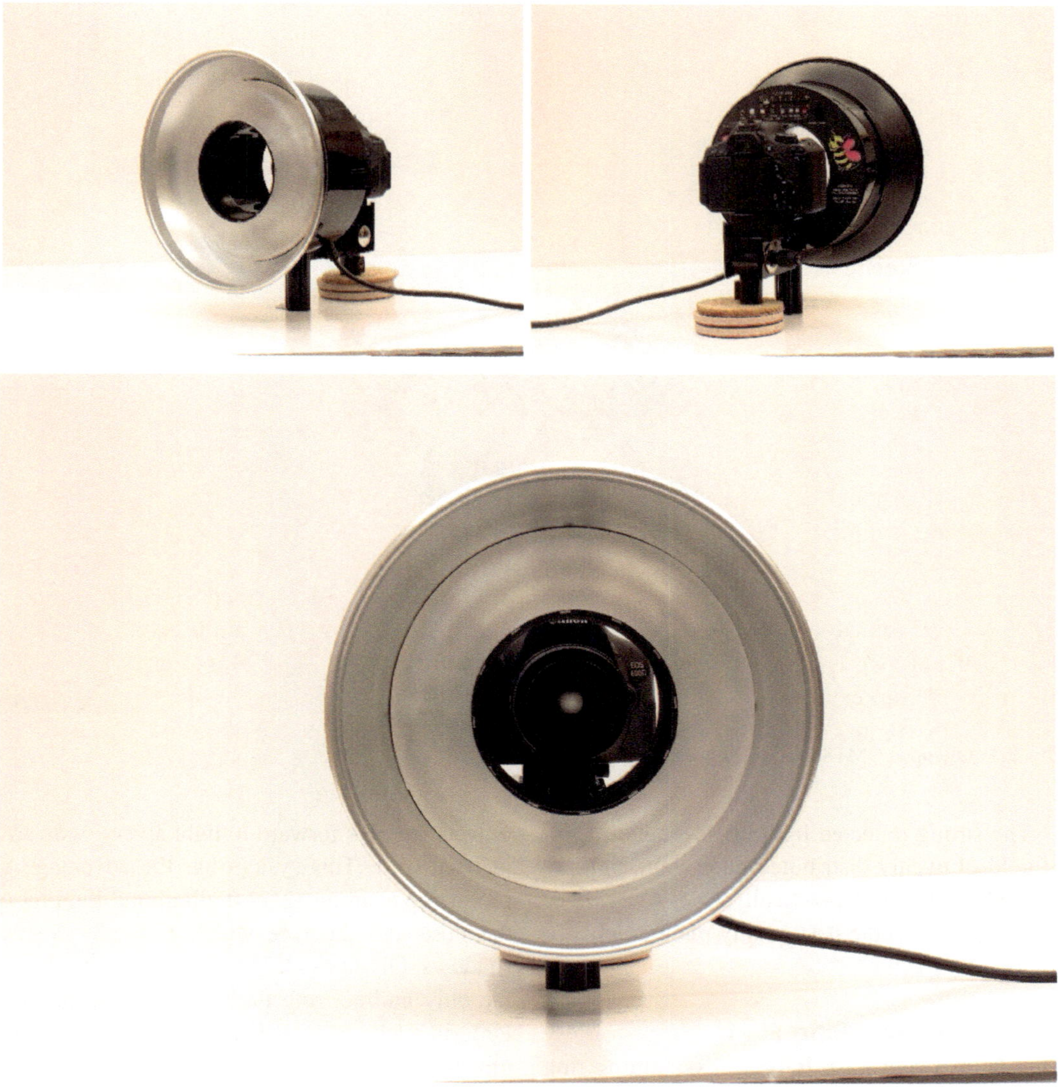

Fig. 9.6 Alien Bees system ABR 800

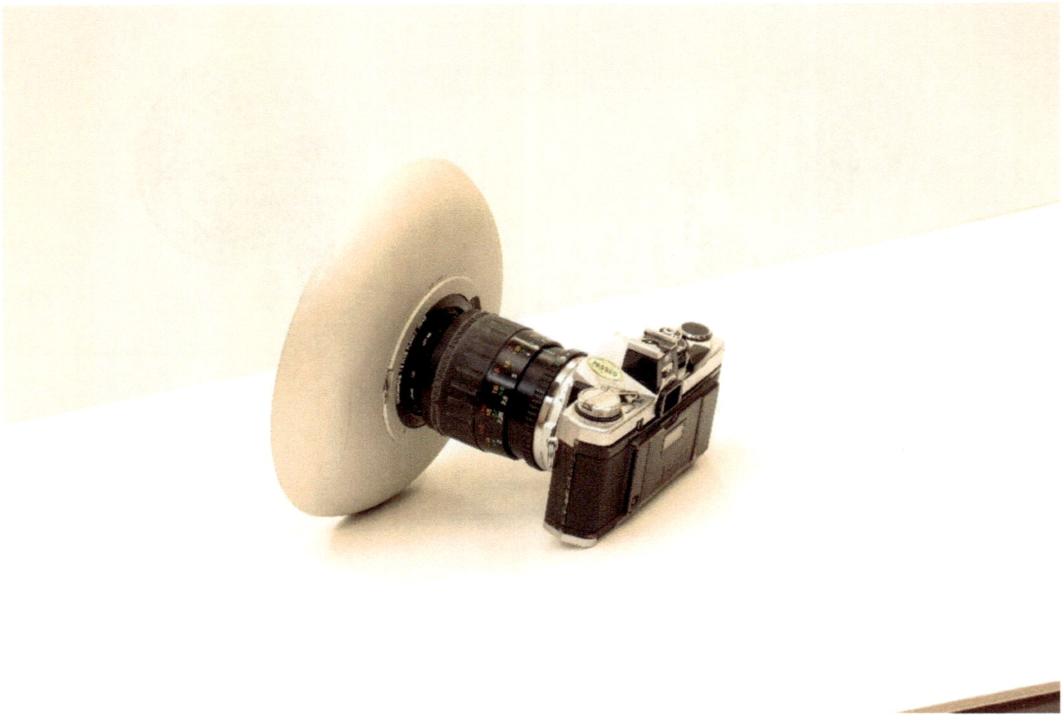

Fig. 9.7 Olympus OMT8 Macro Ring flash

The strong reflected light gives a better depth of field of evenly distributed pure white light.

Technically and practically, the Alien Bees system produces the best quality photographs for rhinoplasty.

9.3.3.3 Indirect Ring Flash

The indirect ring flash is basically a strong ring flash directed backward against a metal dish that reflects the rays forward to light a very wide area in front of it. This system has the advantage of producing a strong yet soft all-around lighting of the nose and the face which is totally free of shadows. Olympus OMT8 Macro Ring flash was the only indirect ring flash system and the best. Unfortunately, it was discontinued by the manufacturer (Fig. 9.7).

Standardization of Rhinoplasty Photography

10

Abstract

Standardization is **the ability** to **reproduce near to identical photographs of the nose and face** taken at different times **for** better **comparison, study, diagnosis** and **follow-up**.

Keywords

Standardization of Rhinoplsty photography · The set up for Rhinoplasty photography · Preparing the patient for photography

10.1 Importance of Standardization

Standardization is **the ability** to **reproduce near to identical photographs of the nose and face** taken at different times **for** better **comparison, study, diagnosis** and **follow-up**.

Standardization includes using the exact clinical **photographic views**, **lighting** and **background**. Care must be taken to ensure that the only **changes** among the clinical photographs taken over time **are in the patient** (Naylar J. R. clinical photography, A guide for clinician J). It is not acceptable to use **photographic digital editing** to enhance the appearance of clinical outcomes (Naylar J. R.).

10.2 Achieving Standardization

To achieve standardization of Rhinoplasty photography, the following is undertaken:

(1) The setup, i.e., place where photographs are taken.
(2) Preparing the patient.
(3) Positioning the camera.

In order to facilitate standardization, repeatability and a speedy flow of photography, **the author has developed a simple protocol**.

10.2.1 The Setup

Organizing the place for photography is made simple so that it can be arranged in an ordinary room in any surgical practice.

The setup includes the **room** and the **chairs** for the patient and the photographer.

10.2.1.1 The Place for Photography

It is amazing how small the place that is needed for photography could be. Any small corner in a room that measures 1.5 x 2 meters is all that is needed. **One sidewall** of the corner must have a **white**, **light gray or magnolia color** to be used

M. H. A. Shafy, *Innovations in Rhinoplasty*,
https://doi.org/10.1007/978-3-030-94573-2_10

as a background. An alternative background is to have a **70 x 100 cm matt white sheet** of thick paper, thin cardboard or artist board which is placed at **85 cm above the floor**.

Any normal room light which is not too strong is acceptable for general room lighting.

Avoid any strong colored light, e.g., fluorescent or LED.

Modern electronic Flashes are powerful enough to negate the effects of room lighting (Naylar J. R.).

10.2.1.2 The Floor Marking Lines

To help standardization of photography, carefully laid out floor lines are strongly recommended. Without these lines, it will be extremely difficult to standardize the positions of the patient and the photographer.

A **150 cm** long **transverse line** is drawn on the floor, exactly **45 cm away from the wall**. This distance is just enough to have the effect of a white or gray background (Fig. 10.1).

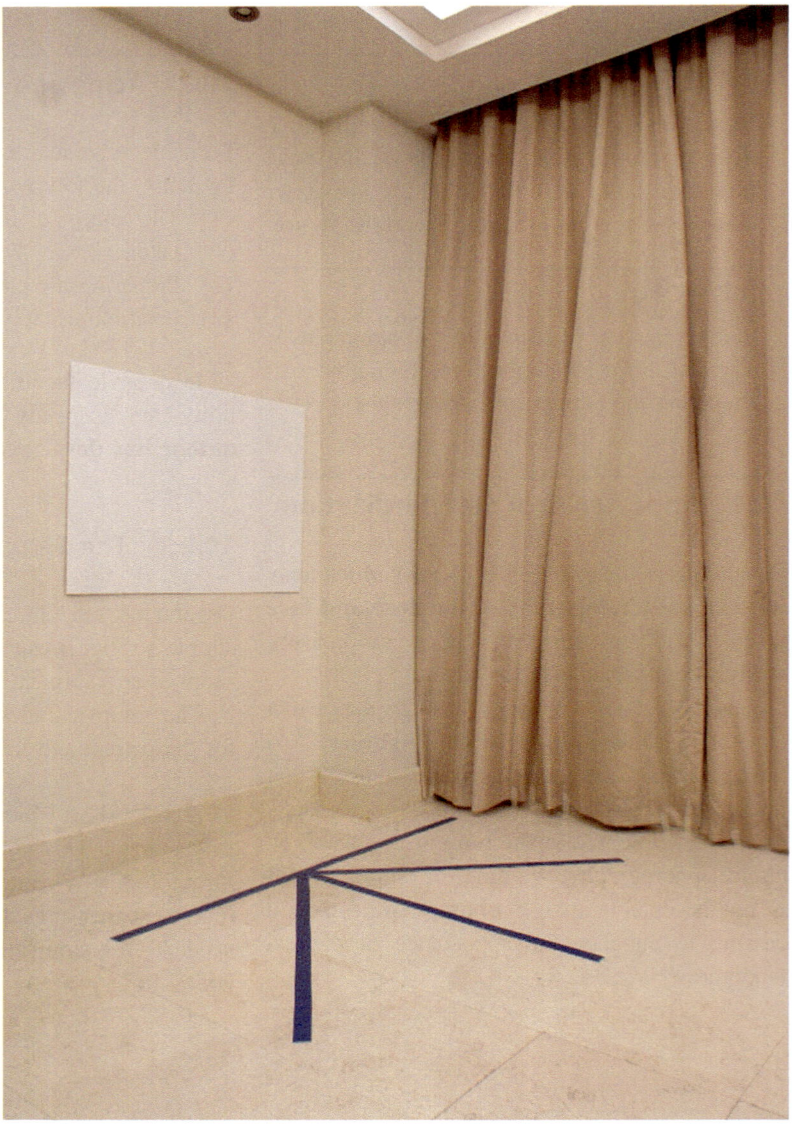

Fig. 10.1 Markings on the floor and a white backboard in an area of 1.5 × 2 m

The chair is placed exactly at the midpoint of the transverse line. From this point, **three 100 cm** long lines are drawn. One **anterior line** at exactly **90 degrees** and **two oblique lines** at **45 degrees** from the transverse line. These lines take the shape of the lower half of the Union Jack, the national flag of the United Kingdom.

Location of the Patient's Chair

The patient's chair is placed over **the point** of meeting of the transverse line with the oblique and anterior lines (Fig. 10.2).

In each view, the patient sits so that his chest and face are in the same direction as the line. Each foot is placed on one side of the floor line, i.e., his feet are straddling the line.

Location of the Photographer's Chair

No fixed point is made for the photographer's chair. He sits in front of the patient on **the anterior line**. The **camera lens must be located directly above the anterior line** at all times. The photographer's chair moves backwards and

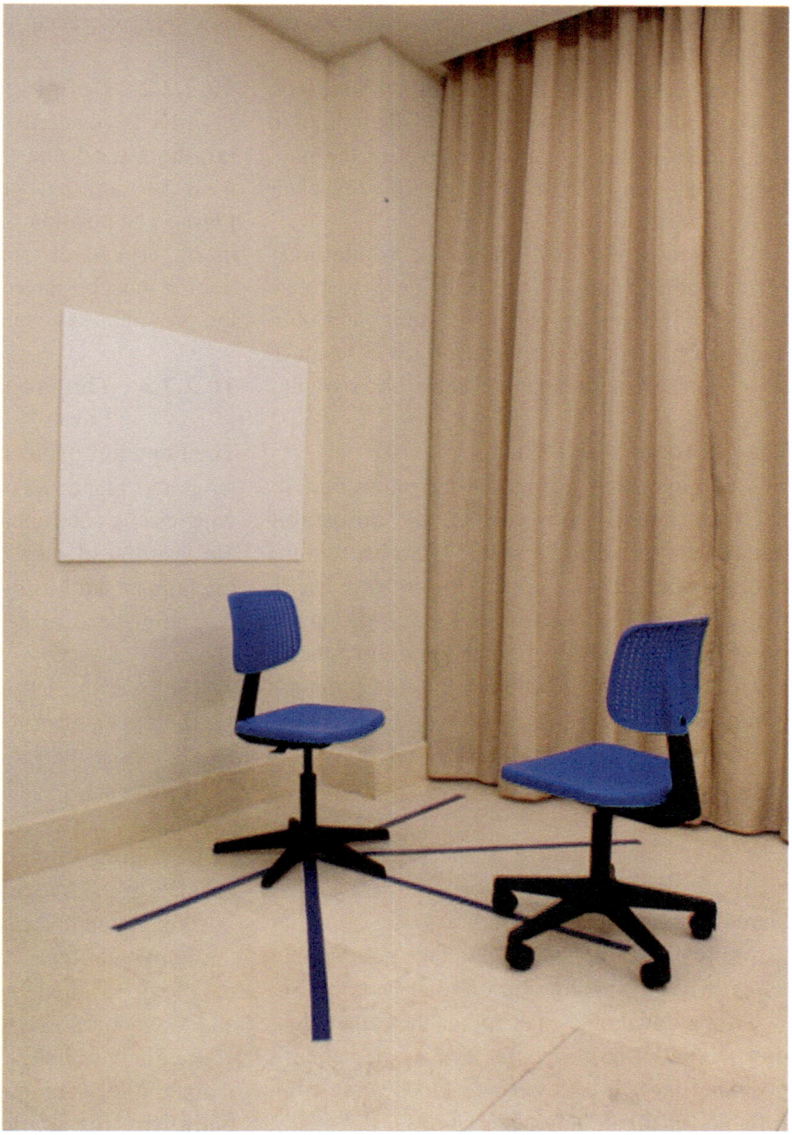

Fig. 10.2 Patient and Photographer's chairs

forwards along **the anterior line** to maintain the focus of the image (Fig. 10.2).

In summary, the location of the patient's chair must be **fixed at one spot in all views** during the whole session of photography. The **photographer's chair** moves along the **anterior line**.

10.2.1.3 The Type of Chairs

The Patient's Chair

The patient's chair must be comfortable, **rotating** with **no wheels** and **of adjustable heights** to accommodate tall and short individuals. The height range 38–48 cm from the floor is reasonable and readily available from the markets.

The **back of the chair** must be **upright** and at a **lower level than the patient's shoulders**. A small cushion is provided for small children to bring them higher to the same level of the photographer's lens and to avoid seeing the chair back.

Rotation of the chair allows the **whole body** of the patient, and not the head only, to rotate around at the same spot for the lateral and oblique views. Rotating the head only will result in poor standardization and inaccurate photographs.

The Photographer's Chair

The photographer's chair must be comfortable, **rotating**, **mobile on wheels**, of **adjustable height** and the back is upright. The wheels in the photographer's chair are only for the easy use of the chair rather than moving it while taking the photographs. The rule is that the **photographer's chair** is in a **fixed position,** while the **patient's chair rotates**.

The photographer must ensure that the camera remains at the same horizontal level as the patient's nose.

Mobility and rotation of the photographer's chair are mainly to move backwards and forwards in the various views.

Many photographers used to take photographs while they are standing up on their feet.

Sitting down on a chair brings the camera lens down to the same horizontal level as the patient's nose and face. It is easier and much more comfortable for the photographer.

10.2.2 Preparing the Patient

The patient's face must not be covered with long hair, head cover, high collars, scarfs or long polo necks. Facial makeup is better avoided or reduced to a minimum. Avoid eyeglasses, and distracting accessories, e.g., earrings, nose beads and jewelry.

10.2.2.1 Positioning the Patient's Head

To ensure standardization, the patient's head must be positioned precisely in the horizontal plane.

It is better for the two ears to be clearly seen, if possible, or at least identified so they can be used as a reference for the horizontal level.

10.2.2.2 Defining the Horizontal Level

In order to standardize photographs of the **frontal**, the **lateral** and the **oblique views**, the face must be adjusted properly in the **horizontal plane**. The position of the head must not vary by tilting backwards, forwards or sideways. Positioning must be carefully applied to all patients in the pre- and post-operative photographs.

10.2.2.3 The Frankfort Plane and Reid's Line

The Frankfort plane, also known as the auriculotemporal plane was established at the world congress on anthropology in Frankfort in 1884 as the anatomical most nearly parallel position of the human skull to the surface of the earth.

The plane is made between **three points:**

- The inferior margin of the left orbit.
- The upper margin of the left external canal.
- The upper margin of the right external canal of the ear (Fig. 10.3).

Benefitting from this fact, the Radiologists decided in the **World Federation of Radiology** in 1962 to define **Reid's Base Line** as a guide for the horizontal level of the skull in conventional radiology, Computerized Tomography (CT Scan) and Magnetic Resonance Imaging (MRI) studies.

Reid's base line is defined as the **line drawn from the inferior margin of the orbit (orbital point) to the center of the orifice of the**

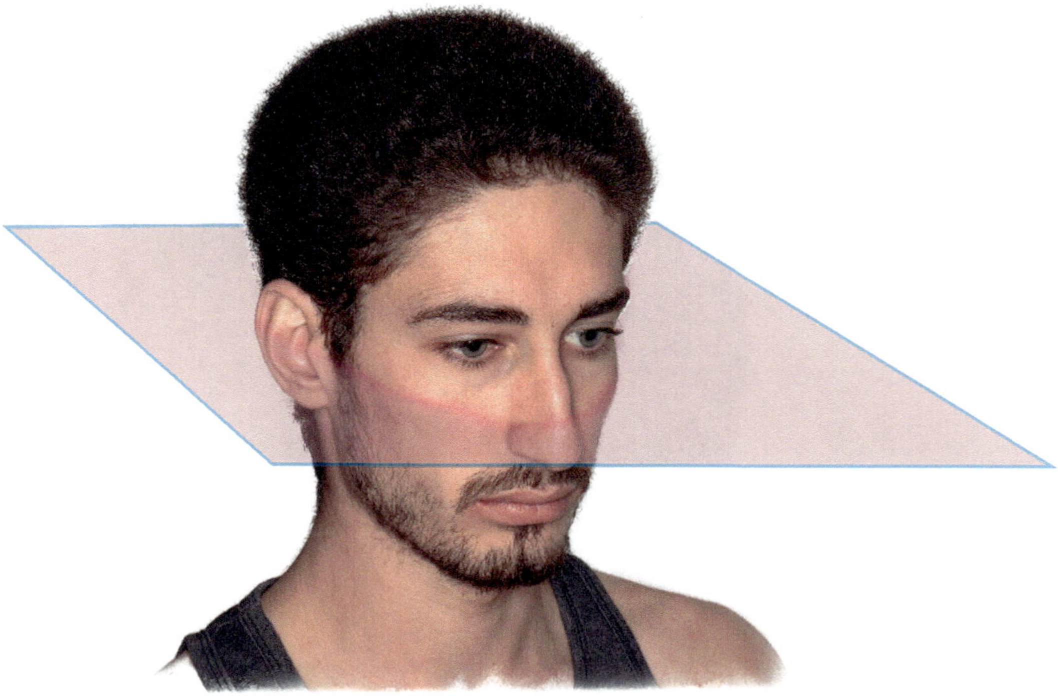

Fig. 10.3 Frankfort horizontal plane

external auditory meatus (auricular point) and extending backwards to the center of the occipital bone (Fig. 10.4). Radiology films are two dimensional, hence the defining method is a line rather than a plane.

Photographs are **two dimensional** outcomes of the **three-dimensional nose and face**. It is therefore important to consider the three-dimensional position of the head while taking the photograph. **Frankfort plane** therefore is more helpful and accurate to consider in patients while taking their **frontal, oblique and lateral views**.

Clinically ensuring the horizontal level of the head while taking photograph is as important as positioning the head in radiology. This is achieved by

- The first step is to draw an imaginary line between **the tragus** and **the infraorbital margin**. This ensures that **the head is not tilted backwards or forwards** away from the horizontal level.
- The second step is to make sure that the **two external auditory canals** are at the same horizontal level, so that **the head is not tilted sideways**.

10.2.3 Positioning the Camera

The **level**, **distance** and **the back orientation** (vertical/horizontal) of the camera's body in relation to the patient's nose and face must be standardized and fixed in all patients in the pre- and post-operative views.

10.2.3.1 The Horizontal Level of the Lens

The horizontal level of the lens in relation to the patient's nose and face must be standardized.

When the photographer maintains the camera over the anterior floor line, the camera is positioned in the correct vertical plane.

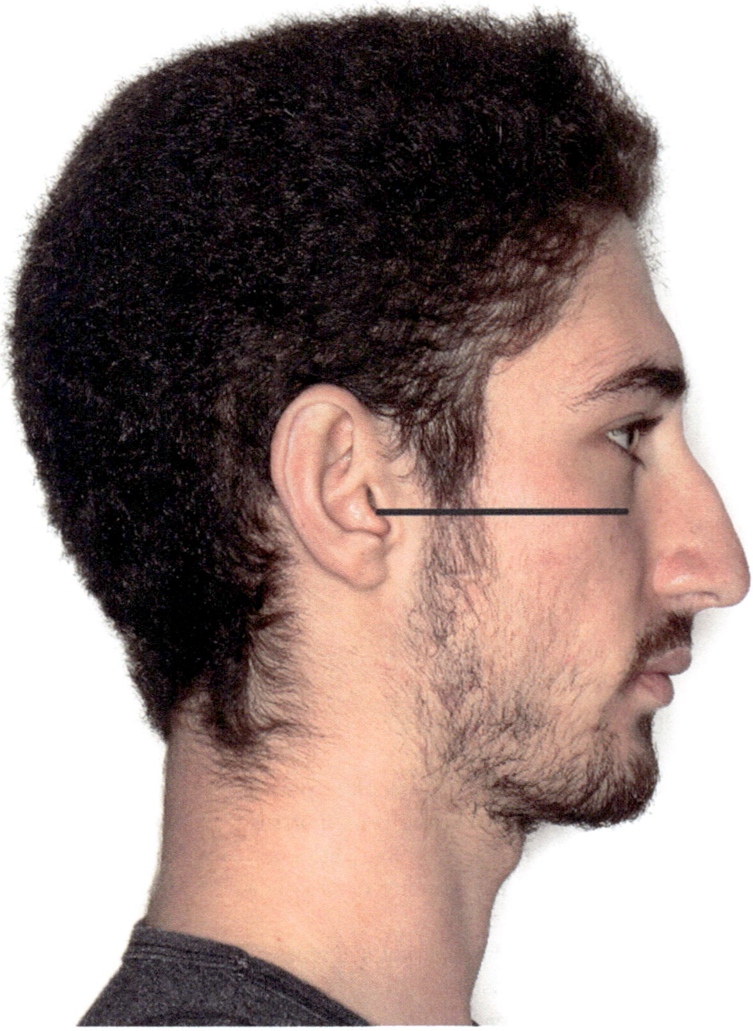

Fig. 10.4 Clinical definition of the Frankfurt Plane: **a** Imaginary line between the tragus and the infraorbital margin. **b** The two external Auditory canals at the same horizontal level

- The lens must be at the same horizontal level of the middle of the nasal dorsum in the following views:
  i. Frontal (Anterior) views
  ii. Lateral views
  iii. Oblique views
  iv. Direct dorsal view
  v. Backward tilting views

- The lens remains at the same horizontal level of the nose in the **basal** and **nasal aperture** views, but focusing is on the **nasal aperture walls**.
- Sometimes, the patient is unable to fully extend the neck backwards. In these cases, the photographer has to come down to be at the same horizontal level with the nasal openings.
- The **overhead views:** in these views, the Patient's chair is rotated to the **transverse line** and the photographer stands behind the patient with his lens **behind** and **above** the patient's head. The patient slides down on the chair seat and is asked to gradually extend the head backwards **till the nasofrontal angle is just seen**.

10.2.3.2 The Distance of the Lens

The **distance** of the lens from the nose must be fixed in order to fix the magnification of the images.

Two distances are used for the different views. The lens is strictly fixed at these two distances in every patient. **No adjustment of the lens focus** to obtain a clearer picture. The **photographer rather moves forwards or backwards**.

(1) The Distance of **60 cm** is used for the standard views:
   i. frontal views.
   ii. lateral views.
   iii. oblique views.
(2) The distance of **40 cm** is used for the specialized views:
   i. Basal views.
   ii. Aperture views.
   iii. Direct dorsal views.
   iv. Backward tilting views.
   v. Overhead views.
   vi. The close-up middle third of the standard views.

10.2.3.3 Orientation of the Camera Back

Orientation of the Camera back is important while taking photographs of the face.

The **long axis of the camera back** is considered differently in the different views.

- A **vertical or portrait orientation,** i.e., the long axis of the camera back is held **vertically**. This is recommended in the full face views and their close-ups, i.e., the **frontal, oblique** and **lateral views**.
  The **natural long axis of the face is vertical**. It is equally natural to take its photograph parallel to its long axis. This maximizes the use of pixels photographically.
- A **horizontal** or **landscape orientation,** i.e., the long axis of the camera back is held **horizontally.** This is recommended in all of the specialized views, i.e., **Basal, Nasal Aperture, Direct Dorsal, Backward Tilting and Overhead views.**

These views are mainly **close-up magnified views** in which details are needed. The whole **extent of the face from side to side** has to be included in the frame ensuring the horizontal level of the eyebrows.

10.2.4 Camera Settings for Photography

The camera, lens and flash settings for full face and close-up views are given below for the Author's equipment. The shutter speed is set to 1/125th of a second.

10.2.4.1 Full Face Photographs

The lens: it is set for the distance of 60 cm (Author's equipment)

The lens aperture:

Omicron f/9 – f/13.
Alien Bees f/14 – f/30.

Camera Back Orientation: Vertical, i.e., Portrait.

10.2.4.2 Close-up Photographs

The lens: it is set for the distance of 40 cm (Author's equipment)

The lens aperture:

Omicron f/9 – f/13.
Alien Bees f/29 – f/36.

Camera Back Orientation: the vertical standard middle third of the face and horizontal for the specialized views.

The Significance of the Light Reflexes of the Nose

11

Abstract

The external skin of the nose is generally hairless, glistening and adherent to underlying structures. This is especially true in the lower two-thirds of the nose.

Keywords

The Significance of the Light Reflexes of the Nose

The external skin of the nose is generally hairless, glistening and adherent to underlying structures. This is especially true in the lower two-thirds of the nose.

On taking photographs to of the nose the flashlight is reflected from the **external nasal surfaces** and the **inferior margins** of the nasal apertures. These reflections appear in the photographs as **lines of Light reflex**. the lines of light reflex have **surgical** as well as **aesthetic** significances.

The light reflexes of the **nasal margins** are of **surgical** significances.

While light reflexes of the external **nasal surfaces** are of **aesthetic** significances.

11.1 The Marginal Light Reflexes

Light reflex of the margins of nasal apertures is a useful guide for **nasal base surgery**. **Three lines** of light reflexes are seen on taking photographs of the nasal apertures. The light lines are seen reflected from the margin of three firm structures, i.e., the **inferior alar margins**, **nasal sill bands** and the **lateral columellar margins**. These firm structures are covered with thin, glistening and hairless skin that reflects the flashlight to produce the lines of light reflex.

The light reflex lines are interrupted by soft skin areas that separate the three firm structures, i.e., the **rim-sill folds**, **flat triangle**s and the **posterior soft fold of columella**.

Not all the light reflexes appear in one photographic view. The flashlight must directly aim at the specific margin in order to elicit the reflex. Each margin is seen in a different view.

11.1.1 Photographic Views of the Marginal Reflexes

i. The **Alar Margin Light Reflex** is best seen at the **nasal aperture views**.
   Margins of the flat triangle may also be seen in these view photographs (Figs. 11.1 and 11.2).
ii. The **Nasal Sill Light Reflex** is best seen in the **oblique views**. Margins of the **flat triangle** may also be seen in these view photographs (Fig. 11.3).
iii. The **lateral crural prominence light reflex** is best seen in the **lateral views** (Fig. 11.4).

M. H. A. Shafy, *Innovations in Rhinoplasty*,
https://doi.org/10.1007/978-3-030-94573-2_11

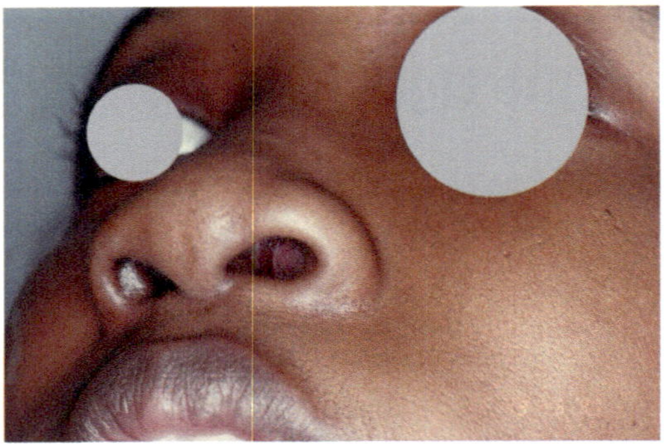

Fig. 11.1 Notice the light reflex at the inferior alar margin. Light reflex is absent from the flat triangle and the rim-sill fold

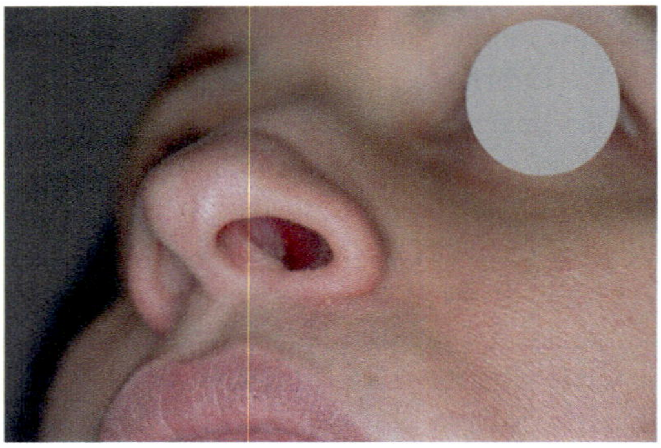

Fig. 11.2 Notice the light reflex at the inferior alar margin and the margins of the left flat triangle. Light reflex is absent from the flat triangle and the rim-sill fold

11.2 The Frontal Surface Light Reflexes

The light reflexes of the frontal external surface of the nose are of great aesthetic significance.

Lines of light reflexes are seen on the nasal dorsum, the nasal tip and margins of the flat triangle. The light reflex in each of these structures is seen in a different photographic view.

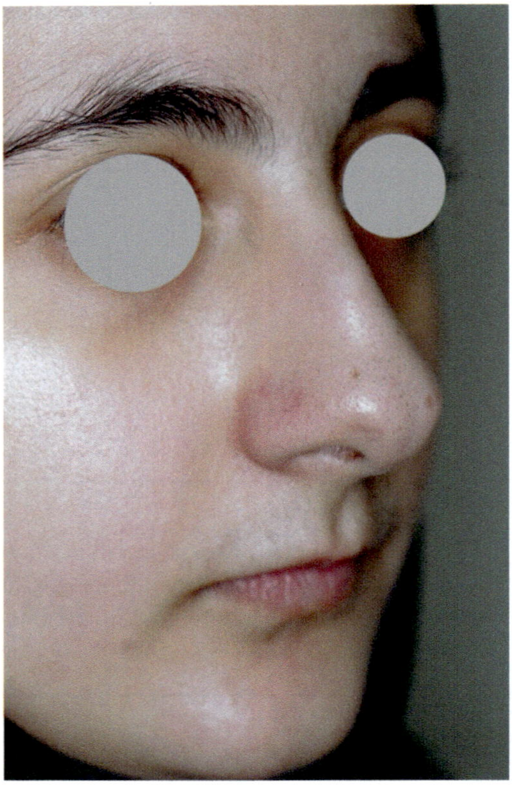

Fig. 11.3 Right oblique view demonstrating the nasal sill light reflex

11.2.1 Photographic Views of the Frontal Surface Light Reflexes

11.2.1.1 Nasal Dorsal Light Reflex

The **Nasal Dorsal light reflex** is best seen in the **direct dorsal view** as the flashlight is directly aimed at the nasal dorsum.

The light reflex is seen as a continuous uninterrupted line from the nasion to the nasal tip. This is especially true in smooth-skinned narrowly rounded dorsum (Fig. 11.5).

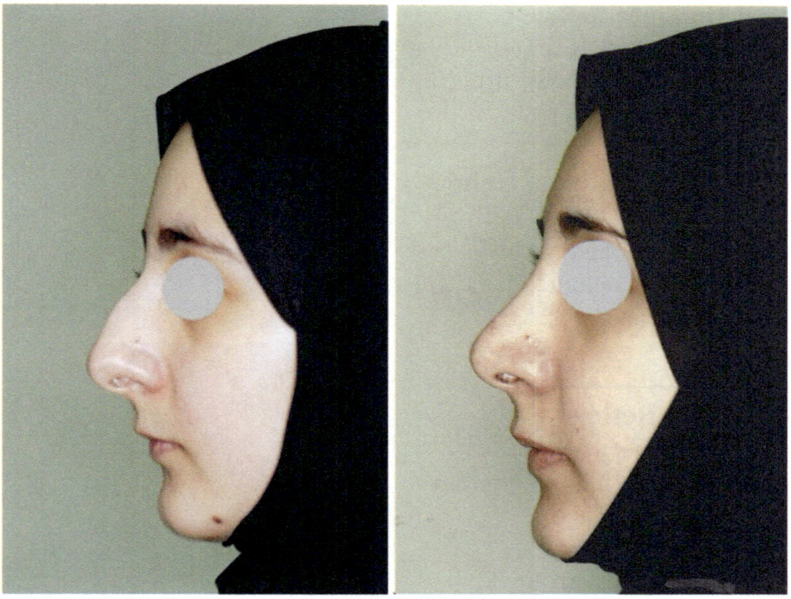

Fig. 11.4 The lateral view demonstrating the lateral crural prominence light reflex pre- and post-operatively

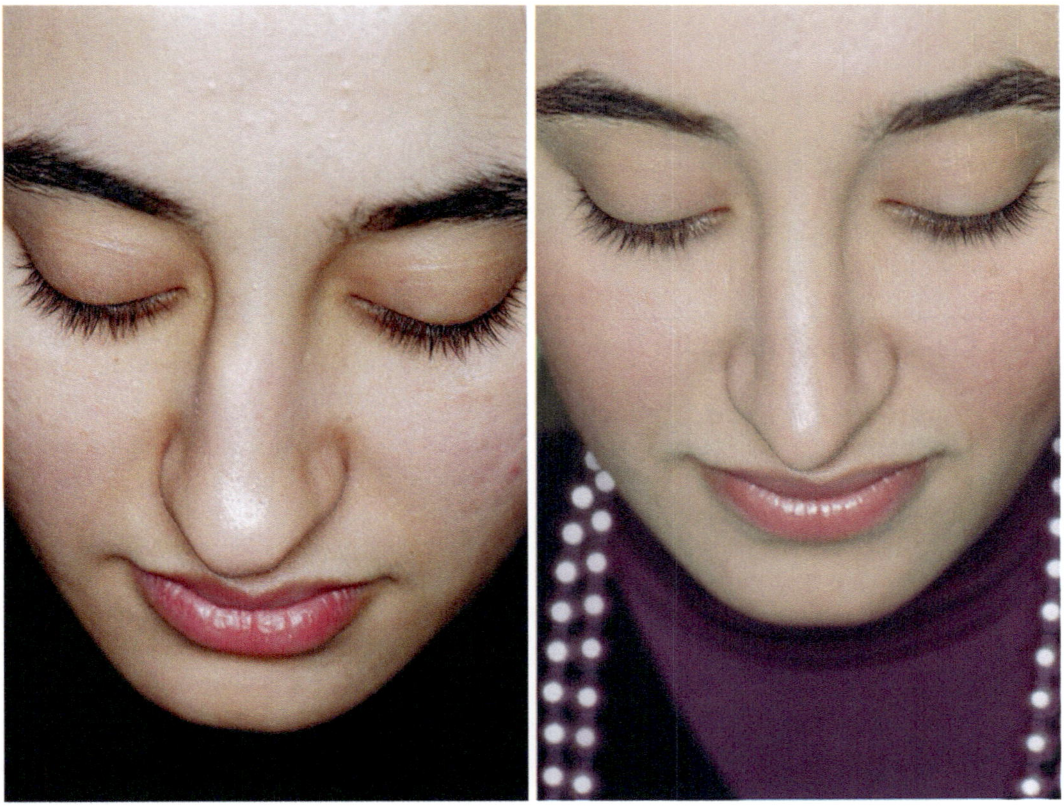

Fig. 11.5 Direct dorsal view demonstrating the nasal dorsal light reflex. The reflex is interrupted pre-operatively due to an irregular dorsum and a wide nasal tip. Post-operatively, the light reflex is continuous from the nasion to the nasal tip

11.2.1.2 Nasal Tip Light Reflex

The **Nasal Tip light reflex** is best seen in the **frontal** and **backward tilting views**. Bifid tip appears as two spots of light reflexes.

11.2.1.3 Flat Triangle Marginal Light Reflex

The **Flat triangle Marginal light reflex** is best seen in **nasal aperture** and **oblique views**. The reflex is clearer in thin-skinned noses.

11.3 Absent Light Reflex

No light is reflected from the following surfaces.

11.3.1 The Weak Areas and Soft Folds

Of the nose, e.g., the flat triangles, the rim-sill folds and the posterior columellar soft folds.

11.3.2 Anatomically Distorted Areas

- Caudally dislocated septum distorts the location of the nasal sill and medial crurae.
- Irregular, crooked, broad or broken nasal dorsum defuses the light and disturbs the light reflex.

11.4 Clinical Use of the Light Reflex

11.4.1 Photographic Pre-operative Assessment

A light reflex is an excellent tool in pre-operative assessment of the different parts of the **nasal dorsum** and **alar base**. Together with the rim-sill test, they demonstrate the exact locations of the alar rims, the nasal sills and the rim-sill folds.

11.4.2 During Surgery

The lines of light reflexes are elicited by shining the strong headlight directly on the nasal margins. They are of great help during surgical alignment of the aperture margins in alar base surgery.

Using the light reflex together with the rim-sill test, the margins of the nasal sill and the alar rim are well recognized. This helps in accurately placing the incision lines and in aligning the two margins in a natural continuity with each other in the closing up stitches (Fig. 11.6).

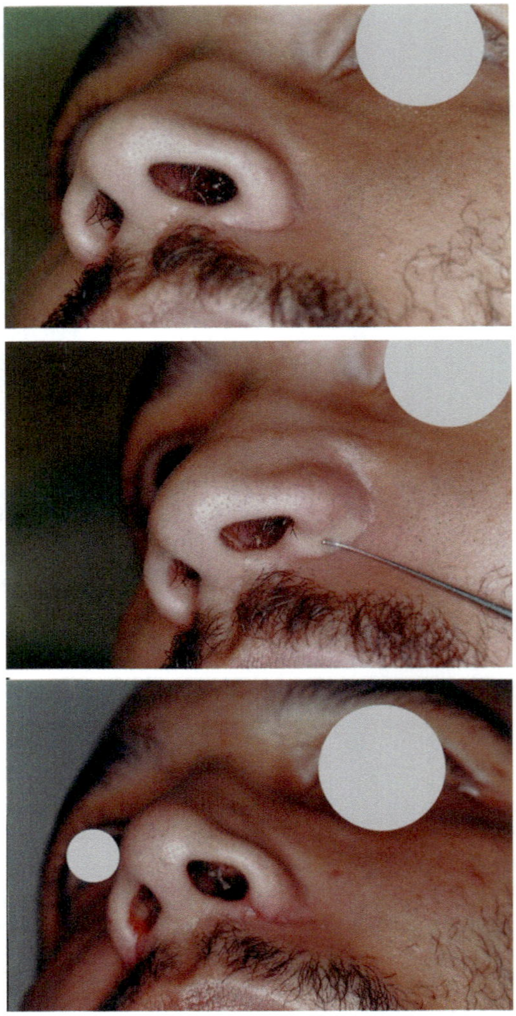

Fig. 11.6 Left alar margin light reflex is absent from the left rim-sill fold which is accurately excised

12 The Rim-Sill Test

Abstract

The rim-sill fold is the surgical target in alar base surgery. It is important to identify its boundaries pre-operatively as well as intraoperatively.

Keywords

The rim-sill test

The rim-sill fold is the surgical target in alar base surgery. It is important to identify its boundaries pre-operatively as well as intraoperatively.

12.1 Defining the Rim-Sill Test

The rim-sill test is a clinical test which demonstrates the anatomical location of the **lateral end of the nasal sill, the posterior end of the alar rim** and their communicating **rim-sill soft skin fold**. The test was performed in **one** or **two** methods in order to demonstrate the **posterior** and the **inferior segments** of the rim-sill folds.

12.2 How to Perform the Rim-Sill Test

While the patient is sitting on the examination chair, his head is gradually tilted backwards so that both nasal apertures are facing the examining physician (Fig. 12.1).

Using a long thin right-angled blunt probe, the posterior end of the **alar rim** is gradually and gently pushed medially. **Two creases** are clearly formed. The **medial skin crease** represents the lateral end of the **nasal sill**, while the **lateral skin crease** represents the posterior end of the **alar rim**. The area between the two creases is the inferior segment off the **rim-sill fold of the skin** (Fig. 12.2).

This method mainly demonstrates the **inferior segment** of the rim-sill fold in a thin or relatively normal nasal skin thickness.

In some individuals, these three anatomical structures are so clearly distinct from each other without the need for a test. This is especially true in a long nasal aperture where there is a sharp change of direction from the alar rim to the nasal sill, i.e., a sharp turn from an antero-posterior to a transverse direction. Nevertheless, this test is useful in cases where the three structures are partly or completely merged into each other in one continuous circular margin.

M. H. A. Shafy, *Innovations in Rhinoplasty*,
https://doi.org/10.1007/978-3-030-94573-2_12

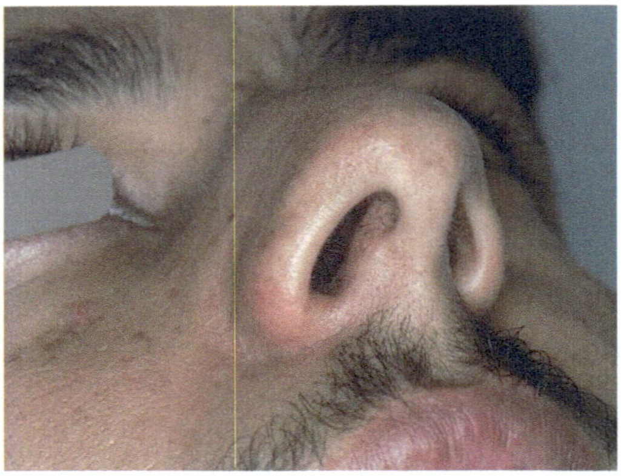

Fig. 12.1 Pre-operative appearance of right nasal aperture. Note the light reflects off the right inferior alar margin, nasal sill, and margins of the flat triangle. It is absent from the rim sill fold area

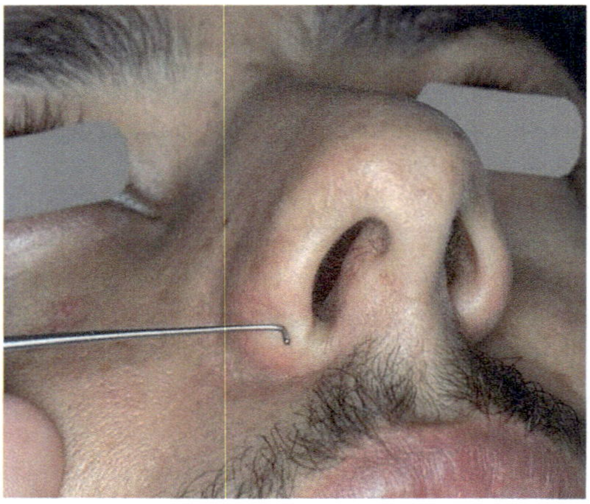

Fig. 12.2 Rim-Sill test demonstrating the inferior segment of the right Rim-Sill fold

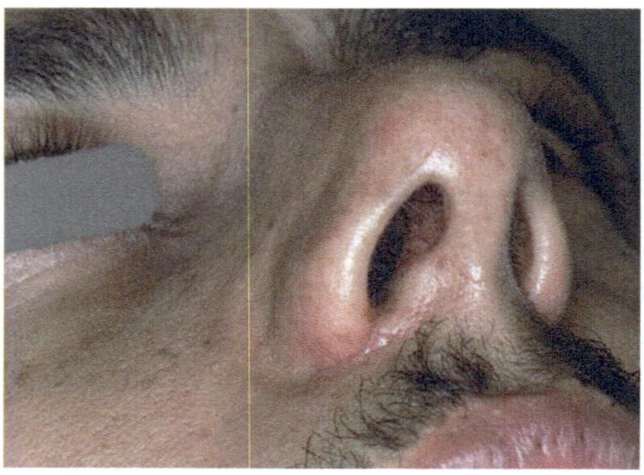

Fig. 12.3 Post-operative appearance of right nasal aperture after excision of the inferior segment of the Rim-Sill fold

12.3 The Rim-Sill Test in Thick Skin

The rim-sill skin fold is sometimes so thick and heavy that it may not bend to make the two creases. In these cases, the probe is placed at the posterior margin of the alar rim, and pushed interiorly instead of direct medially. The **firm** ends of the alar rim and nasal sill appear as **two prominences** at both sides of the **soft** rim-sill fold. The rim-sill fold may look blanched as blood is squeezed out (Fig. 12.4).

This method mainly demonstrates the **posterior segment** of the rim-sill fold (Figs. 12.5 and 12.6).

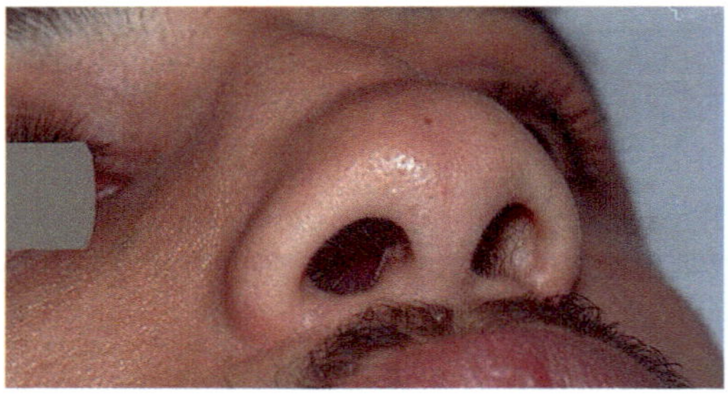

Fig. 12.4 Pre-operative appearance of right thick-skinned nasal aperture

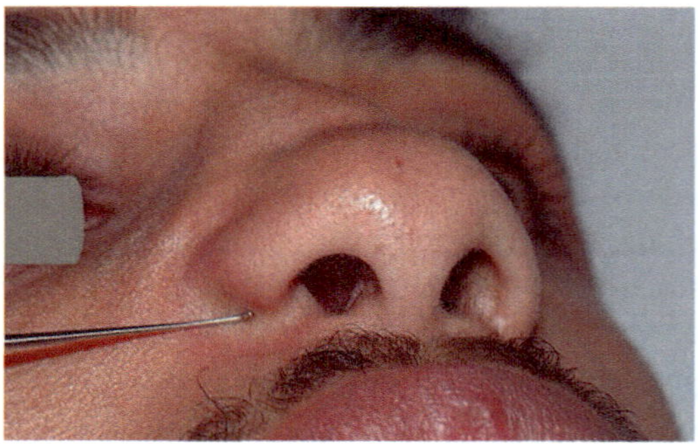

Fig. 12.5 Rim-Sill test in a thick-skinned nose demonstrating the posterior and inferior segments of the Rim-Sill fold. Notice the blanched color of the rim-sill fold

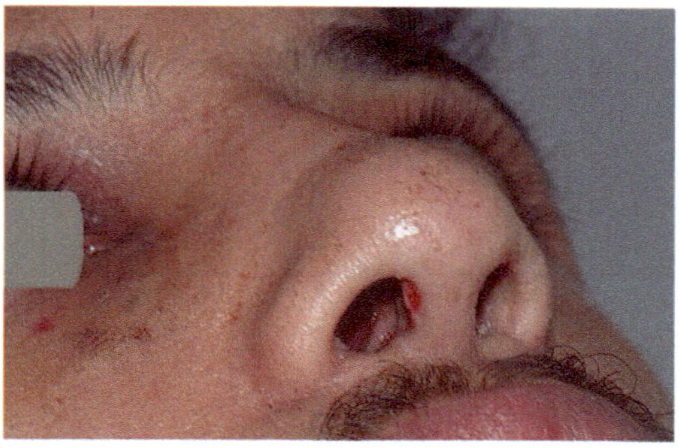

Fig. 12.6 Seven days post-operative appearance of right nasal aperture after excision of the posterior and inferior segments of the Rim-Sill fold

12.4 The Rim-Sill Test in Extremely Thick Skin

A nose may have extremely thick and heavy skin so that no creases could be created at the two ends of the rim-sill fold. In these cases, the probe is pushed just above the posterior alar groove until the **firm** body of the **posterior alar margin** is felt which is distinctly different from the **soft tissue** of the **rim-sill fold** (Fig. 12.7).

A mark is made at this point intraoperatively to delineate the alar side. Similarly, on the floor of the nose, the lateral end of the nasal sill band can easily be palpated.

12.5 Important Points in Performing the Rim-Sill Test

(1) The use of an **appropriate tool,** i.e., a long thin **right-angled** blunt probe.
(2) The **position of the probe** should be at the level of **the firm posterior end of the alar rim** and slightly above the alar margin.
(3) **The pushing force** of the probe should be **gentle** and **adequate** to create the two creases in their anatomical position. Excess force creates creases in the wrong place while inadequate pressure may not be sufficient to create the folds of skin.
(4) **The direction of push**: The direction of the alar rim in relation to the nasal sill may be **variable**, therefore the direction of push of the alar rim may accordingly be variable.
(5) The test can be **repeated** many times until the two creases become as clear as possible. This is especially useful **during surgery** to decide the places of incisions.

12.6 The Clinical Use of the Rim-Sill Test

Pre-operative photographic documentation of the rim-sill folds is of great help in planning for alar base surgery.

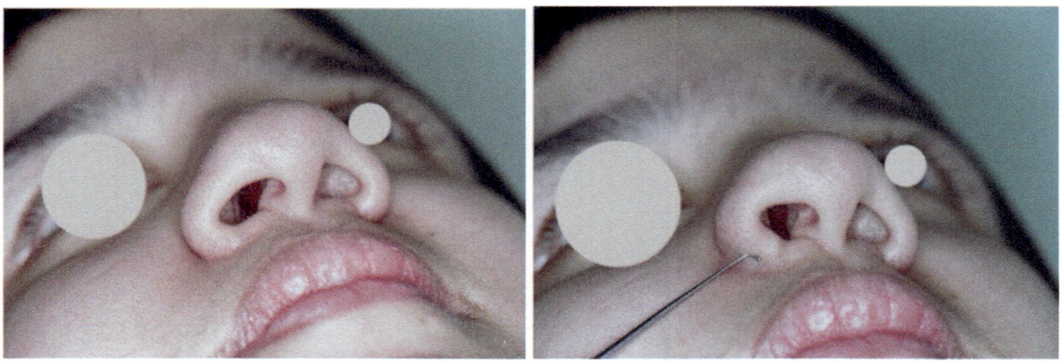

Fig. 12.7 Rim-sill test in extremely thick skin. Note the prominent lateral end of the nasal sill and posterior margin of the alar rim. The skin of the rim-sill fold is blanched

Intraoperative demonstration of the rim-sill fold: Pushing the posterior end of the alar rim in and out repeatedly demonstrates accurately both ends of the alar rim and the nasal sill which in turn helps in locating the sites of the marking, cutting and stitching (see surgery of the Inferior Nasal Wall).

Photographic Views of the Nose 13

Abstract

As a three-dimensional structure, the nose can be seen from a countless number of angles and views. A holistic view of the nose is important. A video recording of the nose and face from all directions seems like an ideal method to cover all of these angles and views. Nevertheless, specific, well-defined angles of photography captured by fixed pictures will give solid documents to every anatomical detail that is targeted by each of these views.

Keywords

Photographic views of the nose · The four standard views · Clinical assessment of the photographs · The four specialized views

13.1 Introduction

As a three-dimensional structure, the nose can be seen from a countless number of angles and views. A holistic view of the nose is important. A video recording of the nose and face from all directions seems like an ideal method to cover all of these angles and views. Nevertheless, specific, well-defined angles of photography captured by fixed pictures will give solid documents to every anatomical detail that is targeted by each of these views.

13.1.1 The Importance of the Standard Views

There are four well-known **standard views** for the nose and face, i.e., the **Frontal**, **Oblique**, **Lateral** and **Basal** views. These are excellent views in showing the **overall appearance of the nose in relation to the face** from the defined different angles.

13.1.2 The Necessity for Specialized Views

Advances in the surgical techniques of Rhinoplasty have led the surgeons into further detailed procedures in the different anatomical areas of the nose. Highlighting the detailed anatomy of each of these areas through more **specialized photographic views** becomes a necessity. New views from different angles are, therefore, introduced.

13.1.3 The Advantages of Photographic Anatomy

Studying the photographs includes a detailed description of the anatomical findings in each view. The correlation between the specific **photographic areas** of the nose and its

M. H. A. Shafy, *Innovations in Rhinoplasty*,
https://doi.org/10.1007/978-3-030-94573-2_13

corresponding **anatomical structures** creates a complete picture of **photographic anatomy** in the surgeon's mind. The normal and the abnormal anatomical areas are recognized, described, hence accurate diagnosis and decisions are greatly helped.

Aesthetic photography of the Nose

In our plan to take photographs of the patient, we must clearly focus on the following two important facts:

(a) The main target is the nose.
(b) The main aim is aesthetics.

Aesthetic views for the nose must aim at taking photographs of the area of interest **at a direct angle** to have a complete view of the true maximal size of this area. Examples of these are:

- The camera directly faces each **nasal aperture** separately in their naturally different angulation in order to see the natural size and appearance of the aperture margins.
- The **nasal dorsum** is best seen by a direct dorsal view where the camera directly faces the nasal dorsum.
- In the oblique views, the camera faces directly the **lateral nasal wall.**

13.2 The Four Standard Views

Standard views are a set of **general overall views of the nose and face**. They are not targeted in certain specific anatomical areas. These views are important for the basic evaluation of **the nose** and **the face** and the aesthetic relations between them.

The most important common factor in the frontal, oblique and lateral views is the **relation between the nose and the rest of the face.**

With the exception of the basal view, all of the other standard views are chosen because they are very much the usual and common views of the photographs taken of the face in our ordinary daily life, e.g., the social occasions of birthdays, weddings, parties, trips and all the official photographs for passport, IDs and graduation.

In some individuals, the nose may be **disproportionately small** or **large** in comparison to the size of the face in general. This may have a negative or detracting effect on the nasal aesthetics. Good examples of these conditions are the Asian and the African noses.

Asians in general have relatively **small noses** as compared to their **large wide cheeks and foreheads**. Anatomic and aesthetic appreciation of the different parts of the nose may be underestimated, unappreciated and even overlooked by the overwhelming sizes and shapes of their surrounding large cheeks, forehead and chin.

Africans are the extreme opposite, as they generally have large flat noses with bulky, wide alae nasi as compared to their relatively small narrow cheeks.

It is for these reasons that as well as the full face photographs, separate **middle third photographs** are taken for the frontal, oblique and lateral views. A **closer look at the nose in isolation from its surrounding facial structures** helps in a better specific appreciation of the nasal aesthetics.

13.2.1 The Frontal Views

The frontal views are also known as the Anterior views. These are **the most important of all views**. They are **the views** used for **identification** in all **official documents,** e.g., passports, schools, colleges and clubs.

People mostly look at themselves in front of a mirror seeing their anterior view. In face-to-face conversations, people look to the front face view of each other. These are the views of the noses and faces as we normally see them in our ordinary daily life.

The nose is seen in its naturally protruding angle of 30–60 degrees forwards. They are the **only views** that show **both sides of the face together** with the **front of the nose**.

It is worth noting that **it is not technically easy to** take a **consistently high**-quality frontal view photograph. The patient's head may be tilted off the horizontal plane, rotated from the vertical axis, or the optical axis of the lens is displaced horizontally or vertically.

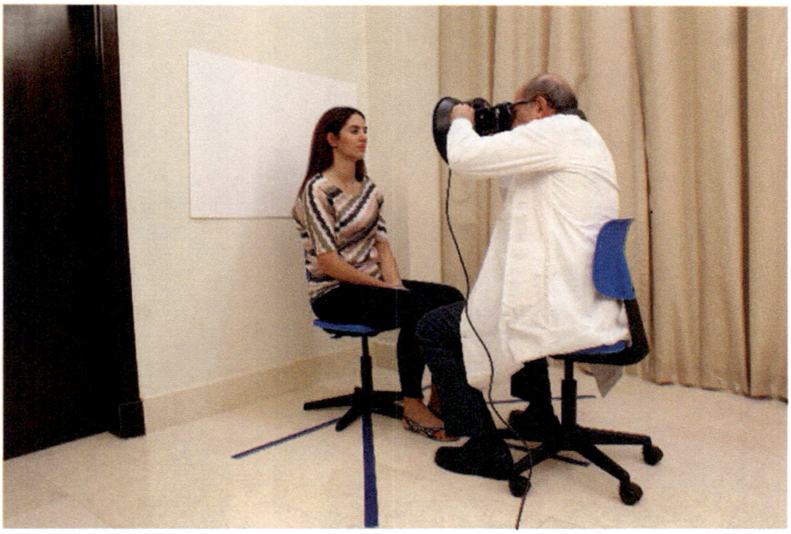

Fig. 13.1 Position of the patient and the photographer in taking the frontal views. Both patient's and photographer's feet straddling the anterior line

13.2.1.1 The Setup

The Patient
The patient sits on his chair with his face and chest looking forward, while his feet are saddling the anterior line (Fig. 13.1).

- The Frankfort horizontal plane is observed.
- A grid in the view finder, if present is helpful.

The photographer
The photographer sits on his chair with his camera setup in front of the patient directly above the anterior line on the floor (Fig. 13.1).

- The camera lens must be at the same level as that of the nose.
- The point of focus is the midpoint of the nasal dorsum.

13.2.1.2 Camera Setting

(a) **Orientation** of the camera back is **vertical**, i.e., **portrait** (Fig. 13.1).
(b) **Lens focus**: at **60 cm** (for the author's equipment).
(c) **Lens Aperture**: adjusted according to the type of flash and skin color of the patient.

Omicron system f/9–f/13.
Alien Bees f/14–f/30.

(d) ISO:

Omicron 400 1/125.
Alien Bees 200 1/125.

13.2.1.3 The Camera View

The view must include the whole face from the hair dawn to the chin. Both cheeks, eyes and ears are shown.

13.2.1.4 Photographs Taken

Non-smiling
Non-smiling natural full face photograph (Fig. 13.2).

Smiling Full
Smiling full face photograph (Fig. 13.3). The patient is asked to smile maximally so that his teeth are shown with his lips and the angles of the mouth are fully stretched sideways. This view demonstrates, among other views, the extent of alar base stretching and widening of the nasal openings.

The Mid Face
A close-up photograph is taken for the mid face, from the level of the eyebrows to the lower lip. The lens is set to 40 cm distance (Fig. 13.4).

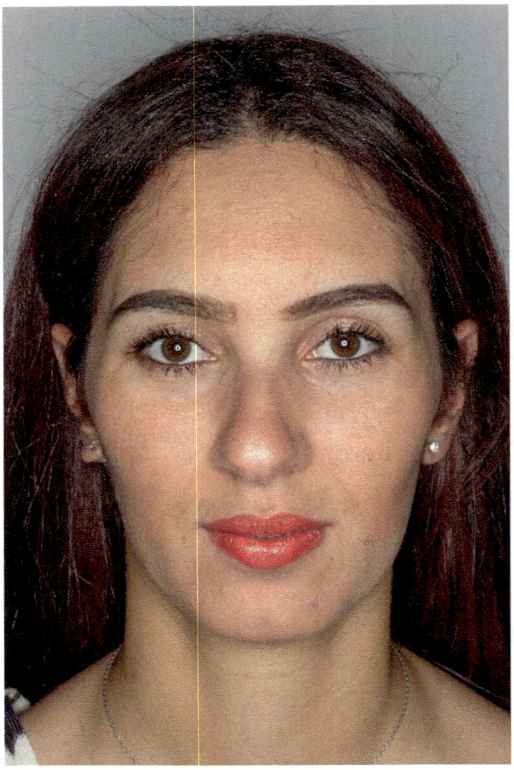

Fig. 13.2 Non-Smiling Full Face Frontal View

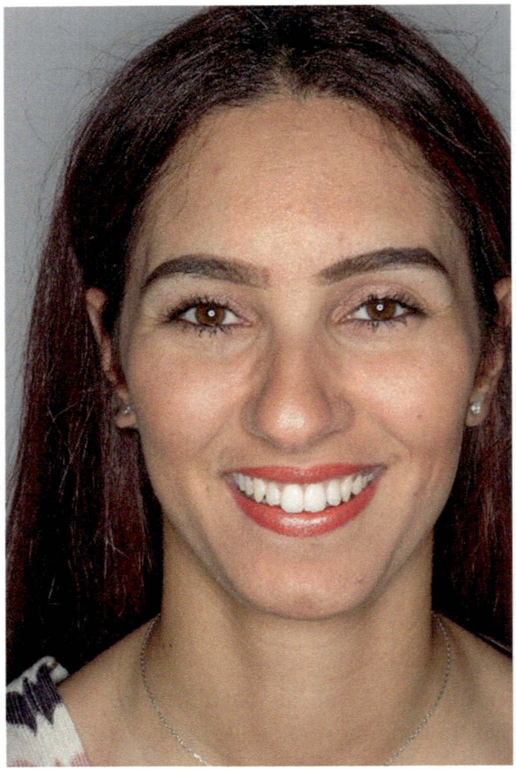

Fig. 13.3 Smiling Full Face Frontal View

13.2.1.5 Clinical Assessment of the Photographs

The smiling and non-smiling views are placed beside each other for direct comparison to see the extent of nasal widening on smiling.

The frontal views are **the first most basic and most important of all views**. As standard views, they are **the best in showing the overall appearance of the face and nose**.They are **the first looked at views** by everybody including the patient himself, relatives, friends and medics.

All other views are for seeing and examining only **one side** or **one area** of the face and nose.

From the **surgical** point of view, the frontal views are quite **unforgiving views**. If the post-operative frontal views are aesthetically unsatisfactory, then the overall result is aesthetically unacceptable, no matter how aesthetically pleasing all other views are. Patients on the other hand may not be unhappy. In fact, they may be quite content, satisfied and happy with the results.

The Nasofacial Relationship:

The proportional appearance of the front of the nose in relation to the face with regards to the **size**, **width**, **length** and **shape** are best shown in the frontal or anterior views (Figs. 13.5, 13.6 and 13.7).

i. **The size**: The size of the nose may be relatively large compared to the size of the face. The large size may affect the area of the bony pyramid, nasal tip, alae nasi or alar base. This is more common in Hispanic, Middle Eastern and African noses. Asians on the other hand have large wide facial skeleton with comparatively small sized and short noses.
ii. **The length:** The proportionate length of the nose in relation to the face is well appreciated and seen in the frontal views.
iii. **The width:** The Frontal or Anterior views are the **only and the best** views that show the general width of the nose in relation to

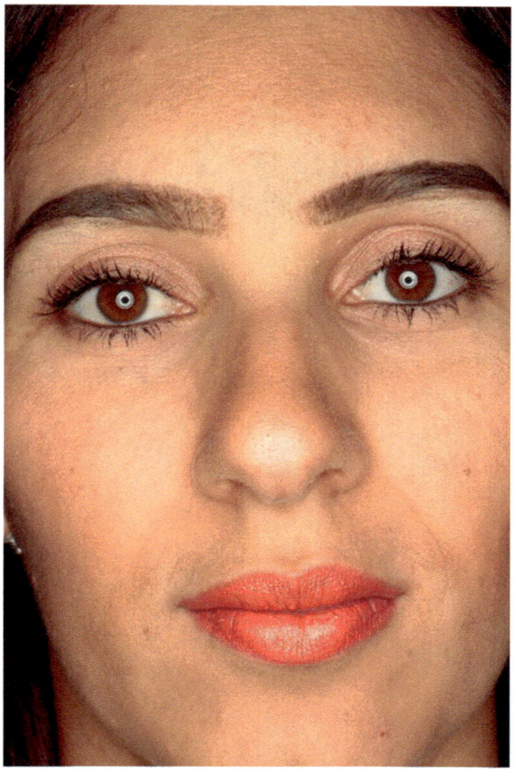

Fig. 13.4 Middle Third Frontal View

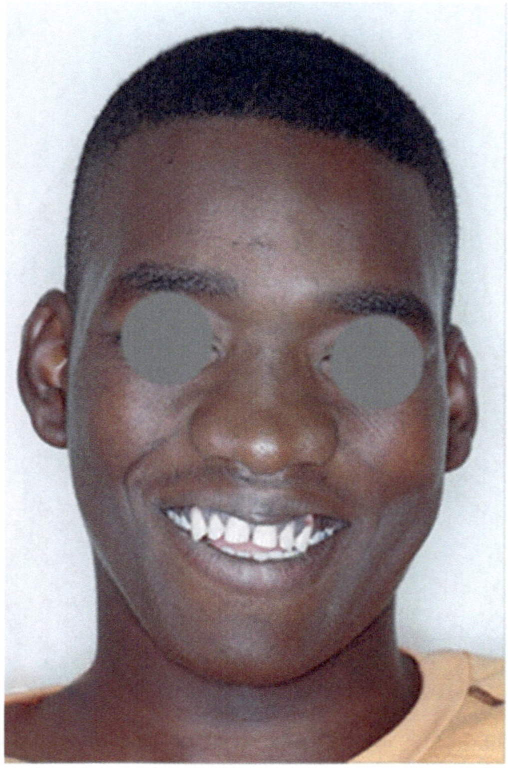

Fig. 13.5 A common African nose occupying a larger area of the face

the rest of the face, i.e., cheeks, lips and eyes. The lower third of the nose is of particular interest and importance, especially with the effects of smiling. That is how the person sees himself in front of the mirror and consequently how his photograph appears and how other people see him or her.

iv. **The Shape:** The overall shape of the nose and its aesthetic match with the faces, eyes, lips and chin are best appreciated in the frontal view.

The Tip-Alar Relationship

The **size** and **shape** of the **nasal tip** in relation to the bodies of the **alae nasi** behind it on each side has a special impact on the nasal aesthetics (Fig. 13.8).

A large bulbous or bulky tip overshadows most of the alar bodies on both sides and **hides** their beautiful contribution to the nasal aesthetics.

The photographic diagnosis of bulbous or bulky tip is of great help clinically. It is a sign of the need to reduce the size or bulk of the tip in order to enhance the aesthetics of both the nasal tip as well as that of the alae nasi.

The Levels of the Nasal Sills

The levels of the nasal sills are seen and compared on both sides. A caudal septal dislocation may push a nasal sill on one side to a lower level than the other (Fig. 13.9). The level of the nasal sill is also affected by facial palsy. It becomes at the lower level in the paralyzed side (Fig. 13.10). Accidental or surgical trauma may have an effect on him location (Fig. 13.11).

The Effects of Smiling on the Face

Smiling is the best and most dramatic way of demonstrating how wide the nose can be. This is the view that the patient sees.

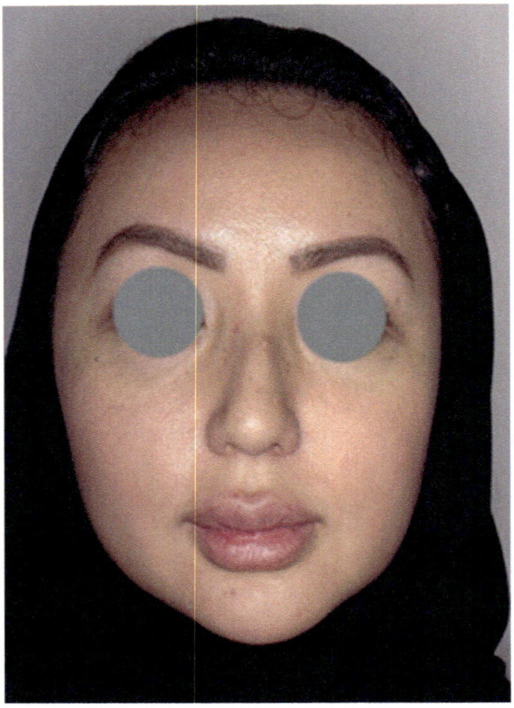

Fig. 13.6 Asian nose is relatively small compared to the size of the face

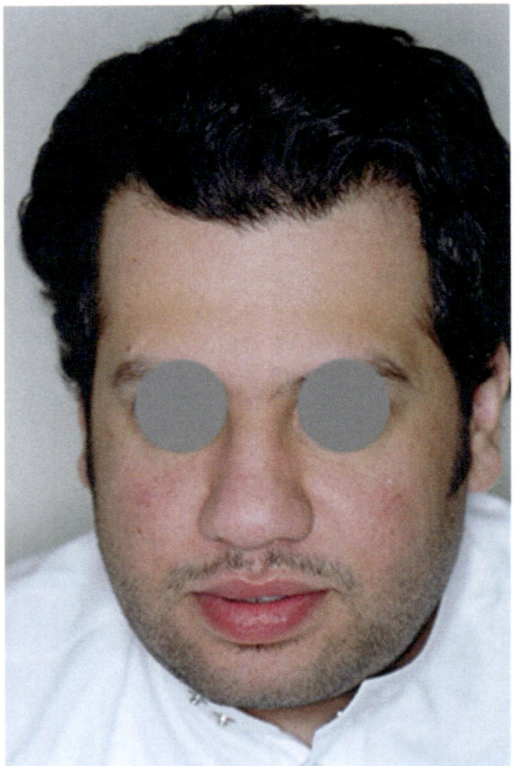

Fig. 13.7 Middle Eastern/Hispanic Nose

A common remark from patients is "I don't like to smile in photographs".

i. Smiling **stretches** the whole of the recoiling **rim-sill folds** of skin. The **alae nasi** expand **upwards and laterally** so that not only the **nasal openings become wider,** but also the aperture tubes, i.e., the whole of the lower third of the nose expands and enlarges in size. Not surprisingly, smiling is one of the **common social embarrassments** that drives someone with a wide alar base to Rhinoplasty (Fig. 13.12)
ii. Depending on the **length of the aperture tube** and the **size of the alae nasi**, widening of the nose on smiling may occupy a **higher** level and a **larger size** than merely the lower third. Hence, the nose may become quite large and occupy a wide area of the face. In these cases, smiling adds more to the size of the nose to make it almost **the most prominent feature of the face.**

If the nasal apertures as well as the alae nasi are small, then they will occupy a smaller area of the nose and face. Smiling in these cases has no unpleasant aesthetic effects on the face.

13.2.1.6 Facial Aesthetic Lines

Two aesthetically important lines are drawn in the non-smiling frontal view photograph.

The Vertical Guidelines for the Alar Base

A **vertical** line from the **inner canthus** of each eye is a useful guide to the **outer limit of the alar nasi**. If the alae nasi bulge outside these lines, then alar base reduction may become necessary. The final decision is made both clinically and intraoperatively (Fig. 13.13).

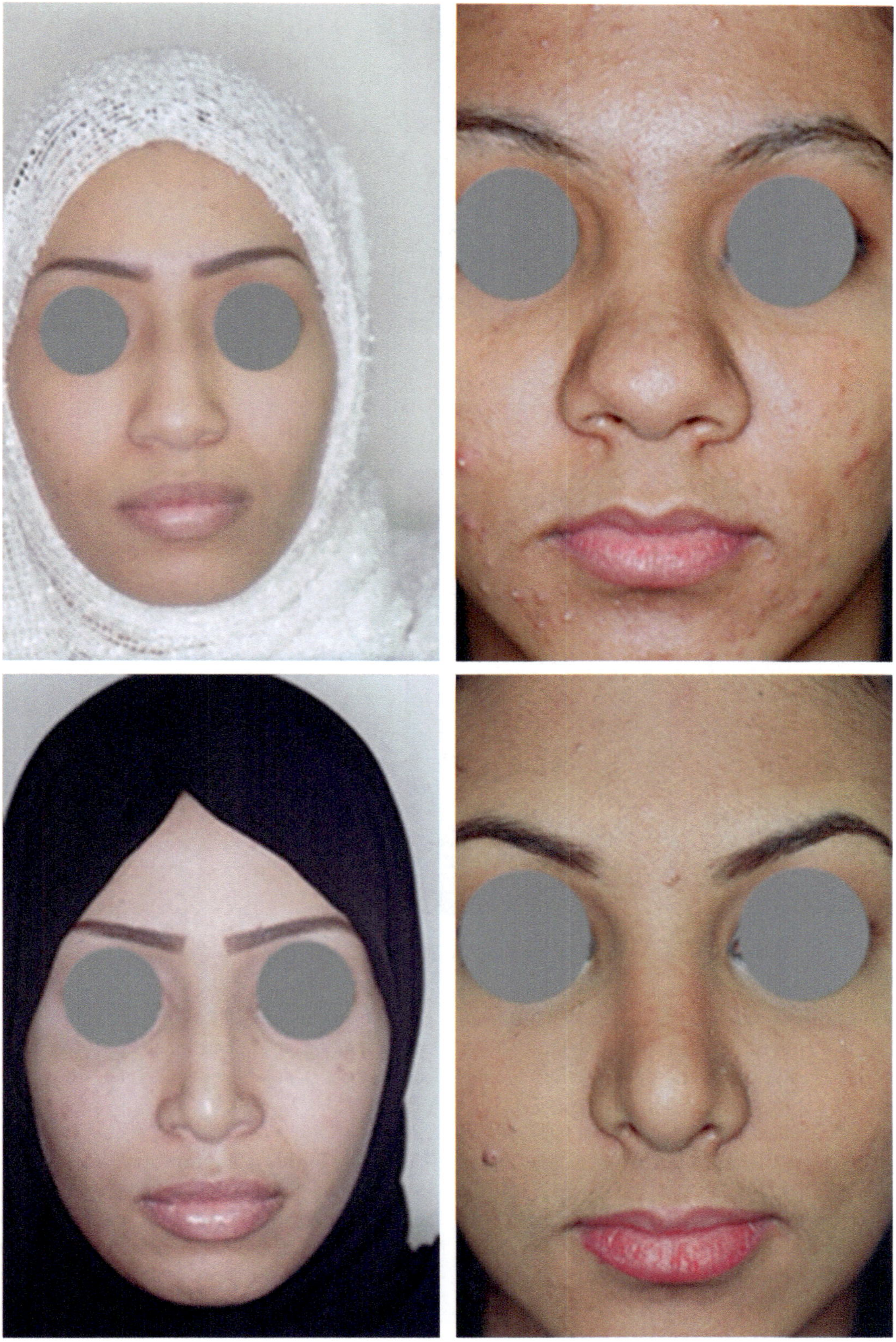

Fig. 13.8 Bulbus tip overshadowing the alae nasi pre-operatively. Post-operatively the alae nasi contribute to nasal aesthetics

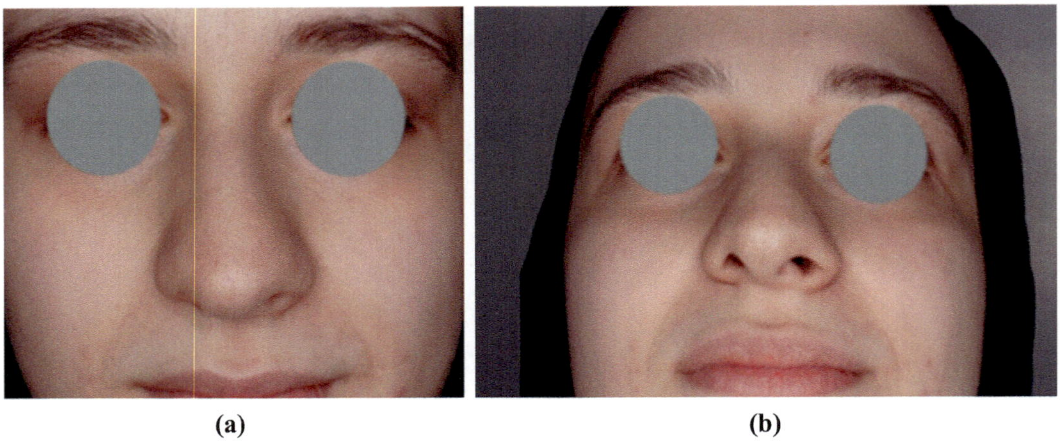

Fig. 13.9 The left nasal sill is at a lower level than the right (**a**) secondary to, left caudal septal deviation (**b**)

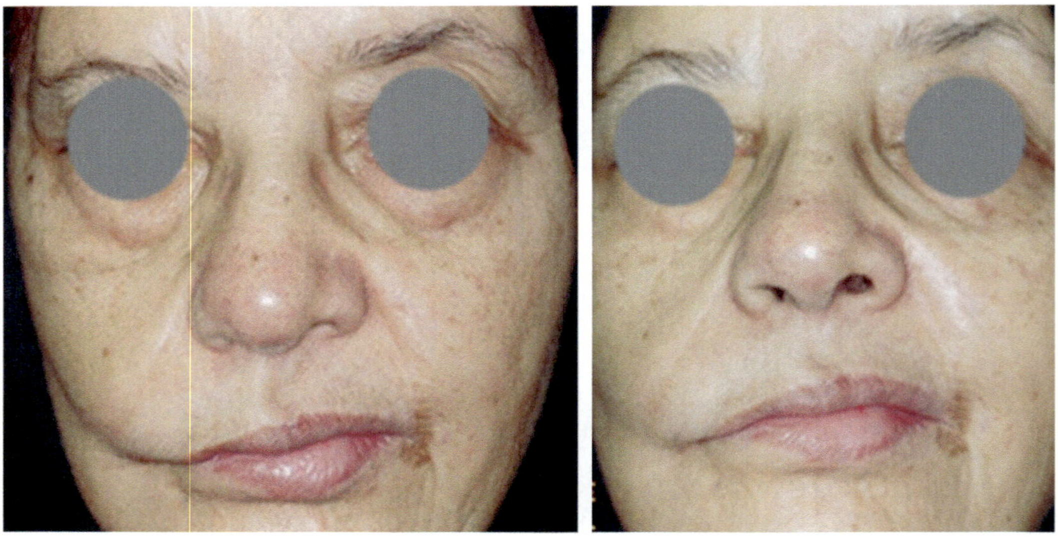

Fig. 13.10 The right nasal sill is at a lower level than the left, due to right facial palsy

The Curved Guidelines for the Nasal Sidewall
This is a **curved**, uninterrupted line that follows the **lower margin of the eyebrow** to the **sidewall of the nose** down to the **alar nasi**.

Each line takes a **C-shape** on the **left side** and an **inverted C-shape** on the **right side** of the patient's face (Fig. 13.14).

Any irregularity or distortion in the integrity of this line indicates the presence of a bony pyramidal unaesthetic feature. An inward curve or an outward bulge signifies an unaesthetic problem in the sidewall of the nose that needs correction, e.g., wide base of the bony pyramid, crookedness or deviation of the nose (Fig. 13.15).

13.2.1.7 Smiling Asymmetry

It is not uncommon to find asymmetrical smiles. Asymmetry may be in the shape and position of the right angle of the mouth as compared to the left angle. The right cheek ball may be different on smiling, from the left cheek ball in size, shape

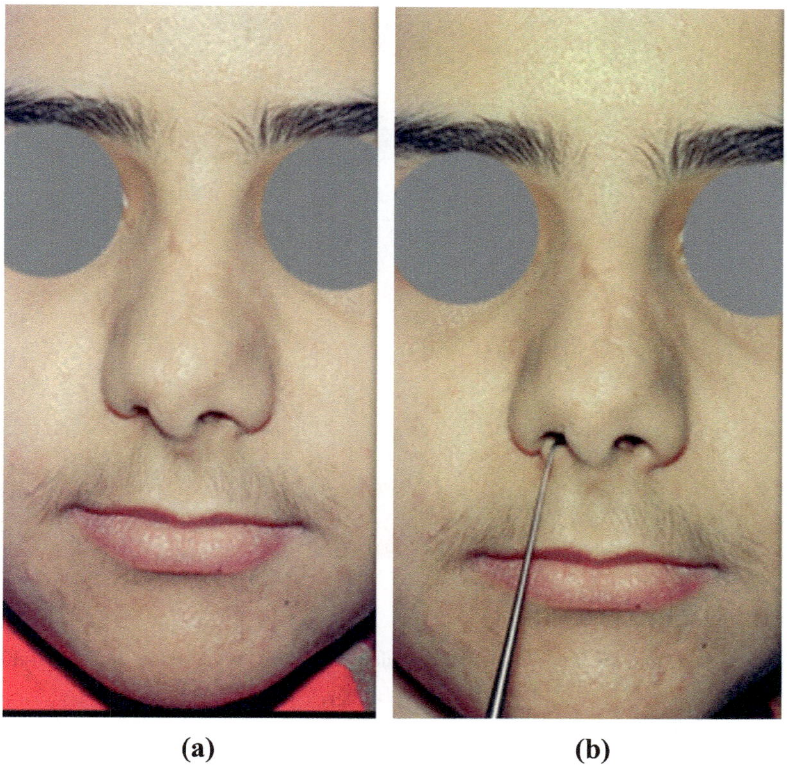

Fig. 13.11 Post-traumatic high right nasal sill (**a**). An angled probe is used to pull down the nasal sill to the same level as that of the left (**b**)

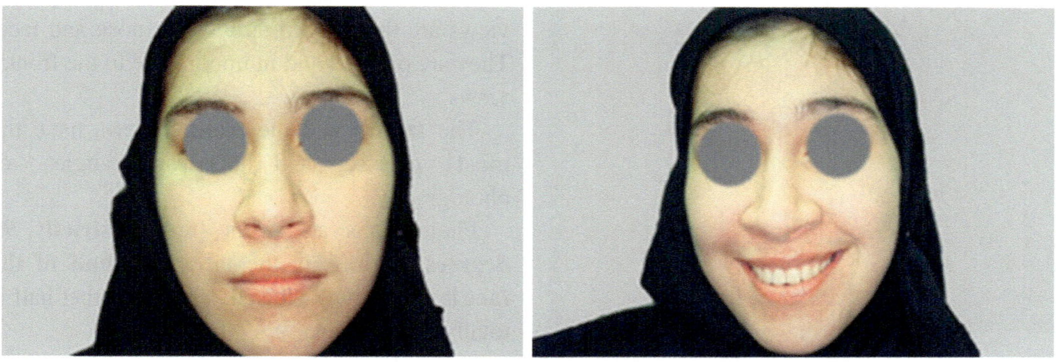

Fig. 13.12 Wide Nasal aperture while smiling is a strong drive for Rhinoplasty

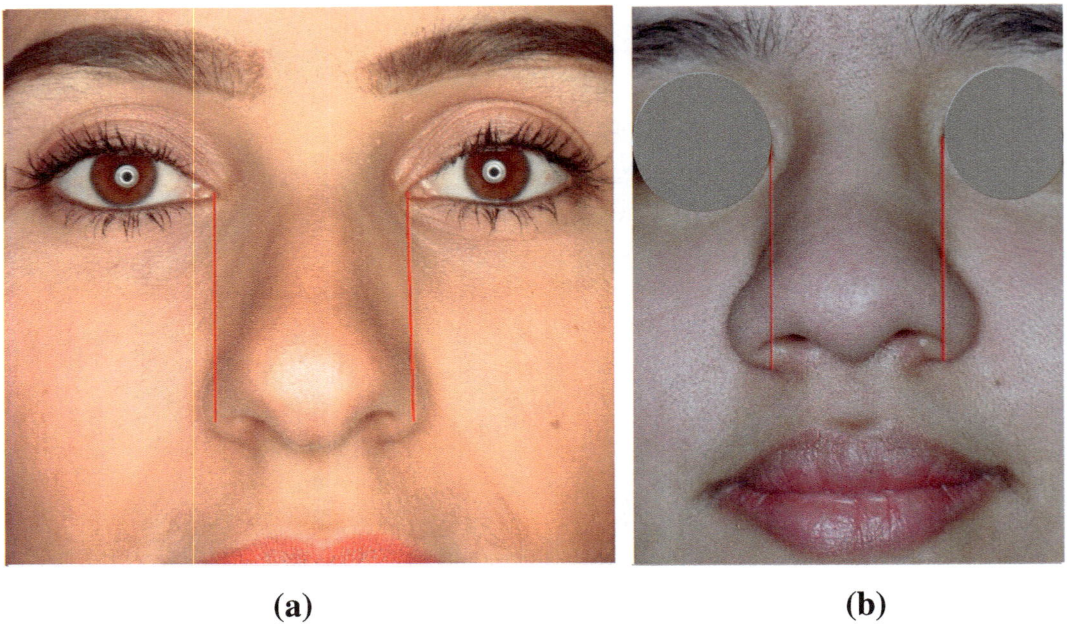

Fig. 13.13 **a** Vertical line from the inner canthus to the ala nasi clearly demonstrates a wide nasal base in case (**b**)

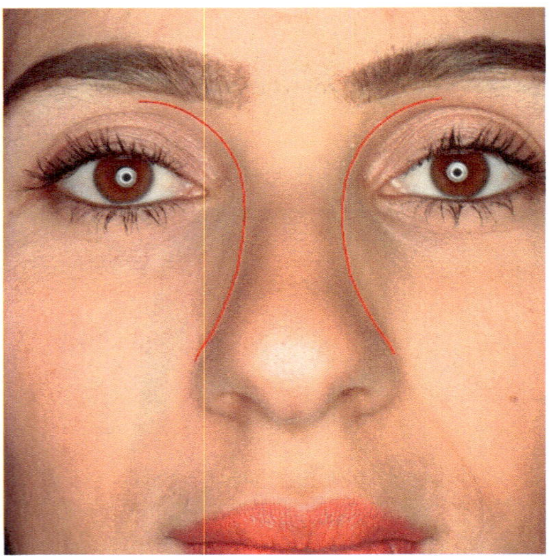

Fig. 13.14 The C and inverted C-shape guideline to the sidewalls of the nose is smooth and almost symmetrical on both sides

and position. Bilateral maxillary asymmetry and social habits may play an important role in smiling asymmetry (Fig. 13.16).

13.2.2 The Lateral Views

These are the profile views. The lateral views are the **second most important** of all views. They demonstrate the true **lateral profile** of the face and nose. As the name implies, these profile views are the **elegant side** of the nose and face. They are only second in importance to the frontal views.

The **lateral** and the **frontal** views have the **most precise** and **accurate** angles of photography.

Photographs are taken from a **strictly 90 degrees angle** from the face. **One half of the face is completely viewed,** while the other half is totally out of view.

The anterior border of the nose is outlined exactly as in the art of **silhouette**. This is the best and most accurate representation of the **dorsal and nasal tip projection**. The nose is viewed exactly at its **maximal height** and **maximal length**.

Measuring the **nasal** and the **paranasal angles** can **only accurately** be measured from

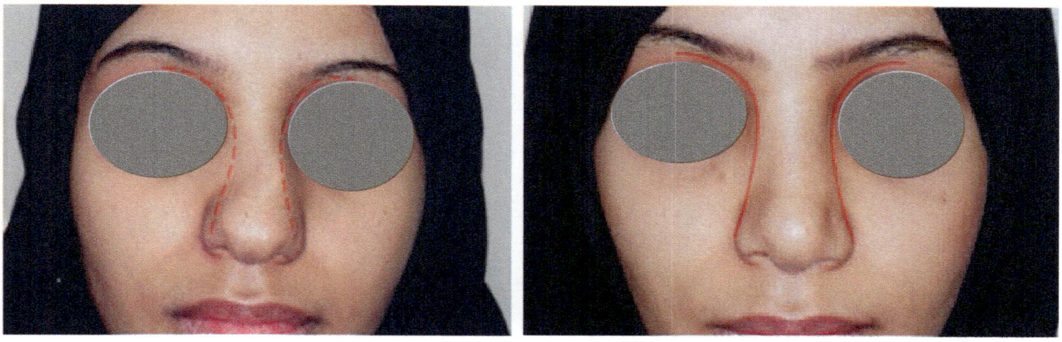

Fig. 13.15 The sidewalls of the nose are away from the C-shaped guidelines. The regular C-shape is regained postoperatively

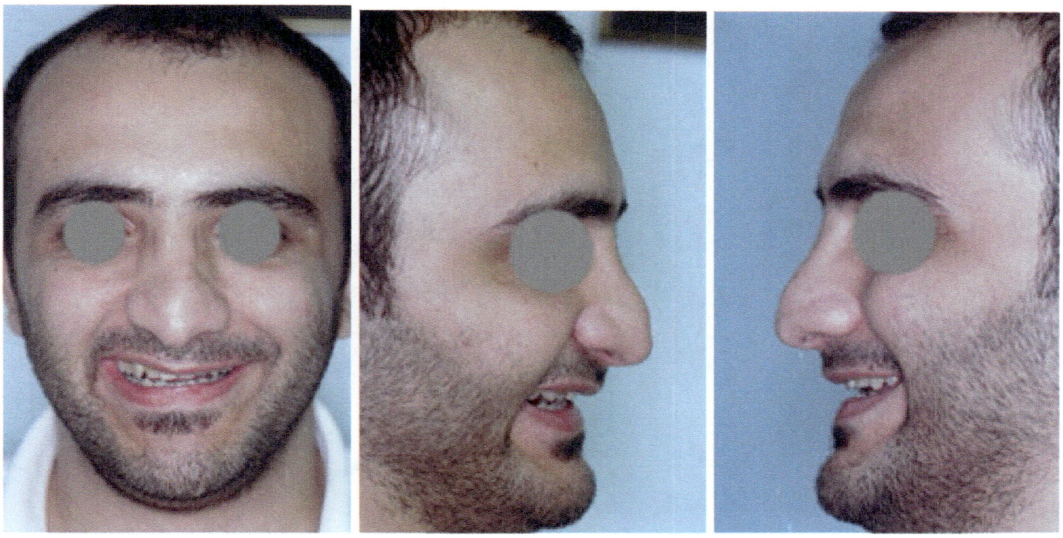

Fig. 13.16 Bilateral asymmetrical smile, there is no facial palsy. Note that the two cheek balls are different in size, shape and position. The left cheek ball is smaller. The right angle of the mouth is wider than the left angle

the lateral views, e.g., the nasal tip, the naso-frontal and the naso-labial angles.

13.2.2.1 The Setup

The Patient

- The patient sits on his chair and is rotated 90 degrees so that his feet straddle **the transverse line** on the floor. His chest and face are along the transverse line (Fig. 13.17).
- The Frankfort horizontal plane is observed.

The Photographer

- The photographer sits on his chair with the camera setup directly above the **anterior** line (Fig. 13.17).
- The lens must be at the same horizontal level as the patient's nose.
- The **point of focus** is the **midpoint of the nasal dorsum.**

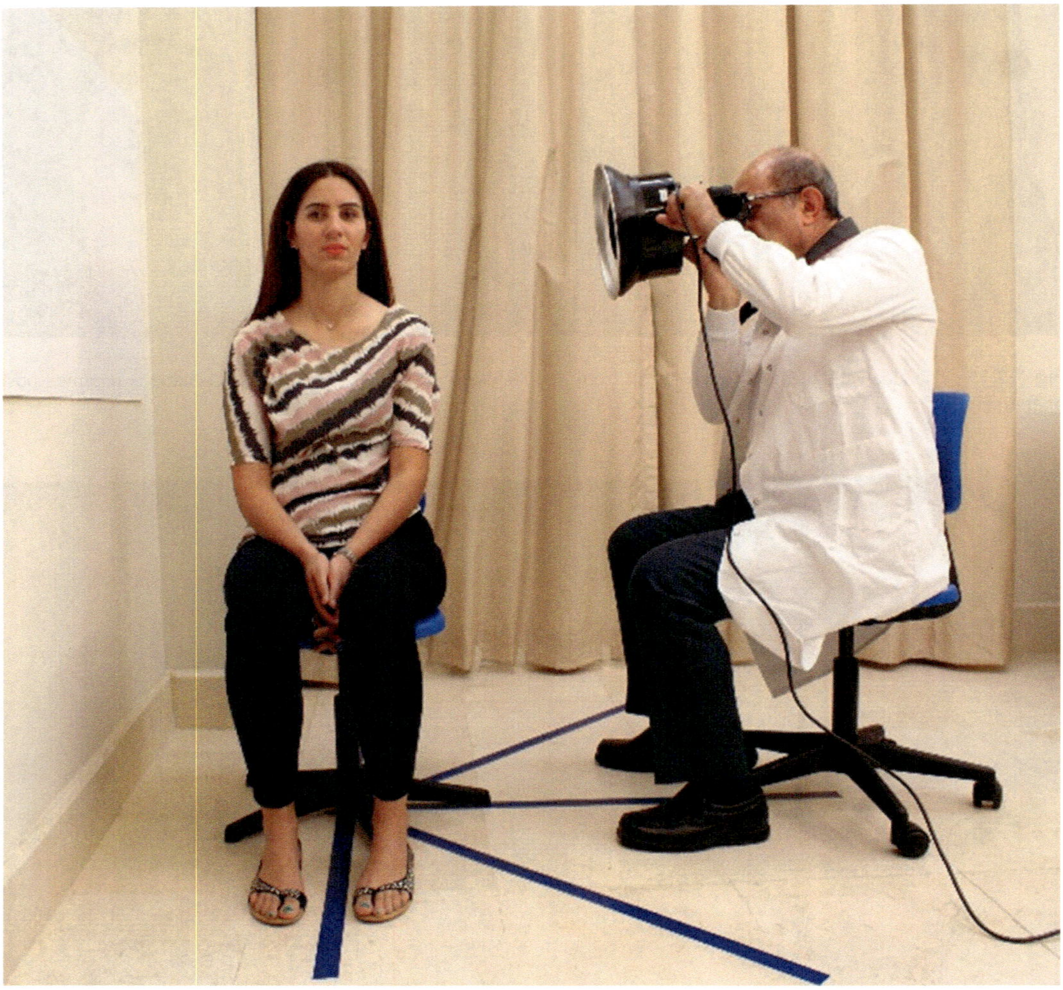

Fig. 13.17 Position of the patient and the photographer in taking the lateral views. The patient's feet are straddling the transverse line and the photographer's feet are straddling the anterior line

13.2.2.2 Camera Setting

- **Orientation** of the camera back: **vertical,** i.e., Portrait (Fig. 13.17).
- **Lens focus**: 60 cm for full face and 40 cm for close-up middle third picture.
- **Lens Aperture**: depending on the type of flash and patient's skin color.

  Omicron f/9–f/13.
  Allien Bees f/14–f/30.

13.2.2.3 The Camera View

The whole side of the face must be included in the view from the hair dawn to the chin. The whole cheek and lower jaw are shown. The ear may or may not be included in the lateral views.

13.2.2.4 Photographs Taken

Full Face Non-smiling

A natural **full face non-smiling** lateral view photograph is taken to the **right** then to the **left** side of the face (Fig. 13.18).

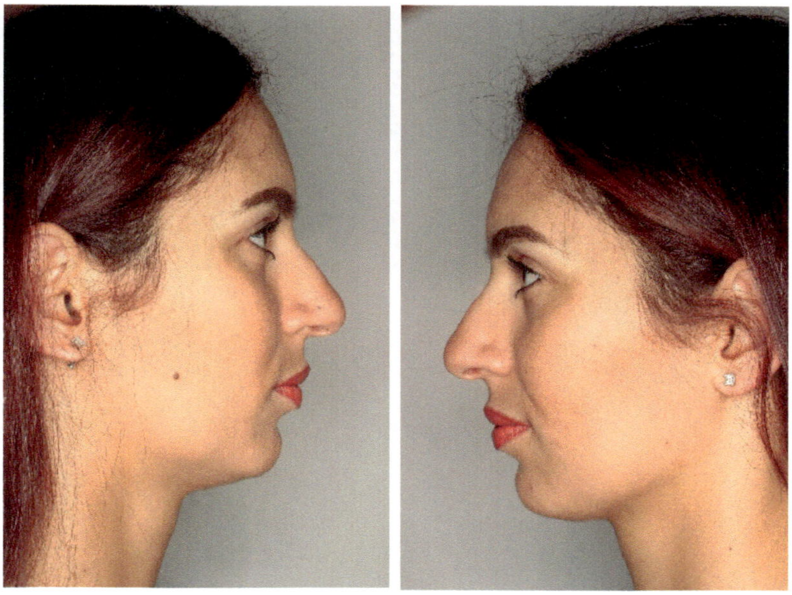

Fig. 13.18 Right and left full face lateral non-smiling views

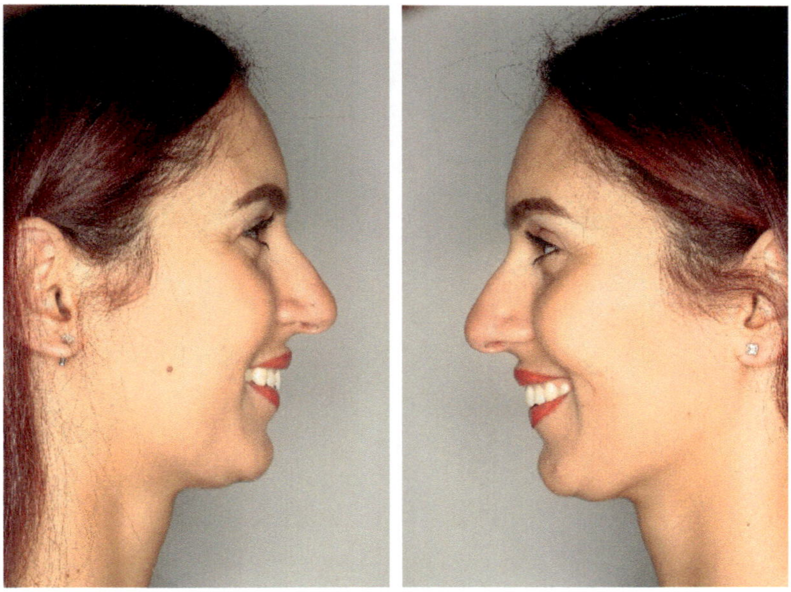

Fig. 13.19 Right and left full face lateral smiling views

Smiling Full Face

A full face smiling lateral view. The patient is asked to smile maximally so that his teeth are shown with the lips and angles of the mouth are fully stretched sideways (Fig. 13.19).

Midface

A close-up view photograph is taken for the midface area from the level of the eyebrow to the lower lip. The lens is set at a 40 cm distance (Fig. 13.20).

13.2.2.5 Clinical Assessment of Photographs

The Nasofacial Relationship

Nasal projection is shown at its **maximum size, height** and **length** (Figs. 13.21 and 13.22) in the

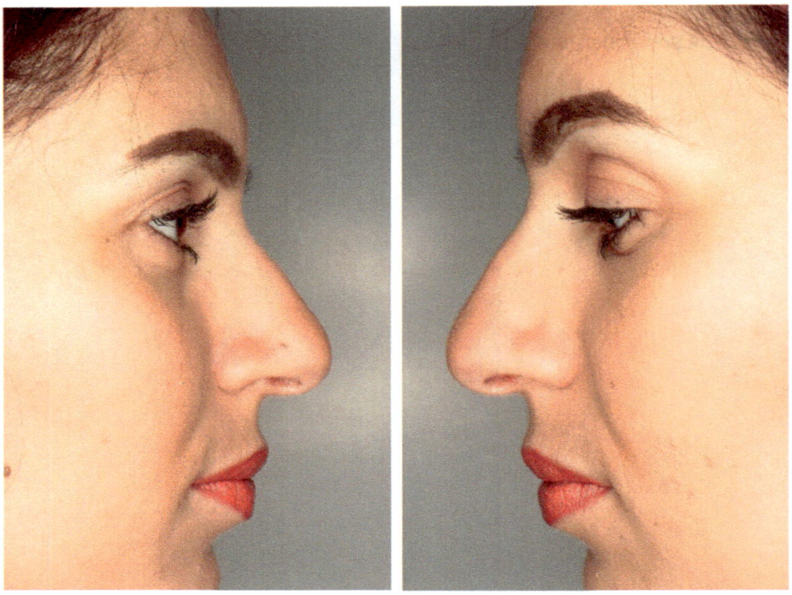

Fig. 13.20 Right and left middle third lateral non-smiling views

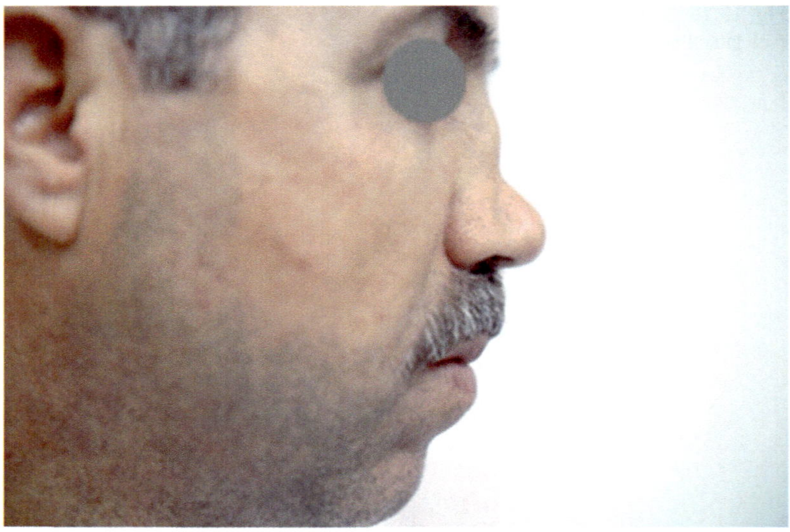

Fig. 13.21 Lateral view demonstrating severe saddling deformity

lateral views. The overall proportionate size, height, length and shape in relation to that of the rest of the face is well demonstrated.

The Size

The nose is shown at its maximum size from the profile angle. This is compared to the overall size of the face.

The Height of the Nasal Dorsum

The maximal dorsal height is most accurately assessed from the lateral views. The location, degree and extent of any increase, decrease or irregularities of the dorsum are best and most accurately assessed from the lateral views. A **saddle deformity** is well located whether it is supratip, midvault or at the bony pyramid

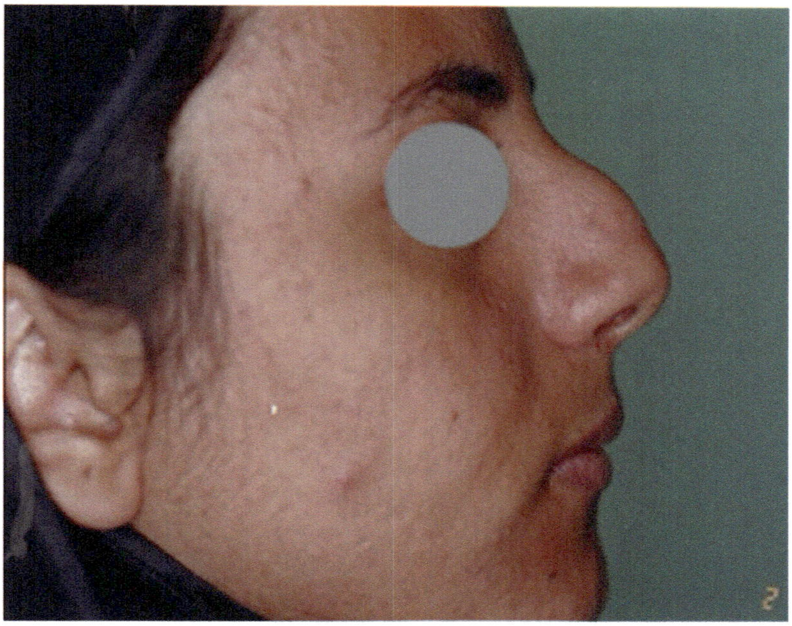

Fig. 13.22 Lateral view demonstrating high osteocartilaginous hump

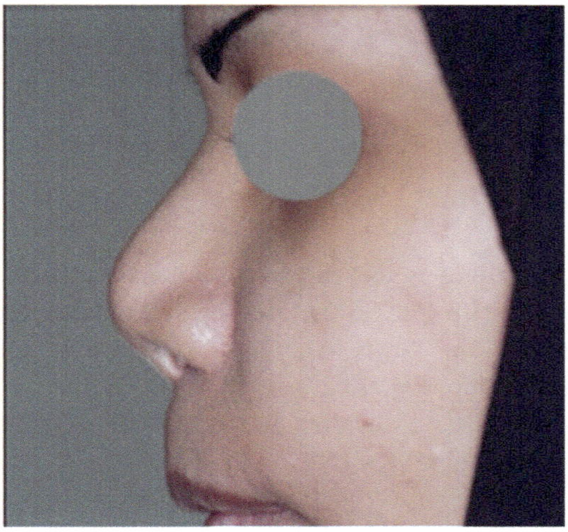

Fig. 13.23 Wide naso-labial angle with shortening of nasal tip

(Fig. 13.21). The extent and depth of depression are well demonstrated. On the other hand, a **hump** may be seen extending over the osteo-cartilagenousarea or at the supratip area (Fig. 13.22). The overall maximum height of the hump is well projected in these views.

The proportionate depression or elevation heights to that of the face is significant aesthetically.

The Length

The length of the nose in relation to the facial length in the profile view has its significant aesthetic value. A well-projected tip at 90 degrees naso-labial angle is ideal. A drooping tip (**Plunging**) or backward turned tip, both conditions contribute to **elongating** and **shortening** the nose successively (Fig. 13.23).

The Shape

The shape of the nose in relation to that of the face in the elegant profile angle is significantly appealing. The type of round angulations of the nasal tip should match with that of the chin and forehead. They should maintain harmonic aesthetic correlation.

The Nasal Tip

The lateral views are the best and most important views, not only to demonstrate, but also to judge and measure the nasal tip projection. To **see the nasal tip** is to **see the lateral views.**

The Tip Projection

Tip projection means the exact **location** and **angulation** of the nasal tip. The nasal tip ideally is located **at the end of the nasal dorsum**. It

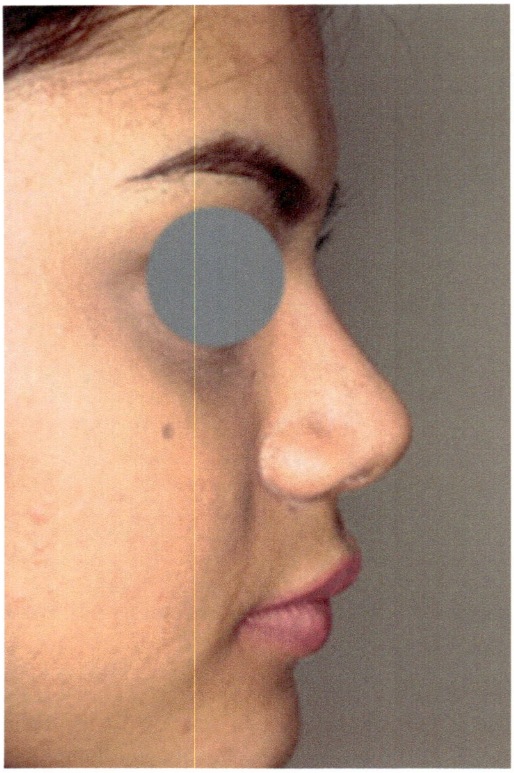

Fig. 13.24 Lateral view is the best for showing the ideal tip projection

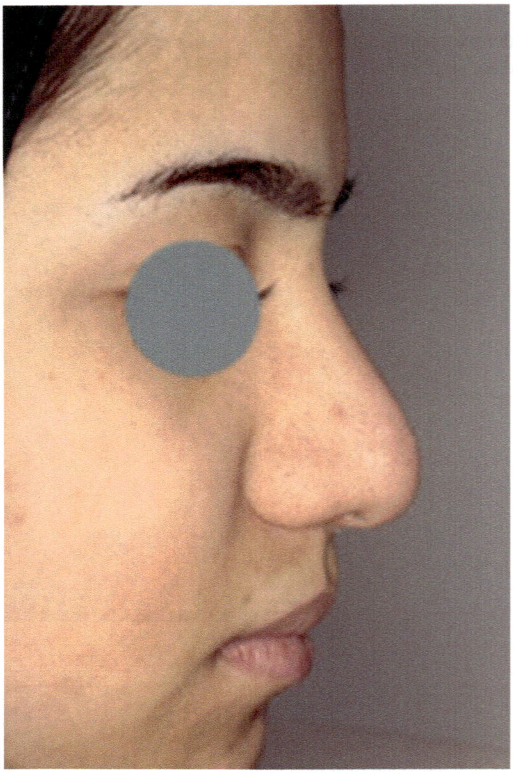

Fig. 13.25 Rounded tip lacking the aesthetic projection

should be **at the same level** or **slightly elevated** than the dorsum. The tip is aesthetically appealing if it is **well defined,** i.e., **tendency to angulation** rather than being rounded (Fig. 13.24). The angle should not be artificially sharp so that it does not give the impression of a surgical nose. It is equally important that the tip is at an **angle of 90–100 degrees with the upper lip** (Fig. 13.24).

The Mobile Tip and the Sliding Tip

The lateral views are the best in demonstrating the exact location of the nasal tip, the direction and the extent of its movement on smiling.

On smiling, the mobile tip moves inferiorly, while the sliding tip moves posteriorly as well as inferiorly (Fig. 13.26).

The direction and the extent of these two movements are best appreciated in the lateral views.

Smiling is the best way to demonstrate the **mobile tip** (Fig. 13.29). **pulling and holding the upper lip** down, May also demonstrate the **sliding** tip (Fig. 13.27).

The lateral views are the best in demonstrating the **plunging tips** (Fig. 13.28).

The Paranasal Angles

As a precise angle of photography at 90 degrees, the lateral view is the only accurate way to assess the nasal and paranasal angles. Two angles are aesthetically significant.

The Nasofrontal Angle

This is the angle between the bony dorsum of the nose and the frontal bone (glabella). Depending on its depth, the angle may be acute or wide in deep or shallow angles successively (Figs. 13.30 and 13.31).

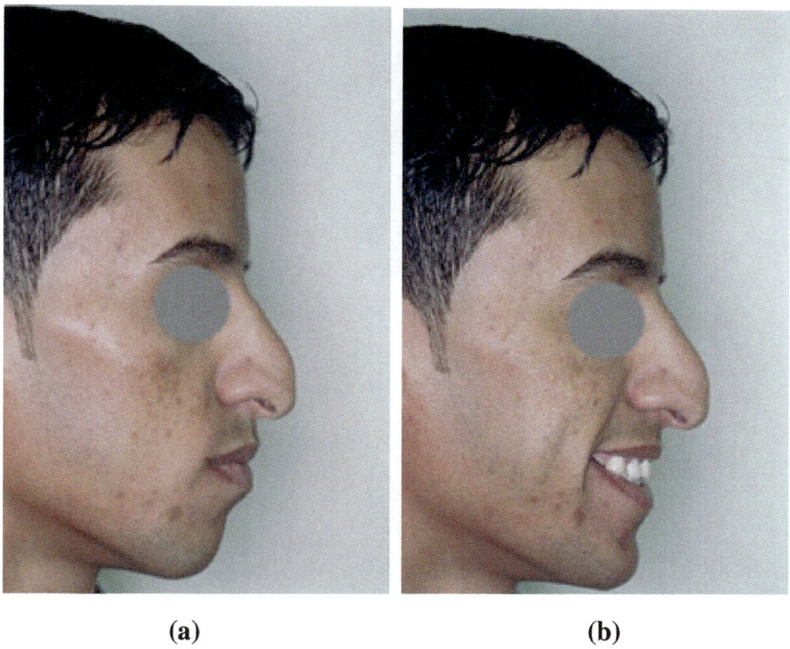

Fig. 13.26 Sliding tip is at a posterior level from the nasal dorsum. Smiling: the tip moves posteriorly as well as inferiorly

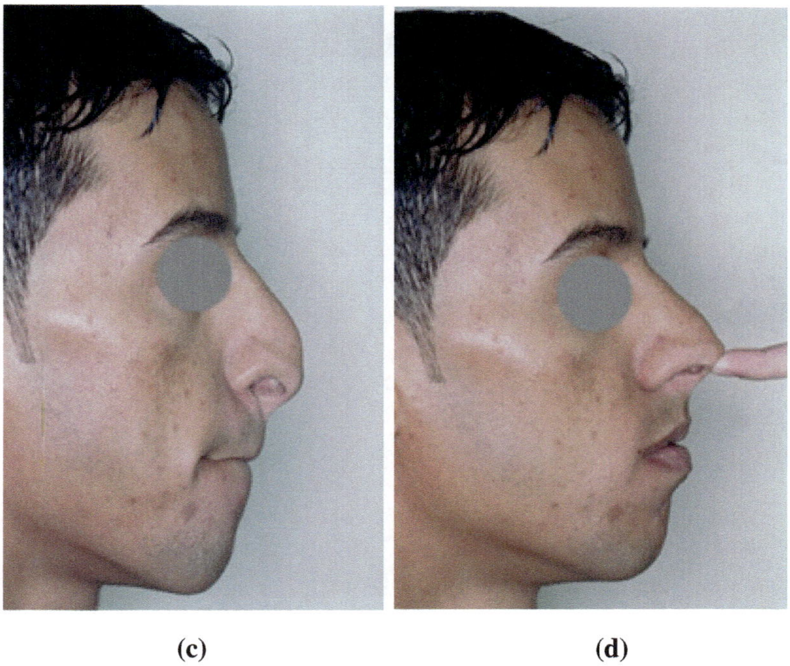

Fig. 13.27 Sliding tip is exaggerated by smiling and by holding the upper lip down. Note the repositioning of the tip in image (**d**)

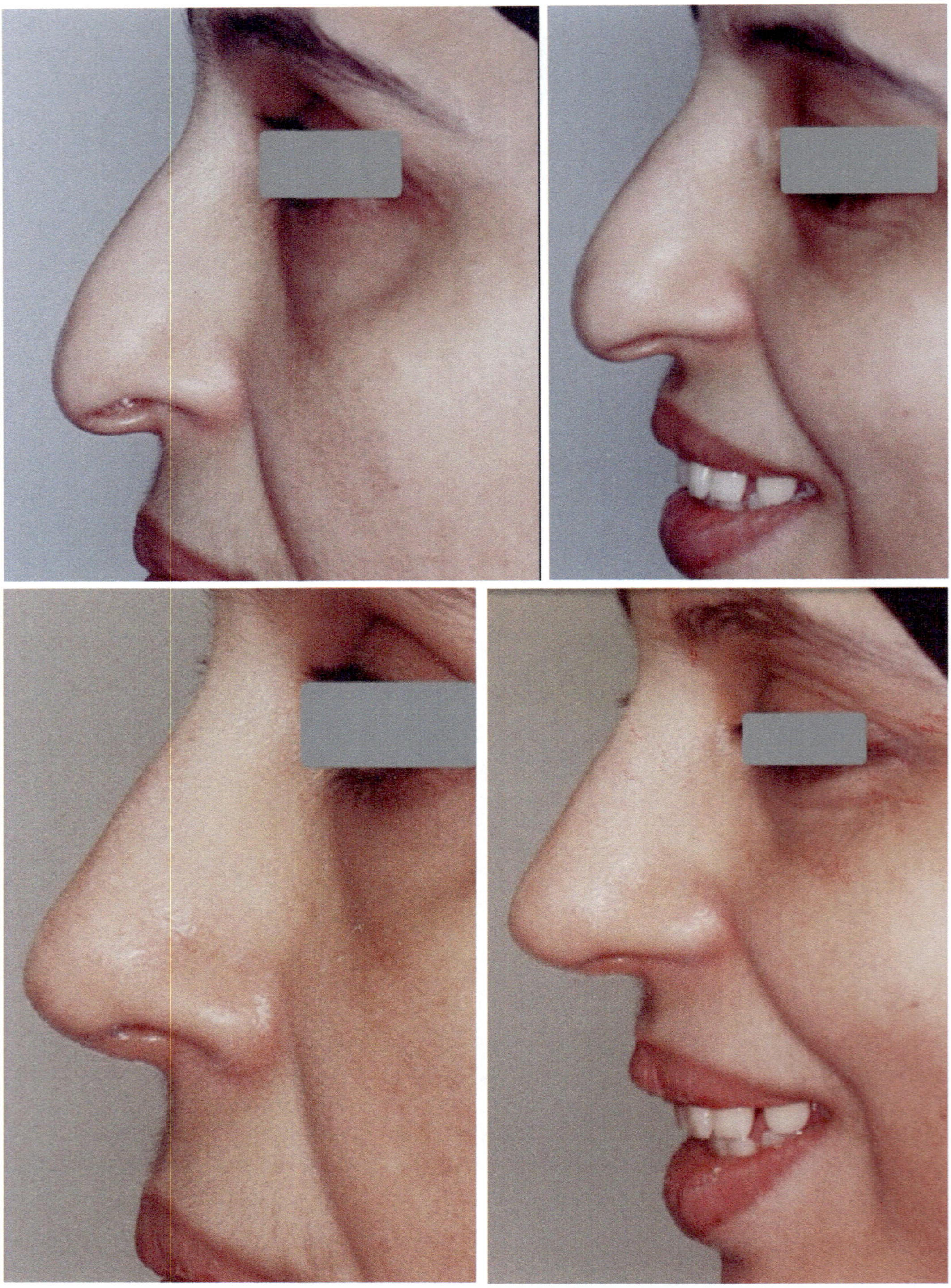

Fig. 13.28 The lateral view is best for demonstrating the plunging tip. This was corrected post-operatively

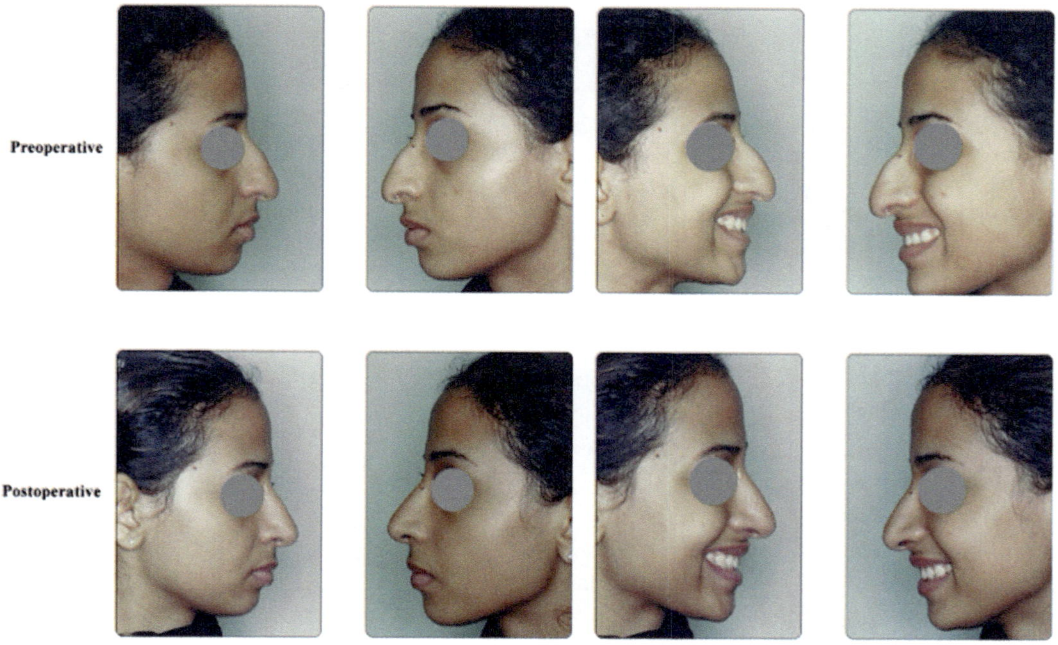

Fig. 13.29 Mobile plunging tip, nasal tip moves inferiorly at the same level of the nasal dorsum

An aesthetically acceptable angle is between 115–135 degrees.

The Naso-Labial Angle

This is the angle between the columella and the upper lip. It is significantly important aesthetically.

A drooping or plunging tip has an **acute angle** and has the effect of a grim-looking face (Fig. 13.29). A wide angle exposes the nostrils which is aesthetically unacceptable.

An aesthetically acceptable angle is between 90–110 degrees.

Alar-Columellar Relationship

The medial columellar margin should just be seen at an inferior level than the alar margin.

High alar margin, large ala nasi (Fig. 13.33), protruding columella and hanging columella (Fig. 13.32) are best seen in the lateral views.

Effects of Smiling

Smiling in the lateral views clearly demonstrate mobile tip, sliding tip, plunging tip, tight lip and gummy smile.

13.2.3 The Oblique Views

These are the **third most important of all views** following the frontal and the lateral views. The oblique views are the beginning of displaying the **naturally different two sides of the nose** and face.

The relationships between each side of the nose and its corresponding side of the face are unique to these views.

The oblique view photographs are quite common in our daily life, e.g., in parties, weddings, holidays, trips, schools and colleges.

A person may say "I don't like a picture taken of me from one oblique side of the face, as it

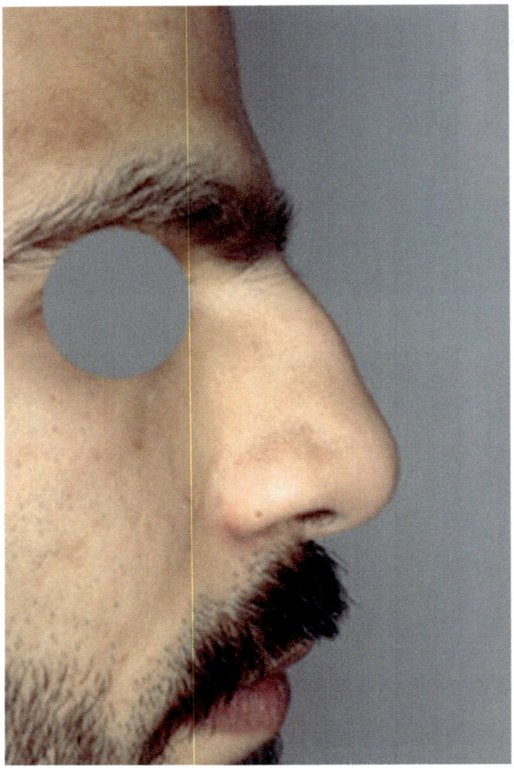

Fig. 13.30 Shallow Nasofrontal angle. The nasal hump gives a false impression of the presence of the Nasofrontal angle

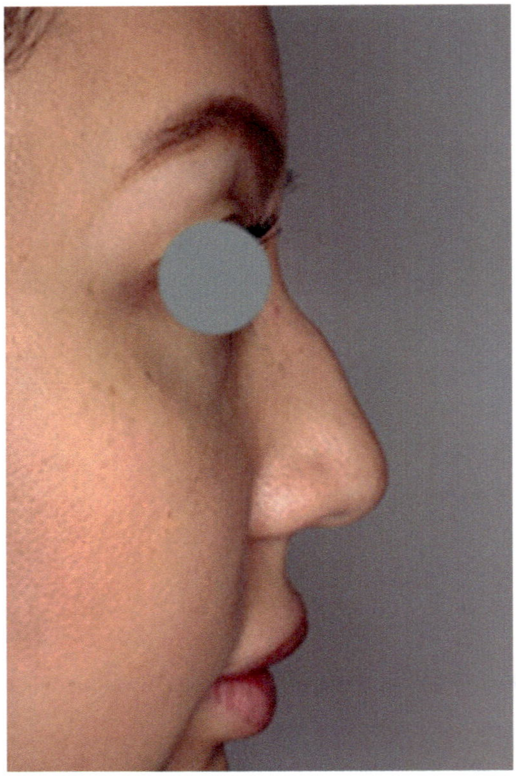

Fig. 13.31 Deep Nasofrontal angle

always shows an exaggerated unaesthetic feature of the nose that does not appear from the other side". A common example of this is a nasal hump, which appears more prominent from one oblique side than the other.

13.2.3.1 The Difficulties of the Oblique Views:

For the purpose of aesthetic Rhinoplasty, an **oblique view** photograph means **a photograph taken directly to the sidewall of the nose**. The angle of the photograph, therefore, varies according to the variation of the obliquity[1] of each sidewall of the nose.

The standardization of the oblique views, therefore, is not quite simple. Considerations are made not only to the rules of **photographic principles**, but also to the **aesthetics** of the nose and face.

The difficulty in standardizing the oblique views is that they deal with **two extremely variable structures,** viz., the **nose** and the **cheeks.** The forehead and chin, are important in facial aesthetics and their relationship to the nose, but they do not have a direct effect on the photographic assessment of the nose.

Both the nose and the cheeks show a wide range of variations that may affect the oblique photographic views:

- Variations in **size** and **shape** of the nose from **one person to another.**
- In the same person, the nose and cheeks may vary in **size** and **shape** in many different ways, for example:
  - Bilateral Variations.
  - Variations Before and after **surgery**.

[1] Footnote: definition according to Meriam Webster deviation from parallelism or perpendicularity.

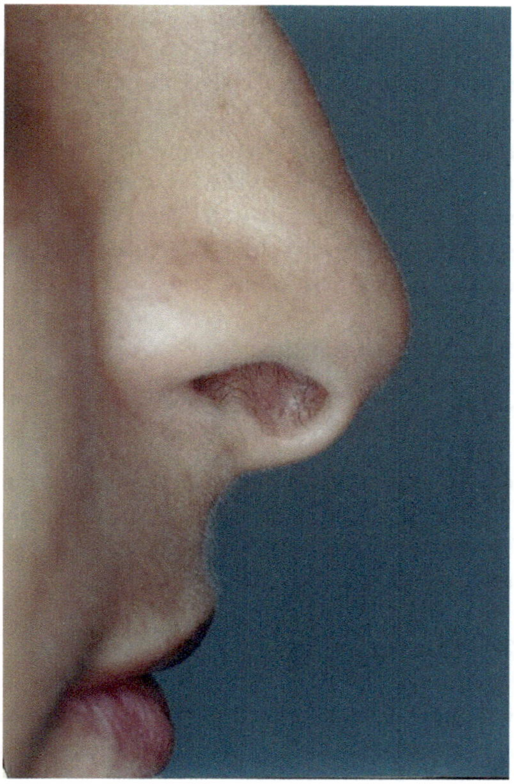

Fig. 13.32 Hanging columella. The body of the medial crus is completely exposed

- Variations Before and after losing or gaining **weight**.
- Variations by the passing of **time** and the process of **aging**.

Variations may appear between one **ethnic group** to another, e.g. , **Asians** have a relatively **small nose** and **wide large cheeks**. **Africans** are the opposite, i.e., with **large noses** and comparatively **small cheeks**.

Two methods are suggested for taking the oblique views photographs:

The Strictly Forty-Five Degrees Technique:

In this method, the patient's chair is rotated to the 45 degrees line. The photographer sits on the anterior line.

Photographs are taken at a fixed angle of 45 degrees to the face and nose regardless of any other considerations, e.g., the size or the shape of the nose and cheek, pre-operative or post-operative.

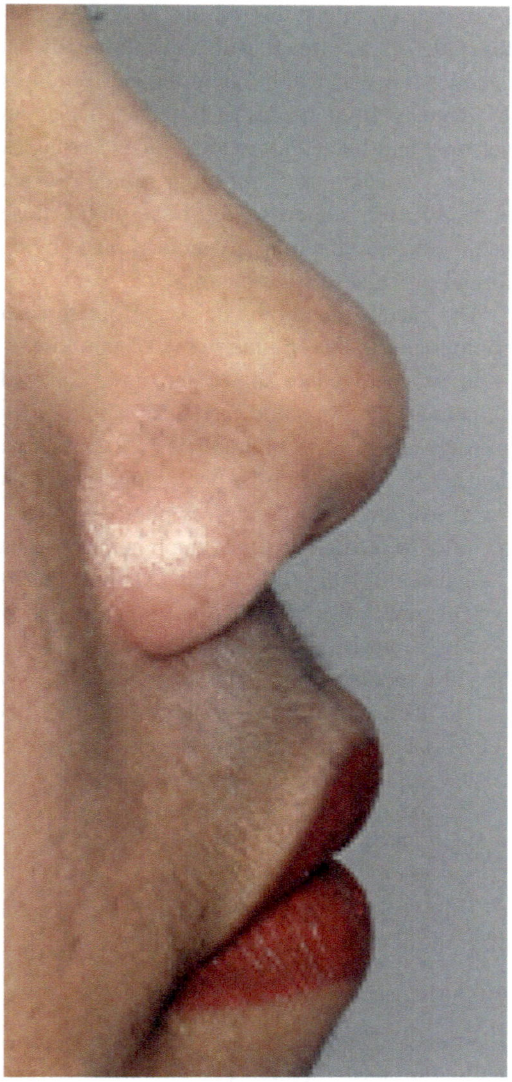

Fig. 13.33 Large ala nasi below the columellar level.

Advantages

Photographically, this is the **most accurate** and the best possible method of **angle fixing** and hence **standardizing the angle** of photography over different time periods.

The Direct Lateral Nasal Wall Technique

Photographs are taken directly to the lateral wall of the nose, i.e., **the camera directly faces the lateral nasal wall** in all of its conditions whether deviated, oblique, pre-operative or post-operative.

A true **oblique view of the nose is a photograph of its lateral wall. Anatomically** the lateral nasal wall is obliquely angled by almost 45 degrees from the sagittal plane. There are personal and bilateral variations of these angles.

The **cheeks** are **photographically** and **anatomically related to the base of the nose,** i.e., the base of the bony pyramid is made by the frontal processes of the maxilla.

The cheeks, therefore, are backgrounds when photographing the oblique views of the nose.

In order to cover all of the nasal sidewall variations, two versatile angles of photography are suggested for the oblique views. In these two angles, the patient and the photographer take the same position as in 45 degrees photographs.

(a) **The first angle**: a photograph is taken of the sidewall of the nose as the **external line of the nasal tip touches the external line of the opposite cheek**, i.e., cheek margin.
(b) **The second angle**: a photograph is taken of the sidewall of the nose as the external line of the nasal tip is **inside** the external line of the opposite cheek by a distance that depends on the obliquity of the nasal sidewalls, i.e., mid cheek.

This versatility covers all the possible variations in the nasal sidewall angulations.

Advantages

The direct lateral wall views are better **anatomically and aesthetically** as they focus directly on the target, i.e., on the lateral nasal walls. They are, therefore, the best method for direct aesthetic standardization. Comparison is better achieved between the two sides of the nose, before and after surgeries, as well as between the different patients.

The angle of photography is almost 45 degrees. It may only slightly change according to the obliquity of the lateral wall so that the accurate photographic rule of 45 degrees is only marginally compromised.

Photographically, the **depth of field is better** as the cheeks are seen farther away from the nose.

In conclusion, the direct lateral wall view is the only angle that shows the **true size, shape and height** of the lateral wall of the nose. A strict 45 degree view may not always be directly facing the lateral wall. This slight angulation may lead to a slightly larger, smaller or even distorted sidewall.Direct lateral wall views are better standardized than the strict 45 degrees both pre-operatively and post-operatively.

13.2.3.2 The Setup

The Patient

- The patient sits on his chair and is rotated to 45degees so that his feet are straddling **the oblique line** (Fig. 13.34).
- Frankfort level is observed.

The Photographer

- The photographer sits on his chair with the camera setup directly above the anterior line (Fig. 13.34).
- The lens must be at the same horizontal level as that of the nose.
- The point of focus is at the mid-dorsal point of the nose.

13.2.3.3 Camera Settings

- The orientation of the camera back is vertical, i.e., portrait (Fig. 13.34).
- The lens is focused at: 60 cm for the full face and 40 cm for the close-up pictures (Author's Setup).
- The lens Aperture: depending on the type of flash and the patient's skin color

Omicron f /9–f/13.
Allein Bees f/14–f/30.

13.2.3.4 The Camera View

The oblique view should include the whole face from the hair down to the chin and back to the angle of the mandible. Ears may or may not be included.

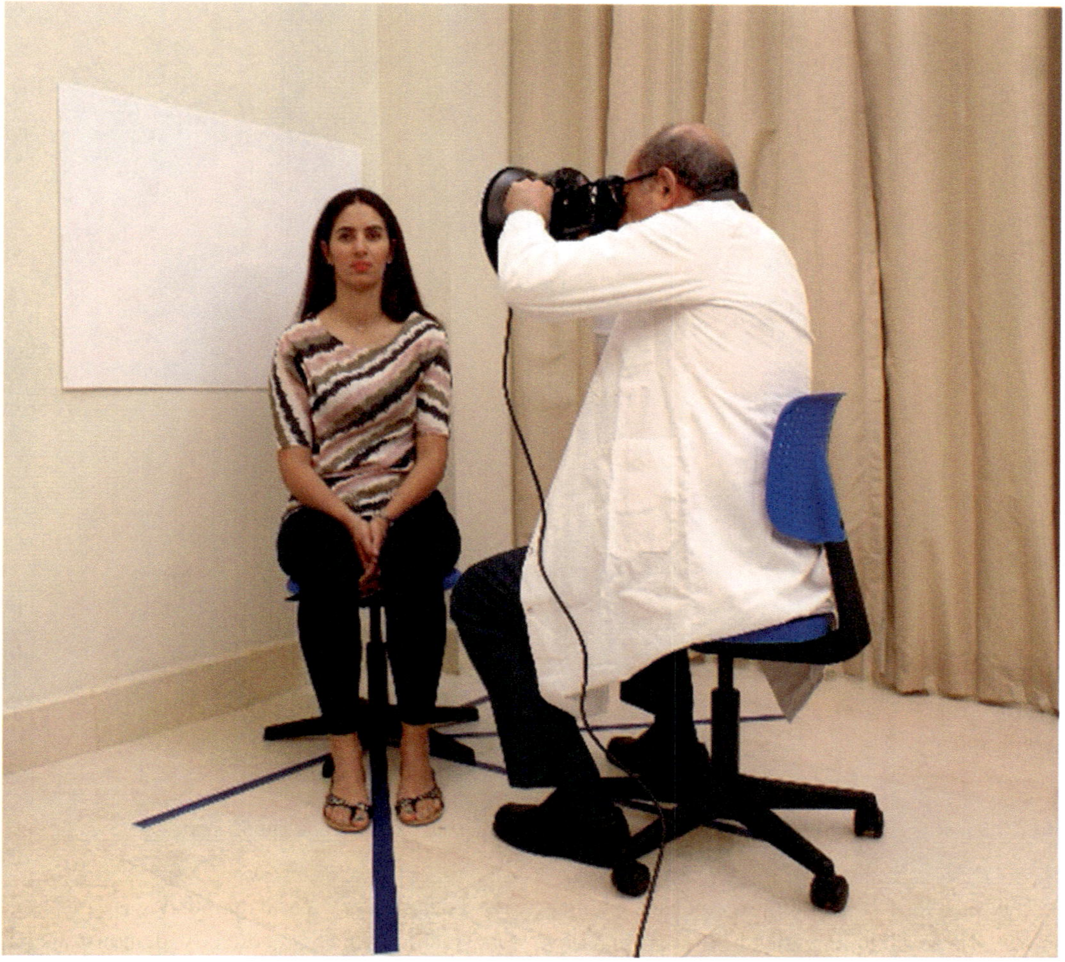

Fig. 13.34 Position of the patient and the photographer in taking the oblique views. The Patient's feet are straddling the right oblique line, photographer's feet are straddling the anterior line

On each side, right and left, a picture is taken with:

(a) The **nasal tip line** is **touching** the **external cheek line i.e cheek margin.**.
(b) The second picture is taken with the nasal tip line is in the **middle of the cheek** away from the cheek line.

13.2.3.5 Photographs Taken

1. Full face right and left oblique Photographs —nasal tip at mid cheek (Fig. 13.35).
2. Full face right and left oblique photographs— nasal tip at cheek margin (Fig. 13.36).
3. Middle third: right and left oblique mid cheek (Fig. 13.37).
4. Middle third: right and left oblique cheek margin (Fig. 13.38).

13.2.3.6 Clinical Assessment of the Photographs

The right and left oblique view photographs are placed beside each other for **direct comparison**. This is the best way to appreciate the aims and benefits of each view.

The Nasofacial Relationship

The oblique views are excellent in showing the aesthetic relationship between each sidewall of the nose and the rest of the face. Only part of the opposite cheek is hidden, otherwise the two sides

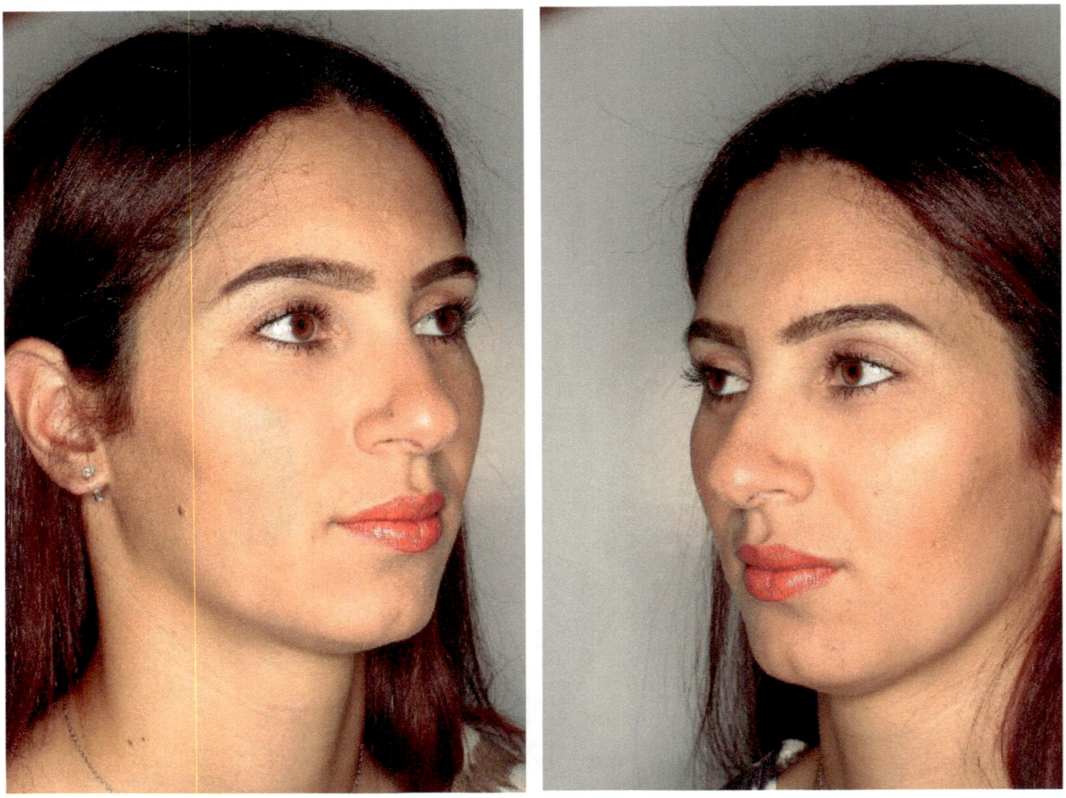

Fig. 13.35 Right and left full face oblique views. The tip of the nose is at the mid-cheek area

of the face are seen in these elegant oblique angles. These oblique angles have a special **elegant appearance** that has a considerable **aesthetic attraction**.

The Sidewall Profile

As a direct nasal sidewall view, this is the best angle that illustrates each of its anatomical components (Fig. 13.39).

The Osteocartilagenous Sidewall

The right and left sidewalls of the bony pyramid and midvault are directly seen as they start to emerge from the face, till they end up anteriorly by making the dorsum of the nose.

The Lower Lateral Cartilaginous Walls

The lateral crurae are directly demonstrated in the oblique views. The lateral sides of the middle crurae, i.e., their profiles are nicely seen.Domal projection, shape and size are compared on both sides of the nasal tip. The degree of domal separation as in bifid tip is observed and compared from the right and left oblique views .

The lateral crural sizes and shapes are almost always different on both sides.

The alae nasi

In no other views are the bodies of the alae nasi and the grooves around them as clearly seen as in these views. The shape, size and position of each

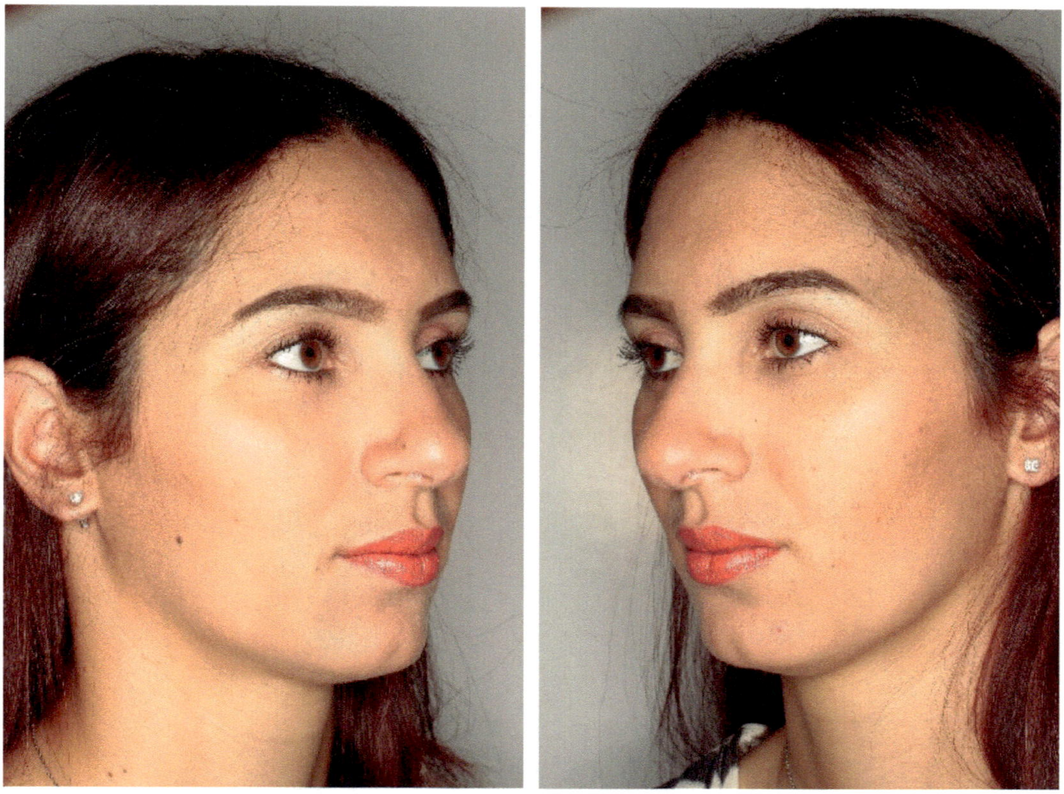

Fig. 13.36 Right and left full face oblique views. The tip of the nose is at the cheek margin

ala nasi, as well as the length and depth of the alar grooves, are clearly seen and appreciated.

Not only do they vary from one patient to another, but also from one side to the other in the same nose.

The Nasal Dorsum

The contribution of each sidewall to the bony and cartilaginous nasal dorsum is clearly seen.

The size, shape, extent and height of each side of the dorsum are best observed in the right and left oblique views.

The nasal hump may look prominently worse from one oblique side than the other. Oblique views taken **from the smaller side** are the ones that usually **look worse** as the ugliness of the larger and higher hump is viewed from its side so that it is totally exposed and projected against the opposite cheek. (Figs. 13.39 and 13.40)

Oblique views taken from the larger side, on the other hand, may not look so unpleasant, as the angle of the photographs is taken **directly** on the summit of the hump and not from the side. They look, therefore, shorter than they really are.

The Neighboring Structures

As well as the lateral nasal wall, it is quite useful to observe the neighboring structures:

Nasal Sills and Lateral Columellar Margins

The **nasal sills** and the **lateral columellar margins** are just seen off the alar margins. They are more apparently prominent in caudal septal deviations. The nasal sill is at a lower level on the deviated side.

Flat Triangles

The **flat triangles** are seen clearly in the oblique views. Both sides are compared in size, shape and position. The relation between them and their neighboring alae nasi, lateral and medial crura are observed.

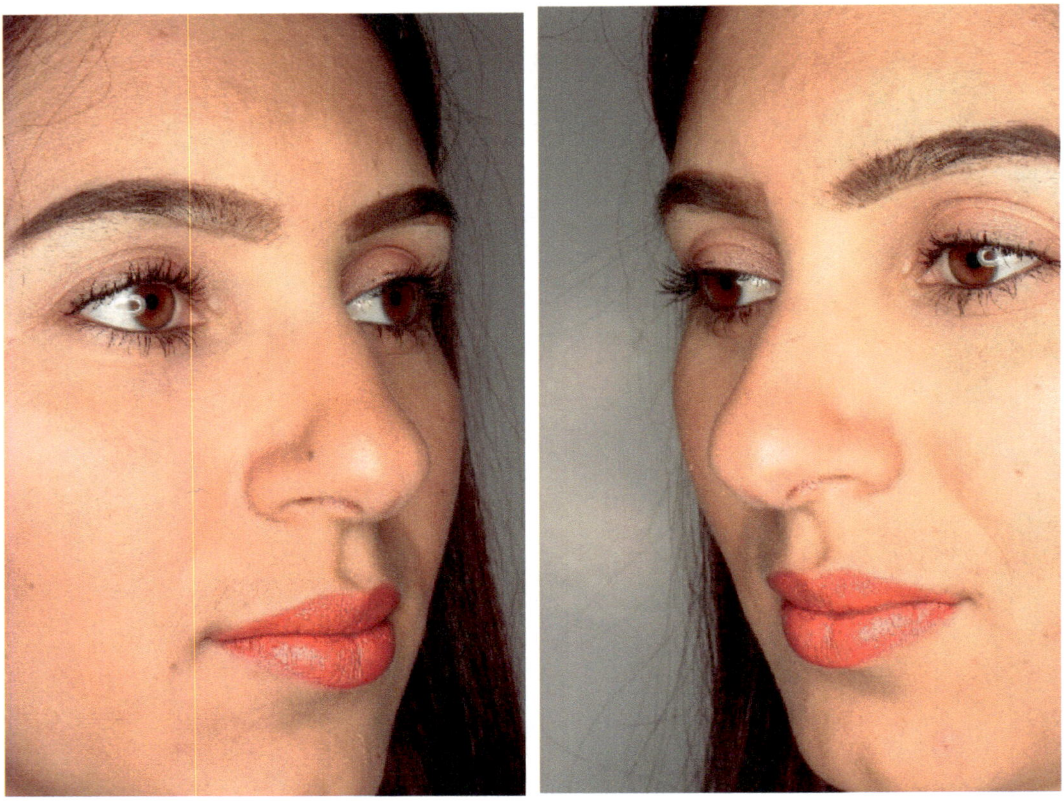

Fig. 13.37 Right and left oblique middle third. The tip of the nose is at the mid-cheek area

13.2.4 The Basal Views

These are the fourth and the last of the standard views. They are specialized views that are designed to show the nasal base. The nasal base includes the alar base, the nasal sills and the rim-sill folds, the flat triangles and the vestibular floors.

Other adjacent structures are also seen, e.g., the nasal tip, the upper lip and the cheeks. Unlike other standard views, the angle of the photographs to the nose is not commonly seen in our daily life.

13.2.4.1 The Setup

The Patient

- The Patient sits on his chair with his **face** and **chest** are looking **forwards** while his **feet** are **straddling the anterior line**.
- The Frankfort horizontal plane is observed.
- The **head** of the patient is **gradually tilted backwards** till both nasal apertures, the columella and the alae nasi are in a strictly vertical position, i.e., in the coronal plane. The nasal tip appears in the middle between the two eyebrows (Fig. 13.41).

If the patient cannot bend his head backwards, because of any neck problems, then the photographer's lens must come at a lower level so that the camera back is parallel to the floor of the nose.

The photographer

- The photographer sits on his chair with the camera setup directly above the anterior line. His feet are straddling the anterior line.
- The lens must be at the same horizontal level as the columella (Figs. 13.41 and 13.42).

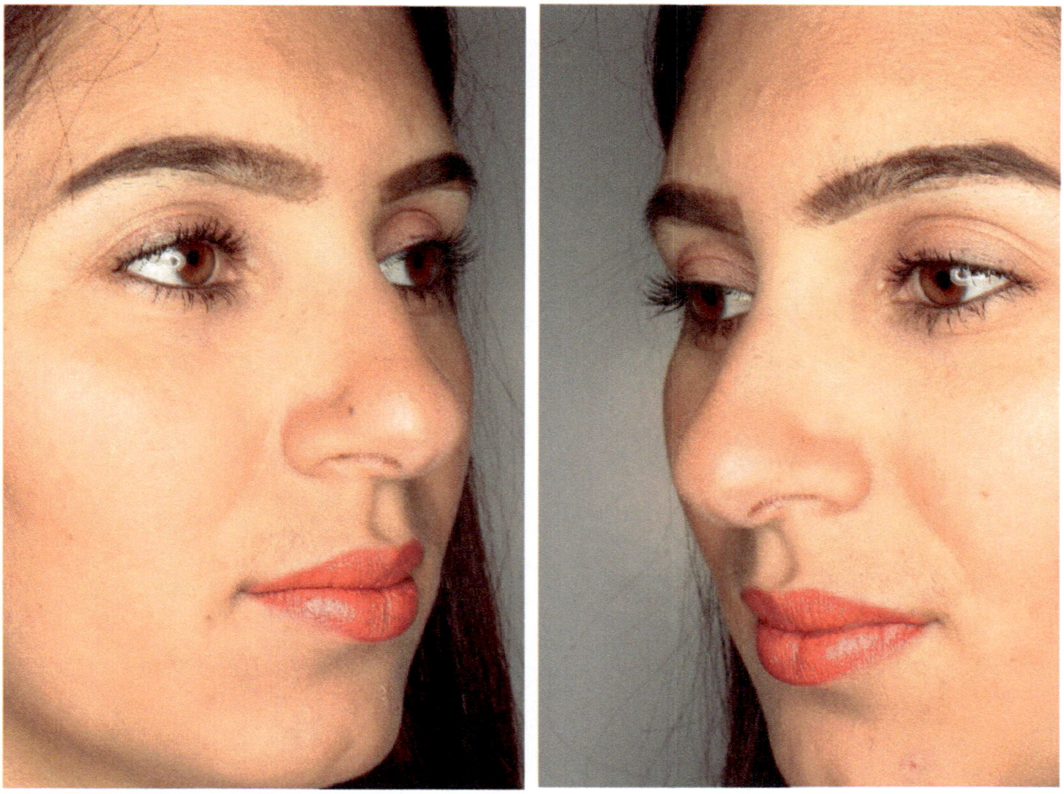

Fig. 13.38 Right and left oblique middle third. The tip of the nose is at the cheek margin

- The point of focus is the midpoint of the columella.

13.2.4.2 The Camera

(a) **Orientation** of the Camera back: **Horizontal,** i.e., landscape (Figs. 13.41 and 13.42).
(b) **Lens Focus**: at 40 cm (for author's equipment).
(c) **Lens Aperture**: adjusted according to the type of flash and the skin color of the patient.

Omicron system: f/9–f/13.
Alien Bees: f/14–f/30.

13.2.4.3 The Camera View

The views in these photographs extend from the lower lip to the top of the forehead. The two sides of the face, i.e., the cheeks and the two sides of the forehead are included.

The **horizontal level** of the patient's head is observed through three horizontal lines:

- The two eyebrows.
- The two nasal sills.
- The line between the two angles of the mouth. The transverse curved line of the upper lip is an additional guide. Having more than one horizontal guideline is because of the anatomical variations in the shapes and sizes of the eyebrows, nasal sills and lips.

13.2.4.4 Photographs Taken

Two basal view photographs are taken (Fig. 13.43).

Non-smiling Basal View

Smiling Basal View

13.2.4.5 Clinical Assessment of the Photographs

The smiling and non-smiling photographs are placed beside each other for direct comparison

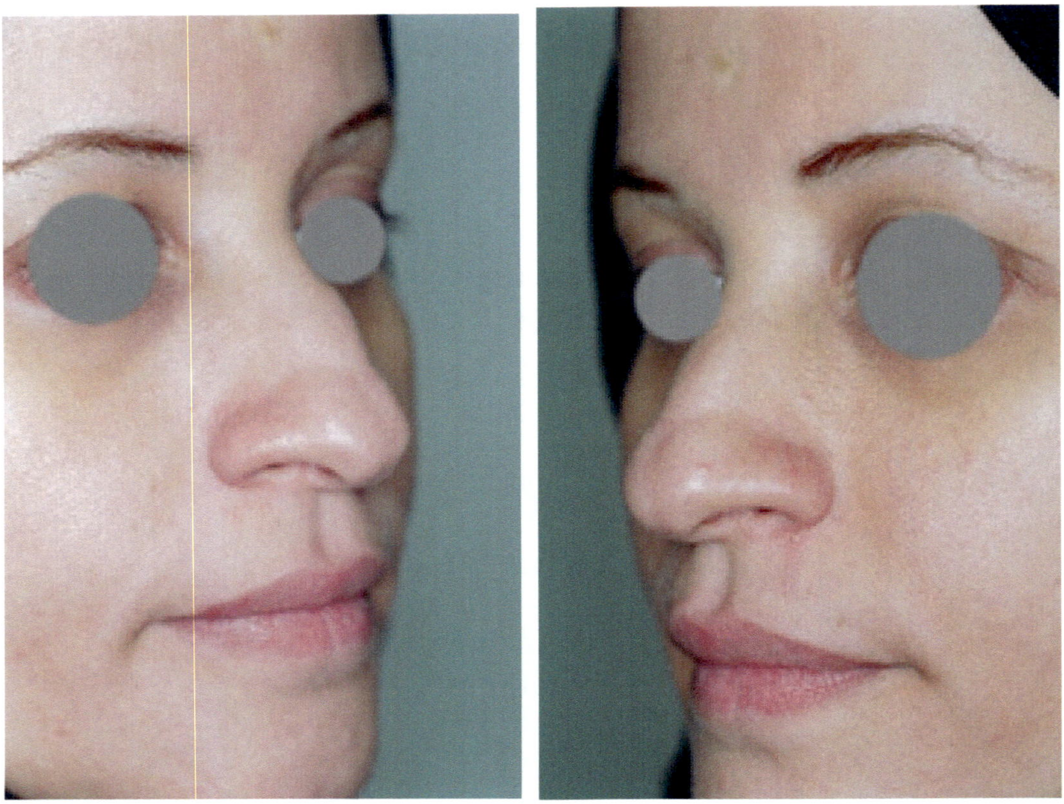

Fig. 13.39 The oblique view is excellent in showing: **a** the size and shape of the domes and lateral crurae. **b** Bifidity of the domes and domal projections. **c** Right sidewall of the nose is larger than the left sidewall. Nasal hump is higher on the right oblique view. **d** The superior and posterior alar grooves as well as the shapes of the alar bodies are well demonstrated. **e** Nasal sills, as well as the flat triangles, are clearly seen

and for the best appreciation of the aims and benefits of surgical planning.

The Nasofacial Relationships

The **sizes** of the **nasal floor** and the **alar base** are compared with the rest of the face. The effect of **smiling** is seen by observing the extent of widening of the alar base and stretching of the rim-sill folds.

- **The cheeks**: The **width** and the **height** of the right and left cheeks are observed. One side may be **high** and **narrow,** i.e., smaller in size as compared to the **wide** and **low** opposite side which is larger in size. This type of maxillary asymmetry reflects itself on the bony pyramid of the nose (Fig. 13.43).
- Smiling basal view may show the different sizes of the cheek balls denoting maxillary asymmetry and/or asymmetrical smile (Fig. 13.43).
- Both eyes, eyebrows and forehead are closely observed in the basal views. It is not uncommon to see the bilateral asymmetry in the shapes and sizes of these structures. This is to be considered during photography and in the pre-operative assessment.

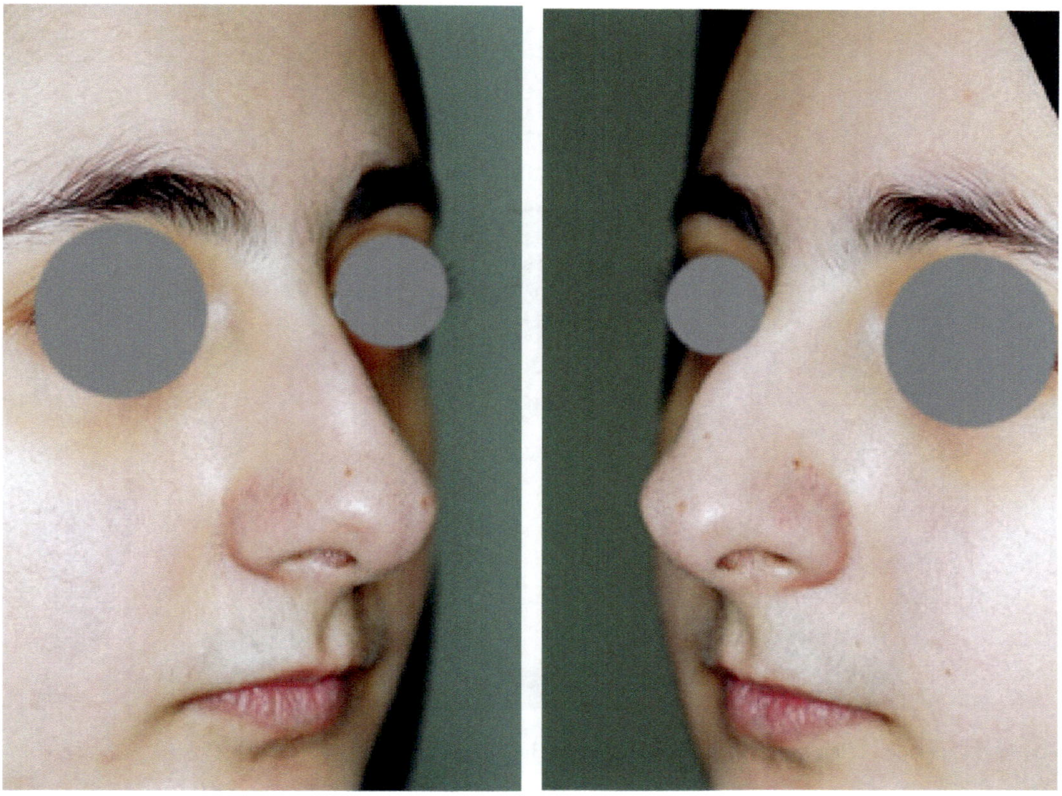

Fig. 13.40 The nasal hump is more prominent in the left oblique view. Bilateral maxillary asymmetry results in a larger left frontal process with the larger left sidewall of the nose

The Nasal Base

The main target of these views is to show the anatomical details of the nasal base that include the alar base, nasal sill bands, rim-sill folds and vestibular sidewalls. The inferior view of the nasal tip is also well demonstrated (Fig. 13.44).

The Nasal Openings

The **size** and **shape** of each nasal opening is seen in these views with a direct comparison between the two sides.

- **Oval-shaped openings** with long **axes** that point to the nasal tip are more aesthetic than the rounded ones.
- **The width** of the alar base, i.e., alar attachment to the upper lip is best seen in these views.
- **Smiling** maximally demonstrates the extent of the expansion of the alar base with the consequent effects on the widening of the nasal openings. The extent of elongation of the rim-sill folds is seen (Fig. 13.44).

The Nasal Tip

The basal views demonstrate the nasal tip from a unique inferior angle. They show the maximum projection of the domes.

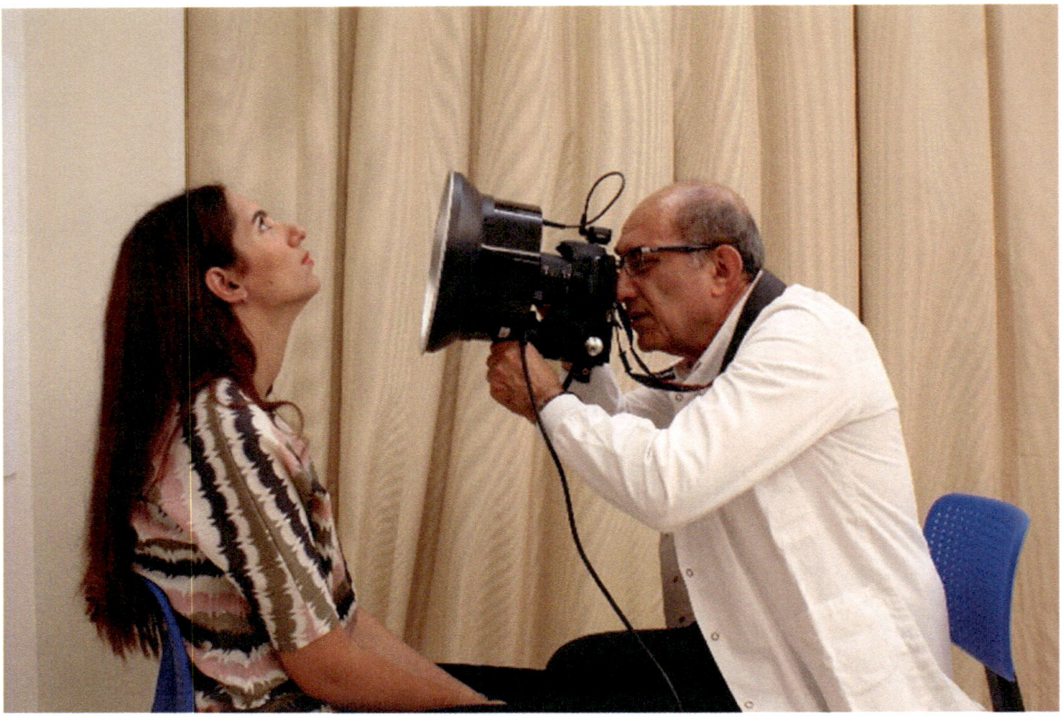

Fig. 13.41 Position of the patient and the photographer in taking the basal view

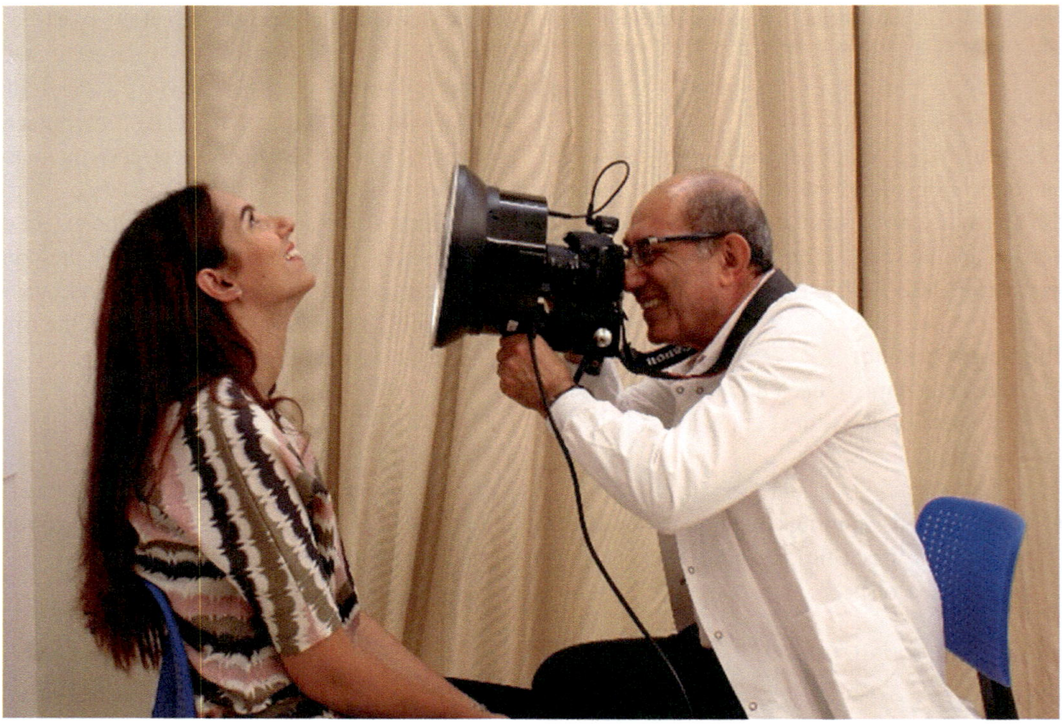

Fig. 13.42 Position of the patient and the photographer in taking the smiling basal view

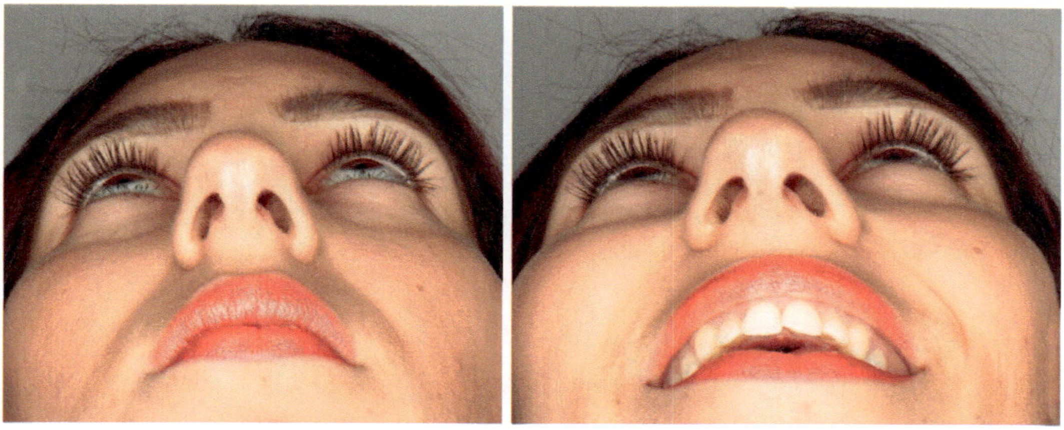

Fig. 13.43 Basal and smiling basal views. The anatomy of the columella, flat triangles, alar margins and nasal sill are clearly seen. Left cheek is larger than the right cheek due to maxillary osteotomies

- The **size**, **shape** and **position** of each dome is observed. Bilateral differences in projection and size of the domes is not uncommon. The extent of separation starts from simple grooving to more extreme bifidity.
- **Mobile tip**: Caudal septal **deviation** to one side, in a mobile tip, is best appreciated in the basal smiling view.

The Columella

The two external components of the columella are observed, i.e., the firm inferior borders of the medial crurae and the posterior soft fold of the skin (Fig. 13.45).

The following must be observed:

(a) Position: the columella should be vertically central between the two nasal openings.
(b) Length: The two medial crurae are the main contributors to the columellar length. The two crura may vary in length so that the left crus may be different in its length than the right crus.
(c) Thickness: The thickness of the columella, vary according to the thickness of the cartilage and the extent of their separation.
(d) The skin: the presence or absence of traumatic or surgical scars are observed.

Factors that affect the columellar position, thickness and shape:

i. Caudal septal deviation: the medial crus is pushed laterally, nasal sill inferiorly and the nasal opening is distorted on the deviated side.
ii. Medial crural prominences: they vary from one side to the other. They are affected by the caudal deviation of the septum.
iii. Traumatic or surgical scars.

The Flat Triangles

They are part of the nasal floor. Both triangles are seen at the same time. Sizes and shapes are clearly demonstrated and compared.

The Alae Nasi

- The **length** of each ala nasi, its curving **shape**, the **thickness** of its wall and finally the **alar lip angle** is best seen and studied from these views.

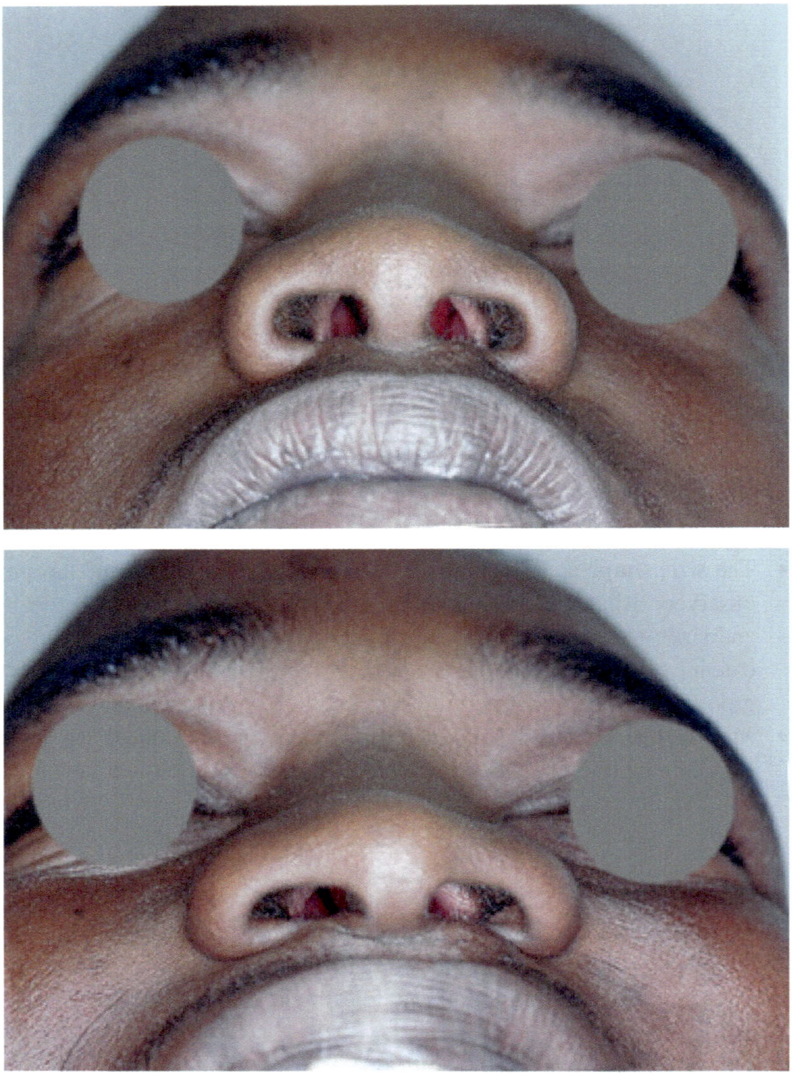

Fig. 13.44 Increased width of the nasal apertures on smiling. The transverse axis of the nasal opening is elongated. The nasal tip projection is reduced

- **The light reflex**: the light is clearly seen reflected from the **inferior margins of the alae** nasi in these views. They are the only margins that have an inferior direction. They reflect the light because the skin is thin, shiny, hairless and tightly adherent to the underlying tough fibrofatty tissues.

The Nasal Sills

The two nasal sills are part of the vestibular floor. The **prominence**, the **transverse level** and the relation between the nasal sills with the **columella** medially and the **rim-sill folds** laterally must all be carefully observed as they are well demonstrated in these views.

The **two nasal sills** should be at the **same horizontal level**. Levels of the nasal sills are disturbed by caudal septal deviation (Fig. 13.45).

The Rim-sill Folds

The inferior segments of the rim-sill folds are clearly seen in the basal views. Only part of the posterior segments is seen.The size, shape, position, thickness of the inferior segments and the extent of their expansion on smiling are all observed.

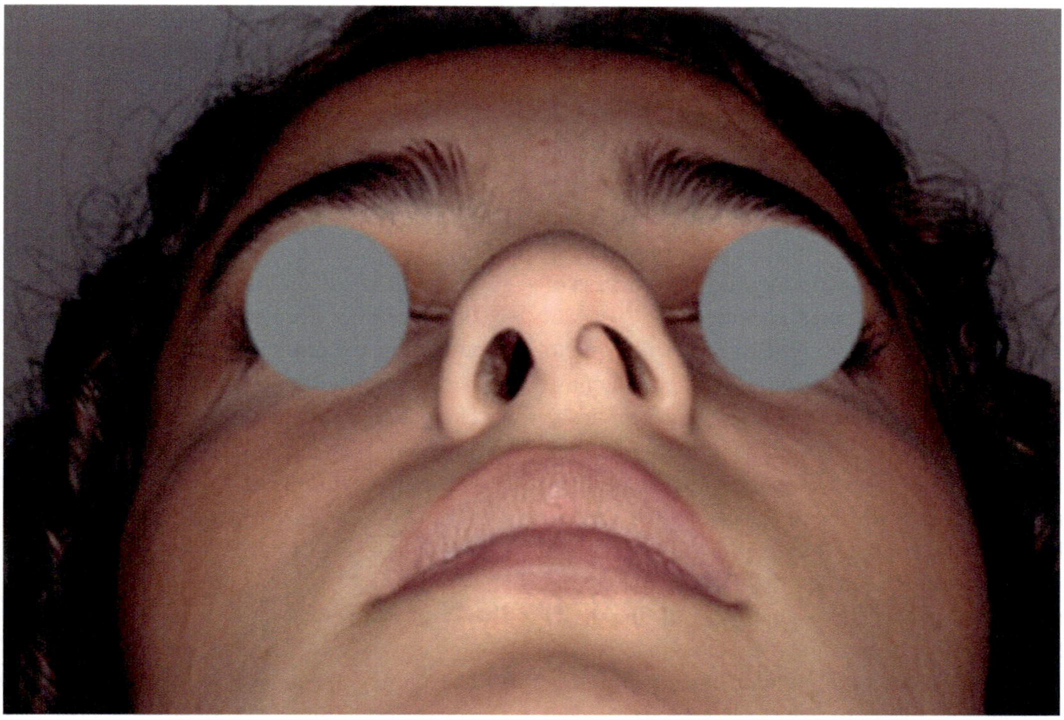

Fig. 13.45 Distorted columella due to left caudal dislocation of the cartilaginous septum. Nasal openings are apparently unequal

13.3 The Five Specialized Views

The standard views are inadequate in showing the detailed anatomy of specific areas like the bony pyramid, nasal dorsum, nasal apertures and cheeks. They need more specialized views.

Each of the newly suggested views is designed to visualize **one specific anatomical area**. Other **adjacent areas** can also be seen from these specialized angles which add more anatomical information to their original specialized view.

Although the Basal Views are standard views, they are specialized views for the base of the nose.

Therefore, there are Five Specialized views. Each view highlights a certain specific anatomical area. These views are:

- The Direct Dorsal Views.
- The Backward Tilting Views.
- The Basal Views.
- The Nasal Aperture Views.
- The Overhead Views.

All these views are taken at a **close-up range** of 40 cm. The **camera setup is the same** for all of these views. The position of the patient's head differs according to the area of interest. The **photographer's position** is always the **same** except for the overhead views.

In addition to the standard and the specialized views, the surgeon must be prepared to take **unconventional views** that are tailored for each individual unusual condition. The surgeon must have a predetermined plan on what to look for in each patient to have the best photographs that not only help him in the pre-operative evaluation, planning and decision- making, but also in the post-operative assessment, comparison and study.

13.3.1 The Direct Dorsal Views

The purpose of the Direct Dorsal views, as the name implies is to highlight the **nasal dorsum**. The nasal dorsum extends from the nasofrontal angle, the nasion, to the anterior septal angle **anatomically**, yet **photographically,** the nasal dorsum is considered from the nasofrontal angle superiorly to the nasal tip inferiorly, regardless of the anatomical structures underneath.

The nasal dorsum is 40–60 degrees **oblique** to the vertical or coronal plane. Looking at the nose from an anterior view, the nasal tip is seen to be more forwardly placed, and therefore, larger than the rest of the nose. Optically and photographically, the nasal tip, being closer to the camera lens, is falsely larger than the rest of the nose.

The anterior view of the face is not a true representation of the actual size of the nasal dorsum, nor is it large and clear enough to see the details of its structural components.

The best and only way to have a true visual assessment of the nasal dorsum is to bring about the whole dorsum to become **at the same distance** from the lens of the camera, i.e., to become strictly vertically positioned rather than oblique.

13.3.1.1 The Setup

The Patient:

- The patient sits on his chair with his face and chest looking forwards, while his feet are straddling the **anterior line**.
- The Frankfort horizontal plane is observed
- The patient is asked to gradually tilts his head down until the nasal dorsum is **strictly in the vertical position,** i.e., down 40–60 degrees, depending on the degree of forward nasal angulation (Fig. 13.46).

The Photographer

- The photographer sits on his chair with the camera setup directly above the anterior line. His feet are straddling the anterior line.

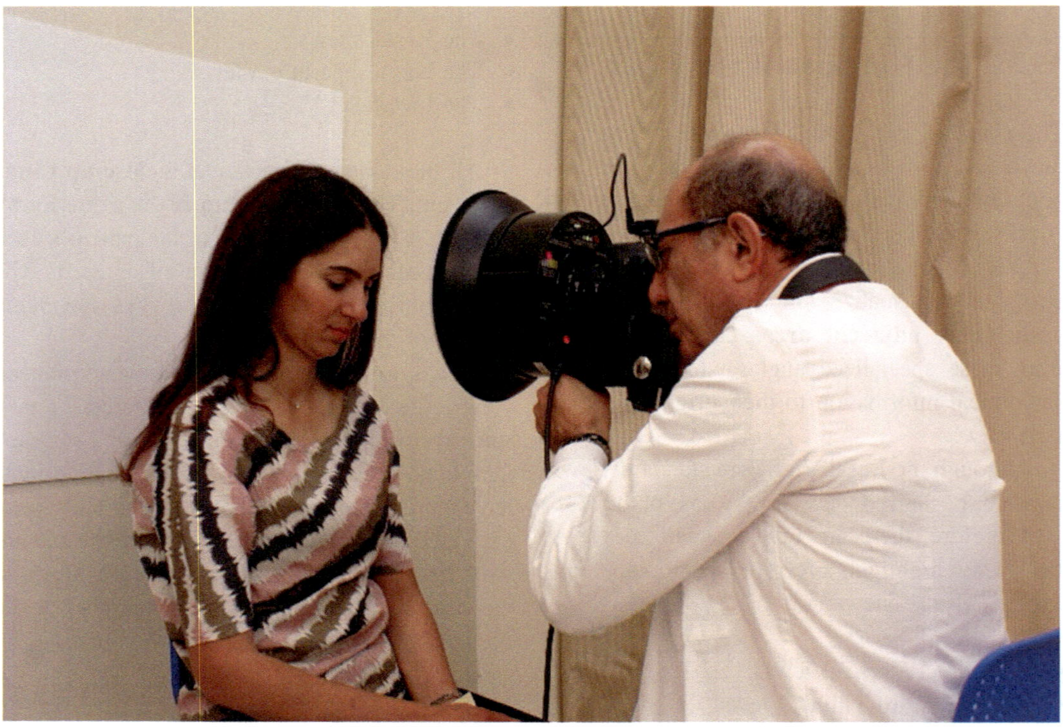

Fig. 13.46 Position of the patient and the photographer in taking the direct dorsal view

- The lens must be at the same horizontal level as the nose
- The point of focus is the midpoint of the nasal dorsum.

13.3.1.2 Camera Settings

(a) **The orientation** of the camera back is **horizontal,** i.e., **landscape** (Fig. 13.46).
(b) The **lens focus**: at 40 cm (for the Author's equipment).
(c) The **lens aperture**: Adjusted according to the type of **flash** and the **skin color** of the patient.

Omicron system: f/9– f/13.
Allien Bees: f/29–f/36.

13.3.1.3 The Camera View

The Direct Dorsal views include the face from the eyebrows downwards. They should include both eyes and cheeks.The horizontal level of the photograph must be observed by watching **the eyebrows**.

13.3.1.4 Photographs Taken

Two photographs are taken:

Non-smiling Direct Dorsal View (Fig. 13.47).

Smiling Direct Dorsal View (Fig. 13.48).

13.3.1.5 Clinical Assessment of the Photographs

The smiling and non-smiling photographs are placed **above** each other for direct comparison and for the best appreciation of the aims and benefits.

The Nasofacial Relationship

As well as the nasal dorsum, these are **direct views** of the cheeks, lower area of the forehead, eyes and the upper lip.

The Forehead

The junction of the forehead with the nose as they meet together is clearly seen.

The Cheeks

The size of each cheek, especially its width, is observed. The smaller cheek has a smaller size of the fat on smiling. The basal attachment of the sidewalls of the nose to the cheeks is directly seen on both sides and compared. This is another view where facial asymmetry is observed.

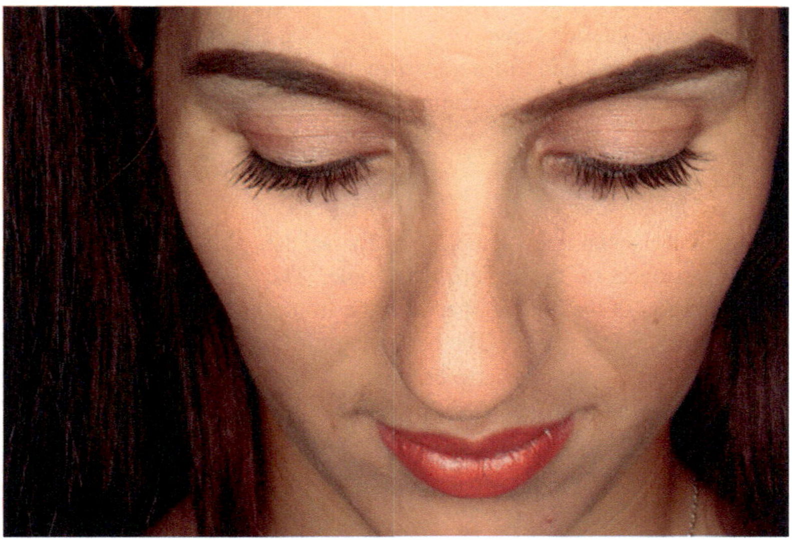

Fig. 13.47 Direct Dorsal View

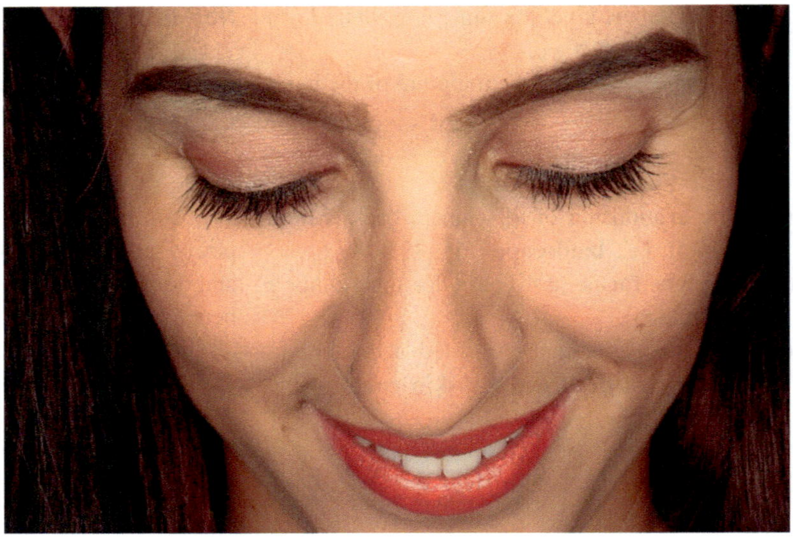

Fig. 13.48 Direct Dorsal Smiling View

The Nasal Features

These are the best views where the whole of the nasal dorsum is directly seen from the nasion down to the nasal tip. The anterior surfaces of the alae nasi are clearly seen.

The Nasal Dorsum

Photographically there are **three distinct components** of the dorsum that are carefully examined, viz., the nasofrontal angle (nasion), the osteocatilagenous dorsum and the nasal tip.

These are the only views that can give **the true length** of the nasal dorsum. The nose being shorter in the anterior view.

There is a direct and true comparison between **the sizes** of the different components of the dorsum.

The Nasion

The Direct Dorsal views look directly at the anterior surface of the nasofrontal angle. The exact location of the junction between the frontal and the nasal areas is seen. The beginning of the C– and inverted C-curve between them on both sides are seen and compared with each side.

The sidewalls of the root of the nose down to the inner cathi are closely observed.

The depth, thickness and irregularities are highlighted.

The Osteocartilagenous Dorsum

The anterior surface and sidewalls of the bony pyramid and midvault are evenly seen in their real sizes.The width, obliquity, deviations, elevations and irregularities are seen in their true proportionate sizes.

The Nasal Tip

The Direct Dorsal views offer a 90 degrees look at the anterior surfaces of the domes and lateral crura of the nasal tip.

The size, bulge and bifidity are clearly seen. One side may be larger or longer than the other.

Special attention must be paid to the width, height and shape of the tip.

- The Width:

The extent of lateral protrusion of the alae nasi is observed from the sides of nasal tip. The relative size and width of the nasal tip as compared to the alae nasi is seen. The depth of the superior alar grooves on both sides are observed and compared. The comparison was also made pre- and post-operatively.

- The Height

The extension of each dome and lateral crura is seen inferiorly and superiorly.The length of the tip inferiorly may vary bilaterally.The relationship between the domes and supra tip area is directly seen. Separation and semi-separation between the two areas is observed.

- The Shape

In some individuals, the domes and lateral crura appear as if they are imprinted through the skin and their exact shapes appear as an external anatomical model.

The Light Reflex

There is a line of light which is reflected from the anterior surface of the whole dorsum down to the nasal tip. The flash is directly aimed at 90 degrees to the nasal dorsum.The light reflex helps in showing the direction and the regularity of the nasal dorsum.

Irregularities, depressions, elevations and deviations are clearly seen.

A **broad irregular** dorsum **defuses the light** (Fig. 13.48), while a **slim smooth skinned** dorsum **reflects one clear line of light reflex,** i.e., narrow smooth dorsal curve reflects the light as compared to the wide irregular dorsal curve that defuses the light (Fig. 13.49).

The Alae Nasi

The anterior surfaces of the two wings of the alae nasi are seen on both sides of the nasal tip and can be compared in shapes, sizes and positions. The depth of the alar grooves is seen and compared.A large nasal tip may overshadow the alae nasi that appear as small protrusions on the sides with shallow alar grooves. Post operatively, after reduction of the nasal tip size, the alae nasi appear larger with deeper grooves.

The Effects of Smiling

Smiling in the Direct Dorsal views affects two areas:

i. The alae nasi expand laterally.
ii. The nasal tip moves downwards in a mobile tip.

13.3.2 The Backward Tilting Views

By the backward tilting views, we mean to look at the nose and face from below as the head is gradually tilted backward.

These are unique angles where the nose appears **as near as possible to a three dimensional structure** in a two dimensional photograph. The two sidewalls, the dorsum, the nasal tip and the nasal apertures can all be seen in these views.

13.3.2.1 The Setup

The Patient

- The patient sits on his chair with his face and chest looking forwards, while his feet are straddling the **anterior line**.
- The Frankfort horizontal plane is observed.
- The patient's head is gradually tilted backwards in order to have an inferior view of the nose and face (Fig. 13.50).

With the gradual backward tilting, both the nasal openings will come into view, as well as the nasal tip and the sidewalls of the nose. The patient continues to tilt his head backwards till just before the nasofrontal angle (nasion) disappears from view (Fig. 13.51).

The Photographer

- The photographer sits on his chair with the camera setup directly above the **anterior line**.
- The lens must be at the same horizontal level as the nasal tip.
- The point of focus is the midpoint of the nasal dorsum.

13.3.2.2 Camera Settings

The orientation of the camera back is **horizontal,** i.e., **landscape** (Figs. 13.50 and 13.51).

The lens focus: at 40 cm (for the author's equipment).

The **lens aperture**: adjusted according to the type of flash and the skin color of the patient.

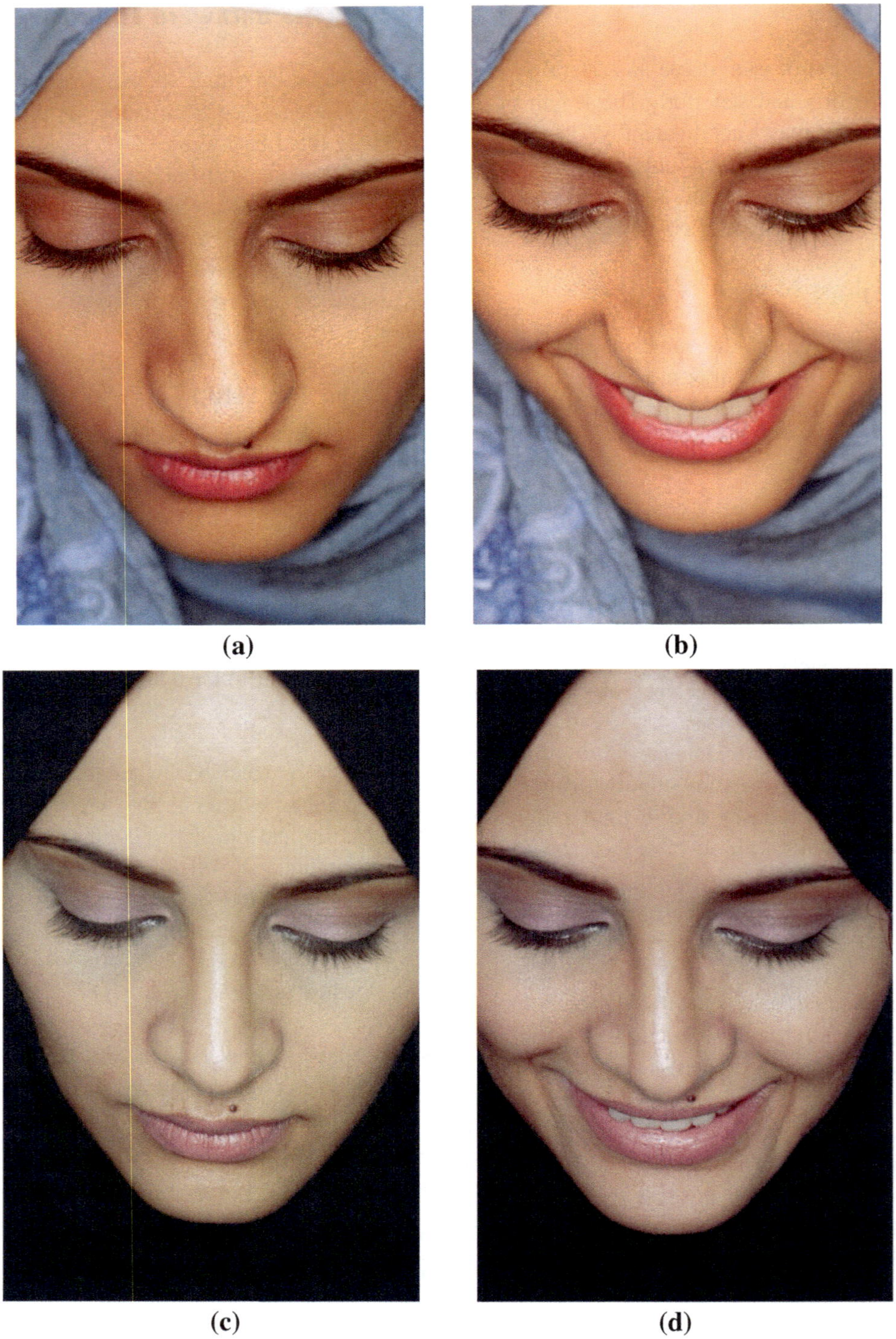

Fig. 13.49 The right base of the bony pyramid is wider than the left and the nose is slightly deviated to the left due to maxillary asymmetry. The large fronto-lateral walls are over shadowing the alae nasi. Mobile tip, the tip moves down on smiling. The dorsal light reflex is diffused pre-operatively (**a** and **b**) The light reflex is a straight line post-operatively (**c** and **d**)

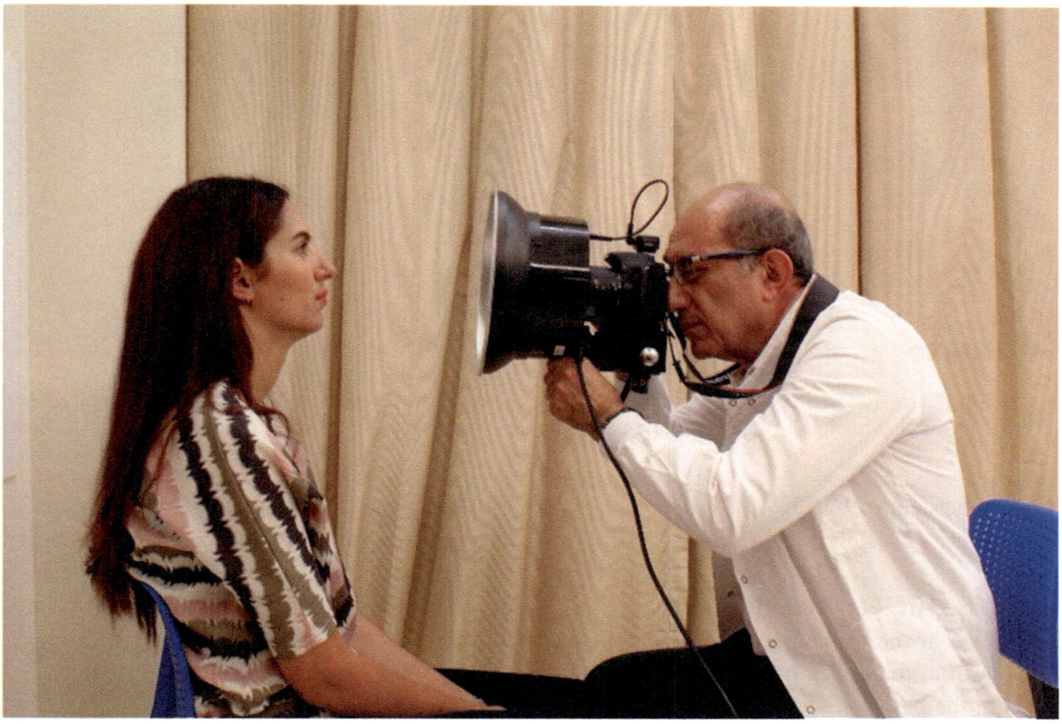

Fig. 13.50 Position of the patient and the photographer in taking the backward tilting view

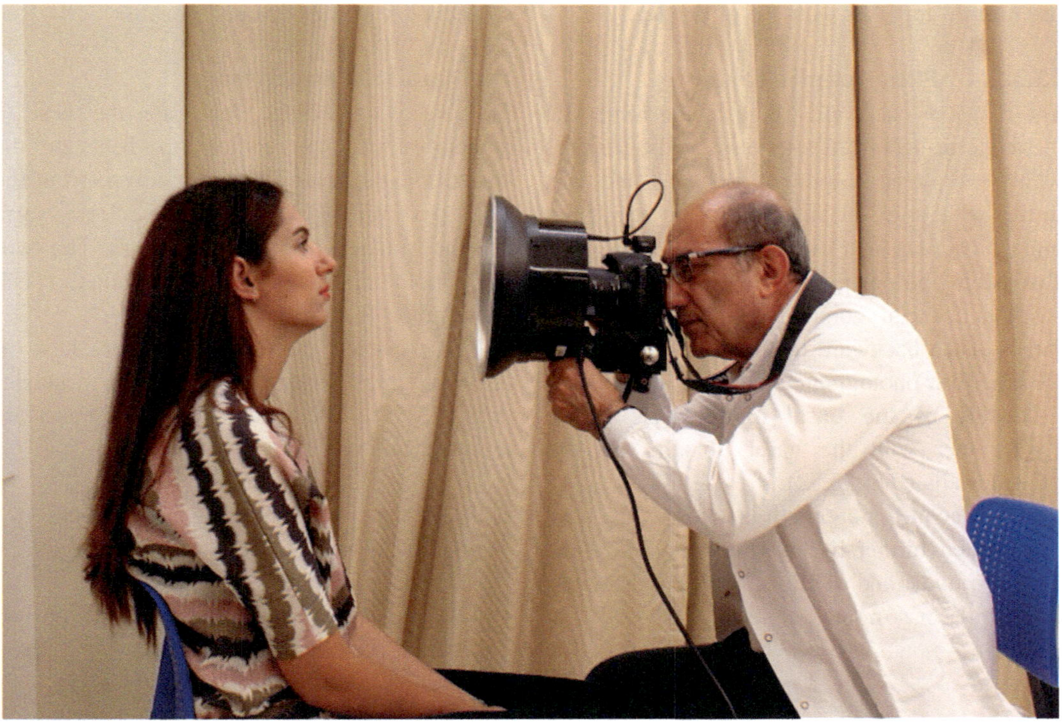

Fig. 13.51 Position of the patient and the photographer in taking the steeper backward tilting view

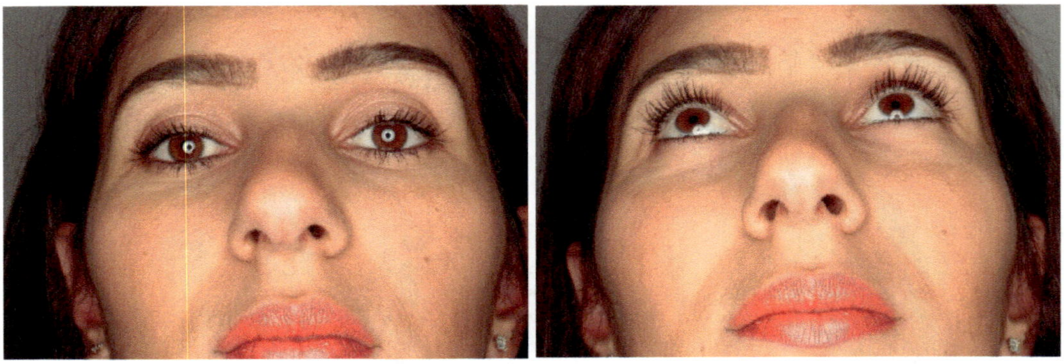

Fig. 13.52 Backward and Steeper Backward Tilting Views. These views demonstrate the following: The light reflex of the nasal tip and flat triangles. Anatomy of the nasal apertures, nasal dorsum, sidewalls of the nose and both cheeks

Omicron system: f/9–f/13.
Alien Bees: f/29–f/36.

13.3.2.3 The Camera View

The views in these photographs should include the area from the **lower lip to the eyebrows**.

As in the basal views, the **horizontal level** of the patient's head is observed through the three horizontal lines, i.e., the **eyebrows**, the **two nasal sills** and the **line between the angles of the mouth**, together with the **upper lip**.

13.3.2.4 Photographs Taken

The range of backward tilting of the head, i.e., the angle of backward rotation is wide. It varies with the different anatomy of each nose and face. In this wide angle of backward tilting, two photographs are taken at two consequent steps. This **Two step photography** is needed to show the nasal and facial contours from two different stages of the backward rotation of the head.

(a) The **first** photograph is taken **as soon as the inside of the nasal openings** is shown together with the nasal dorsum and the sidewalls (Fig. 13.52).
(b) The **second** photograph is taken as the head is tilted further backwards, **just before the disappearance of the nasion** off the view, i.e., the nasofrontal angle (Fig. 13.52).

Three-step photography is occasionally needed in case of multiple combined abnormalities of the nose and cheeks, e.g., large nasal hump severe crookedness and extreme bilateral maxillary asymmetry.

13.3.2.5 Clinical Assessment of Photographs

The two-step photographs are placed one above the other for direct comparison for the best appreciation of the aims and benefits.

The Nasofacial Relationship

The backward tilting views are the best in demonstrating the relationship between the **cheeks** and the **nose**. The **commencement of the bony pyramid** from the cheeks is clearly seen, i.e., the frontal processes of zygomas. The two-step photographs illustrate the gradual cheek contribution from below upwards.

These views, therefore, are the best in demonstrating **bilateral maxillary asymmetries** (Fig. 13.53). The two-step photographs are excellent in showing:

- The contours of the two cheeks from two different degrees of head rotation. Asymmetrical smile is seen in these views.
- The sidewalls of the bony pyramid from two different degrees of head rotation.

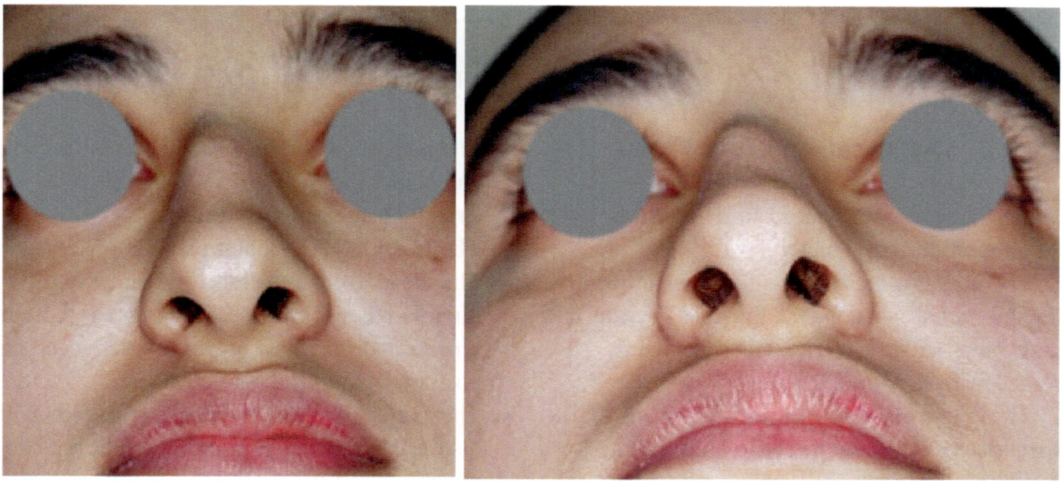

Fig. 13.53 In bilateral Maxillary asymmetry, the left maxilla is wide and low while the right maxilla is narrow and high (in consideration of the view). The left frontal process is larger than the right, leading to, right deviation of the bony pyramid and a prominent hump. The beginning and the end of the osseocartilagenous hump are well demonstrated in these views

In these cases, the cheeks are **narrow and high** on one side, while **wide and low** on the other side. The **bony pyramid** is **deviated toward the smaller cheek bone**.

The Nasal Features

The two-step photographs are great in showing the two sides of the nose simultaneously from below upwards (Figs. 13.52 and 13.53).

The Nasal Apertures:

i. These are **the only views** where the **vestibular floor**, **vestibular sidewalls** and **posterior vestibular margins** are seen in most cases.
ii. The columella, nasal sills, rim-sill folds, alar margins and the flat triangles can be seen and compared on both sides from these angles.
iii. Aesthetic consequences of caudal septal dislocation:

- Distortion of the **flat triangle** in the contralateral side of caudal septal deviation are clearly seen in the backward tilting views.
- The **nasal sill** is pushed down on the same side of the caudal deviation.
- The **medial crus** is pushed laterally and the **nasal opening** is distorted and may look apparently smaller than on the dislocated side of the septum.

The Nasal Dorsum

- These are unique views of the nasal dorsum from the nasion to the nasal tip.
- Irregularities, deviation, crookedness, depressions elevations and humps are seen from below upwards on both sides simultaneously.
- The height, the deviation and the extent of a **nasal hump** is seen from its exact beginning inferiorly till it ends superiorly. The depth and extent of any **depression** is clearly observed in these views.
- The nasal tip and its relation with the supra tip area, i.e., elevation or depression are clearly observed in these views.

The Sidewalls of the Nose

The **whole surfaces** of the two nasal sidewalls are simultaneously seen from below upwards as they emerge from the face. Deviations, crookedness and irregularities are clearly demonstrated. Bilateral maxillary asymmetries are best observed in these views.

13.3.3 The Nasal Aperture Views

These views are introduced to demonstrate each nasal aperture individually.

The need for these views becomes imperative for the increasing demand for **nasal septal** and **alar base** surgeries. The latter is mainly concerned with the rim-sill folds.

These are **the most important of all of the specialized views** for the following reasons:

- They are the only views that look directly at the nasal apertures.
- There are many types of highly specialized surgeries that may take place in this area, e.g., caudal septal and alar base surgeries.

The **membranous septum** and the **rim-sill folds** are the main targets in these views.

13.3.3.1 The setup

The Patient

- The patient sits on his chair with his face and chest looking forwards, while his feet are straddling the **anterior line**.
- The Frankfort horizontal plane is observed.
- The head of the patient is gradually **tilted backwards** till both nasal apertures, the columella and alea nasi are in a strictly vertical position, i.e., at the coronal plane.
- The patient is then **gradually rotated**, with his chair, to one side, right then left, until **the nasal aperture is directly facing the lens** (Fig. 13.54).

The angle of rotation **varies** from one patient and from one nostril to the other. This depends mainly on the degree of nasal flare, i.e., the upward, backward and lateral position of the alae nasi.The **nasal tip** is seen projected against the **opposite eye** (Fig. 13.55).

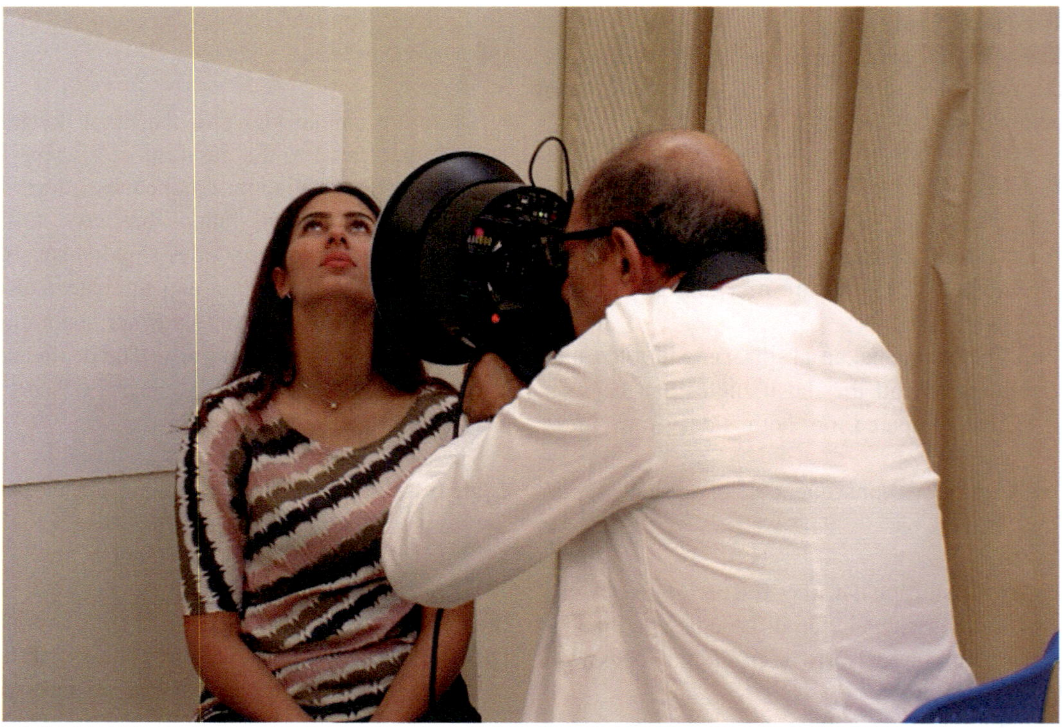

Fig. 13.54 Position of the patient and the photographer in taking the left nasal aperture view

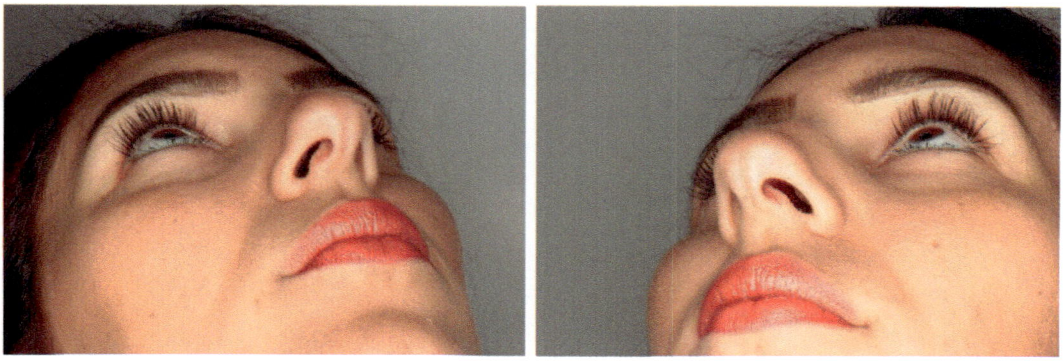

Fig. 13.55 Right and left nasal aperture views. This view demonstrates the light reflex of the alar margins and margins of the flat triangles. The columellar bifidity, lateral crural prominences and the nasal sills are clearly seen

The Photographer

- The photographer sits on his chair with the camera setup directly above **the anterior line**.
- The lens must be at the same horizontal level as the nasal aperture (Fig. 13.54).
- The plane of focus is the margin of the nasal aperture.

13.3.3.2 Camera Settings

- **The orientation** of the camera back is **Horizontal,** i.e., **landscape** (Fig. 13.54).
- The **lens focus**: at **40 cm** (for the author's equipment).
- The **lens aperture**: adjusted according to the type of flash and the skin color of the patient.

Omicron system: f/9 – f/13.
Alien Bees: f/29 – f/36.

13.3.3.3 The Camera View

The view in these photographs includes the nasal aperture of one side of the nose with its walls, the nasal tip which is projected against the opposite eye, the lips, the cheek, the eye, the sidewall of the nose and the forehead of the same side of the nose.

13.3.3.4 Photographs Taken

Four photographs are taken:

1. Right Nasal Aperture (Fig. 13.55).
2. Left Nasal Aperture (Fig. 13.55).
3. Right Rim-sill test.
4. Left Rim-sill test (Fig. 13.56).

It is to be noted that the **angle** for the right nasal aperture view may be different from the left, therefore, the projection of the nose against the opposite eye may not be the same on each side (Fig. 13.57).

13.3.3.5 Clinical Assessment of the Photographs

These views demonstrate the details of the nasal apertures as well as their adjacent areas.

The right and left photographs are placed beside each other for direct comparison and for the best appreciation of the aims and benefits.

The Nasofacial Relationship:

The **cheek** and the **sidewall of the nose** are seen and compared from the right and left sides.

Irregularities, depressions, bruises and fractures individually and uniquely are observed from these angled views to the sidewalls.

Bilateral asymmetrical differences in the cheeks with their contributions to the bony pyramid and dorsum are observed.

The lips, eyes, eyebrows and forehead are also seen.

Anatomical Structures of the Nasal Aperture:

The rim-sill folds and the membranous septum are two fundamentally important areas in rhinoplasty for which these views are specially and

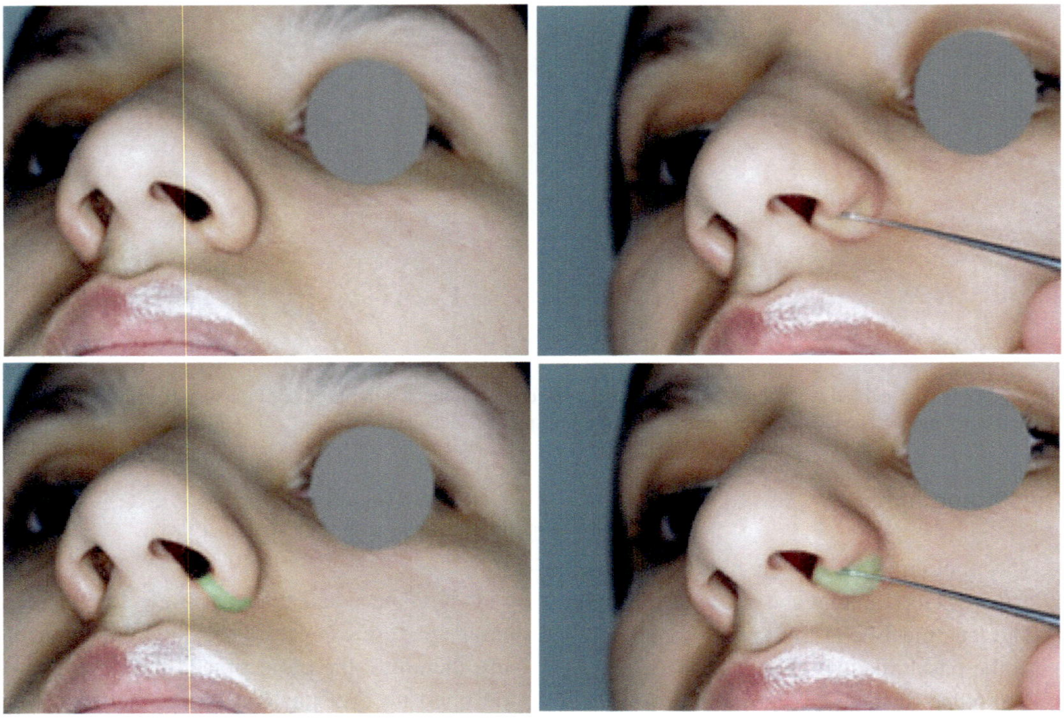

Fig. 13.56 Left rim-sill test in a thick skinned nose demonstrating the inferior and posterior segments of the left rim-sill fold

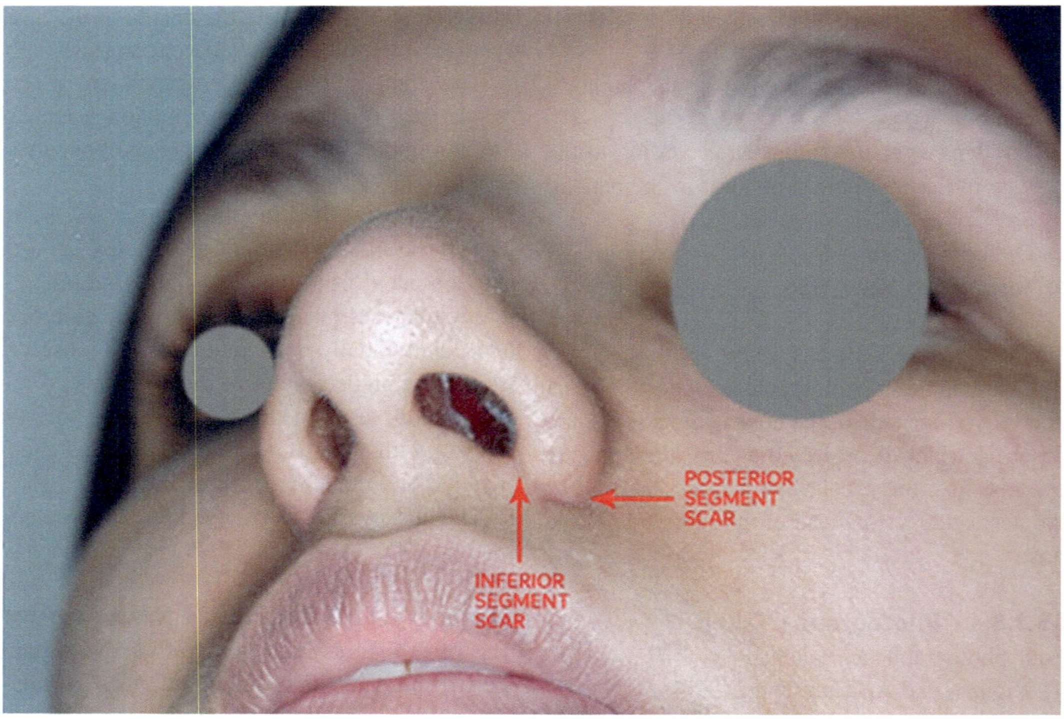

Fig. 13.57 The inferior and posterior segments of the left rim-sill fold are excised

specifically introduced. The angle of the photographs and the close-up magnification helps in demonstrating the detailed anatomy of each of these areas

The Rim-Sill Folds

Both the posterior and inferior segments of the rim-sill folds are best seen and studied in these views. The rim-sill tests help in identifying the limits of the folds, i.e., the locations of the alar margins and nasal sills (Fig. 13.56).

The membranous Septum

These are the only views that show the membranous septum from the right and left sides.

These are especially useful in cases of caudal septal deviation.Minimal caudal deviation may only be spotted by comparing the right and the left views of the membranous septum.Even the slightest deviation of the caudal margin off the midline will drive the whole of the membranous septum to the same side.As the deviation increases, the **medial crus** of the lower lateral cartilage is driven into the aperture space.In more severe deviations, the caudal margin itself is seen through the nasal opening as a free margin.

In these cases, the membranous septum either partially or totally **disappears** from the aperture view photographs of the **opposite side** as the caudal and membranous septum are driven away from the midline.

Other Nasal Structures

- **The Nasal openings**: these are more **direct views** of the nasal openings than the basal views. The true shape and size of each nasal opening with a direct comparison between the two sides are well demonstrated.

The two sides may be naturally different in size and/or shape or secondary to previous surgery or caudal septal deviation.

- **The Nasal Sill:**

The **whole course** of the **nasal sill band** is seen from this angle of photography (Fig. 13.55). It becomes more prominently clear if the patient is asked to **pull down his upper lip and hold it** using his lower lip. The nasal sill band is straightened, more prominent and is clearly seen as it continues from the floor of the nose to the columella around the posterior, then superior margins of the medial crus, i.e., the full course of the sill band.

The upper lateral fold of the nasal sill, if present, can also be seen.

- **The light reflex**: light may be seen reflected from all margins of the alar nasi, nasal sill and lateral columellar margin.
- **The Flat Triangle**: its actual size and shape is seen from this **direct angle of photography**. The two sides can be directly compared.
- **The Nasal Tip**: each dome is directly seen above the flat triangle on each side. The projection of the opposite dome is also seen.
- The **columella** is observed for its thickness, position, bifidity and scars.

13.3.4 The Overhead Views

The overhead views are looking at the nose from above and slightly anterior angle. They demonstrate the anatomy of the nasal dorsum and how the nose relates to both cheeks.

13.3.4.1 The Setup

The patient

- The patient sits on his chair and is rotated 90 degrees so that his feet are straddling the transverse line. His face and chest are along the transverse line (Fig. 13.58).
- The Frankfort horizontal plane is observed
- The patient is asked to slightly slide down in his seat
- The head of the patient is then gradually tilted backwards till the nasal tip, dorsum and finally the nasofrontal angle comes into view.
- The degree of backward tilting depends on the forward nasal angulation and the depth of the nasofrontal angle.

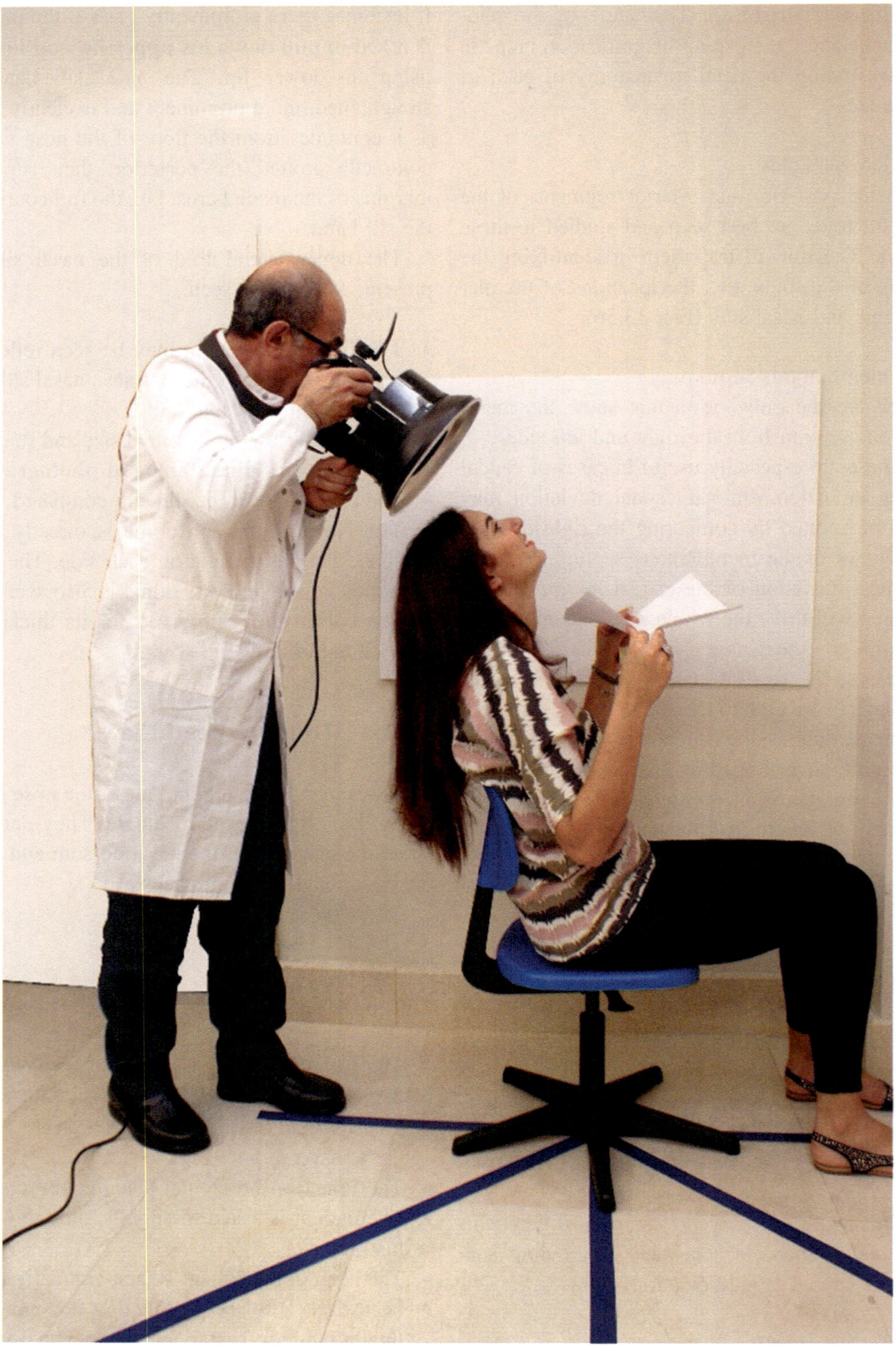

Fig. 13.58 Position of the patient and the photographer in taking the overhead views. The photographer's and patient's feet are straddling the transverse line. Note that the white paper held by the patient is used as a standard background for the overhead views

The Photographer

- The photographer stands behind the patient with his feet straddling the transverse line (Fig. 13.58).
- The camera set is held above the patient's head.
- The camera lens is at a superior angle from the horizontal line. The angle varies according to the degree of the backward tilting and the depth of the nasofrontal angle.
- The point of focus is the **midpoint** of the nasal dorsum.

It is possible to demonstrate these views if the **patient's head** is turned downwards, while the **photographer** is sitting in front of the patient. **Both** are facing each other at the **anterior line** with their feet straddling it.

The disadvantage of this method is that the **cheeks tend to sag down** with gravity, especially in older individuals. This distorts the anatomy of the cheeks and the sidewalls of the bony pyramid.

13.3.4.2 Camera Settings

The orientation of the camera back is **horizontal,** i.e., landscape (Fig. 13.58).

The **lens focus**: at 40 cm (for the author's equipment)

The **lens aperture**: adjusted according to the type of flash and the skin color of the patient.

Omicron system: f/9 – f/13.
Alien Bees: f/29 – f/36.

13.3.4.3 The Camera View

The views include the eyebrows, the nose from the nasofrontal angle to the tip, the eyes and cheeks. Parts of the chin may come into view.

The horizontal level of the patient's head is observed by leveling the **eyebrows** (Figs. 13.59 and 13.60)

13.3.4.4 Photographs Taken

Two photographs are taken.

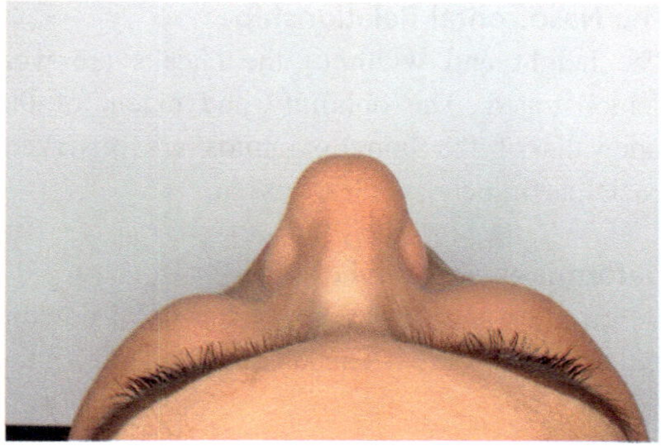

Fig. 13.59 Overhead View, the nose and cheeks are considerably compressed and shorter. The height and width of both cheeks are compared

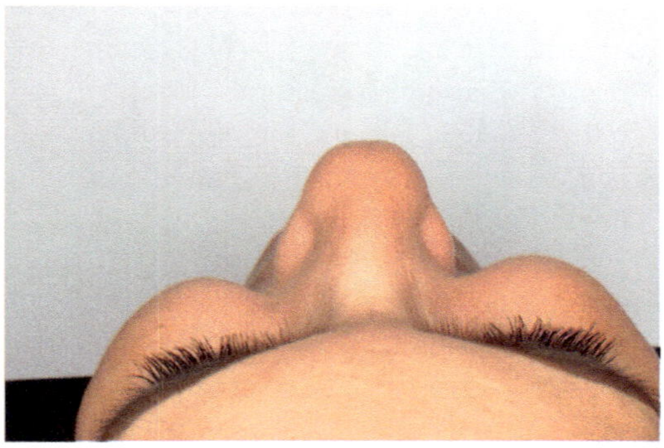

Fig. 13.60 Overhead Smiling View. Note that the higher right cheeks are compared to the left. The right cheek ball is bigger than the left on smiling

Non-smiling

Standard **non-smiling** backward tilting view (Fig. 13.59).

Smiling

Smiling backward tilting view (Fig. 13.60).

13.3.4.5 Clinical assessment of the photographs

The two photographs are placed **above** each other for direct comparison and the best appreciation of the aims and benefits.

The nose and cheeks in these photographs look **considerably shorter** than their real length. This has the advantage of **intensifying** any abnormality or deformity.

The Nasofrontal Relationship

The height and width of the cheeks are well demonstrated. The obliquity and extent of the sidewalls of the bony pyramids are observed. Facial asymmetry is clearly seen.

Deformities and Deviations

Deformities and deviations of the nasal dorsum and tip are observed. The lateral extensions of the alae nasi and the effect of smiling on alar widening and tip movement are observed.

The sidewalls of the bony pyramid are seen at their attachments to the face. The two sides are compared in size, obliquity and deviation.

The Workflow of Photography Taking, Filing and Displaying

14

Abstract

Photography plays a pivotal role in Rhinoplasty. It is essential for pre-operative diagnosis, intraoperative guidance, post-operative assessment, long-term feedback, academic studies and research work. The whole process of photography must be well organized in a simple stereotyped routine. Establishing this routine reduces the time taken for the photographic procedures and avoids missing any of the standard, specialized and other views. It is important to **take all the views in every single case**, no matter how simple it is. It is not uncommon to have to go through a totally unplanned procedure due to unexpected findings, changes or mishaps during an apparently straight forward Rhinoplasty. The session of taking photographs must be **accurate** and **brisk**. The **simple setup** and the **specific order** of taking the photographs have made it a fast routine. Photographs are then **transferred into computer** to be saved. One or more safe **backup systems** must be arranged. Photographs may then be retrieved and reviewed.

Keywords

The work flow of photography · Taking · Filing and displaying

14.1 Introduction

Photography plays a pivotal role in Rhinoplasty. It is essential for pre-operative diagnosis, intraoperative guidance, post-operative assessment, long-term feedback, academic studies and research work. The whole process of photography must be well organized in a simple stereotyped routine. Establishing this routine reduces the time taken for the photographic procedures and avoids missing any of the standard, specialized and other views. It is important to **take all the views in every single case**, no matter how simple it is. It is not uncommon to have to go through a totally unplanned procedure due to unexpected findings, changes or mishaps during an apparently straight forward Rhinoplasty. The session of taking photographs must be **accurate** and **brisk**. The **simple setup** and the **specific order** of taking the photographs have made it a fast routine. Photographs are then **transferred into computer** to be saved. One or more safe **backup systems** must be arranged. Photographs may then be retrieved and reviewed.

The suggested method of **photographic display** has made it easy to study the **photographs in a glance**.

M. H. A. Shafy, *Innovations in Rhinoplasty*,
https://doi.org/10.1007/978-3-030-94573-2_14

14.2 Photographic Workflow

The process of photography must carefully be taken care of for the sake of better documentation, studying and finally the short and long-term educational and research benefits.

Photographic workflow goes through the following chronological phases.

14.2.1 Phase I: Taking the Photographs

Photographs are taken in a specific order, that is **stereotyped**, **simple** and **fast**.

The Order of Taking Photographs

The order of taking photographs that is suggested below makes the photographic session quick and easy in such a way that no single view is missed. Experienced photographers may prefer to use their own routine.

1. **From Left to Right complete half circle**

Full face 60 cm Photographs are taken in the following order:

i. Left lateral views—non-smiling then smiling: two photos.
ii. Left oblique views cheek margin then mid cheek: two photos.
iii. Frontal views, non-smiling then smiling: two photos.
iv. Right oblique views mid cheek then cheek margin: two photos.
v. Right lateral views non-smiling then smiling: two photos.

2. **From Right to Left complete half circle**

Middle Third close up 40 cm Photographs are taken in the following order:

i. Right lateral view: one photo.
ii. Right oblique views cheek margin then mid cheek: two photos.
iii. Frontal view: one photo.
iv. Left oblique views mid cheek then cheek margin: two photos.
v. Left lateral view: one photo.

3. **From Above Downwards**

Specialized views close up 40 cm Photographs are taken in the following orders:

i. Direct Dorsal views non-smiling then smiling: two photos.
ii. Backward Tilting views in two to three steeper steps: two to three photos.
iii. Basal views non-smiling then smiling: two photos.
iv. Nasal Aperture views right then left: two photos.
v. Rim-sill tests right then left: two photos.
vi. Overhead views non-smiling then smiling: two photos.

The floor is marked by lines that accurately locate the photographer's chair, the patient's chair and the angles of patient's rotation (Figs. 14.1, 14.2 and 14.3).

14.2.2 Phase II: Downloading to the Computer

Photographs are downloaded from the camera memory card to the computer. These photographs must be backed up.

14.2.3 Phase III: Editing and Saving

Photographs may be edited and "save as" to a new folder. Good filling system helps to have an easy access to the photographs. Folders are filed according to:

- Patient's name.
- File number.
- Date of photographs.
- Type and condition, i.e., large, bulky crooked, deviated, fractured, fitness, child and revision Rhinoplasty.

Table 1: Order of Photography

Standard Views: Camera Orientation = Vertical Lens focus = 60cm Aperture = f11

Order	View	Patient's chair	Point of focus	Example
1	Photo of the patient's record card: Name, patient number, diagnosis and date of photography			
2	Left lateral	Lt. Lateral Line	Mid Nasal Dorsum	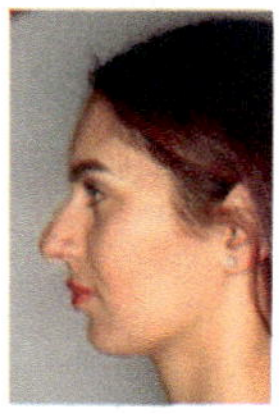
3	Left lateral smiling	Lt. Lateral Line	Mid Nasal Dorsum	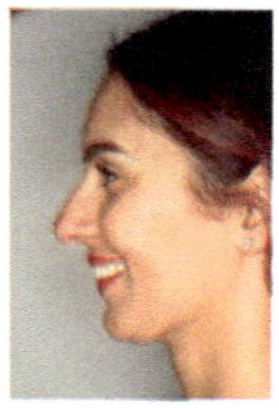
4	Left oblique cheek margin	Lt. Oblique Line	Mid Nasal Dorsum	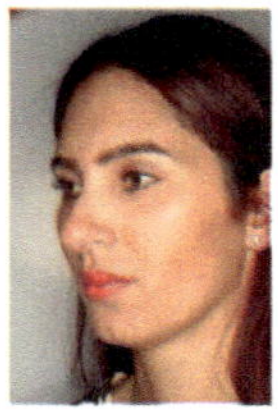
5	Left oblique mid-cheek	Lt. Oblique Line	Mid Nasal Dorsum	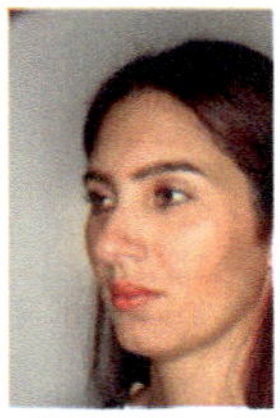
6	Frontal	Anterior Line	Mid Nasal Dorsum	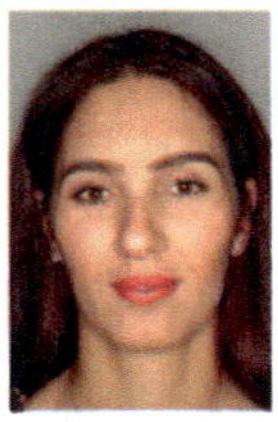
7	Frontal smiling	Anterior Line	Mid Nasal Dorsum	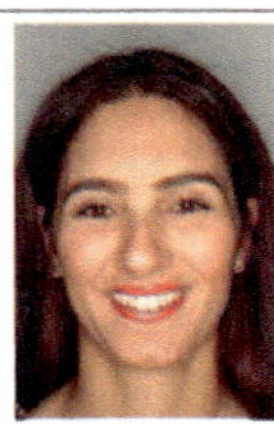

Fig. 14.1 The order of taking photographs with the corresponding pictures

Standard Views: Camera Orientation = Vertical Lens focus = 60cm Aperture = f11

Orde r	View	Patient's chair	Point of focus	Example
8	Right oblique mid-cheek	Rt. Oblique Line	Mid Nasal Dorsum	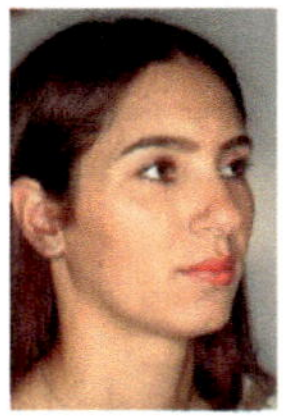
9	Right oblique cheek margin	Rt. Oblique Line	Mid Nasal Dorsum	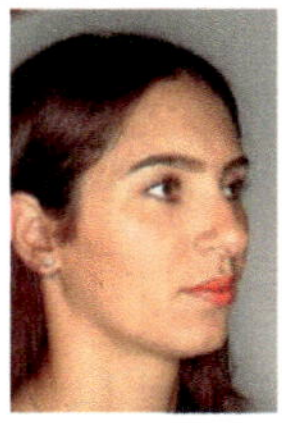
10	Right Lateral	Rt. Lateral Line	Mid Nasal Dorsum	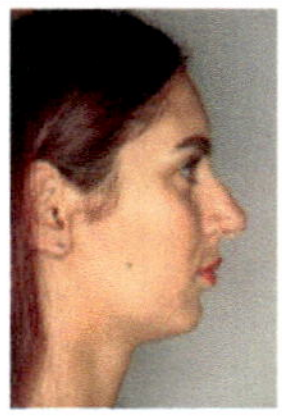
11	Right Lateral smiling	Rt. Lateral Line	Mid Nasal Dorsum	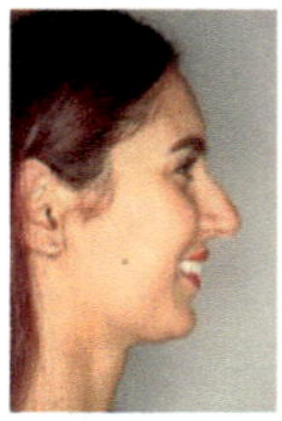

Fig. 14.1 (continued)

– Ethnic group: Asian, African, Caucasian and Middle Eastern or Hispanic.

14.2.3.1 Backing up of the Stored Photographs

Backing up should be to the photographs from:

(A) The **original photographs** from the memory card of the camera, i.e., **camera file**.

(B) The **edited photographs**.

Backup (A) and (B) can be on the same storage device, but preferably in **different folders**.

Backup can be:

- **Option 1** to an **external storage device** attached to the computer such as an external hard drive (onsite storage).
- **Option 2** to a **storage system over the internet** such as Google Drive, Microsoft One Drive or a cloud-based system (offsite storage).

Option 1 is simpler but a disaster could damage the main storage and backup storage as they are likely to be in the same premises.

Middle Third Views: Camera Orientation = Vertical Lens focus = 40cm Aperture = f16

Order	View	Patient's chair	Point of focus	Example
12	Right lateral	Rt. Lateral Line	Mid Nasal Dorsum	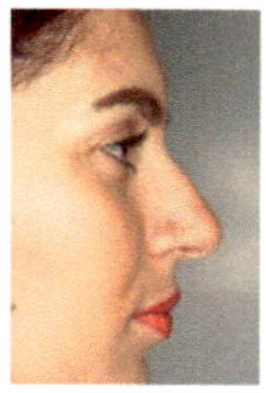
13	Right oblique cheek margin	Rt. Oblique Line	Mid Nasal Dorsum	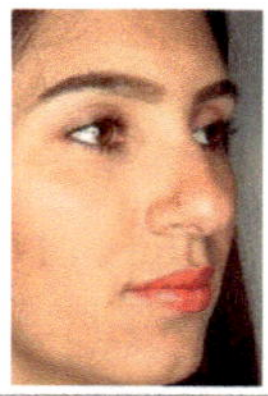
14	Right oblique mid-cheek	Rt. Oblique Line	Mid Nasal Dorsum	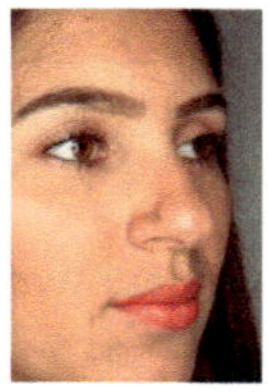
15	Frontal	Anterior Line	Mid Nasal Dorsum	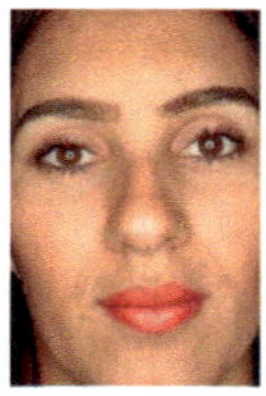
16	Left oblique mid-cheek	Lt. Oblique Line	Mid Nasal Dorsum	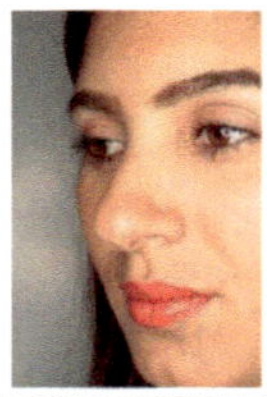
17	Left oblique cheek margin	Lt. Oblique Line	Mid Nasal Dorsum	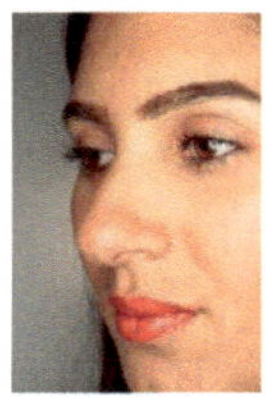
18	Left lateral	Lt. Lateral Line	Mid Nasal Dorsum	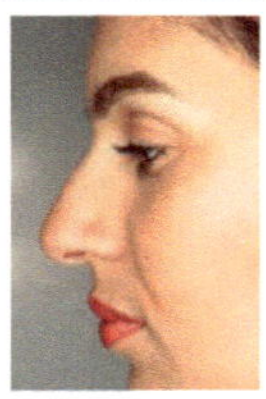

Fig. 14.1 (continued)

Specialized Views: Camera Orientation = Horizontal Lens focus = 40cm
Aperture = f16

Orde r	View	Patient's chair	Point of focus	Example
19	Direct Dorsal	Anterior Line	Mid Nasal Dorsum	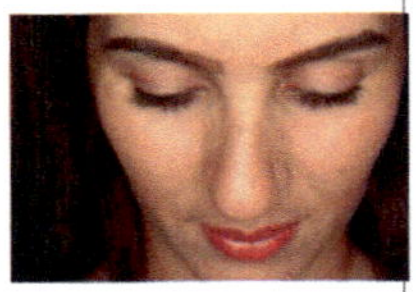
20	Direct Dorsal smiling	Anterior Line	Mid Nasal Dorsum	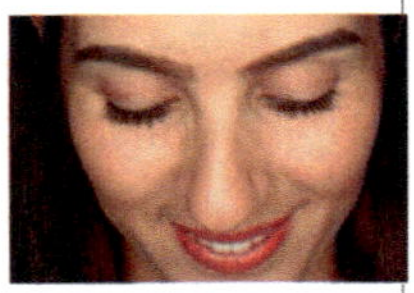
21	Backward tilting	Anterior Line	Mid Nasal Dorsum	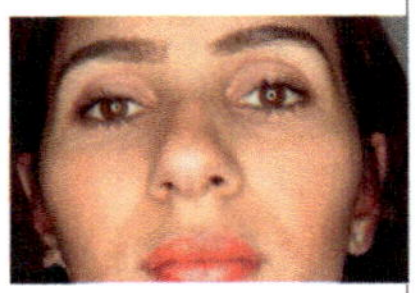
22	Steeper backward tilting	Anterior Line	Mid Nasal Dorsum	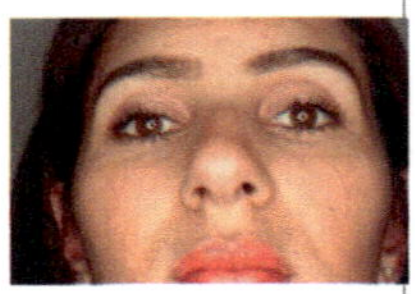
23	Basal	Anterior Line	Columella	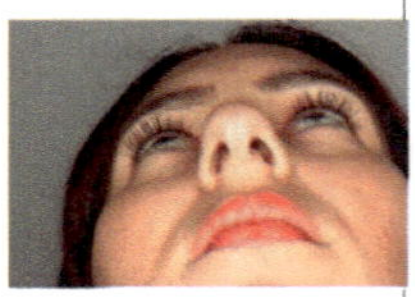
24	Basal smiling	Anterior Line	Columella	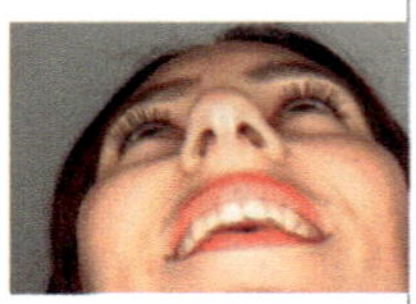

Fig. 14.1 (continued)

Specialized Views: Camera Orientation = Horizontal Lens focus = 40cm Aperture = f16

Orde r	View	Patient's chair	Point of focus	Example
25	Right nasal aperture	Lt. Oblique Line	Aperture Margins	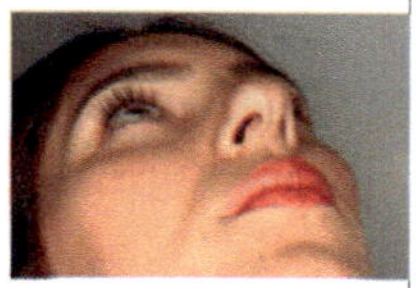
26	Right nasal aperture Rim Sill Test	Lt. Oblique Line	Aperture Margins	
27	Left nasal aperture	Rt. Oblique Line	Aperture Margins	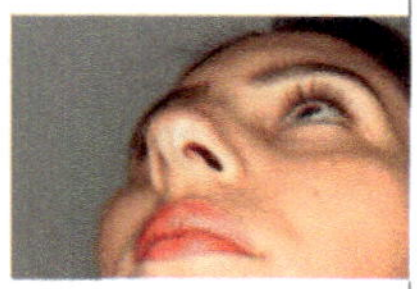
28	Left nasal aperture Rim Sill Test	Rt. Oblique Line	Aperture Margins	
29	Overhead	Anterior Line	Mid Nasal Dorsum	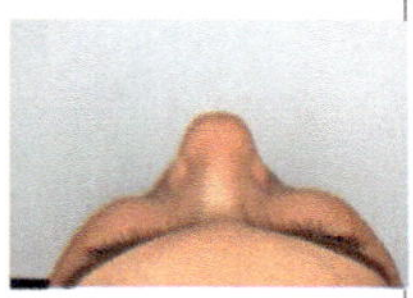
30	Overhead smiling	Anterior Line	Mid Nasal Dorsum	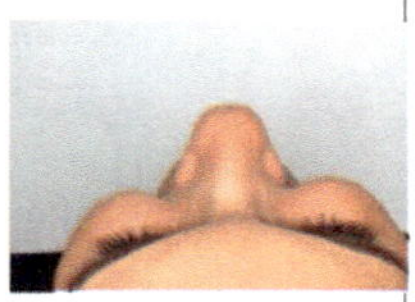

Fig. 14.1 (continued)

Table: Order of Photography

Order of Photography		View	Shorthand code for the view	Patient's chair	Camera back Orientation	Lens Focus	Lens Aperture
1		Photo of the patient's record card showing patient number and date of photography					
2	Standard Views	Left lateral	Lt.La	Lt. Lateral Line	Vertical	60cm.	Omicron f/9-f13 Alien Bees f/14-f/30
3		Left lateral smiling	Lt.La.s	Lt. Lateral Line			
4		Left oblique mid cheek	Lt.Ob1	Lt. Oblique Line			
5		Left oblique cheek margin	Lt.Ob2	Lt. Oblique Line			
6		Frontal	Fr	Anterior Line			
7		Frontal smiling	Fr.s	Anterior Line			
8		Right oblique mid-cheek	Rt.Ob1	Rt. Oblique Line			
9		Right oblique cheek margin	Rt.Ob2	Rt. Oblique Line			
10		Right Lateral	Rt.La	Rt. Lateral Line			
11		Right Lateral smiling	Rt.La.s	Rt. Lateral Line			
12	Middle Third Views	Right lateral	Rt.La	Rt. Lateral Line	Vertical	40cm	Omicron f/9-f13 Alien Bees f/14-f/30
13		Right oblique mid-cheek	Rt.Ob1	Rt. Oblique Line			
14		Right oblique cheek margin	Rt.Ob2	Rt. Oblique Line			
15		Frontal	Fr	Anterior Line			
16		Left oblique mid-cheek	Lt.Ob1	Lt. Oblique Line			
17		Left oblique cheek margin	Lt.Ob2	Lt. Oblique Line			
18		Left lateral	Lt.La	Lt. Lateral Line			
19		Direct Dorsal	DD	Anterior Line	Horizontal	40cm	Omicron f/9-f13
	Specialised Views						
20		Direct Dorsal smiling	DD.s	Anterior Line			Alien Bees f/14-f/30
21		Backward tilting	BT	Anterior Line			
22		Steeper backward tilting	BT.s	Anterior Line			
23		Basal	Ba	Anterior Line			
24		Basal smiling	Ba.s	Anterior Line			
25		Right nasal aperture	Rt.NAp	20° to Rt side of the Anterior Line			
26		Right nasal aperture Rim Sill Test	Rt.NAp.rst	20° to Rt side of the Anterior Line			
27		Left nasal aperture	Lt.NAp	20° to Lt side of the Anterior Line			
28		Left nasal aperture Rim Sill Test	Lt.NAp.rst	20° to Lt side of the Anterior Line			
29		Overhead	OH	Anterior Line			
30		Overhead smiling	OH.s	Anterior Line			

Fig. 14.2 The order of taking photographs with the corresponding camera set up

Order of taking photographs		Order of viewing
Lt.La → Lt.La.s → Lt.Ob1 → Lt.Ob2 → Fr → Fr.s → Rt.O1 → Rt.O2 → Rt.La → Rt.La.s	Full Face	Fr Fr.s; Fr; OH OH.s; DD DD.s
Rt.La → Rt.O1 → Rt.O2 → Fr → Lt.O1 → Lt.O2 → Lt.La DD → DD.s BT1 → BT2 Ba → Ba.s Rt.NAp → Rt.NAp.rs Lt.NAp → Lt.NAp.rs OH → OH.s	Close up	BT1 BT2; B Bs; Rt.NAp Rt.NAP.rs; Lt.NAp Lt.NAP.rs
	Full Face	Rt.O1 Lt.O1; Rt.O2 Lt.O2
	Close up	Rt.O1 Lt.O1; Rt.O2 Lt.O2
	Full Face	Rt.La Lt.La; RtLs Lt.La.s
	Close up	RtL LtL

Fig. 14.3 The order of taking photographs with the corresponding order of their display. Lt. Lat.& Lt.Lat.S—Left Lateral & Left Lateral Smiling; Lt Ob1&2—Left Oblique mid-cheek & cheek margin; Fr.—Frontal; Fr. s—Frontal smiling; Rt.O1&2—Right oblique mid-cheek and cheek margin; Rt. Lat. & Rt.lat.S—Right Lateral & Right Lateral Smiling; OH & OH.s—Over Head & Over Head smiling; DD—Direct Dorsal / BT1& BT2 = Backward Tilting & Backward Tilting steeper; Ba & Ba.s—Basal & Basal smiling; Rt. &Lt.NAp.—Right & Left Nasal Aperture views; Rt.& Lt.NAp. rs—Right & Left Nasal Aperture views with rim-sill test

Option 2 is slightly more complicated and more expensive, but the digital images will be safer and also available online (Fig. 14.4).

14.2.4 Phase IV: Retrieval and Display of Photographs

This is the final and most important phase as it is the objective of the whole photographic process.

Retrieval of the photographs is easier with a good filing system. According to their needs, photographs are displayed in a very specific manner that makes it easy to review.

14.2.4.1 The Large Number of Photographs

For accurate and comprehensive pre-operative photographic assessment, each patient needs a large number of photographs. At least 30 photographs are needed. As well as the standard views, there are newly introduced editions to them, which added extra clinical significance. In addition, the specialized views are useful in scrutinizing each specific area of the nose.

The Standard Views

The four standard views are:

- Frontal view: one photo.
- Oblique views, right and left: two photos.

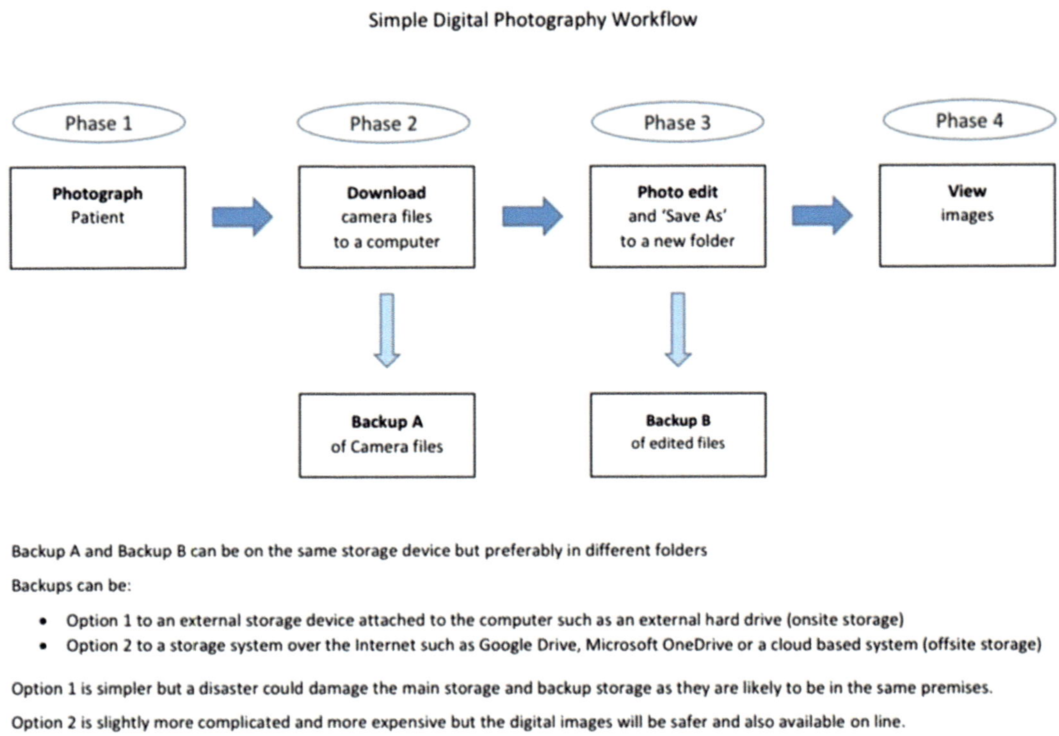

Fig. 14.4 The Four Phases of Photographic Work Flow

- Lateral views, right and left: two photos.
- Basal view: one photo.

New Editions to the Standard Views

- The smiling full face, frontal view: one photo.
- The smiling full face, right and left lateral views: two photos.
- The oblique mid cheek and cheek marginal views: two photos.
- The middle third views:
  - Frontal view: one photo.
  - Oblique views, right and left mid cheek and cheek margins: four photos.
  - Lateral views right and left: two photos.
- Smiling basal view: one photo.

Specialized Views

- Overhead views: two photos.
- Direct dorsal views: two photos.
- Backward tilting views: two to three photos.
- Nasal aperture views, right and left: two photos.
- Rim-sill tests, right and left: two photos.

Thirteen new views are added to the six standard views. The newly suggested specialized views are 10–11 views.

The total number of photographs needed for pre-operative assessment is 30 photographs. Additional views are improvised in some individual cases.

14.2.4.2 Advantages of the Large Number of Photographs

It is of great advantage to have the general appearance of the nose and face as well as the detailed study of every anatomical component of the nose.

The introduced new method of photographic display makes it easy for the surgeon to see all these details in an organized systematic way.

The display of two photographs beside each other to compare the pre-operative with the post-operative is good enough to show, specific angle of the nose and face, but it is not sufficient to study all areas of the nose that are involved in the surgery.

Arrangement of the photographs must make it easy for the eyes of the surgeon to directly study and compare. The following must be clearly seen on displaying the photographs:

- Easy recognition of the **abnormal anatomical areas** versus the normal areas.
- Direct comparison between the **right** and **left sides** of the face and nose.
- The **effects on smiling** on the nose, nasal base, cheeks and eyes. Comparison is made before and after surgeries.
- Observations of the **immediate, long-term** and **post-traumatic** changes on the nose and face.

14.2.4.3 Methodology of Displaying the Photographs

Displaying photographs is made for many purposes:

- **Pre-operative** assessment and study.
  Twenty nine photos or more are displayed.
- **Post-operative** comparison.
  58–60 photos are displayed.
- **Tertiary study** as in cases of multiple surgeries, long-term changes or trauma. More than 70 photos are displayed.

<u>Displaying the Pre-operative Photographs</u>

For clear and direct display of pre-operative photographs many of the **comparative** or **sequential** anatomical areas of the nose and face must be seen closely **beside each other**. This is especially true in the following views:

- The **non-smiling** and **smiling** views are placed beside each other in order to give the direct visual impression of the anatomical changes that takes place after smiling. This is seen in the **frontal**, **lateral**, **basal**, **direct dorsal** and **overhead views**.
  The right and left smiling lateral views are especially good example to see the extent of nasal tip animation.
- The **right** and **left oblique views** must be seen side by side facing each other in the display. This is the best demonstration and comparison between the right and left side of **nasal dorsum**. Nasal **hump** is more prominent on one side in cases of maxillary asymmetry.
- The **right** and **left lateral views** must be seen side by side facing each other to directly compare profiles, paranasal and nasal angles as well as alar grooves and columella.
- The two or three steps of the **backward tilting views** are placed beside each other for direct observation.
- The right and left **nasal aperture views** are beside each other.
- The right and left **rim-sill tests** must be seen beside each other.

<u>Displaying the post-operative and tertiary photos</u>

The post-operative photographs, one or more sets, are arranged in exactly the same pattern as the pre-operative ones. The two comparative and sequential photographs are placed beside each other. Each post-operative photograph is then placed **below** the corresponding pre-operative photograph.

The final presentation of the display is that the two comparative pre-operative photos are beside each other and the corresponding two post-operative photos are below them. **All four photos** are clearly seen in one place at a glance. In cases of a third set of photographs, i.e., second post-operative condition, photos are placed in a **third row below the previous photographs**.

Examples of this is having the pre-operative full face frontal non-smiling and smiling photos above their equivalent post-operative non-smiling and smiling photos. It is, therefore, possible to see the effect of smiling on the nose and face pre-operatively and the effects of surgery post-operatively, all at the same time.

Another example is the pre-operative right and left rim-sill tests beside each other while their post-operative resection photos below them.

14.2.4.4 The Order of Photographic Display

Photographs are displayed in the order of their clinical significance which in turn reflects the extent of benefits.

Arrangement of the views is made in the following order:

- The Frontal views full face and mid-third.
- The Overhead views.
- The Direct Dorsal views.
- The Backward Tilting views.
- The Basal views.
- The Nasal Aperture views.
- The Rim-sill tests right and left.
- The Oblique views full face, middle third, mid cheek and cheek margins.
- The Lateral views full face and middle third.

14.2.4.5 The Display of the Text

The easy stereotyped display of photographs is associated with an equally easy stereotypes display of text. Each case is studied in exactly the same systematic pattern as follows:

- Relevant history.
- Surgical analysis.
- Surgical plan.
- Surgical procedure.
- Post-operative analysis and commentary.

In each case, the surgical analysis, plan and procedure are discussing the four areas of the nose and the corresponding four Rhinoplasty surgical procedures.

The four areas and their corresponding four surgeries of the nose are:

1. The frontolateral walls.
2. The bony pyramid and midvault.
3. The medial wall, including the columella and nasal septum.
4. The nasal base including the alar base, vestibular floors and flat triangle.

14.3 Conclusion

The simple stereotyped pattern of the display of the photographs and the text makes them easy to view and read at a glance.

Bulky Tip in a Small Nose

Preoperative Assessment

1. Frontolateral walls
   a. Bulky and large Nasal tip as compared to the overall size of the nose. The bulky tip overshadows the alae nasi (Frontal , Direct Dorsal and Overhead views).
   b. The lower third of the nose is disproportionally large. In the lateral view, it occupies the lower half of the nose. In the frontal view, however, its size and bulk are overwhelming.
   c. The right ala nasi is larger than the left.

2. Medial Wall
   Nil of note
3. Bony pyramid
   a. Short and low. The boney pyramid occupies the upper 1/5th of the nose rather than the usual 1/3rd.
   b. The dorsum, made by the bony pyramid and midvault, is quite low compared with the lower half of the nose made by the frontolateral walls.

4. Alar base
   a. Wide alar base due to long inferior segments of rim-sill folds.
   b. Thick alar base due to thick posterior segments of the rim-sill folds, i.e., the flat tire appearance (Backward Tilting, Basal and Nasal Aperture Views).
   c. The right ala nasi is larger than the left (Frontal Views)

Aims of Surgery

1. Reduce the bulk and size of the frontolaretal walls, to make it proportionate with the rest of the nose.

Display of photos

FRONTAL VIEW (F.V.)	FRONTAL VIEW SMILING (F.V.S.)	FRONTAL VIEW MIDDLE THIRD (F.V. 1/3)	
DIRECT DORSAL VIEW (D.D.V)	DIRECT DORSAL VIEW SMILING (D.D.V.S.)	OVERHEAD VIEW (O.H.V.)	OVERHEAD VIEW SMILING (O.H.V.S)
BACKWARD TILTING VIEW 1 (B.T.V. 1)	BACKWARD TILTING VIEW 2 (B.T.V. 2)	BASAL VIEW (B.V.)	BASAL VIEW SMILING (B.V.S.)
RIGHT APERTURE VIEW (R. A. V.)	RIGHT APERTURE VIEW RIM SILL TEST (R.A.V. R.S.T.)	LEFT APERTURE VIEW RIM SILL TEST (L.A.V.R.S.T.)	LEFT APERTURE VIEW (L.A.V.)
OBLIQUE VIEW 1 RIGHT (O.V. 1 Rt.)	OBLIQUE VIEW 1 LEFT (O.V.1 Lt.)	OBLIQUE VIEW 2 RIGHT (O.V. 2 Rt.)	OBLIQUE VIEW 2 LEFT (O.V. 2 Lt.)
OBLIQUE VIEW 1 MIDDLE THIRD RIGHT (O. V.1 1/3 Rt.)	OBLIQUE VIEW 1 MIDDLE THIRD LEFT (O.V.1 1/3 Lt.)	OBLIQUE VIEW 2 MIDDLE THIRD RIGHT (O.V. 2 1/3 Rt)	OBLIQUE VIEW 2 MIDDLE THIRD (O.V.2 1/3 Lt)
LATERAL VIEW RIGHT (L.V.Rt.)	LATERAL VIEW LEFT (L.V. Lt.)	LATERAL VIEW SMILING RIGHT (L.V.S.Rt.)	LATERAL VIEW SMILING LEFT (L.V.S. Lt.)
LATERAL VIEW MIDDLE THIRD RIGHT (L.V.1/3 Rt.)	LATERAL VIEW MIDDLE THIRD LEFT (L.V. 1/3 Lt.)		

2. Elevation of the nasal dorsum.
3. Reduction of the size and bulk of the alar base.

Surgical Plan

1. Frontolateral walls
   a. DDD includes the weak triangle.
   b. Cephalic trim of lateral crurae.

2. Medial wall
   Nil of note
3. Bony pyramid.
   a. Osteotomies and medialization of the lateral bony walls.
   b. Dorsal augmentation by graft using septal graft.

4. Alar base
   Bilateral excision of the inferior and posterior segments of the rim-sill folds.

Surgical Procedure

a. As per surgical plan.
b. A double layer of osteocartilaginous graft was used to augment the nasal dorsum. The bony septum was used for the deeper layer. The latter was scored longitudinally to give it a rounded appearance simulating the natural dorsum.
c. A noticeable depression appeared just above the right lateral crus area during surgery. Trimming of the lateral crurae was used as a graft to fill this depression. This depression was noticed in the preoperative frontal views.

Post-Operative Analysis

1. Frontolateral Walls

a. Tip definition improved: the tip is slimmer and well defined from the surrounding alae nasi on both sides. The alae nasi came into view to share in nasal aesthetics (Frontal, Direct Dorsal, Overhead, Backward Tilting, Basal and Nasal Aperture Views).
b. Tip projection: The nasal tip is at is high at the end of the nasal dorsum with good aesthetic and angle, coupled with aesthetic nasolabial angle (Lateral and Oblique Views).
c. Tip Light Reflex: light is seen as one spot off the nasal tip (Frontal and backward tilting views).

2. Medial Walls
Nil of note.

3. Bony Pyramid

a. Bony pyramid: the nasal dorsum is straight and the side walls are smooth and narrow (all views except the Basil views).
b. Dorsal light reflex is seen as an uninterrupted line off the nasal dorsum (Directed Dorsal views).

4 . Alar and Base

a. The superior alar groove aesthetics improved, they are deeper and longer (Oblique, Lateral, Nasal Aperture, Direct Dorsal and Overhead Views).
b. Posterior alar groove aesthetics improve by defatting as well as excising the posterior segments of rim-sill folds. The flat tire appearance is no longer present (Backward tilting, Basal and Nasal Aperture views).
c. The inferior segment of the rim-sill fold was surprisingly short, i.e., only 2 mm long. It was the thickness of the posterior segment that mainly contributed to the bulky alar base.
d. Alae nasi aesthetics improved. They are pulled medially, better scene and smaller in size.
e. Nasal aperture aesthetics improved by defatting and excision of the rim sill folds. The size of the aperturers are smaller. Nasal apertures transformed from wide rounded with transverse axes to small triangular with long axes (Backward tilting, Basal and Nasal Aperture Views).

Commentary:

a. The four areas of Rhinoplasty were addressed i.e. frontolateral walls, the bony pyramid and alar base.

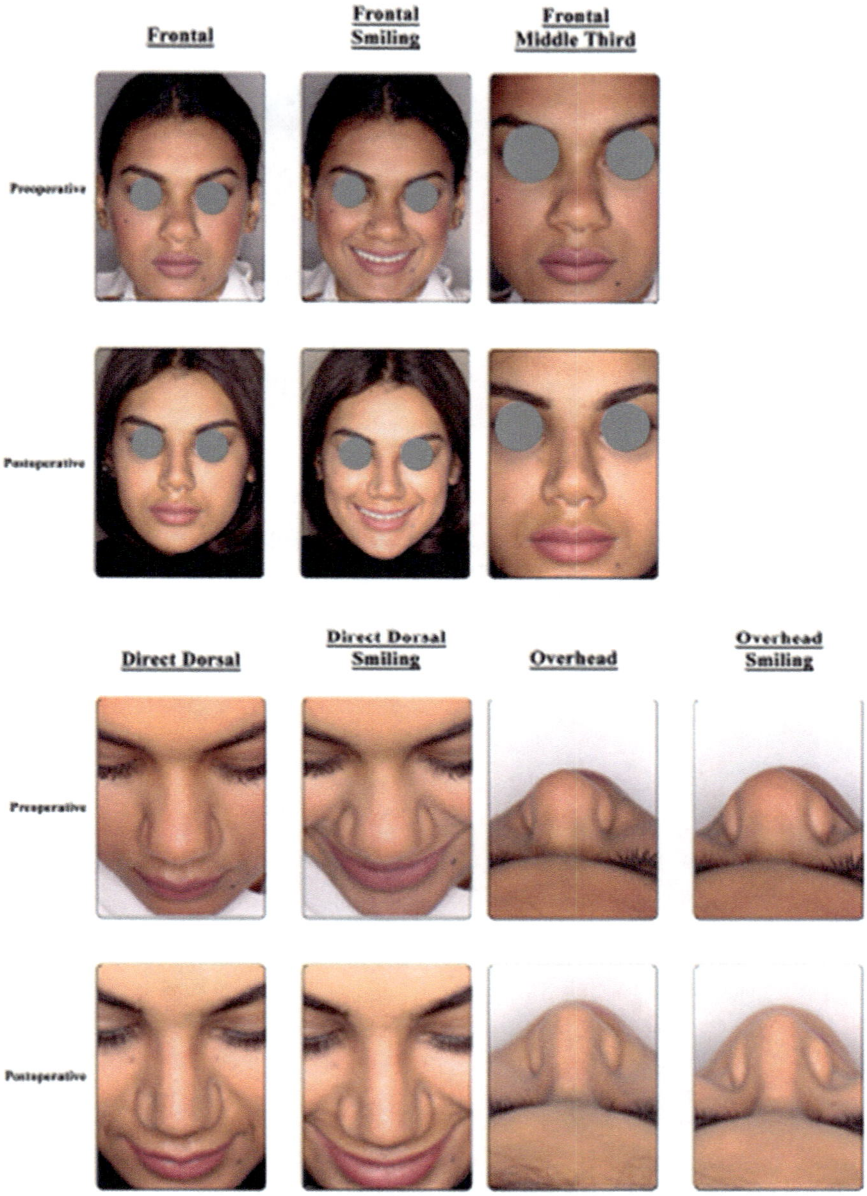

b. The drumstick appearance of the nose totally disappeared. The lower third is integrated with the upper 2/3 in an attractive double empathy.

c. No tip drafts and no direct crural stitching. The nasal tip and the columella maintain their natural softness and normal physiological roles.

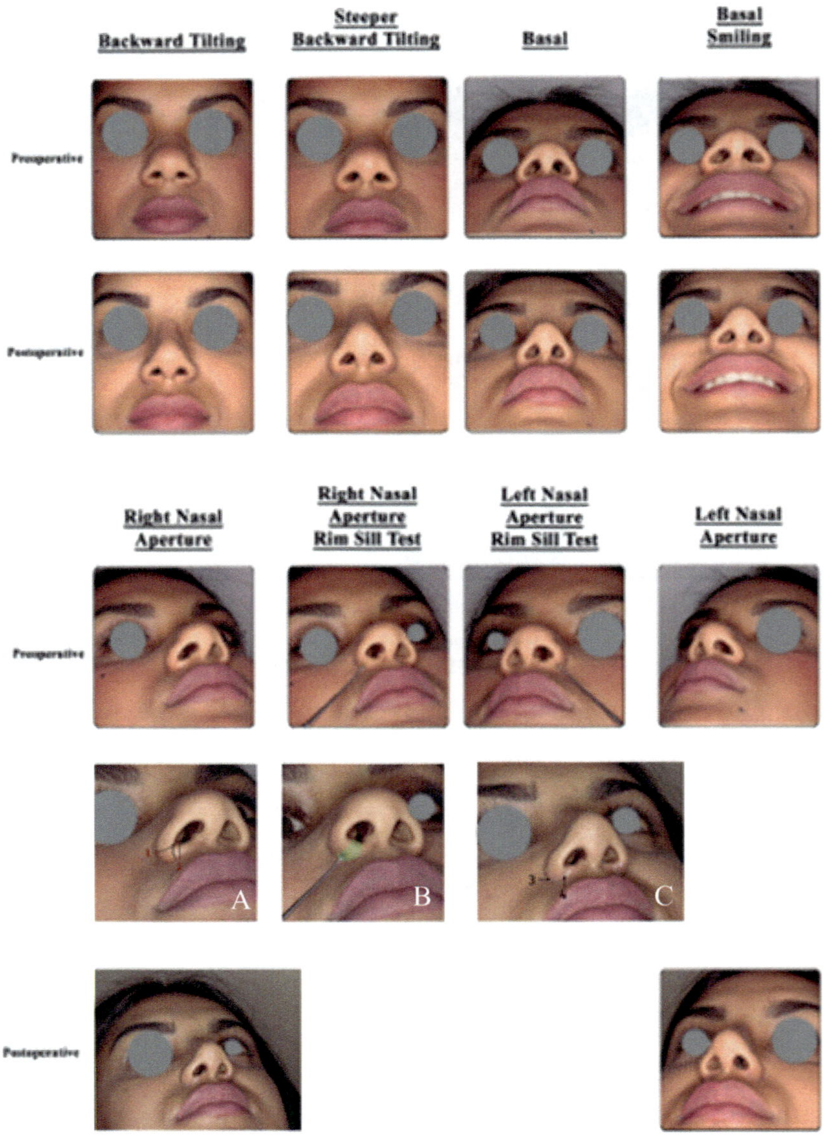

A - The posterior (1) and inferior (2) segments of the rim sill fold.
B - The rim sill test for thick skin demonstrating the two segments.
C – The posterior segment excision scar (3) and the inferior segment excision scar (4).

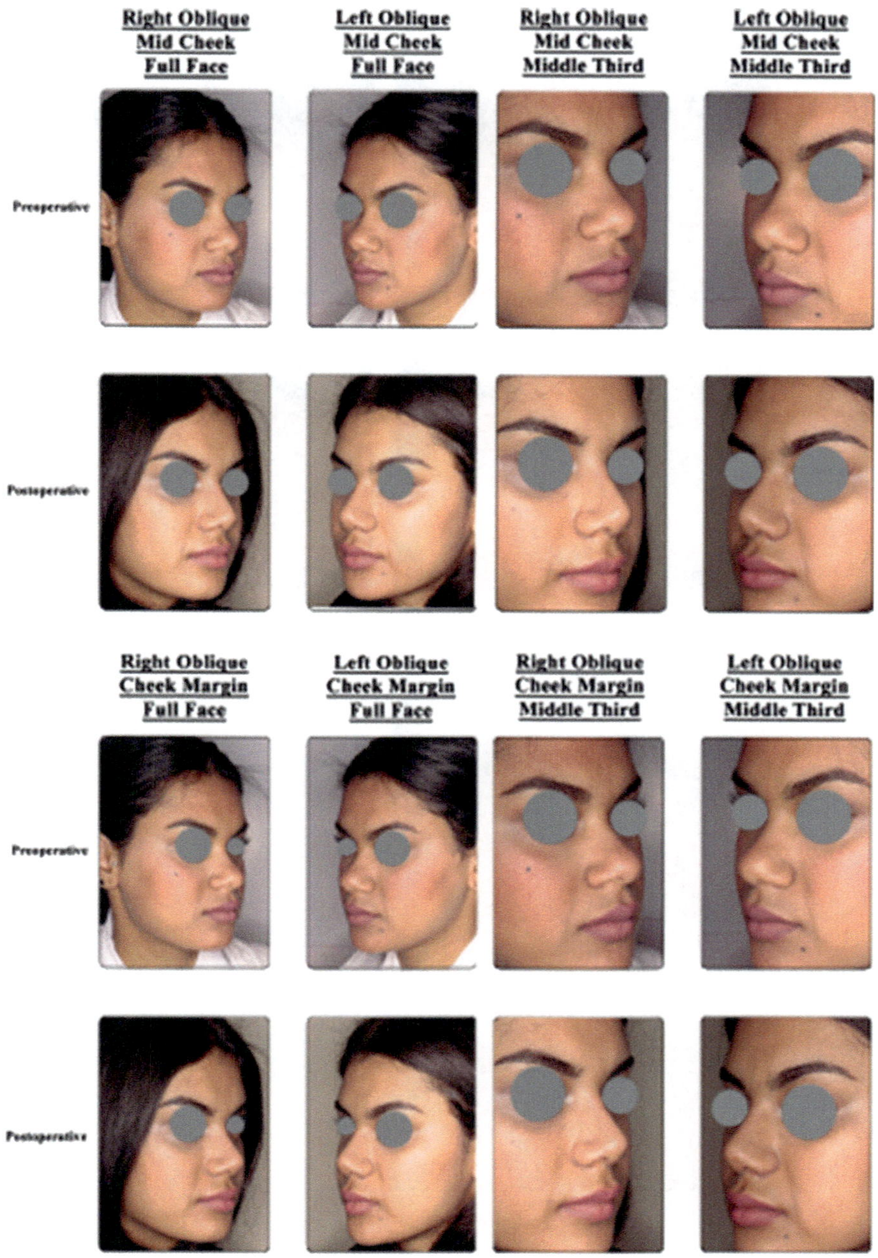
Right Oblique
Mid Cheek
Full Face
Left Oblique
Mid Cheek
Full Face
Right Oblique
Mid Cheek
Middle Third
Left Oblique
Mid Cheek
Middle Third
Preoperative
Postoperative
Right Oblique
Cheek Margin
Full Face
Left Oblique
Cheek Margin
Full Face
Right Oblique
Cheek Margin
Middle Third
Left Oblique
Cheek Margin
Middle Third
Preoperative
Postoperative

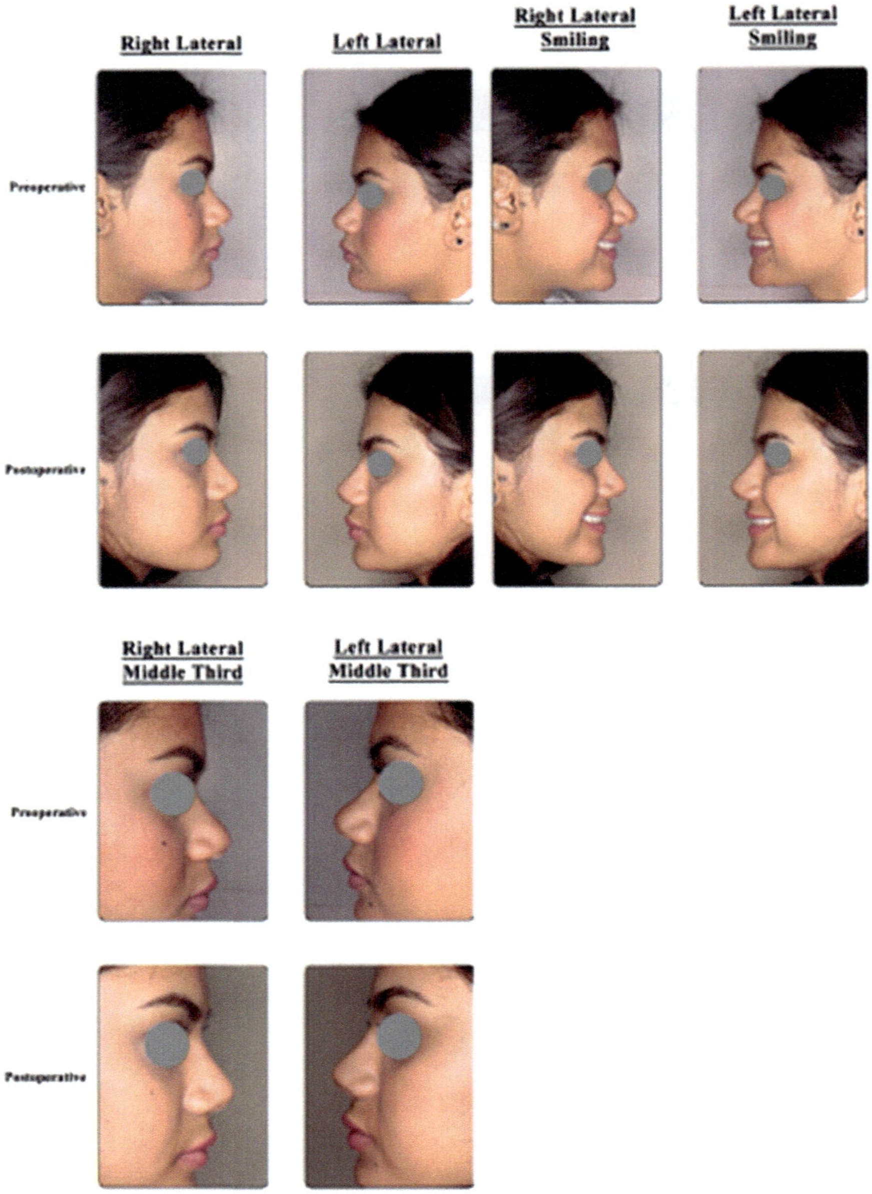
Right Lateral
Left Lateral
Right Lateral Smiling
Left Lateral Smiling
Preoperative
Postoperative
Right Lateral Middle Third
Left Lateral Middle Third
Preoperative
Postoperative

Part III

Surgical Techniques

Closed Versus Open Rhinoplasty an Academic Approach

15

Abstract

The internal or endonasal and external or open approaches to Rhinoplasty are terms that are commonly used for the closed and open Rhinoplasty. They are two different approaches for two totally different different surgical objectives.

Keywords

Closed versus open rhinoplasty · History of open rhinoplasty · The weak triangle and the weak area of the nose · Physiology of the columella · Surgical anatomy of the columella · Consequences of the open approach · A visible columellar scar

The internal or endonasal and external or open approaches to Rhinoplasty are a terms that are commonly used for the closed and open Rhinoplasty.

The dialogue between the **external** and the **internal** approaches for Rhinoplasty has never been objectively made on clear academic grounds. They are **not** two different approaches for the same operation. They are **two very different approaches for two very different objectives**.

As well as its clear aesthetic significance, the anatomical and physiological roles of the **columella** are currently poorly understood and its importance in the three-dimensional structure of the lower third of the nose is greatly underestimated.

15.1 A Preservative incisional approach versus an Invasive surgical procedure

The **closed or internal approach** is **a direct exploratory incision,** in which the intercartilaginous incisions directly explore the upper two thirds of the nose. The **marginal incisions** to the lower lateral cartilages are **a choice** that can be made only if surgery is needed in this area.

The **open or external approach** is **not** a direct exploratory incision. It is **a surgical procedure** that starts by the external columellar incision. The **crural marginal incisions** are **a must** that is linked to the columellar incision. Incisions are followed by **a dissection process** within and around the lower lateral cartilages before exploration is finally accomplished.

This is one, of many basic differences, between the two approaches that will be discussed in this chapter.

15.2 History of Open Rhinoplasty

External Rhinoplasty was first introduced in 1921 by Rethi. The transcolumellar approach was suggested to gain access to the nasal tip. Jacques Joseph (1865–1934) was an

M. H. A. Shafy, *Innovations in Rhinoplasty*,
https://doi.org/10.1007/978-3-030-94573-2_15

innovator of modern plastic surgery including Rhinoplasty in the early 20th century. He was followed by generations of excellent surgeons who made great progress in the art and science of *Rhinoplasty*. Their work included the details of anatomy, definitions of surface anatomy, photography identification of aesthetics and unaesthetic of the nose. Many techniques were described. The art of specific pre-operative analysis and diagnosis was enhanced by the fact that almost all surgeons were pursuing the endonasal approach.

In the last half of the twentieth century, Rhinoplasty becomes more popular and acceptable procedure. Demands for the surgery increased rapidly for many reasons, including the increased awareness, successful results, the entertaining business and the appearance of celebrities and the increase number of surgeons.

The wide variations in nasal shapes demanded correction of more than just simple deformities, e.g., nasal humps and crooked noses. Both patients and surgeons become more ambitious for further refined and finesse work especially on the most important part of the nose, i.e., the nasal tip. Unfortunately, the progress in endonasal tip surgery was not parallel to patient's and surgeon's ambitions. Gradually more surgeons shifted to external approach technique, which achieved better results in nasal tip surgeries.

At the end of 1980s and beginning of 1990s, the external approach gained more popularity for the following reasons:

a. New generation of excellent surgeons who succeeded in modifying the external approach with additional techniques that had good results.
b. Widespread of the rapidly progressing technique has led the newer generations of surgeons to primarily adopt external approach.
c. Parallel to the rapid progress of the external approach, the endonasal *Rhinoplasty* made very slow progress and failed to make noticeable change especially to the nasal tip.
d. The pioneer of the art of endonasal approach, in the previous three to four decades, was not followed by newer generation that advances the techniques.
e. Slow progress in the basic knowledge of anatomy of the lower third of the nose.

For the best interest of understanding the **consequences** and **effects** of open and closed approaches, the following basic fundamental facts are discussed.

I. **The Three-Dimensional Structure of the Lower Third of the Nose.**
II. **The Structural and Aesthetic Roles of the Skin of the Lower Third of the Nose.**
III. **The Columella**: Anatomy, Aesthetics and Physiology.

15.3 The Three-Dimensional Structure of the Lower Third of the Nose

Maintaining the three-dimensional structure of the external nose, preventing it from collapse and restoring the structure are major concerns in Rhinoplasty.

The three-dimensional structure of the upper two thirds of the nose is fairly simple. The lower third of the nose is made of soft **delicate tissues** that have more **sophisticated anatomical structure and physiological role**. The three-dimensional structure is maintained by the equally **delicate columella**.

15.3.1 The Solid Upper Third

The three-dimensional structure of the three-walled upper third of the nose is **made** and **supported** by the solid walls of the **bony pyramid** and **bony septum**.

15.3.2 The Firm Midvault

The three-dimensional structure of the three-walled middle third of the nose is **made** and **supported** by the firm structures of the **upper lateral cartilage** and the **cartilaginous septum**.

15.3.3 The Soft Lower Third

The four-walled lower third of the nose, from the anterior angle of the caudal septum down to the nasal tip is **made by** the membranous septum, the lower lateral cartilages, the alae nasi and the two vestibular floors. The three-dimensional structure is mainly **supported by** the **columella**.

The three-dimensional structure in the lower third of the nose is maintained by a totally different mechanism than the upper two thirds.

15.3.4 The Weak Triangle and the Weak Area of the Nose

The weak triangle is located in the supratip area in the transitional area between the solid three-walled upper two third and the relatively mobile four-walled lower third of the nose.

It is bounded superiorly by the two sides of the inferior border of the upper lateral cartilage and inferiorly by the superior borders of the two middle crurae.

This **weak junction** between the **upper two thirds** and the **lower third** of the nose is present **externally** as well as **internally.**

Intranasally, the upper lateral cartilage and cartilaginous septum (the middle third of the nose) are separated from the nasal tip and columella (lower third) by a **gap** that is filled by the **loose soft structure less membranous septum** (see chapter Soft and Weak Areas). This is an area of severe lack of support, i.e., the **weak area of the nose**. It corresponds to the **weak triangle** externally.

15.3.5 The Superior and Inferior Supports of the Lower Third

The lower third of the nose is supported by the **caudal cartilaginous** septum superiorly and the **columella** inferiorly. Between these two structures lies **the weak area of the nose,** i.e., the soft structure less membranous septum. The fronto-lateral walls, i.e., nasal tip and lateral crurae, are mainly supported by the columella.

Collapse of the columella inferiorly will consequently lead to **collapse of the lower third of the nose** starting from the level of the caudal cartilaginous septum down to the nasal tip.

15.3.6 The Hard, Firm and Delicate Principle

The nose goes from its **hard solid bony pyramid** at its root to the **firm** cartilaginous **midvault** and finally ends in its **soft delicate lower third.** This delicate end has an equally **delicate supportive structure,** i.e., the **columella.**

The principle of having an organ that goes from being **large**, **hard** and **strong** at its origin and gradually becomes **smaller**, **softer** and **more delicate** is quite true in humans and plants.

The arms and legs are strong and large at the shoulders and hips then gradually become more delicate till the hands and feet are reached. The hands and feet have more delicate structures and smaller muscles and tendons. They are the most important parts of the arms and legs.

The same with the tree that needs a strong support by a large heavy trunk and roots. As it grows higher up, the supportive branches become smaller till they reach the leaves and flowers, which are the final and the best parts of the tree. Flowers and leaves only need minimal support with very thin branches.

The delicate lower lateral cartilages only need the delicate support of the delicate columella.

15.4 The Structural and Aesthetic Roles of the Skin of the Lower Third of the Nose

The skin of the lower third of the nose has fundamental **structural** as well as **aesthetic** roles (see Skin section). This is quite unlike the skin of the upper two third of the nose.

15.4.1 The Paradox of the Nasal Skin

The upper two thirds of the nose has soft skin and hard skeleton, while the lower third has firm skin and soft skeleton.

15.4.2 The Paradox of the Nasal Walls

The walls of the **upper two thirds** of the nose are **solid**, **firm** and **uninterrupted**, while the walls of the **lower third** are **soft**, **pliable** and **interrupted** by weak areas and soft folds.

15.4.3 Skin Cover of the Lower Third

15.4.3.1 Skin Cover of the Alae Nasi

The alae nasi are covered externally by thick, firm, greasy and immobile, i.e., fixed skin. Internally they are covered by the equally adherent thin hairy vestibular skin.

The external thick greasy **epidermal** layer is directly adherent to the thick fibrofatty **dermal** layer. The alae nasi have **no subdermal layer**. Aesthetically, the **shape of the alae nasi** is purely **made** and **maintained** by their dermal and epidermal skins.

15.4.3.2 Skin Cover of the Middle and Lateral Crurae

The middle and lateral crural skin has a totally different role.

Aesthetically, the shape of the frontolateral wall of the lower third of the nose is **determined** by the **shapes of the middle** and **lateral crural cartilages**. **Maintaining** the shapes of these cartilages needs the support of the external skin.

On their own, the lower lateral cartilages are too soft to maintain their shapes.

The skin cover of the **middle** and **lateral crurae** has thick greasy **epidermis**, thick fibrous **dermis** and thick fibrofatty **hypodermis**. The three components are tightly bound together to make one thick firm layer of skin. The skin is attached to the middle and lateral crurae via its **hypodermis**. Multiple **fibrous bands** pass from the deep dermal surface, through the hypodermal fat, to be attached to the **capsular walls** of the crural fat cover. In this way, the **external skin is fashioned and contoured** to the shapes of the middle and lateral crurae.

Together, the crural cartilages and the skin make one thick and firm wall that has the **exact same shape** of the middle and lateral crural cartilages, i.e., the nasal tip and lateral crurae only in a **larger scale**, **thicker wall** and **firmer consistency**. The frontolateral wall is made stronger by the **three thick layers of the external skin**, the **crural cartilages** and the **vestibular skin**. The nasal tip and lateral crurae are now firm enough to maintain their **three-dimensional structure**.

15.4.4 The Importance of the Hypodermal Fatty Layers

The key to the bond between the **skin** and **crural cartilages** is in the structure of the hypodermis. The latter is made of **two** neatly arranged **layers of fat**. The **first one** is a thick **capsular layer of fat** on the outer surfaces of the middle and lateral crurae. The capsules are attached to the crural margins, so that the fat capsules are of the same shape of the well-padded crurae. There are **multiple fibrous bands** between the outer capsules and the deep surface of the thick dermal layer. Between these bands lies the **second layer** of fat. The fatty tissues are loculated in these tightly organized chambers. From the crural capsules of fat, the **bands pull on the external skin and fashions it to the same shapes and contours of the middle and lateral crurae**.

15.4.5 The Three-Step Exploration of the Hypodermal Layer

The two hypodermal layers of fat should always be clearly seen on exploring the lower lateral cartilages.

Exploration must follow the anatomical locations of the lower borders of the crural cartilages.

A three-step exploratory procedure is the best anatomical method of exploring and observing these layers. Starting from the most obvious lower border of the lateral crus, then the medial crus and finally the middle crus (refer to the Surgical section).

In conclusion, aesthetically, **the shapes** of the nasal tip and lateral crurae are **determined by the middle and lateral crural cartilages** while **maintaining** these shapes is accomplished by the **nasal skin** (see Anatomy section).

Partial or complete excision of the subdermal fat has great contribution to nasal tip aesthetic. The post-healing fibrous tissues after defatting are strong enough to still maintain the shapes of the frontolateral wall of the nose, including the nasal tip.

15.5 The Columella

Columella, in Latin means little or small column. The columella is a unique anatomical structure that contains **cartilages**, **bands** and **muscles,** i.e., the **medial crurae**, the **Inferior Vestibular Bands** (IVBs) and the **Depressor Septi muscles**. Through the inferior vestibular bands, the columella is directly attached to the Orbicularis Oris muscle.

It is important to understand the detailed anatomy, physiology as well as aesthetics of the columella. This will enable us to appreciate the columella's structural **supportive role** as well as its importance in the **vascularity of the nasal tip**.

The columella is characterized by being **firm**, **flexible** and **mobile**. All these versatile characteristics are important for the physiology, aesthetics and supportive roles of the columella.

15.5.1 Physiology of the Columella

As part of the lower third of the nose, the columella shares in facial movements and facial expressions.

On its own, the columella has limited range of movements, but together with the upper lip and the lower third of the nose, it shares in movements like speech and articulation, mastication, smiling, snarling, whistling and other facial expressions. The columellar body with its firm yet maliable texture can move and bend with the different nasal kinetic movements. The **Depressor septi** muscles are attached to the medial crurae. The **inferior vestibular bands** I.V.B., on each side of the nose, passes from the nasal sill, at the floor of the nose, to the columella medially. Each band passes posterior then superior to the corresponding medial crus (see Histology of the Inferior Vestibular Band). The nasal sill bands, as parts of the I.V.B.s are firmly attached to the **Orbicularis Oris muscle**.

The columella, therefore, moves freely with the upper lip in all its movements, i.e., sideways, upwards, downwards, forwards and backwards. The columella is indirectly affected by movements of the alae nasi.

There are abundant elastic fibers in parallel bundles, in the membranous septum just inferior to the caudal cartilaginous margin. Thus, the columella is dynamic, moving posteriorly by muscle contraction and anteriorly by elastic recoil (Paul J.O. Keefe).

The medial crurae and consequently the columella are the most mobile crurae of the lower lateral cartilages.

15.5.2 Surgical Anatomy of the Columella

The detailed anatomy of the columella is discussed in the Anatomy section. The columella has two components, a **firm anterior segment** and a **soft posterior fold** (see Anatomy section).

15.5.2.1 The Firm Anterior Segment

This segment of the columella is in the form of an inverted T-shaped structure, which is made by adjoining of the **lower halves of the two medial crurae**. They are covered by the **vestibular** and the **external nasal skins**. The columella contains several structures that are **tightly bound** together by connective tissue bonds. The vestibular and the external skins are holding the medial crurae in a **tight grip**. The conjoined convex medial surfaces of the medial crurea are adherent together by fibrous tissues. **Inferiorly** the two bodies of the medial crurae curve are laterally away from the midline and from each other. The medial crurae end in **laterally directed inferior margins** that project intranasally as the **lateral columellar margins**. The curvatures of the medial crural bodies result in the following consequences:

i. The medial crurae end in laterally directed, and not inferiorly directed, inferior margins.
ii. As the inferior margins curve laterally, the **medial** surfaces of the lower halves become **inferior** or external surfaces. The latter adhere to the **external nasal skin** by tough adherent connective tissues. The **lateral** surfaces of the medial crurae become **superior** surfaces and are covered by **vestibular skin**.
iii. The posterior margins of the medial crurae project laterally and appear as the posterior columellar prominences.

15.5.2.2 The Soft Posterior Fold

This is the **posterior segment of the columella,** which is made of a soft fold of skin. It acts as a delicate transition between the firm bodies of the **medial crurae** and the actively mobile **Orbicularis Oris muscle**.

15.5.3 Skin Cover of the Columella

The **lateral surfaces** of the medial crurae are **totally intranasal** and are covered by the thin, hairy and adherent **vestibular skin**. Exactly at the **inferior crural margins,** the **vestibular skin ends** and the **external skin begins**. The **external skin** covers the inferiorly directed **medial surfaces** of the medial crurae. In contradistinction to the vestibular skin, the external skin is thick, hairless and has a subdermal layer of tough connective tissue.

15.5.4 Contents of the Columella

The columella is a **skin envelope** that contains the following structures:

a. The **lower halves** of the two **medial crurae**.
b. The two vertical segments, right and left, of the **inferior vestibular bands**, IVBs (see Histology section). The horizontally located nasal sill band (part of IVB) ends medially by passing backwards then upward posterior than superior to the medial crus on each side.
c. The **Depressor Septi muscles** are attached to the posterior and inferior ends of the medial crurae and the caudal septum. They then pass through the soft segment of the columella before gaining insertion from the incisive fossae of maxillae on both sides.

15.5.5 Blood Supply of the Columella

The columella has a **pair of columellar arteries.** They are branches of the **superior labial arteries,** which are branches of the **facial arteries.**

The columellar arteries reach anteriorly to the **nasal tip**. They are major contributors to tip skin blood supply (R. Daniel and P. Palhazi).

15.5.6 How the Columella Supports the Lower Third

The anatomical structure and the physical characteristics of the columella provide enough strength to make it **the major support of the nasal tip and the lower third of the nose**. The body of the columella possesses outstanding qualities. The anterior columellar segment is firm yet maliable while the posterior columellar fold is soft, pliable and stretchable. Both components are mobile and movable with lower third of the nose and the upper lip.

The columella maintains the three-dimensional structure of the **nasal tip** and the **lower third of the nose** in the most delicate, versatile and dynamic way.

There are **internal** and **external factors** that help the columella to keep its three-dimensional stabilizing effects.

15.5.6.1 Internal Factors

The medial crurae are tightly adherent by connective tissue bonds in three surfaces:

i. Intercrural surfaces medially.
ii. Vestibular skin laterally.
iii. External skin inferiorly.

15.5.6.2 External Factors

i. The **arc-shaped** construction of the two **medial**, **middle** and **lateral crurae** with their characteristic cartilaginous bodies is an important contribution to the three-dimensional structure.
ii. **The grip**: the columella is like the stems of a bunch of flowers that are grasped together by the grip of a hand. The grip here is represented by the external and the vestibular skins.
iii. The **Firm Frontolateral Dermocartilaginous Structure**: The thick skin that covers the middle and lateral crurae is attached to them by a well-structured subdermal fatty layer (see anatomy). Together they make a firm frontolateral structure that holds the two domes of the middle crurae anterior to the columella as well as the lateral crurae.

15.5.7 Why the Columella is not a Single Solid Structure

A stiff cartilaginous or bony columella would mean a rigid inflexible columella, which is immobile and poorly connected with the medial crurae and the domes. It would not be attached to the Depressor Septi and Orbicularis Oris muscle and, therefore, unable to share with facial and oral movements. It would end up being just a monumental structure.

The unique structural anatomy of the columella with its contents and attachments enables it to achieve its multipurpose role **aesthetically**, **functionally** and **anatomically**.

15.6 Surgical Steps for Open Rhinoplasty

Open Rhinoplasty is **not** just a simple **external skin incision** that directly explores nasal structures. It is an **invasive surgical procedure** that starts from the **external columellar skin** and the **marginal vestibular skin** in order to explore the lower lateral cartilages, then the midvault and finally the bony pyramid.

The **columellar**, the **middle** and the **lateral crural skins** are dissected away and elevated. **Transcolumellar** and **trans-membranous septum** dissections are made before the exploration for Rhinoplasty is finally accomplished.

15.6.1 The Surgical Steps

15.6.1.1 The Columellar Incision

- An inverted v-shaped or stepladder incision is made in **external skin** at the posterior end of the firm segment of the **columella**.
- The incision then passes sideways bilaterally across the laterally directed **inferior margins** of the medial crurae.
- On each side, the incision proceeds for a short distance into the **vestibular skin** on the lateral surface of the corresponding medial crus.
- From the medial crus, each incision then **passes forwards** to meet with the inferior marginal incision.

15.6.1.2 The Inferior Marginal Incisions

These are two incisions that are made at the **inferior margins** of the right and left **middle** and **lateral crurae** and are communicated with the columellar incision on both sides.

It is noteworthy that the inferior margins of the medial crurae correspond to the inferior nasal aperture margins, while the inferior margins of the middle and lateral crurae are inside the nose farther away from the alar margins.

15.6.1.3 Dissection and Exploration

i. The columella

Dissecting off the columellar skin is not an easy task. Both the external and vestibular skins are tightly adherent and have a firm grip on the underlying cartilages.

The following planes are opened in this step:

- The skin is dissected off:
  - The inferiorly faced lateral surfaces of the medial crurae.
  - The laterally directed inferior margins.
  - Part of the vestibular surfaces of the medial crurae.
- The intercrural connective tissues are divided.

ii. The Lower Third of the Nose

- The two layers of the membranous septum are dissected and separated from each other.
- The skin is dissected and totally separated off the middle and lateral crurae.

15.7 Consequences of the Open Approach

The immediate skin closure after external surgical approach, i.e., open and immediate closure, without any surgical procedures, will lead to instant and delayed consequences.

15.7.1 Dismantlement of the Columella

The extent of tissue dissection and exploration will lead to total dismantlement of the internal and external stabilizing factors of the columella.

- There is almost **total degloving** of the columella off its covering external and vestibular skins.
- **Complete vertical transaction** of the columellar skins, external and vestibular, at the junction between its anterior firm segment and the posterior soft fold.
- The **firm anterolateral skin** is dissected off the middle and lateral crurae.
- The **two medial crurae are separated** from each other by dividing the inter-crural connective tissue bond.
- The **membranous septum** is further **weakened** by dividing the connective tissue layer between the two midline vestibular skin layers.

15.7.2 Loss of Crural Support by the Columella

- The **columella loses its ability** to **support** the nasal tip and the lower third of the nose. The **grip** and bonds of the **interstructural connective tissues** have all been severed. Losing the support of the columella will expand the weak area of the nose. It will extend from the caudal septal cartilage to the nasal tip.
- The lower lateral cartilages become:

- **Disoriented**: the lateral cartilages are displaced from their natural location.
- **Collapsed**: the crural bodies are weakened by the loss of the supporting grip of skin, bands and connective tissue bonds. The arc effect is greatly weakened.
- **Distorted**: the natural curves and twists in their bodies change and unfold.

15.7.3 The Effects on Nasal Tip and the Three-Dimensional Structure

- **Tip projection**: the nasal tip recedes instantly backwards and it loses its original height. The tip continues to recede further as the columellar scar contracts.

- **The Three-Dimensional Structure:** There is total collapse of the three-dimensional structure of the lower third of the nose, starting from the caudal septum down to the nasal tip.

15.7.4 Division of the Columellar Arteries

The columellar incision deprives the nasal tip of a good source of blood supply. Collaterals are quite rich, but there is a definite compromise that has two consequences:

a. Ischemia: total defatting of the anterolateral walls or reducing the thickness of the fibrous dermal layer carries the risk of ischemia and perhaps sloughing of the nasal tip.
b. Infection: there is increased risk of infection of the nasal tip area post-operatively due to reduced blood supply.

15.7.5 Prolonged Swelling and Delayed Healing

Due to extensive tissue dissection, the use of grafts and the reduced blood supply, swelling of the nose takes weeks, months and sometimes years before settling down to the final shape.

15.8 Surgical Procedures that Follow Open Rhinoplasty

The surgical procedures that follow the external approach or open Rhinoplasty have two phases:

15.8.1 Reconstructive Phase

The reconstructive phase means all procedures that must be done to restore the three-dimensional structure of the lower third. These procedures include: **medial crural strut**, **septal extension graft** and **tip graft.**

15.8.2 Aesthetic Phase

The aesthetic phase means all other procedures that modify the shape of the nose. These procedures include tip grafts, tip stitching, lateral crural grafts, alar graft as well as the aesthetic procedures in the upper two thirds of the nose.

The two phases may be done synchronously. Surgeons are obliged to go through **structural** and **physiological** reconstructive steps together with the **aesthetic** procedures.

i. <u>Columellar Strut</u>

The first step the surgeons have to do is to **secure a columellar support**. A **columellar strut** is made using a cartilaginous graft. Alone, this graft is not sufficient to regain the three-dimensional structure of the nose. Long-term results were disappointing. Grafts gradually appeared as unpleasant protrusions through the skin.

To regain the three-dimensional structure of the lower third, further grafts are needed to the **weak area of the nose** and the **nasal tip**.

ii. <u>Septal Extension Graft</u>

Clinically this is the supratip area of the nose. Anatomically it is the weak triangle and weak area of the nose.

A **septal extension graft** is used to support the weak area between the caudal cartilaginous septum and the nasal tip.

iii. <u>Tip Graft and Shield's Graft</u>

The domes recede backwards due to lack of columellar support. They are not sufficiently projected to produce a prominent tip. A **tip graft** or **shield's graft** are necessary. The graft is better camouflaged with further soft tissue grafts, e.g., perichondrium, or fibrofatty tissues.

Some surgeons proceed to directly narrow the curves of the middle crurae, i.e., **direct domal stitch.**

iv. Spreader Grafts

The walls of internal valves of the nose are weakened secondary to the disrupted three-dimensional structure. **Spreader grafts** are almost always necessary to support the midvault.

v. Lateral Crural Grafts

- **Discrepancies** between the two lateral crurae become apparent especially after direct surgical maneuvers on the middle crurae. These are natural normal findings or iatrogenic.
- The lateral crurae become comparatively **weak**, **distorted** and **disoriented** especially after using multiple rigid grafts in the neighboring nasal tip, columella and supra tip area.
- The lateral crurae may be weakened from previous surgery.

In all or some of these conditions grafting of lateral crurae become necessary.

vi. Alar Marginal Grafts

One of the techniques to narrow nasal tip is by direct stitching of the domes. Consequently, the sidewalls of the middle and lateral crurae are pulled medially leaving the lateral skin walls unsupported. It appears as an external depression or defect at the alar margins next to the nasal tip. **Grafts** are required to support to fill these defects.

vii. Soft tissue grafts

Soft tissue grafts, e.g., perichondrium, fatty tissues and fascias, are frequently needed to camouflage the sharp edges of the hard cartilaginous and bony grafts.

Areas of defects and depression may appear during surgery. Common areas are the nasal dorsum, midvault and supra tip. Soft tissue grafts are suitable for filling these defects.

The Nasal tip graft is especially important to camouflage as the external skin thins out in the long term and hard grafts become unpleasantly prominent under the skin.

viii. Effects on Alar Base

Lateral crural grafts **stretch the floor of the nose,** i.e., the rim-sill folds are elongated. This has the unpleasant effect of **enlarging the overall size of the nose**. The alar grooves are flattened and nasal apertures are widened.

Alar resection helps to reduce the aperture size but not the overall size of the nose that remains large.

15.9 Open Rhinoplasty is a Graft-Dependent Surgery

Surgeries that follow open or external approach Rhinoplasty predominantly need grafts to accomplish their goals. This is to compensate for the weakening of the three-dimensional structure of the lower third of the nose.

Structural reformation and modification of the lower third rely on the use of grafts.

The skin paradox is lost or even reversed. Internally the soft crurae of the lower lateral cartilages are replaced but the hard inflexible grafts. Externally the skin cover remains as thick and as tough as before the surgery.

15.10 Pitfalls of Grafts

In open Rhinoplasty, surgeons must have sufficient and efficient grafts.

The **bony cartilaginous** septum, if available, is the best source of grafts.

Even in primary surgeries, nasal septal materials are always harvested. Cartilages of the **ear** and **ribs** may also being used.

- **Graft material highly variable**

Grafts vary according to their source, i.e., nasal septum, ear cartilages and ribs. They are extremely variable in their texture due to many factors including, the normal natural variability, age, trauma and previous surgery.

If grafts are not the same, then results will never be the same, i.e., surgical outcomes are less predictable.

• **Variable Availability of Grafts**

Septal grafts are not always available, e.g., cases of secondary Rhinoplasty or following trauma.

Ear and rib grafts are less advantageous than septal grafts.

• **Unpredictable Results**

Short and long-term results have extremely variable predictability even with the best grafts and the best surgeries. It is fair to say that results may sometimes be idiosyncratic.

• **Unnatural consistency and function of the nose**

The consistencies of grafts are never the same as the natural nasal tissues especially these of the lower third of the nose. Natural movement of the columella with speech eating and facial expressions is affected.

15.11 A Visible Columellar Scar

The **columellar incision** is not in a natural fold or crease, e.g., alar crease.

Patients perceive the external **columellar scar** with varying degrees of reservation and uncertainty. This is especially true in cases of primary Rhinoplasty, females, celebrities, young age and thin skinned individuals.

Scars are not always invisible. There is a possibility of secondary infection, gaping as well as long-term contraction.

15.12 Indications for Open Rhinoplasty

Open Rhinoplasty is an invasive exploratory procedure that causes instability of the three-dimensional structure of the lower third of the nose. It is, therefore, a graft-dependent surgery.

Open Rhinoplasty is excellent in reconstructive procedures, i.e., in bad cases of secondary and multiple revision surgeries. Cases of severe malformations, e.g., hairlip, have better results with open approach Rhinoplasty.

15.13 New Advances in Endonasal Techniques

New anatomical discoveries have led to more understanding of the detailed anatomy of the four walls of the lower third of the nose. The walls include the middle crurae of the nasal tip anteriorly, the nasal base inferiorly, the alae nasi and lateral crurae, laterally and the columella and the membranous septum medially.

There are more detailed knowledge of the frontolateral wall skin layer of the lower third of the nose, the weak and soft folds that separate the lower lateral cartilages, the inferior vestibular bands and the alae nasi.

These informations and others have made it possible to control and reshaping the four walls of the lower third of the nose. The columella is preserved, i.e., the three-dimensional structure of the lower third of the nose is not compromised. Modifications in the nasal tip do not rely on the use of grafts. It mainly relies on the combined modifications of the skin cartilage relationships in the lower third (see Surgery section).

There is no fear of infection or ischemia of the tip skin. The advantages of this technique are that the natural normal anatomy is preserved. The shapes of the frontolateral walls of the lower third of the nose, including the nasal tip, are dictated by the shapes of the patient's own lower lateral cartilages.

The inferior wall and alar base surgeries have greatly improved. They are no longer limited to simple reduction in the size of nasal apertures.

New techniques have developed as a result of the progress in anatomical knowledge, e.g., aesthetic enhancement of nasal and alar base as well as the reduction in their sizes and bulk.

The nose continues to preserve the exact shapes of the cartilages externally even after the surgical modifications of both the skin and cartilages. The outcome is an ideal aesthetic result:

- Patients maintain their own original natural image, i.e., their **own nasal prints**.
  The original natural **skin paradox** is maintained in the lower third, i.e., the soft

cartilages are inside while the firm skin is draping them outside.

- Noses, look and feels **naturally soft** and the normal movements with **facial expressions** and eating are not affected.
- The physiology of nasal respiration is maintained.
- Other surgeries to the soft folds, e.g., rim-sill folds at the alar base are additional enhancements to nasal tip aesthetics.

Enhancement of skin Aesthetics: The skin thickness is completely under control. Not only the thick-skinned noses but also the minimally thick and even thin noses can be thinned out in a controlled way to enhance its aesthetic. Thickness of the hypodermal fatty layer is controlled without the fear of infection, ischemia or necrosis.

15.14 Preservation Incisions in Closed Rhinoplasty

Preservation is mainly to the shapes of the lower lateral cartilages.

It is important to preserve the deep ligament of Pitanguy. The interdomal and intercrural ligaments are superficial ones. Post-surgical healing tissues bind the domes and the crurae together. Healing of intercartilaginous incision makes the scroll area stronger. The telescopic relation between upper lateral cartilage and lateral crurae does not get loose with age nor with pregnancy.

The bulky fats are reduced with or without reduction of the thickness of the fibrous dermal layer. The three preservative incisions are:

- Intercartilaginous incisions.
- Septal incisions.
- Marginal incisions.

Other incisions may be the alar wounds in alar base surgery and the external osteotomy stab wounds.

16 Clinical Subdivisions and Clinical Varieties of Rhinoplasty

Abstract

Rhinoplasty is not a simple, stereotyped or straightforward procedure. Each operation must be personalized to each particular nose and face. Rhinoplasty is four different operations for the four anatomical areas of the nose.

Keywords

The four areas of Rhinoplasty · Varieties of noses presenting for Rhinoplasty

16.1 Introduction

Rhinoplasty is not a simple, stereotyped or straightforward procedure.

It is a detailed and complicated surgery. Despite the well-known anatomy, each nose has its own unique structural and anatomical differences. Each operation must be **personalized** to each particular nose and face.

What is applicable on one nose may not be the same for another nose, even the other half of the same nose.

16.2 The Four Areas of Rhinoplasty

Aesthetic Rhinoplasty is not a single operation. Rhinoplasty is four **different operations**; one in each of the four anatomical areas of the nose.

Each one of the four surgeries is **a totally different procedure** that has different guidelines and techniques. The outcome of all **four surgeries must** produce a harmonized, **aesthetically attractive nose**. These four surgeries are:

i. **Anterior and Lateral wall surgery** for the Nasal tip and lateral crurae
ii. **Medial Wall Surgery** for the Nasal septum, the medial crurae and columella
iii. **Surgery of the Bony Pyramid** and **Mid Vault**
iv. **Alar Base Surgery** for Rim-sill folds and the vestibular floor.

16.3 Varieties of Noses Presenting for Rhinoplasty

Patients seeking Rhinoplasty present with various nasal shapes and conditions. Each of these conditions required **combined regional surgeries** in one or more of the four areas of the nose. The common clinical presentations are:

(1) **Large Nose**
(2) **Bulky Nose**
(3) **Crooked Nose**
(4) **Deviated Nose and oblique nose**
(5) **Fractured Nose**
(6) **Finesse Rhinoplasty**
(7) **Secondary Rhinoplasty**
(8) **Ethnic Nose**
(9) **Children**
(10) **Special clinical conditions**:

M. H. A. Shafy, *Innovations in Rhinoplasty*,
https://doi.org/10.1007/978-3-030-94573-2_16

i. Developmental and Congenital anomalies, e.g., dermoid cyst, Waardenburg syndrome.
ii. Large Alae Nasi.
iii. Sliding tip.

In each of these conditions, the same basic surgical techniques are pursued. Special attention is paid to each special case. Each of the major groups will be studied in further details.

16.4 Clinical Assessment of Rhinoplasty Patient

Getting to see a person who is thinking of or willing to have Rhinoplasty has its own characteristics and considerations. Although not sick, the candidate is a clinical condition that seeks surgery. The surgery is a highly sophisticated type that has many details in the different small areas of the nose. The outcome of the surgery is a new shape of the external nose. This results in a new image of the face that has substantial physical and psychological effects.

In the interest of best results, a Rhinoplasty candidate is managed professionally as a patient. This ensures a thorough and accurate clinical assessment. In addition, there must be a social and psychological assessment. The surgeon must be aware of the reasons and psychological status of the patient.

Should any alarming signs in the history or behavior of the patient, the surgeon must consider the help of a psychiatrist without any hesitation.

If the patient is already under the care of a psychiatrist, then he must be approached and asked about the patient's ability to take this type of surgery.

16.5 Clinical Assessment

16.5.1 History

(a) Patient's name, age, sex and ethnicity are taken.
(b) The Patient must have complete freedom to express himself about when, why and what.
   - When did he first think about Rhinoplasty?
   - Why would he like the change? Is it a personal own wish or there are psychological, social or professional obligations.
   - What does he like and dislike about his nose? What is the mental vision of the expected changes that he wishes for? What does it mean to him to have the surgery?
(c) Trauma
   - Accidental trauma: trauma that causes nasal deformity must be a considerable one. It causes severe bleeding, hospitalization and possible surgery.
   - Surgical: Previous Rhinoplasty or any other plastic surgery on the face or body.
   - The date(s) of trauma and the number of surgeries are reported.
(d) History of psychological or mental illness. The intake of any antidepressants, sleeping pills or similar drugs.
(e) Sinonasal symptoms and diseases, e.g., nasal airway, smell disturbance, halitosis, anterior or posterior nasal discharge. History of sinus infection, allergy or polyps. History of sinus or septal surgery.
(f) General illness, e.g., diabetes, hypertension, asthma or other systemic diseases.
(g) Family History:
   History of Rhinoplasty or any type of plastic surgery to any member of the family, close relative or friends.
   Family history of mental or psychological illnesses or general diseases, e.g., allergy, diabetes or hypertension.

16.5.2 Examination

Examination of a candidate for Rhinoplasty must include general, local, psychological and photographic.

16.5.3 General Examination

The patient must be generally fit for the surgery. According to the history, the patient may be referred to a specialized doctor if necessary to see if fit, or may need further treatment.

Listening to patient's chest and taking his blood pressure are two basic general examinations that can be done in the clinic.

16.5.4 Nasal Examination

Examination of the nose must include the **four areas of Rhinoplasty**. The functioning part of the nose is inseparable from the external nose and must be examined as well. This includes the nasal turbinates, nasal septum, postnasal space and eardrums.

16.5.4.1 The Frontolateral Walls

The frontolateral walls anatomically include the middle and lateral crurae and the alae nasi. The latter are surgically more related to the alar base. Clinically this area is mainly concerned with the nasal tip and its sidewalls. The examination includes the size, shape, position and thickness of the skin. Ethnicity has an effect on the skin, the size and the shape of the anterolateral walls.

Size and Shape:

The tip is seen whether large and bulbous or thick and bulky. The patient may have combinations of these. A deformity, scars or grafts under the skin are observed.

Position:

The tip should be the highest point of the nose. The tip is observed if projected, depressed, deviated or drooped, i.e., plunging.

16.5.4.2 The Medial Wall

The medial wall includes the **columella** and the **nasal septum**.

The Columella

The columella is examined for its length, thickness, bifidity, position and scars from previous surgery.

The position of the columella is the most significant aesthetically so that the columella may be:

- Oblique to one side.
- Retracted, protracted or hanging.
- The naso-labial angle is observed.

The Nasal Septum

i. The vestibular septum:

The caudal septal cartilage with its inferior margin, anterior and posterior angles is examined for its length, position and deformity.

Oblique, deviated, dislocated or a broken caudal septum may deform the shape of the columella and nasal apertures. Both nasal apertures will be **unequal** in size and shape. The naso-labial angle will be affected. The medial crural prominence, as well as the location of the nasal sill bands, will be affected.

ii. The Internal Respiratory septum:

The internal part of the septum that is beyond the nasal vestibule is covered by respiratory mucosa. The bony and cartilaginous parts are examined for deviation and their ability to contribute to nasal stability.

16.5.4.3 The Bony Pyramid and Midvault

The bony pyramid and midvault, anatomically, aesthetically and surgically, are closely linked to each other. They both share in the formation of the osteocartilagenous three-walled structure of the upper two-thirds of the nose.

The midvault usually follows the bony pyramid in its anatomical shape and its surgical changes.

Before examining the detailed anatomy, it is important to see the presence of **bilateral facial asymmetry**. The latter affects the rest of the anatomy and aesthetics of the bony pyramid.

The bony pyramid and midvault are examined for their size, shape and position.

Size and Shape

The bony pyramid has a base, top and overall size. Observation must include all three.

- The bony base may be wide, unequal, or narrow.
- One side of the bony pyramid may be depressed as a result of trauma.
- The top of the pyramid may be depressed, elevated making a hump or irregular.
- The overall size may be proportionately large, or small as compared to the overall size of the face.
- In facial asymmetry, one side of the bony pyramid is larger than the other. The pyramid is, therefore, deviated and oblique to one side.
- Both maxillae and cheeks are observed for their sizes, width and height. Bilateral maxillary asymmetries are not uncommon in deviated and crooked noses.

Position

The bony pyramid may be central, deviated to one side, oblique or crooked.

16.5.4.4 The Alar Base

The size, shape and skin thickness are examined.

The size and shape

The nasal apertures may be wide, distorted, scarred or narrowed.

The sizes and shapes of the two openings are seen and compared with each other. Unequal openings may be natural or secondary to unequal medial crural prominence, caudal septal deviation or previous surgery.

Both openings may be different in shape but equal in size.

The Rim-sill Folds

The rim-sill folds are examined for their length, thickness and obliquity.

The nasal sill bands are seen and compared for their length, thickness and position.

One side may be displaced inferiorly by a long caudal septum, secondary to unilateral facial weakness or previous surgery.

1. **Photographic Assessment**

This is an essential part of the assessment procedures for the patients (Refer to photographic section).

2. **Consent for Surgery**

Clear consent must be signed after discussing the details of the surgery. All the pros and cons are explained. Avoid high expectations and living unrealistic dreams of outstanding results. Professional legal advice must be sought. Legal consent may differ from one person or one country to another.

3. **Consent for Photography**

Consent for photography may be included in the general consent or it may be separate.

As a general rule, informed consent should always be obtained before photography is undertaken.

Each patient must understand the important need for photography and documentation.

Clinicians must spare good time to answer all the questions and concerns of the patient. A well informed written consent has three levels (Institute of Medical Illustrators IMI):

1. Consent for Medical use.
2. Consent for use in teaching health care staff.
3. Consent for publication. This should be for specific single use only or for general release in journals, books and electronic media. Patients should be warned that once published the consent cannot be withdrawn. This is especially for internet publication.

4. **Investigations**

Pre-operative operating room screen tests include the following:

- Complete Blood Count, CBC.
- HCV, HIV, HbsAg.
- PT, PTT, INR.
- For patients over thirty years, additional Chest X-ray and ECG are done.
- Other investigations depend on the general condition of the patient, e.g., Fasting Blood Sugar, Creatinine and liver function tests.

17 Clinical Assessment of Rhinoplasty Patient

Abstract

Getting to see a person who is thinking of or willing to have Rhinoplasty has its own characteristics and considerations. Although not sick, the candidate is a clinical condition that seeks surgery. The surgery is a highly sophisticated type that has many details in the different small areas of the nose. The outcome of the surgery is a new shape of the external nose. This results in a new image of the face that has substantial physical and psychological effects. In the interest of best results, a Rhinoplasty candidate is managed professionally as a patient. This ensures a thorough and accurate clinical assessment. In addition there must be a social and psychological assessment. The surgeon must be aware of the reasons and psychological status of the patient. Should any alarming signs in the history or behavior of the patient, the surgeon must consider the help of a psychiatrist without any hesitation. If the patient is already under care of a psychiatrist, then he must be approached and asked about the patient's ability to take this type of surgery. Clinical Assessment: History: Full medical, personal and family history, psychiatric history assessment. Examination: All four areas of the nose are examined. Photographic assessment: Consent for photography is of three levels • Taking photographs for teaching purposes and finally • For publication in book, journal and internet. Investigations: include blood tests, chest X-ray and ECG.

Keyword

Patient assessment for Rhinoplasty · Clinical assessment · Photographic assessment · Consent for surgery · Consent for photography

17.1 Clinical Assessment

17.1.1 History

(a) Patient's name, age, sex and ethnicity are taken.

(b) The patient must have complete freedom to express himself about when, why and what.

- When did he first think about Rhinoplasty?
- Why would he like the change? Is it a personal own wish or there are psychological, social or professional obligation.
- What does he like and dislike about his nose? What is the mental vision of the expected changes that he wishes for? What does it mean to him to have the surgery?

(c) Trauma

- Accidental trauma: trauma that causes nasal deformity must be a considerable one. It causes severe bleeding, hospitalization and possible surgery.

M. H. A. Shafy, *Innovations in Rhinoplasty*,
https://doi.org/10.1007/978-3-030-94573-2_17

  - Surgical: previous Rhinoplasty or any other plastic surgery in the face or body.
  - The date(s) of trauma and the number of surgeries are reported.

(d) History of psychological or mental illness. The intake of any antidepressants, sleeping pills or similar drugs.

(e) Sinunasal symptoms and diseases, e.g., nasal airway, smell disturbance, halitosis, anterior or posterior nasal discharge. History of sinus infection, allergy or polyps. History of sinus or septal surgery.

(f) General illness, e.g., diabetes, hypertension, asthma or other systemic diseases.

(g) Family history:
History of Rhinoplasty or any type of plastic surgery to any member of the family, close relative or friends.
Family history of mental or psychological illnesses or general diseases, e.g., allergy, diabetes or hypertension.

17.1.2 Examination

Examination of a candidate for Rhinoplasty must include general, local, psychological and photographic.

17.1.3 General Examination

Patient must be generally fit for the surgery. According to the history the patient may be referred to the specialized doctor if necessary to see if fit or may need further treatment.

Listening to patient's chest and taking his blood pressure are two basic general examinations that can be done in the clinic.

17.1.4 Nasal Examination

Examination of the nose must include the **four areas of Rhinoplasty**. The functioning part of the nose is inseparable from the external nose and must be examined as well. This includes the nasal turbinates, nasal septum, post-nasal space and ear drums.

17.1.4.1 The Frontolateral Walls

The frontolateral walls anatomically include the middle and lateral crurae and the alae nasi. The latter are surgically more related to the alar base. Clinically, this area is mainly concerned with the nasal tip and its sidewalls. Examination includes the size, shape, position and thickness of the skin. Ethnicity has an effect on the skin, the size and the shape of the anterolateral walls.

Size and Shape:

The tip is seen whether large and bulbous or thick and bulky. The patient may have combinations of these. A deformity, scars or grafts under the skin are observed.

Position:

The tip should be the highest point of the nose. The tip is observed if projected, depressed, deviated or drooped, i.e., plunging.

17.1.4.2 The Medial Wall

The medial wall includes the **columella** and the **nasal septum.**

The Columella

The columella is examined for its length, thickness, bifidity, position and scars from previous surgery.

The position of the columella is the most significant aesthetically so that the columella may be:

- Oblique to one side.
- Retracted, protracted or hanging.
- The nasolabial angle is observed

The Nasal Septum

i. The vestibular septum:

The caudal septal cartilage with its inferior margin, anterior and posterior angles is examined for its length, position and deformity.

Oblique, deviated, dislocated or a broken caudal septum may deform the shape of the columella and nasal apertures. Both nasal apertures will be **unequal** in size and shape. The nasolabial angle will be affected. The medial crural prominence as well as the location of the nasal sill bands will be affected.

ii. The Internal Respiratory septum:

The internal part of the septum that is beyond the nasal vestibule is covered by respiratory mucosa. The bony and cartilaginous parts are examined for deviation and their ability to contribute to nasal stability.

17.1.4.3 The Bony Pyramid and MidVault

The bony pyramid and midvault anatomically, aesthetically and surgically are closely linked to each other. They both share in the formation of the osteocartilaginous three-walled structure of the upper two thirds of the nose.

The midvault usually follows the bony pyramid in its anatomical shape and its surgical changes.

Before examining the detailed anatomy, it is important to see the presence of **bilateral facial asymmetry**. The latter affects the rest of the anatomy and aesthetics of the bony pyramid.

The bony pyramid and midvault are examined for their size, shape and position.

Size and Shape

The bony pyramid has a base, top and overall size. Observation must include all three.

- The bony base may by wide, unequal, or narrow.
- One side of the bony pyramid may be depressed as a result of trauma.
- The top of the pyramid may be depressed, elevated making a hump or irregular.
- The overall size may be proportionately large, or small as compare to the overall size of the face.
- In facial asymmetry, one side of the bony pyramid is larger than the other. The pyramid is, therefore, deviated and oblique to one side.
- Both maxillae and cheeks are observed for their sizes, width and height. Bilateral maxillary asymmetries are not uncommon in deviated and crooked noses.

Position

The bony pyramid may be central, deviated to one side, oblique or crooked.

17.1.4.4 The Alar Base

The size, shape and skin thickness are examined.

The size and shape

The nasal apertures may be wide, distorted, scarred or narrowed.

The sizes and shapes of the two openings are seen and compared with each other. Unequal openings may be natural or secondary to unequal medial crural prominence, caudal septal deviation or previous surgery.

Both openings may be different in shape but equal in size.

The Rim-sill Folds

The rim-sill folds are examined for their length, thickness and obliquity.

The nasal sill bands are seen and compared for their length, thickness and position.

One side may be displaced inferiorly by a long caudal septum, secondary to unilateral facial weakness or previous surgery.

17.2 Photographic Assessment

This is an essential part of the assessment procedures for the patients. (Refer to photographic section)

17.3 Consent for Surgery

A clear consent must be signed after discussing the details of surgery. All the pros and cons are explained. Avoid high expectations and living in unrealistic dreams of outstanding results. Professional legal advice must be sought. Legal consent may differ from one person or one country to another.

17.4 Consent for Photography

Consent for photography may be included in the general consent or it may be separate.

As a general rule, informed consent should always be obtained before photography is undertaken.

Each patient must understand the important need for photography and documentation.

Clinicians must spare good time to answer all the questions and concerns of the patient. A well-informed written consent has three levels (Institute of Medical Illustrators IMI)

1. Consent for medical use.
2. Consent for use in teaching health care staff.
3. Consent for publication. This should be for specific single use only or for general release in journal, books and electronic media. Patients should be warned that once published the consent cannot be withdrawn. This is especially for internet publication.

17.5 Investigations

Pre-operative operating room screen tests include the following:

- Complete blood count, CBC.
- HCV, HIV, HbsAg.
- PT, PTT, Inr.
- For patients over 30 years, additional chest X-ray and ECG are done.
- Other investigations depend on the general condition of the patient, e.g., fasting blood sugar, creatinine and liver function tests.

18 Immediate Pre-operative, Operative and Post-operative Rhinoplasty

Abstract

Both the patient and the surgeon must be prepared for the surgery. The patient is prepared psychologically and physically. No matter how **experienced** is the **surgeon** or how **simple** is the **surgery,** surgeons must have a **written plan for the proposed surgery**. The plan must be written clearly in definitive chronological steps.

Keywords

Preparing the patient for surgery · Preparing the surgeon for the surgery

18.1 How the Surgeon Prepares Himself for the Surgery

18.1.1 Review Patient's History and Photographs

18.1.1.1 Written Plan for Surgery

No matter how **experienced** is the **surgeon** or how **simple** is the **surgery,** surgeons must have a **written plan for the proposed surgery**. The plan must be written clearly in definitive chronological steps.

The written plan includes:

(a) **Surgical assessment**.
(b) **Aims of surgery**.
(c) **Surgical plan**.

All of the **four areas of rhinoplasty** must be included in the analysis and the surgical plan.

The written plan is placed in the operating room where it can be seen by the surgeon and his assistants.

> **Your mind is for having ideas, not holding them.** (David Allen)

Plans might be modified or changed during surgery, but having them helps in **going smoothly through the surgery** both by the **surgeon** and his **assistants**. Nurses and assistants are **better organized**, while the surgeon is able to **concentrate on the techniques of surgery** rather than worrying about the next step or what is missed.

At the end of the procedure, the surgeon, assistant and nurses must check that the written plan is completely fulfilled.

> **By failing to prepare, you are preparing to fail.** (Benjamin Franklin)

18.2 Preparing the Patient for Surgery

18.2.1 Preoperative Discussion

- Explanation: in simple terms, the details of the provisional plan for surgery are explained to the patient.
- Length of procedure and duration of hospitalization are reassuring facts.

M. H. A. Shafy, *Innovations in Rhinoplasty*,
https://doi.org/10.1007/978-3-030-94573-2_18

- Pain control: It is of great psychological value to reassure the patient about the post-operative pain control plans in the immediate and subsequent days.
- Timeline: The look of the nose in the immediate post-operative and the time it takes for complete settling down. Although it was discussed in the previous interviews, yet it is important to re-emphasize these facts immediately before surgery.

18.2.2 Preparation of the Operating Theater

18.2.2.1 Display of Photographs

Photographs of the patients are displayed on **a table or a screen in front of the surgeon**. Areas of interest are particularly displayed clearly.

It is not always necessary to display all views. The **standard views are always displayed,** i.e., frontal, basal, oblique and lateral. **Each individual case may have its necessary views** that help the surgeon during the procedure, e.g., **smiling lateral** views are displayed in cases of **mobile tip, aperture views** in **alar base** surgery and **backward tilting** views in cases of **wide bony pyramid** and **columellar deformities**.

At the end of the procedure, it is extremely helpful to see **the result of the surgery** and compare the post-surgical outcome with the pre-operative photographs.

18.2.2.2 Position of the Patient and the Operating Table

The patient is placed on the operating table in a **reverse Trendelenburg position**. The **upper half of the table is further raised** and the **head is slightly elevated**. This helps to **reduce the nasal blood flow**, and in the meantime, the nose is at the **best position and height** that enables the surgeon pursuing the surgery.

A suitable size firm, but not hard, **horse shoe** or a **head ring** is placed under the occiput. To avoid post-operative discomfort and sometimes pain, it is advisable to put a cushion under the knees and a smaller one just above the heals.

18.2.2.3 Placing the Anesthetic Tube

In case of general anesthesia, the **oral anesthetic tube must be placed in a central position**. Fixation of the tube should be away from the lower lip to avoid undue pulling of the angle of the mouth. Connections of the anesthetic tube are secured at a **lower level than both lips**, so that they do not come in the way of the surgeon hands. Bulky connections or filters are diverted sideways by a suitable T-shaped connecting tube.

18.3 The Surgery

18.3.1 Preliminary Surgical Preparation

18.3.1.1 Shaving of the Vestibular Hair

Vibrissae of the nasal vestibules can be thick, dense and heavy. They tend to hide the anatomy of the vestibular walls especially if alar base surgery or delivery of the lower cartilages is planned. Close shaving is, therefore, a useful basic routine preparation of the nose for surgery.

The vestibular walls may vary in their shapes, density of their hair contents and the condition of the skin. The vestibule may have thick, heavy condensed vibrissae and dry crusty skin or exactly the opposite, i.e., scanty, thin, vibrissae with greasy or wet skin.

In cases of dry skin or dense vibrissae, it is better to paint the skin with any type of **ointment** using a cotton bud before shaving. A No 15 blade is best used for shaving. The side of the knife is coated with a thin film of ointment so that the vibrissae stick to the blade rather than falling inside the nasal cavity. The ala nasi is stretched using a sharp alar retractor to facilitate the shaving process. The area of the **flat triangle** has to be **everted** and gently shaved to avoid injury of the skin. Finally, the slope of the vestibular floor is easily shaved from side to side (Fig. 18.1).

18.3.1.2 Additional Local Anesthesia

Local anesthesia is used in addition to the general anesthesia to favor hemostasis. One in one

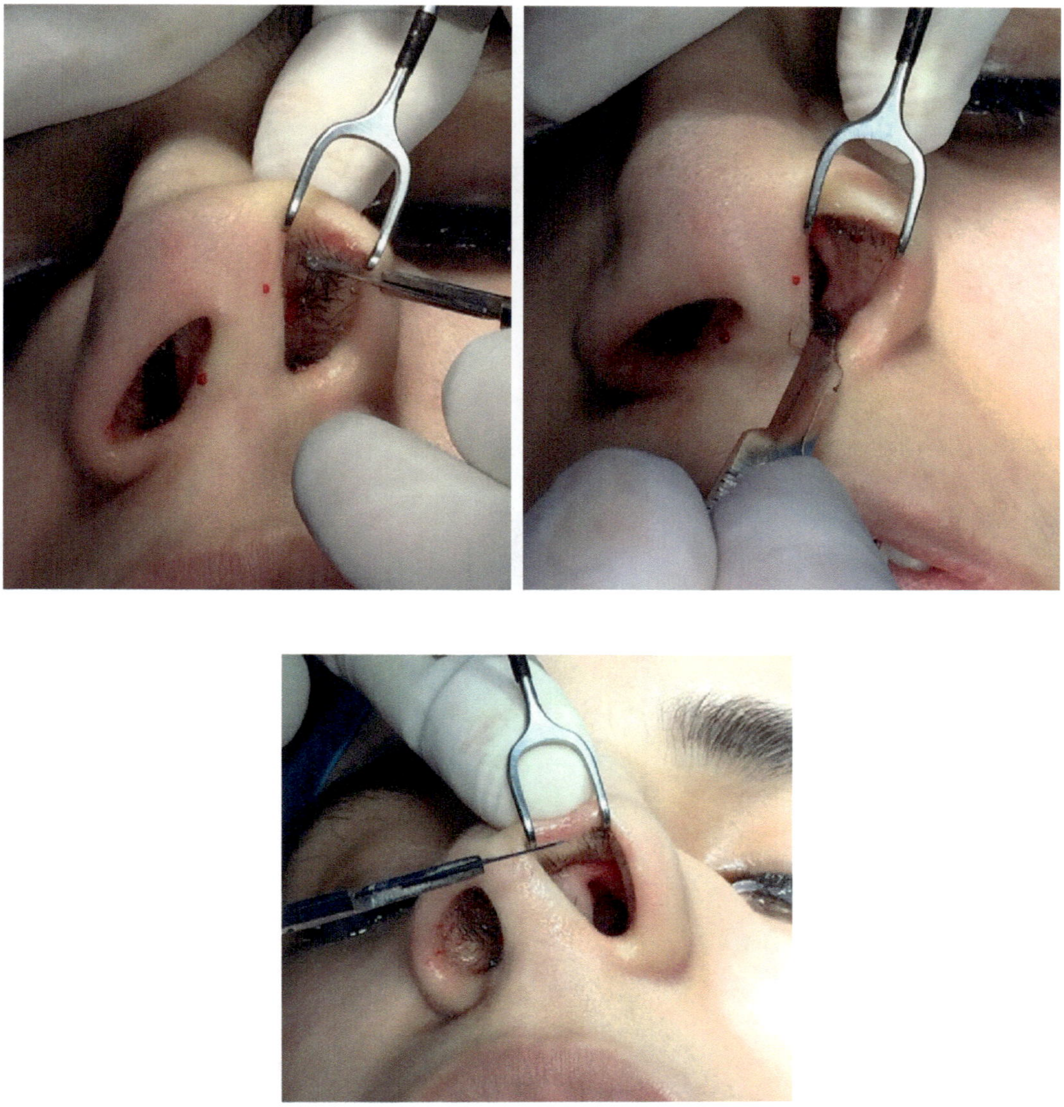

Fig. 18.1 Shaving of the lateral and inferior vestibular walls

hundred thousand (1:100,000) of adrenalin mixed with Lidocaine 1–2% is used. A total of almost 5ml is more than sufficient.

A fine subdermal insulin needle and syringe is used. For higher injections around the bony pyramid, a longer fine needle is used. Only a few milliliters are injected in the following places:

- Intercartilaginous folds.
- Columella exactly at the midpoint between the inferior margins of the medial crurae.
- The inferior margins of the medial and lateral crurae.
- The inferior margins of the lateral crurae (Fig. 18.3).
- The rim-sill folds, should alar base surgery be anticipated (Fig. 18.2).
- The membranous septum (Fig. 18.4).
- The nasal dorsum (Fig. 18.5).
- The base of the bony pyramid at the osteotomy lines.

Surgery starts 5–10 minutes after the injections in order to allow for the full effect of local

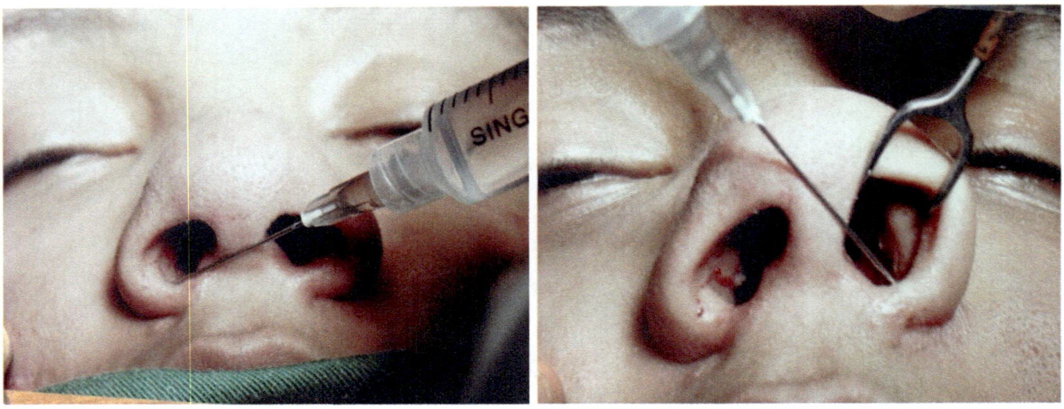

Fig. 18.2 Local anesthesia of the rim sill folds

Fig. 18.3 Local anesthesia of the inferior margin of the lateral crus

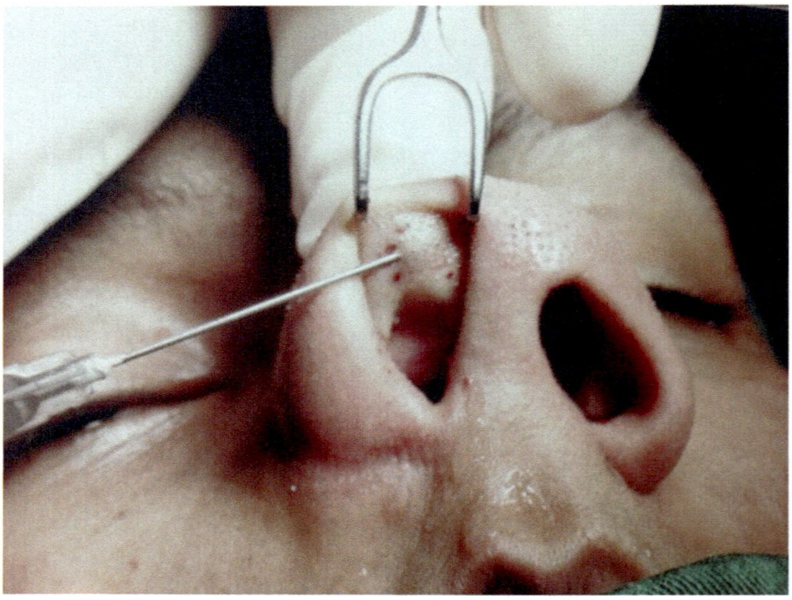

anesthesia to take place and for the swollen areas of injection to settle down.

18.3.2 Incisions and Skeletonization

18.3.2.1 The Intercartilaginous Incisions

A no. 15 blade is used in a Burt Parker handle for making the initial fresh incision. An intercartilaginous incision is made in the gutter between the lower margin of the upper lateral cartilage and the body of the lateral crus. The incision should be **as close as possible to the** medial side of the gutter to avoid injury to the folded overlap of the lateral crus (Fig. 18.6).

Incisions on both sides are gradually deepened in an upward, **sawing like action**, till the **lower borders of the nasal bones** are reached. Undermining should be **as close as possible to the cartilage**, to minimize damaging the small muscles of the nose.

Note that the limen nasi, i.e., the mucocutanous junction is located exactly at the inferior margin of the upper lateral cartilage.

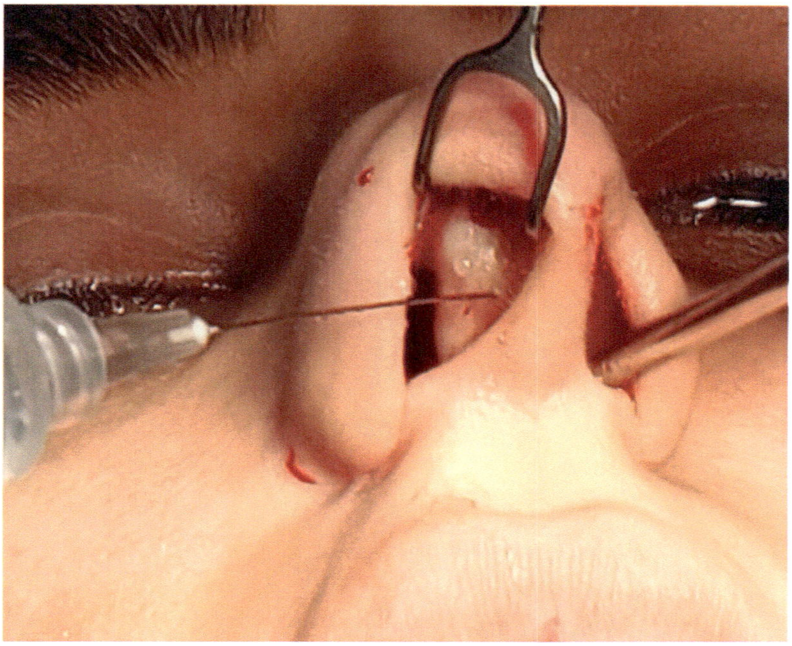

Fig. 18.4 Local anesthesia of the membranous septum

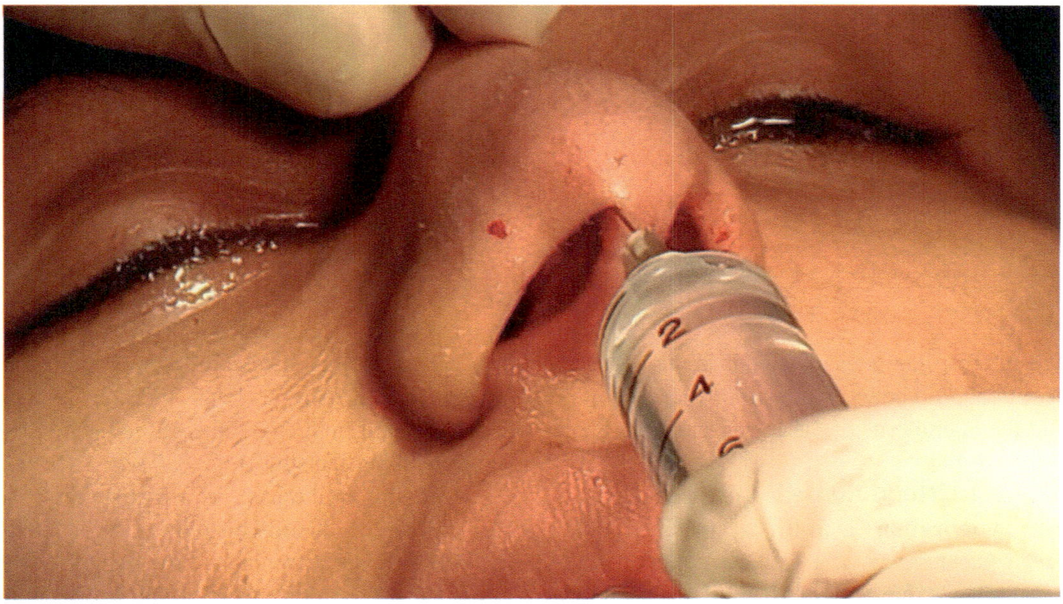

Fig. 18.5 Local anesthesia of the nasal dorsum

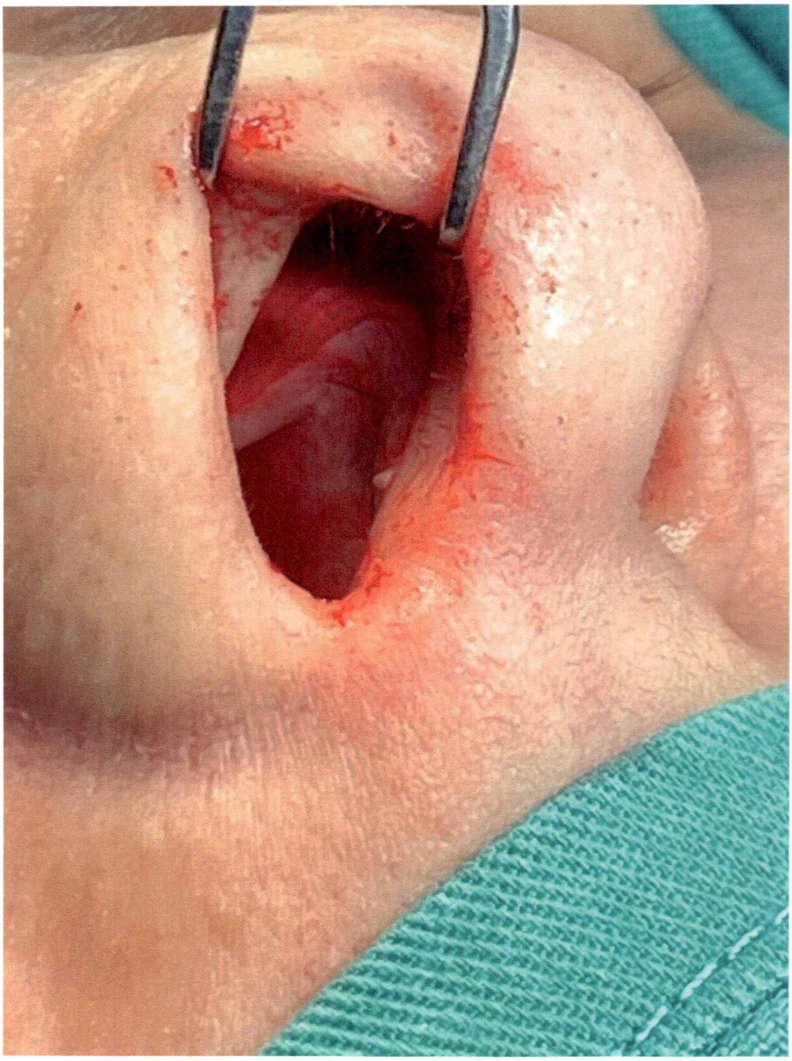

Fig. 18.6 The intercartilaginous incision

The intercartilaginous incision is in the vestibular skin lined fold between the upper lateral cartilage and the lateral crus of the lower lateral cartilage.

18.3.2.2 The Columellar Incision

The **membranous septum** is **stretched** inferiorly using toothed or a Cottle's columellar forceps. The inferior border of the **caudal cartilaginous septum** becomes apparently clear. A **second transfixing incision** is made at the caudal margin of the septum. It is better to start this incision as **two separate ones** on both side of the caudal margin. Each incision is then deepened until both are connected to each other, i.e., transfixing incision (Fig. 18.7).

Depending on the plan for septal surgery, the incision may be a **hemitransfixing** one, i.e., only reaching halfway between the two angles, i.e., the anterior and posterior angles of the cartilaginous septum. It is better to avoid complete transfixing incision. Septoplasty can be made by extending the excision on one side of the septum only.

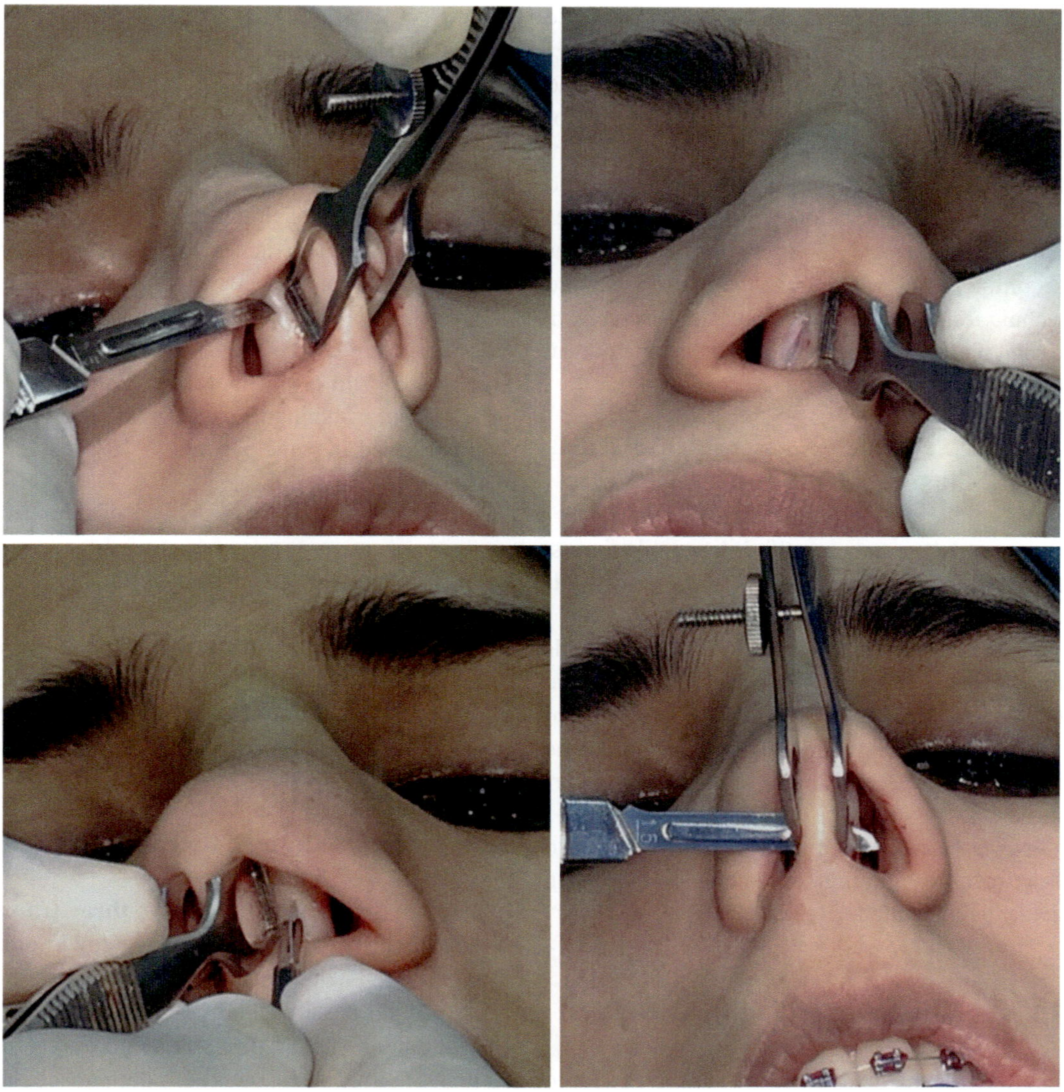

Fig. 18.7 Transfixing columellar incision

18.3.2.3 Communicating the Incisions

The columellar incision is communicated with the intercartilaginous incisions on both sides, **inferior to, and avoiding the anterior angle of the internal nasal valve** (Fig. 18.6).

18.3.2.4 Skeletonization

A periosteal elevator is introduced via the intercartilaginous incision. The periostium is elevated off the nasal bones, i.e., only over **the top midzonal area of the bony pyramid.** Special attention must be paid to **start exactly at the lower edges of the nasal bones**, where the **procerus muscles** are attached. They are **detached together with the periostium** in this step.

Periostial elevation and skin undermining **must not extend too far laterally** over the frontal processes of the maxillae. The sides of the bony pyramid should remain attached to the skin for better stability of the bony pyramid.

Elevation of the periostium continues superiorly **till the nasofrontal angle** is reached, i.e., the nasion. Here the elevator has to go deeply to scrape the periostium off the bottom of the angle and its two sides superiorly and inferiorly.

Now exposure of the nose is complete and the nose is ready for the different techniques of rhinoplasty according to the predetermined plan. Each part of the nose has its own dynamics and anatomical considerations. Surgical techniques have to be adapted for each of the four areas accordingly. Nevertheless, there are standard techniques in each of these areas that serve as a basic guide in dealing with its special anatomical and aesthetic specifications.

18.4 Closure of Wounds

Rhinopalsty wounds are the **intercartilaginous**, **columellar**, **marginal**, **septal**, **external osteotomy** and **alar** wounds.

Generally speaking, many of these wounds may come back to their natural anatomical location without gaping. Delicate stitching of these wounds using fine stitches enhances the natural appearance of the nose as well as securing them.

Nevertheless, any of these wounds are seen to be **unstable**, **gaping** or **prone to bleeding** demands meticulous closure.

18.4.1 The Intercartilaginous Incision

The intercartilaginous incisions are better closed by one or two absorbable stitches. If omitted protrusion of the upper lateral cartilage may come into view, with possible external depression.

18.4.2 The Columellar Incision

Even in the smallest hemitransfixing columeller incision, it is better secured with 3 or 4 zero vicryl stitches on each side of the incision.

As the columellar incision is continuous with the intercartilaginous incision, both incisions must be seen to be safely and securely away from the anterior angle of the nasal valve. The columellar incision may have the following special situations:

i. The complete transfixing incision: It is a long wound that needs to be closed. Each side is closed separately using four zero vycril stitches.
ii. Transcolumellar Stitches:
iii. Inter-sill band stitches may be needed in cases of prominent or unequal medial crurae. No 3 zero proline stitches in a straight needle are used.
iv. Caudal trim of the **septal cartilage** with or without trimming of **excess vestibular skin** is needed in some patients.

18.4.3 The Marginal Incisions

Although very stable and secure wounds, it is better to have a stitch or two at the lower margins of the lateral or medial crurae using five or six zero vycril stitches.

18.4.4 Trans-septal Stitching

In cases of septal surgery, **two or three trans-septal stitches** are taken from above downwards to avoid septal hematoma as well as avoiding the need for tight nasal packings.

Light nasal packing may still be necessary for nasal stability and securing the vestibular wounds.

18.5 Final Dressing of the Nose

Special attention and care must be given to the final dressing of the nose. It is as important step as the surgery itself. Defatting leaves a potentially large space between the skin and the underlying soft tissues which are mostly weakened by surgery. Most of the fibrous bands between the domes as well as anterior angle of septum are all served.

The external dressing helps to eliminate the dead space and hold the lower lateral cartilages together so that their main support now is the external skin. The cartilages are quite soft and malleable and that the nasal tip can easily be molded by the external dressings.

The sidewalls of the bony pyramid are secured in their new medial position, after osteotomies by the solid external support, i.e., Plaster of Paris.

The external dressing needs to be tailored to support each part of the surgery, i.e., the bony pyramid, nasal dorsum and the nasal tip.

The external dressing is made in three steps:

18.5.1 Preparing the External Skin

The nasal skin needs to be dried up off its grease to allow for the dressing to stick and remain tightly held against it.

Skin of the forehead and cheeks needs to be dried up as well to allow for the external fixation of the plaster with adhesive tapes.

Compound tincture of Benzoin or pure alcohol solution is used to dry the skin of the nose, cheeks and forehead. Care is taken to protect the eyes and the nasal cavity.

18.5.2 Steri-strip Dressing

A light intranasal pack is placed, to have an internal support to the vestibular skin.

A square piece of gauze swab is placed over the nose. The excess accumulated blood under the skin is gently squeezed out.

It is quite essential to have a good type of steristrip to fit tightly on the nose. The author uses a soft type of steri-strip is used, e.g., proxistrip 0.5 × 10 cm. A long stripe is placed in the form of a U-shaped around the nasal tip inferiorly then along the sidewalls of the nose.

Transverse stripes are then placed across the nose from below upwards. Shorter stripes of only 5 cm or less are needed for the midvault and bony pyramid.

Continuous gentle external pressure and squeeze of the nose to avoid recollection of subcutaneous blood.

Then final new shape of the nose is now seen.

18.5.3 Plaster of Paris Dressing (POP)

Plaster of Paris is important not only to secure and maintain the medialized sidewalls of the bony pyramid but also to maintain the new shape of the soft tissues in the lower thirds of the nose especially the nasal tip.

Five stripes of plaster are prepared one 0.5 cm × 10 cm and four 0.5 cm × 5 cm.

1. The first long stripe is placed in the form of a U-shaped around the nasal tip inferiorly (just like steri-strip dressing).
2. One short stripe is placed along the nasal dorsum.
3. Two stripes are placed across the bony bridge and the midvault.
4. One final stripe is placed across the nasal tip holding the two sides of the U-shaped inferior nasal tip stripe.
5. The dorsum and the two sides of the plaster are securely held by the index, middle finger and the thumb of the surgeon while the assistant index finger gently support the nasal tip upwards till the plaster hardens up. This secures the bony pyramid and helps shaping the nasal tip.
6. The T-shaped plaster is then placed over the forehead and the nose. The forehead part of the plaster is necessary to stabilize the nasal part and keep it in place.
7. POP is fixed in place by two transverse adhesive tapes. One on the forehead and the second across the nasal tip bridge.

Other materials than P.O.P. may be available in local markets.

All of these dressings including the P.O.P. are removed after 1 week. The steri-strip layer can easily be peeled off the face by the use of the rounded blunt side of a Jobson Horn probe.

Difficulties Associated with Rhinoplasty

19

Abstract

According to the American Society of Plastic Surgery, Rhinoplasty is the **most popular elective plastic surgery** for patients in many ethnic groups, e.g., Anglosaxons, Africans, Asians and Hispanic or Middle Eastern. Not every individual with a deformed nose is readily prepared to have Rhinoplasty and not every competent surgeon is readily prepared to perform Rhinoplasty. There are difficulties before during and after the surgery of Rhinoplasty.

Keywords

Difficulties associated with Rhinoplasty

19.1 Introduction

According to the American Society of Plastic Surgery, Rhinoplasty is the **most popular elective plastic surgery** for patients in many ethnic groups, e.g., Anglosaxons, Africans, Asians and Hispanic or Middle Eastern.

Aesthetic Rhinoplasty is not an easy operation. In fact, it is one of, if not the most difficult aesthetic surgeries. (Rees and Latrento).

Not every individual with a deformed nose is readily prepared to have Rhinoplasty and not every competent surgeon is readily prepared to perform Rhinoplasty.

Patients must be ready physically, mentally and emotionally.

Rhinoplasty demands a high level of knowledge, aptitude, training and the ability to think in three dimensions with imagination. There is an element of artistry in the surgery that needs fine motor skills. Surgeons must have the talent, right attitude and be well balanced mentally and emotionally.

Rhinoplasty demands detailed, comprehensive preparation before the surgery from the surgeons and the patients.

19.2 Difficulties Before the Surgery

19.2.1 Difficult Pre-operative Assessment

In many cases, nasal deformities are clearly seen, e.g., nasal deviation, hump or depressed areas. The plan for management may equally be quite clear, yet a totally unexpected deformity, defect, deviation or other distortion may appear in the course of the routine surgical procedure. These intraoperative surprises may take place no matter

M. H. A. Shafy, *Innovations in Rhinoplasty*,
https://doi.org/10.1007/978-3-030-94573-2_19

how experienced and well prepared is the surgeon.

As the surgeon acquires more experience, he or she becomes more capable of dealing with these situations as they arise.

The unpredictable situations that cannot be foreseen in the pre-operative assessment are:

19.2.1.1 Defective Areas

Areas of defects may appear, despite the absence of previous trauma. They are common especially in facial asymmetries and localized angulations at the nasal dorsum or sidewalls.

Common areas of defects in order of ambiguity and prevalence are:

i. One side of the **midvault**.
ii. One side or the middle of the **supratip area**.
iii. **One side of the bony pyramid** may be smaller and slightly more depressed than the other side.
iv. The **nasofrontal angle** and the most superior part of the bony dorsum.

19.2.1.2 Nasal Aperture Discrepancies

i. The size of nasal openings:
   During the course of surgery, normal-sized nasal openings may become unaesthetically wide after reduction surgery. An unplanned decision for reduction alar surgery can only be taken during the course of surgery.
ii. Similarities of the nasal openings:
   Intraoperatively each of the nasal openings may become **different** in **size** and/or **shape**, e.g., after defatting.
   It is important to maintain bilateral near to equal **sizes**. The bilateral differences in **shapes** may be quite natural.
iii. Aesthetics of the nasal openings:
   During the course of surgery, the nasal openings that were previously aesthetically acceptable may **become unaesthetic,** e.g., the alae nasi become everted, inverted, elevated or lowered. An intraoperative decision for alar surgery becomes necessary.
iv. Developmental differences
   The two nasal openings may be naturally different in many individuals with quite acceptable overall aesthetic outlook.
   During the course of surgery, the differences between the two sides become noticeable and aesthetically unpleasant. Alar surgery is required to minimize these differences.

19.2.2 Difficulties of Standardized Photography

Photography, as an important pre-operative assessment tool, is not quite a simple procedure. It needs a well-equipped surgeon with the appropriate tools and training for taking standardized photographs.

Standardization of photographs includes the camera, lens, lighting, patient orientation and the background.

Should a professional medical photographer is available then a very close communication between the surgeon and photographic department must be well established. Having good **standardized photographs** is the main target at the end of the day to help out in the pre-operative assessment.

19.2.3 A Lack of Holistic Approach to Nasal Assessment

When a patient presents to the surgeon he or she always has **one** major disturbing unpleasant part of the nose, e.g., nasal hump, wide nostrils, crookedness, etc. It is the job of the surgeon to have a more professional look at the nose and study other areas that may consequently require adjustment. All anatomical areas of the nose must be considered.

If the surgeon only addresses one disturbing problem, the result might be disappointing, e.g., removal of a nasal hump and overlooking wide alae or thick-skinned anterolateral walls. Postoperatively, the patient will have a trumpet like nose.

19.2.4 Many Factors Affect the Surgical Technique

Many factors are considered in order to have a good aesthetic result, e.g., Ethnic origin, trauma, gender, facial asymmetry, previous surgeries, congenital anomalies and most importantly nasal airway and the physiology of nasal respiration.

19.2.5 Psychological Readiness of Surgery

Rhinoplasty has a very strong psychological impact on the patient. Psychology of the patient is a major concern. This is especially true in females' young age and revision. (Refer to Chapter of Psychology).

19.3 Difficulties During Surgery

19.3.1 Different Tissues in a Small Organ

The nose is a small organ composed of **different tissues,** i.e., **bones, cartilages** and **fibro fat** and is covered with **seven types of different skins**. Each of these structures has special surgical considerations.

The different tissues are attached to each other in many different ways:

- Sutures between bones.
- Overlap between cartilages and bone.
- Overlap between two cartilages.
- Fibrous bands connecting skin and cartilage.

19.3.2 Rhinoplasty is of Four Surgeries

Rhinoplasty is not a single operation. It is rather multiple variant surgeries in the different areas of the nose.

There are **four areas** in the nose. These four areas are:

i. The **Frontolateral walls** include the nasal tip and lateral crurae.
ii. The **Medial wall** includes the nasal septum, medial crurae and columella.
iii. The **bony pyramid** and **the midvault.**
iv. The **Nasal Base** including the alar base.

Each of these areas has its own detailed **anatomical** structure that requires a totally **different** surgical technique. Not only **skill** is needed in the surgery for each of the four areas but also excellent judgment is essential in **harmonizing** between them, so that they finally integrate into an aesthetically attractive nose.

19.3.3 Nasal Stability

The pyramidal shape of the nose, as a three-dimensional structure must be sustained throughout the whole surgical procedure. Care must be taken to **avoid collapse** of any part of the nose, e.g., total collapse of the **bony pyramid, midvault, supratip** or the **nasal tip**. This may lead to varying degrees of **saddle deformity**, **depressed**, irregular or crooked areas in the osteocartilaginous dorsum or the nasal tip.

The main contributors to nasal stability are:

<u>The Nasal Septum:</u>

The nasal septum is a major stabilizing structure of the nose.

Partial disruption, especially at the anterior and inferior margins, leads to immediate corresponding depression at the dorsum or columella successively.

Sudden dorsal collapse may take place if there is a disruption anterior to the line between the osteocartilaginous junction, at the nasal dorsum, and the anterior nasal spine.

Dislocation, loss by infection, surgical or accidental trauma may lead to a total or partial collapse of the nasal dorsum. The overall outcome is varying degrees of saddle deformity and or columellar retraction.

The Bony Pyramid:

The bony pyramid is the primary framework of the upper third of the nose. Over-reduction of the nasal hump may lead to varying degrees of saddle deformities.

Overzealous dissection of the skin off the sides of the bony pyramid may lead to its collapse after osteotomies.

The Upper Lateral Cartilage:

Surgical, accidental or natural defects may affect one side, or, less commonly, both sides of the upper lateral cartilage.

Dividing the sides of the upper lateral cartilage from the nasal septum is better avoided in patients who had previous septal surgery, especially if parts of the cartilaginous septum were excised.

The Columella

The firm grip of the vestibular skin on both sides of the lateral surfaces of the medial crurae as well as the intercrural connective tissues give the columella strength to keep up the **lower third of the nose** including the nasal tip. (See the chapter of Closed Versus Open Rhinoplasty).

19.4 Difficulties After the Surgery

19.4.1 The Paradox of Tissue Healing

Although the nose is a small external organ, yet it is made of several smaller subunits. Each of these subunits has its own **anatomical** and **histological** makeup. They vary from thin to thick bones, cartilages, skin and subdermal tissues. Each of these tissues requires **different techniques for surgery** and **heals in different ways** at different **speeds**.

Although soft tissues, in general, heal faster than bones and cartilages, the subdermal tissues of the nasal tip may take many months or may be a year before reaching their final aesthetic shape.

Edema and swelling in the soft cartilaginous and subdermal tissues take longer time than the hard bones to settle in their **final sizes and shapes** especially in the nasal tip area.

It is something of a **paradox** that even though **bones** are hard yet they heal and take their final shape **faster** than the **soft tissues of the nasal tip**, which includes thick skin, subdermal fat and lateral cartilages.

19.4.2 Variability of Post-operative Outcomes

Despite excellent surgical techniques and the almost perfect result on table at the time of surgery, results may not be equally perfect after removing the plaster cast.

Some cases may have perfect immediate postoperative results but disappointing long-term results. These vary from minor deformity to more disappointing deviations, depressions or elevations.

Tissue healing, graft resorption and skin condition are variable factors between patients that affect the long-term results.

19.4.3 Psychological Factor

One of the important factors that has great consideration is patient's psychological condition. The change of the facial image is not to be taken lightly especially in young females.

The psychological impact of an unpleasant looking nose, true or perceived is variable from one person to another. Details are discussed in the section of Psychology.

20 Psychology of Rhinoplasty

Abstract

A deformed nose, actual or perceived, may have varying degrees of emotional and psychological effects on people, especially those who decide to seek surgery. The surgeons attitude should be supportive and informative. Most patients go through five psychological stages

Keywords

Psychology of Rhinoplasty

20.1 Introduction

A deformed nose, actual or perceived, may have varying degrees of emotional and psychological effects on people, especially those who decide to seek surgery.

Rhinoplasty not only has **physical** effects but more importantly is associated with varying degrees of **emotional** and **psychological** overlay.

The impact of surgery on a person whether successful or unsuccessful is equally profound regardless of age, sex, ethnicity, social or educational status.

The person's age is not the sole determining factor for surgery. They have to be psychologically, emotionally and mentally ready.

Considering change and modifying the shape of someone's own nose and consequently the facial image is the outcome of various physical, psychological and emotional reactions of a person who finally decides, by his own will, to go through this experience. He may express his wishes to a close relative or a friend. In some individuals, this may remain totally within themselves as their own private affair.

The decision is not a simple or an easy one. It carries the complexities of both the **emotional** and **physical** changes that affect someone's image and face forever. There are varying degrees of **uncertainties** despite the great need for surgery and the trust in surgical success. This is especially true if the surgeon is well known to the individual. The feeling of being a normal person who decides to go through the pains of surgery in a hospital, which is a place for sick people, is associated with varying degrees of **fear**.

20.2 Surgeon's Attitude During Patient Assessment

It is better, especially during the first consultation, that the doctor takes a **neutral** and **unbiased attitude**, i.e., listening more than suggesting. He should **avoid any strong views** and reserve them for later, after long periods of listening carefully, patiently and sometimes repeatedly to the patient's own views.

M. H. A. Shafy, *Innovations in Rhinoplasty*,
https://doi.org/10.1007/978-3-030-94573-2_20

Professional views are only made after complete personal and clinical judgment. The person himself must be the one who **wishes** for the surgery **for his own satisfaction** and not under any other social or familial obligations. Consideration is made for those few who have insight. Insight is the degree of awareness that he is ill and worthful of treatment.

The doctor may reassure the person in certain areas of success of the surgery, and the probabilities in the areas of uncertainties. A nasal hump may be well excised, yet asymmetry or crookedness may not be completely corrected. The patient's psychological stability is assessed. Only experience can be the best judge in these situations. Psychological testing, by a psychiatrist, can rule out or confirm the possibility of underlying **mental illness**.

Normal Individuals and NOT Patients

People seeking rhinoplasty are not sick individuals. They cannot be called or referred to as patients. They only become patients if and when surgery is indicated. Dealing with these cases by the surgeons is partly informal and partly formal.

A lady with a large nose is very much like a pregnant lady. Both are not sick. They cannot be called patients. They become patients if and when surgery is indicated.

20.3 Consent and Patient Psychology

A very clear consent must be taken. The consent may change according to each condition and the personality of the patient. Areas of uncertainty in surgical outcomes must be realistically and clearly written down, even if it means that the surgery may have to be dismissed altogether. This is a true and crucial test of the patient's will, psychological stability and strength to accept what might be unexpected.

20.4 The Five Stages of the Patient's Psychology

To understand and appreciate the patient's emotional reactions, one must start from the very beginning of the patient's awareness of his nose. There are usually five stages of a patient's psychological reaction:

20.4.1 The Stage of Discontent

The patient is unsatisfied with the look of the nose. There is no parallel relation between the nasal deformity and that feeling. A person may be obsessed with a minor deformity and vice versa, i.e. quite content with a severe deformity. Traumatic deformities, in general, have a less psychological impact, than natural developmental deformities.

20.4.2 The Stage of Decision

As the feeling of discontent gradually grows stronger, patients finally decide for the change. Plastic surgery is now common knowledge available to the public, especially via social media. Relatives, friends and public figures are commonly seen having these surgeries.

20.4.3 The Stage of Action

This is the active stage which is further subdivided into four important substages:

20.4.3.1 Searching for a Surgeon

The patient starts the journey of searching for the right surgeon that he may trust to make his surgery. The patient may see more than one surgeon at this stage. During this stage, the patient may decide to either back off or proceed to the next stage.

This stage and the previous two stages are usually bypassed by someone who has a close relative or a friend that went through the rhinoplasty experience successfully. It makes the idea closer to the patient's mind so that the decision is earlier for the surgery and the selection of the surgeon. This patient has fewer mental and emotional stresses.

Many members of one family and their next generation may all, one after the other, have a nose job even if it is only for minor changes. They mostly choose the very same surgeon.

20.4.3.2 The First Consultation

This is a very big psychological step for the patient. It is the first step of decision and real action to be taken by the patient. Patients vary in their abilities to express their feelings, wishes and hopes.

They may be still indecisive, hesitant or quite unsure of their goals and decisions.

20.4.3.3 Setting a Date for Surgery

When the patient is convinced of the idea and the surgeon, a date is set for the time of surgery. This is another important psychological step on the way to having surgery. Consequently, photographs are taken and the consent form is signed. During this period the emotional curve climbs speedingly high. The patient becomes progressively under the stress of mixed feelings of excitement and anxiety.

20.4.3.4 The Day of Surgery

At this point, patients need a lot of psychological, emotional and mental support. Mutual confidence and trust in the surgeon play a major role in reassurance. Pre-operative sedation is of great help.

At any point during the previous stages, patients may decide not to proceed any further. These patients may come back at a later date having overcome their fears and other reservations.

20.4.4 Immediate Reaction After Removing the Cast

Patients are in desperate need of reassurance. Surgeons must reassure their patients as soon as they recover from anesthesia. The idea of taking intraoperative post-surgical photographs of the nose is not a successful method of reassuring patients. Noses usually are swollen and the result after removing the cast is always better.

After discharge from the hospital till the day of removing the cast patients will have numerous mixed feelings of tension, curiosity, fear and rarely depression.

Few patients are so curious that they may remove the cast ahead of time and then replace it. This is seen in obsessed patients.

20.4.5 Stage of Facing Reality

This stage starts from the decisive moment of removing the plaster cast by the doctor. From this moment onwards most patients go into a series of emotional and psychological reactions.

It is the final step of the patient's long ordeal and the climax of all of his emotional, mental and psychological reactions.

Patients' reactions are quite variable, but generally, three reactions are present, i.e. **positive, paradoxically negative** and a **frozen** reaction depending on the degree of tension, personality and the outcome of the surgery.

(a) **The Positive Reaction:**
Despite the clear apprehension, the patient is willing to look into a mirror to see the result of the surgery. The reaction is parallel to the surgical result or exaggerated in variable degrees. There is a combined sense of relief and happiness, filled with joy and appreciation. These reactions may be overwhelming from the start.

(b) **Paradoxically Negative Reaction:**
Very few patients who are normally well adjusted may surprise the surgeon and the relatives with an unusual and totally unexpected severely, negative reaction. Males and females may have these reactions but it is more common in females. Age has no bearing.
Despite the satisfactory and even excellent results, their reaction is paradoxically in the opposite direction in a very strong emotional reaction. The patient is desperate to look into a mirror and see the result. At first, usually feels numb, stunned amazed and shocked. Then there is a strong verbal and physical reaction of complete refusal of the new look of the nose. Some patients clearly recognize that the nose looks beautiful, but as one patient said, "I cannot cope with all these changes in my face. I would rather only have minimal changes in my nose". As if he is delusional and his false and fixed belief has not changed.

(c) **The Numb Frozen Reaction:**
Having gone through this long, exhausting procedure, patients may come to this final moment totally drained mentally, psychologically, emotionally and physically.
They are frozen and numb mentally and emotionally. They feel so empty and don't have the words or feelings to truly express themselves. They are totally stunned by the whole situation. On removing the cast they prefer to be quiet, as they are in an indifferent state.
They prefer not to look into a mirror now despite all the encouraging remarks from all surrounding individuals. They prefer to have this emotional moment to themselves at home. It is a more private and personal emotional state.
Generally, all these emotional reactions may only last a few days. Occasionally they may last for a few weeks before the patients finally settle, calm down and come to reality. The patients regain their normal senses and are able to see and feel the outcome of the surgery. Some patients decide to visit a psychiatrist to help them to cope with their emotions.
It is quite suitable here to emphasize the fact of keeping the patient's own image in the same nasal print during the surgery, i.e. the art of improving the patient's own nose rather than creating a new shape of the surgeon's making, i.e. surgical nose. This has the best psychological and emotional response from the patients.

20.5 Successful Rhinoplasty

Successful aesthetic results stabilize and boost the overall psychological and emotional state of patients. They are more confident and the overall behavior improves in parallel with the improved image.

There is a better attitude that positively affects their social and professional lives. As a result of surgery, some patients decide to change their career to another one that depends on their new external appearance, e.g. representative, TV introducer or other entertainment business.

20.6 Relationship with the Mirror "Mirror Sign"

As the patient acknowledges the new change in the nose and face, she or he usually looks at the mirror more frequently. They thoroughly and literally examine each and every part of their nose. They used to look into their mirror to observe their abnormal nasal shapes before surgery. After surgery, they look almost ten times more frequently than before and more critically.

20.7 Unsuccessful Surgeries

Failure to achieve a satisfactory result of varying degrees has quite the opposite effect. Patients are severely disturbed, withdrawn and tend to hide. They avoid socializing and may quit school or college to avoid the remarks and comments of people.

Unsuccessful surgery in the eyes of the surgeon may be quite acceptable by the patient and vice versa. The patient may be quite unhappy with fairly minor deformities in the nose which can only be seen by the critical eyes of the patient. Psychological and psychiatric management is highly recommended at this stage.

20.8 The Surgeon's Attitude Post-Operatively

The main role of the surgeon is support and reassurance. The patient needs this support during all stages of the surgery, i.e.

Preoperatively
On the day of surgery
The immediate post-operative days
At the time of removing the cast
The near and late results and expectations

The surgeon must not pass any negative remarks about the result of surgery. Patients may be quite happy, content and satisfied with the result.

From the surgeon's point of view, they may feel that there is room for improvement. **Perfection is always the biggest enemy**.

20.9 The Unpleasant Terms and Patients' Psychology

Some terms are commonly used among rhinoplasty surgeons to describe certain nasal deformities, e.g. "polly beak", "Parrot beak" and "pig snout".

These terms are written in many renowned rhinoplasty books. To the surgeon's mind, these terms describe specific anatomical abnormalities that need no further detailed explanations. They are used by the surgeon with minimum or even no sensitivity. They don't have any unpleasant impact. The sad fact is that these terms are strongly unpleasant and quite offensive to ordinary people, especially when it comes to the pig snout expression. As they reach the patients, these terms have a quite negative impact on them. In addition to the state of dissatisfaction from their nasal condition, they become severely disturbed and unhappy to hear these terms. "**It is best to be sensitive when describing peoples' physical appearance**" (Elizabeth Pope). Surgeons must be careful in using more acceptable descriptive words for their patients. With the clear advancement in anatomical knowledge, these deformities could be described using more appropriate phrases. These terms are totally avoided in this text and hopefully from all future textbooks.

Surgery of the Four Areas of the Nose 21

Abstract

The **anterior wall surgery** is the surgery which involves the **middle crura**, while the **lateral wall surgery** is that which involves the **lateral crura** as well as the **alae nasi**. The median wall surgery involves the columella, the medial cruise and the nasal septum. The inferior wall surgery involves the nasal base i.e the alar base, the vestibular floor and the flat triangle.

The middle and lateral crurae are **linked surgically** as they are both explored via the same surgical incision and share the same surgical steps.

The **alae nasi** on the other hand are made of solid fibrofatty tissue and have totally different approach for their surgery.

Keyword

Preservation surgery of the lower lateral cartilages · Delivery of the lower lateral cartilages · Surgery of the alar nasi · Surgery of the columella · Surgery of the nasal septum · Nasal septal deviation · The membranous septum · Alar base surgery · Surgery of rim sill folds

Part I: The Anterior and Lateral Walls Surgeries

The **anterior wall surgery** is the surgery which involves the **middle crura**, while the **lateral wall surgery** is that which involves the **lateral crura** as well as the **alae nasi**.

Although the middle and lateral crurae are in **different anatomical walls** and have **different aesthetic** roles, yet they both are **continuous with each other** and **sandwiched by the same two skin layers**, i.e., the adherent vestibular skin and the fibrofatty external skin.

21.1 Innovative Preservation Surgery of the Anterolateral Walls

It is important that the surgeon is **capable of exploring all parts of the four walls** of the nasal aperture in order to make the surgical changes in each and every wall as well as their communicating folds.

The **middle and lateral crurae** are completely **sandwiched** by the two skin layers of the nasal aperture walls. Their full separation and **exploration** enable the surgeon to directly deal with any necessary alterations. It also allows exploration of whole of the subdermal **fibrofatty layer**.

The detailed knowledge and training of the surgeon to explore and **deliver the lower lateral cartilages** is therefore essential to fully command the surgery of the lower third of the nose.

M. H. A. Shafy, *Innovations in Rhinoplasty*,
https://doi.org/10.1007/978-3-030-94573-2_21

Although the **middle crural surgery** is usually carried out as part of the lower lateral cartilaginous surgery, the aesthetic outcome is uniquely individual for **each nose** and **each wall**. The fact remains that they both contribute to the beauty of each other in an integral way.

The surgical procedures that involve the anterolateral walls are of two types:

21.1.1 Structured Aesthetic Surgery

Structured Aesthetic Surgery: which involves the use of cartilaginous tip grafts to cover the original middle crural cartilages of the nasal tip, e. g. tip graft, shield's graft and lateral crural grafts.

21.1.2 Preservation Aesthetic Surgery

Preservation Aesthetic Surgery: which involves the reshaping of the anterior wall components, i.e., the middle and lateral crural cartilages. This goal is achieved by direct approach and stitching of the crural cartilage.

In this text, the author introduces a new method of a purely natural anatomical preservation surgery to the frontolateral walls. It is based on understanding the anatomy of the two hypodermal fibrofatty layers of the middle and lateral crurae and their surgical significance. In this technique:

- There is no need for grafting.
- There is no need for direct interference in the shapes of the crurae by stitching.

The natural own shapes of each person's cartilages are preserved and untouched. The outcome is a thinner skin nose that has the very same shape and the exact patient's own image, i.e., exact nose print. This technique is known as the Delivery and Defatting technique. (Defatting is discussed in the chapter on the Bulky Nose).

21.1.2.1 Delivery of the Lower Lateral Cartilages

The lower lateral cartilages are totally subcutaneous structures. **On the vestibular side** they can be both seen and palpated, as the covering vestibular skin is delicately **thin, adherent** and **hairy**. The only exception is the lateral crurae which are usually covered with hairless thin adherent vestibular skin.

Externally the bodies of the middle and lateral crurae as well as the inferior margins of the medial crurae are all subcutaneous structures.

Definition of Delivery

Delivery of the lower lateral cartilages is defined as the full dissection and **freedom** of the **external surfaces** of both lower lateral cartilages so that they can be **brought out** of both nasal apertures like a bucket handle.

They remain attached at their two ends medially and laterally. The vestibular skin remains closely adherent to their inner surfaces.

The Surgical Technique

Preparation

The nose must be prepared before surgery in order to have clear, clean and bloodless field.

Shaving the Nasal Vibrissae

In order to have a clean and clear field for surgery the vestibular hair, vibrecae, is **closely shaved** using a No 15 blade.

A sharp double-pronged alar retractor is used to elivate the lateral alar wall. The middle or ring counter-pushes the middle and lateral crura from outside to expose their vestibular surface for surgical exploration and shaving.

For smoother shave, the vestibular skin is thinly painted with a layer of any type of skin cream or ointment. The sides of the blade are similarly painted so that the knife will cut the hair smoothly off the skin with minimal injury or bleeding and the hairs will stick to the sides of the knife, rather than falling inside or outside the nasal cavities.

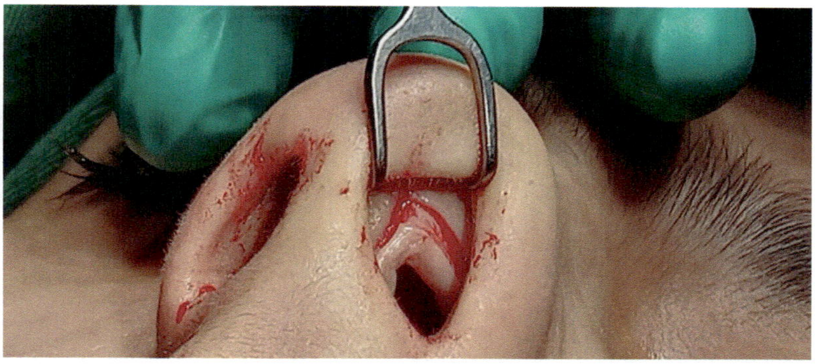

Fig. 21.1 Rhinoplasty incisions and location of the anterior valve angle. The intercartilaginous and columellar incisions are superior and inferior to the anterior valve angle

Local Anesthesia Iinjection

Lidocaine with adrenalin diluted 1:200,000 is used. A thin insulin needle is a good choice for this purpose. Injections are made in the interior margins of the medial, middle and lateral crurae. The intercartilagenous fold is infiltrated with local anesthesia. Other areas of the nose are infiltrated with local anesthesia according to surgical plan.

Intercartilaginous Incision

The ala nasi is elevated by an alar retractor. Incision is made as close as possible to the inferior border of the upper lateral cartilage. The cut is deepened superiorly in sawing movements till the dorsum of the nose is reached (Fig. 21.1).

The Marginal Incisions

These are the **exploratory incisions**. Exploring the lower lateral crura is only possible through these incisions. They are **more difficult** technically, than the intercartilaginous incisions, as the **lower border of each of the three crura has its own special surgical anatomical considerations**. The inferior border incision for **each crus** has to be pursued separately. Once the **three incisions** are completed, they are connected with each other to become **one inferior border incision**. From this incision, exploratory dissection and delivery of the whole body of the lower lateral cartilage becomes then possible.

The Lateral Crus Incision:

The lateral crus should be the **first crus to be explored** in the lower lateral cartilage. A rough guide to the inferior border of the lateral crus is the **hair line,** as the vestibular skin over the lateral crural body is usually smooth and devoid of hair. Only occasionally it may extend beyond this line (Fig. 21.2).

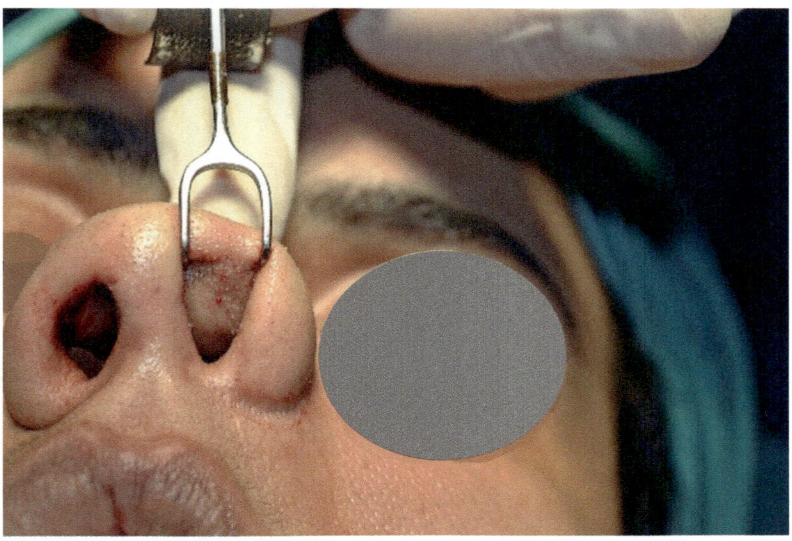

Fig. 21.2 Exploration of the lateral crus, the infrior margin is seen at the junction between the hairy and non-hairy vestibular skin

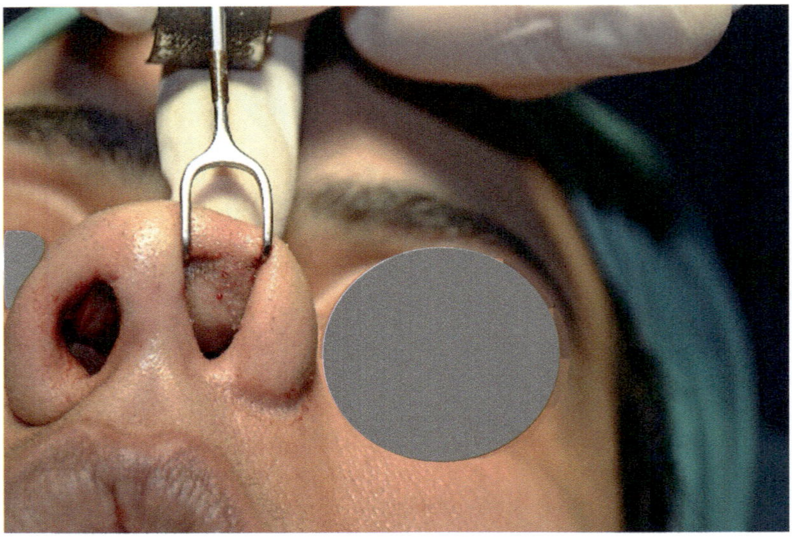

Fig. 21.3 The handle of the knife is rolled against the lateral vestibular wall to determine the edge of the inferior margin of the lateral crus

A sharp double-pronged alar retractor is used to elevate the alar margin and explore the lateral alar wall. The smooth rounded lower end of a Bard Parker knife handle is used to palpate the lateral alar wall by sliding it against the vestibular skin from below upwards, i.e., from the alar margin inwards (Fig. 21.3).

The inferior margin of the lateral crus is felt as an **elevated firm step** on the vestibular surface. It is usually located at the hair line where the hair begins to disappear from the skin over the lateral crural body.

Using a No. 15 blade an incision is made at the margin. As the skin is extremely thin, the knife must be held and used extremely gently as if drawing a line with a pen (Figs. 21.4 and 21.5). A right-angled sharp hook (neuro-surgical epidural hook) is used by the assistant to elevate the cut margin of the vestibular skin by pulling it posteriorly. The glistening white inferior cartilaginous margin now comes into view (Fig. 21.7).

The sharp thin tips of Joseph's scissors are then introduced inside the wound just anterior to the cartilage. The two blades are opened to expand the wound.

Following the inferior margin of the lateral crus, the vestibular skin is cut by the scissors and

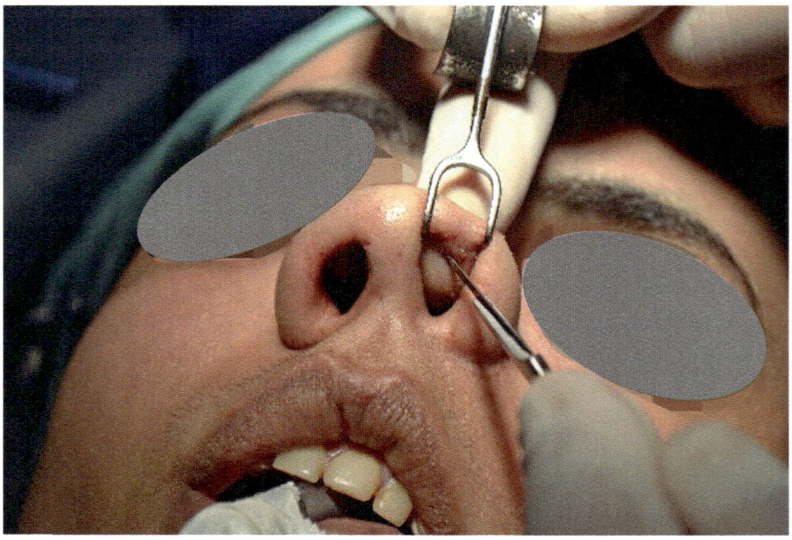

Fig. 21.4 A very shallow incision using a number 15 blade is made at the inferior margin of the lateral crus

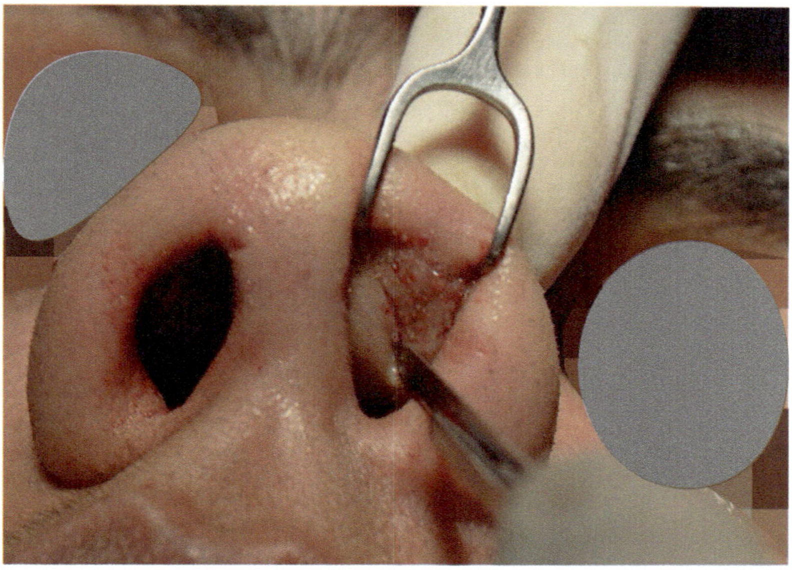

Fig. 21.5 The incision reaches to the posterior end of the inferior margin at the junction between the hairy and the hair free vestibular skin

the incision is extended **laterally** till it ends at the upward curving of the lower border.

Medially the incision ends at the lateral angle of the flat triangle where the inferior margin is hidden under its soft skin fold.

The curved Joseph's scissors is then used to **free the external surface** of the lateral crus by cutting through the fibrous bands in the loose fibrofatty layer (Fig. 21.8).

The dissection ends **laterally** when the whole body of the lateral crus is exposed, while **medially** it continues till the beginning of the middle crus.

The Medial Crus Incision:

The medial crus should be the **second crus to be explored** after the lateral crus and not the middle crus.

The inferior margin of the medial crus is located **at the junction** between the **vestibular** and the **external skin** (see anatomy section).

No retractors are needed here. Between the surgeon's thumb and index fingers, the lower

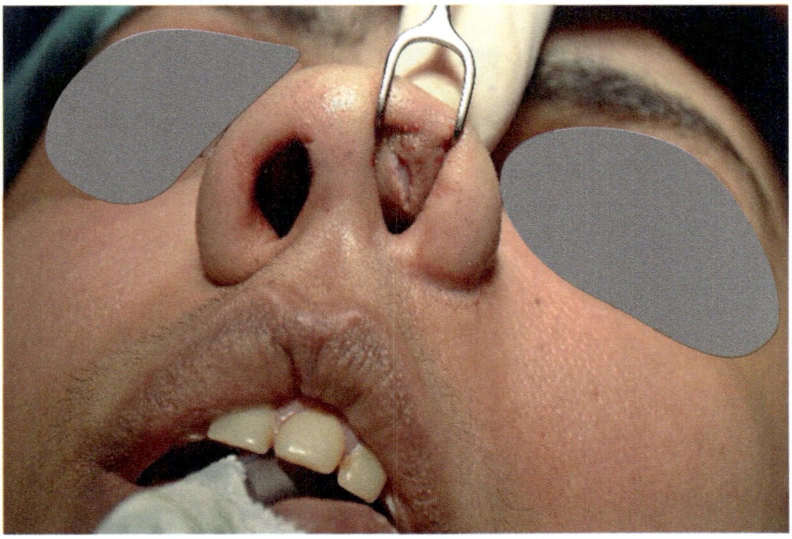

Fig. 21.6 The inferior margin of the lateral crus together with its adherent hairless skin are separated from the hairy vestibular skin

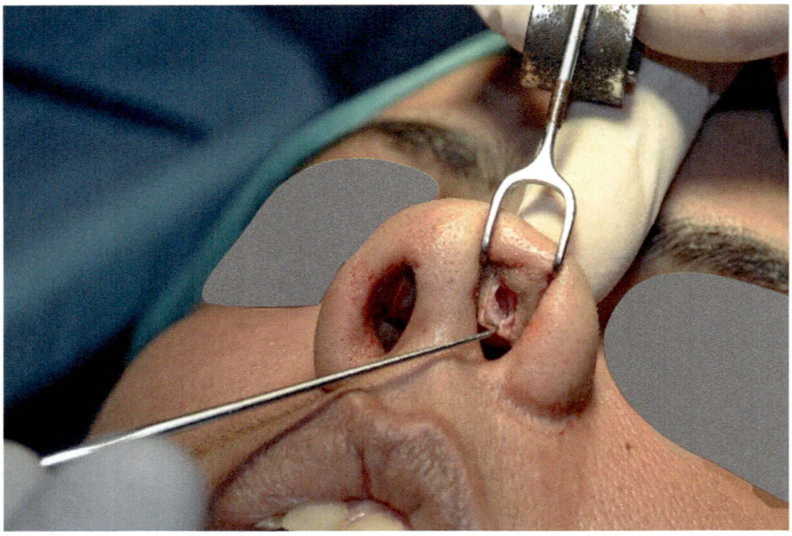

Fig. 21.7 The inferior margin is pulled posteriorly using a neurosurgical epidural hook

third of the nose is held by its sidewalls at the supratip region. The **columella** is now **fixed** and **protruded** in the middle between the squeezed two alae nasi (Fig. 21.9).

Using No 15 blade the knife is held by the second hand. The sharp curved **edge** of the blade is aimed at the **junction between the external and the vestibular skin** at the lateral columellar margin. The external skin is **pushed aside** by **the side** of the blade of the knife, while the **edge of the blade** is making a **very small incision**, which is almost a stab wound, exactly at the junction between the two skins **just next to the margin** (Figs. 21.9 and 21.10).

A right-angled neuro-surgical hook is used to pull on the vestibular skin superiorly thus exploring the white glistening inferior margin of the medial crus that comes immediately into view (Fig. 21.7).

The incision is then extended for very short distances both anteriorly and posteriorly following the inferior crural margin.

The tips of the sharp curved scissors are used to free the **medial** crural surface by cutting through the intercrural connective tissues. Some surgeons prefer to use angles scissors.

The **scissors** may be used from the start **after the first stab wound**. The tips are introduced just

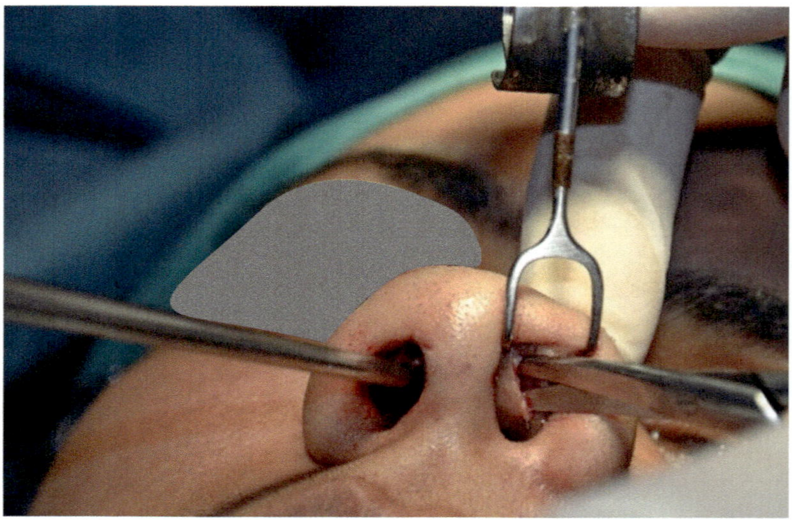

Fig. 21.8 The remainder of the lateral crus is dissected and explored using a pair of scissors

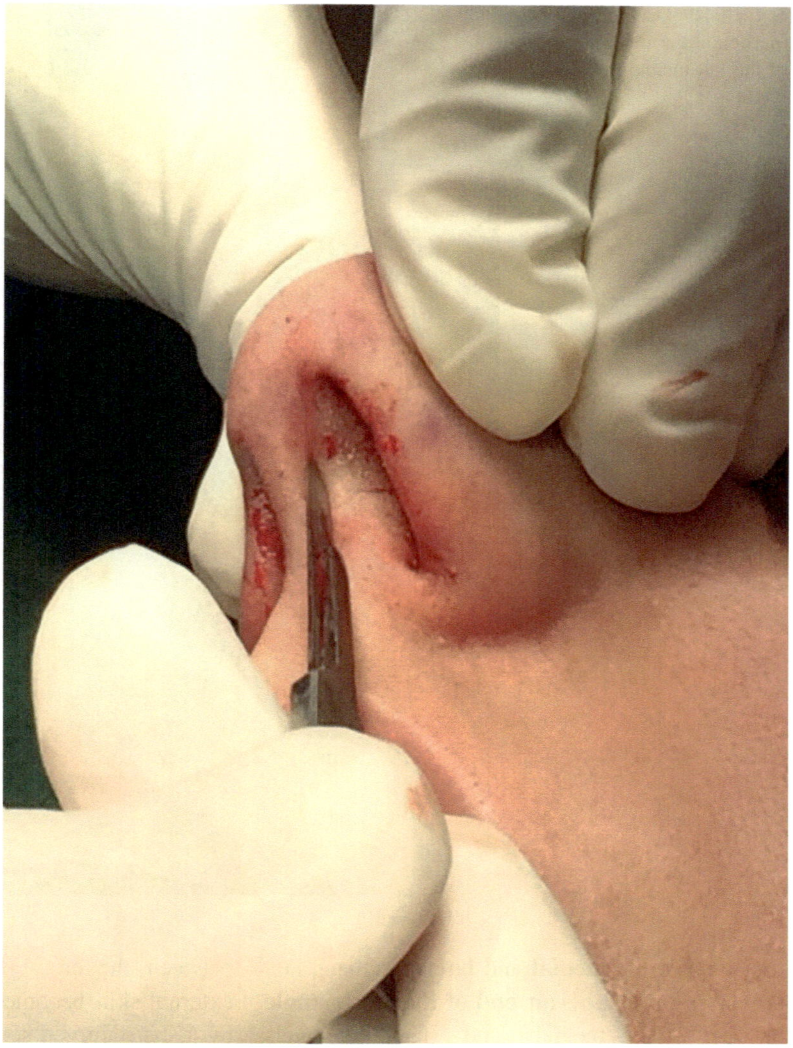

Fig. 21.9 The columella is fixed by holding the two lateral walls of the nose thus it becomes prominent and immobile. The side of the knife pushes the external skin medially, while its edge is directed at the junction between the external and vestibular skin exactly at the inferior margin of the left medial crus

inside the medial crural margin and then **opened** in a gradual process of dissection of the fibrous layer of the lateral surface.

The medial crus incision therefore starts from the **posterior end** of the inferior margin of the medial crus and continues until it ends **anteriorly** at the medial angle of the **flat triangle**.

The Middle Crus Incision:

The middle crus is **the last crus to be explored**, as it has an **inferior border** which is **deeply buried** under the backwardly folded **flat triangular** soft skin.

The two prongs of a sharp alar retractor are placed at the anterior ends of the marginal incisions of the lateral and medial crurae, i.e., at the lateral and medial angles of the flat triangle.

A right-angled neuro-surgical hook is used by the assistant to pull down the inferior margin of the **lateral crus** posteriorly together with its vestibular skin cover, as it appears at the lateral incision.

The inferior margin of the middle crus is now clearly seen as a **prominent step** in the vestibular skin between the **two ends of the marginal**

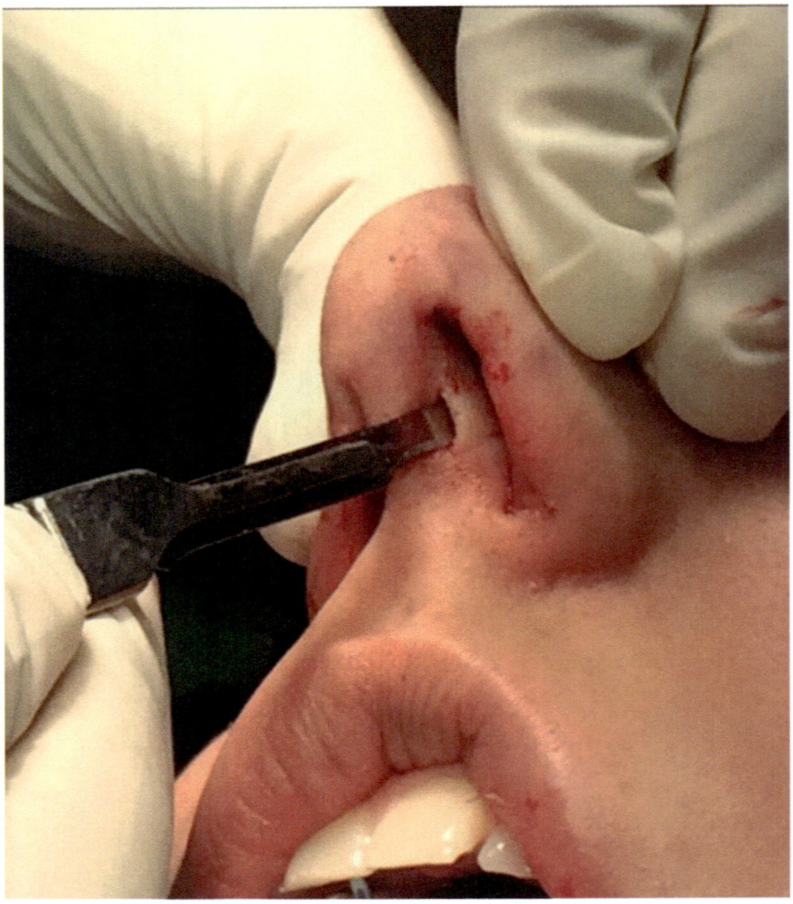

Fig. 21.10 Deepening the incision at the inferior margin of the left medial crus using the knife

incisions of the **medial** and **lateral crurae,** i.e., **traversing the superior end of the flat triangle** between its medial and lateral angels (Fig. 21.13).

The marginal **incision** for the middle crus is now made using a knife or a curved scissors. Care must be taken to avoid nipping the **cartilaginous margin** or encroaching upon the vestibular **skin of the flat triangle** (Fig. 21.14).

The medial and lateral crural incisions are now communicated by the middle crural incision and they are all joined to become **one inferior marginal incision** for the lower lateral cartilage.

Exploration of the whole of the lower lateral cartilage is now possible.

As the alar margin is elevated, **the middle crus** is counter pulled down using the neurosurgical right-angled hook. The **fibrous bands** between the crural fibrofatty capsule and the external skin become taut and are gradually cut by a sharp curved scissors.

Dissection continues **superiorly** till the superior margin of the lateral crus is reached at the **inter-cartilaginous incision** (Fig. 21.15).

The Technique of Delivery

The **whole body** of the **lower lateral cartilage** is now **completely explored** and can be **delivered**.

The right-angled hook is introduced into the nasal aperture. The sharp pointed end is moved forwards in a strictly anterior direction till it penetrates the middle crus, exactly at the **mid-domal point**. The whole of the lower lateral cartilage is dislodged and pulled down to be delivered outside the nasal aperture. It looks like a **bucket handle** (Fig. 21.16).

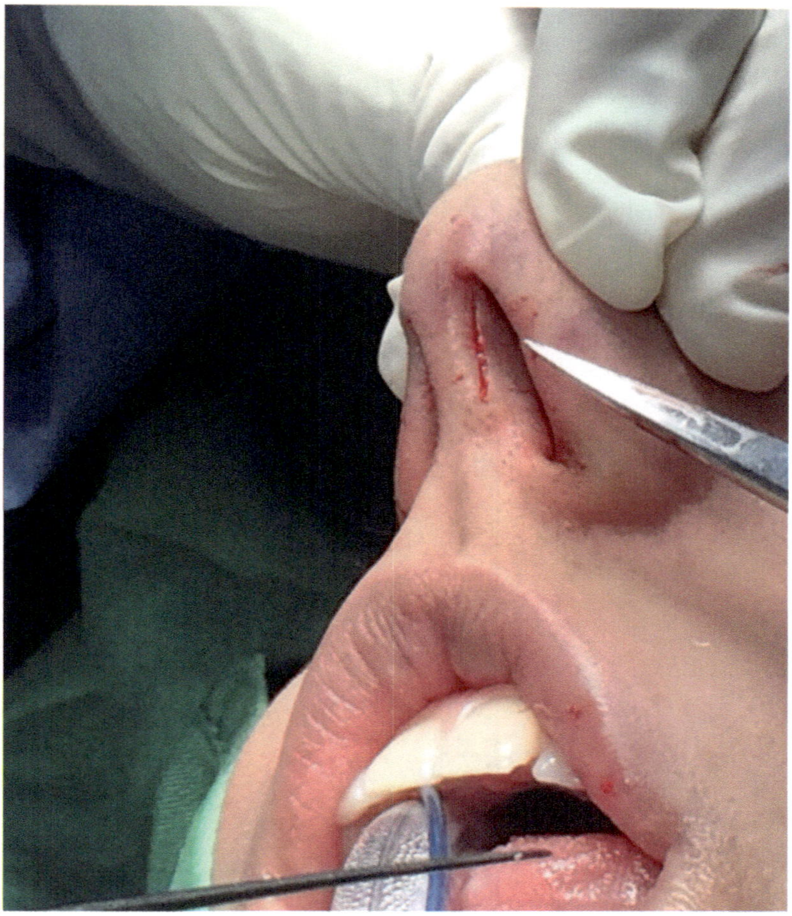

Fig. 21.11 The medial crural incision is complete

For easier surgical manipulation and fixation, an elevator, e.g., Freer's or Cottles's, is introduced under the domal curve, while the alar margin is counter elevated in the opposite direction.

Procedures that Follow the Delivery:

Now delivery of the lower lateral cartilages is completed, which means the **complete exploration** of the **inner** surface of the external skin walls and the **outer cartilaginous surfaces** is achieved.

Both are now amenable and ready for surgical reforming. The surgical procedures in these two areas may be a combination of one or more of the following processes:

Defatting of the lower and upper lateral cartilages as well as the area of the weak triangle.

Reshaping the lower lateral cartilage. This may be in the form of **cephalic trim of the lateral crura**, **cross hatching of the middle crura** to weaken the domes or **excision of a bulky area of overlap** between the upper and lower lateral cartilages.

Details of defatting procedure are discussed in detail in the chapter of The Bulky Nose.

The commonest combinations are **Delivery**, **Defatting** and **Dome** weakening, i.e., **D.D.D.** This is usually followed by cephalic trim of lateral crurae.

Dressing of the Antrolateral Walls

The dead space between the crural antrolateral walls and the external skin should be secured both internally and externally

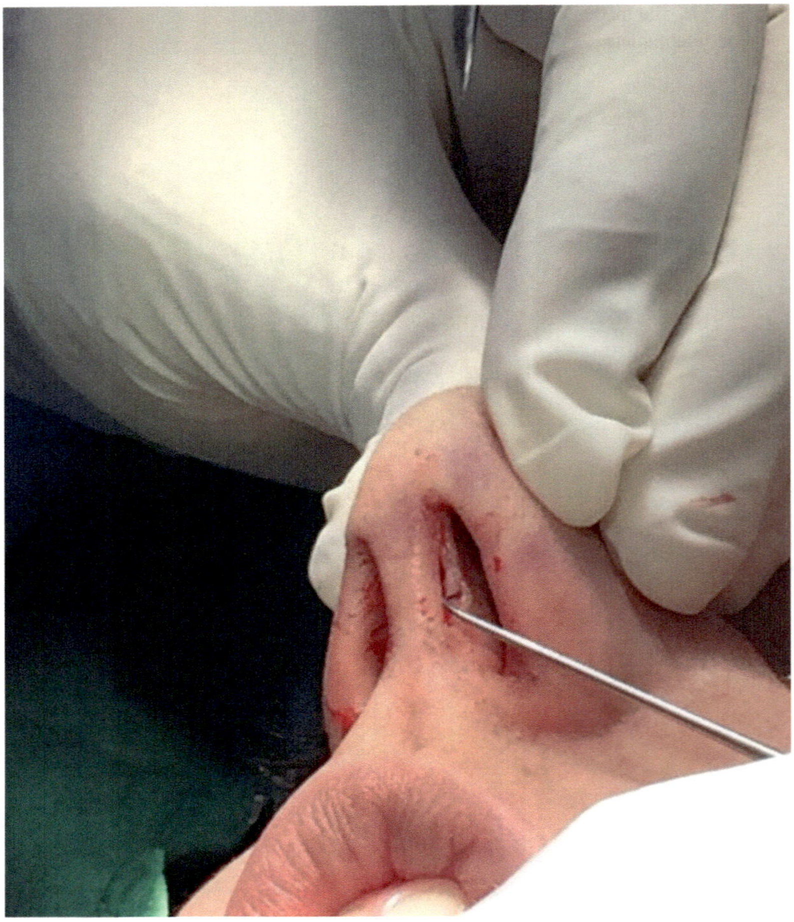

Fig. 21.12 Retracting the inferior margin of the medial crus by an epidural hook. Further deepening of the incision using Josephs scissors

i. Internally
  - The marginal wounds are secured by one or two Vicryl absorbable stitches.
  - Thick short intranasal splints are placed abutting the columella and membranous septum on both sides. They should be high enough to reach both domes of the middle crurae. The splints are then secured by a transcolumellar proline stitch as they remain for one week.
  - Light nasal packing is placed for 24 h.

ii. Externally
  - A good quality sterístrip layer is placed after thoroughly drying the skin with pure alcohol or tincture bezoini. The author uses proxistrip 12mmx100mm.
  - Plaster of Paris or similar materials that takes the shape of the external nose before it becomes firm.
  - An external elastoplasts to fix the cast to the face. All external and internal supports are removed after one week.

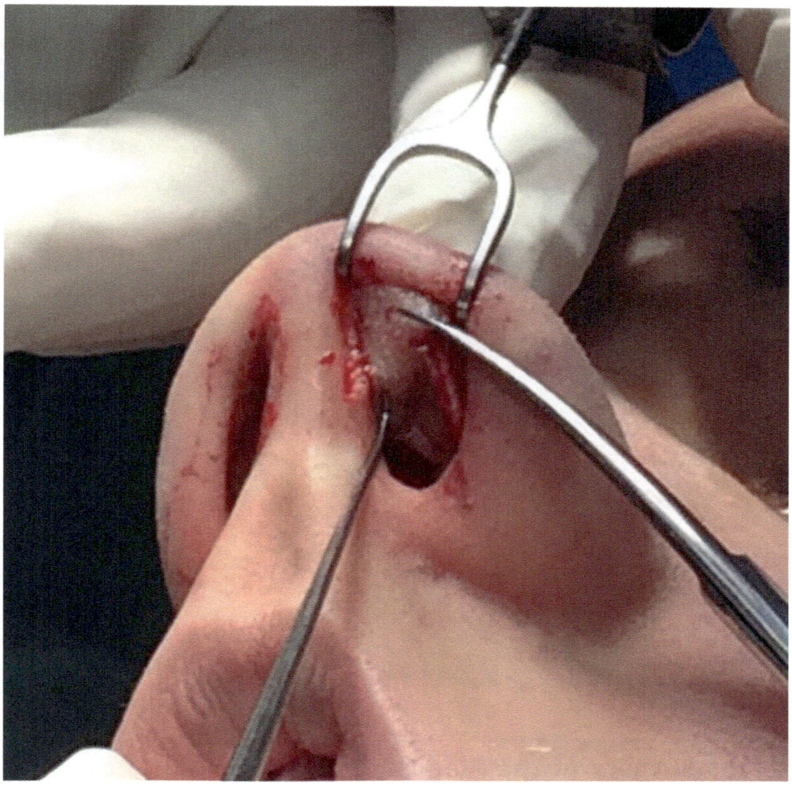

Fig. 21.13 Cutting of the vestibular skin at the inferior margin of the middle crus

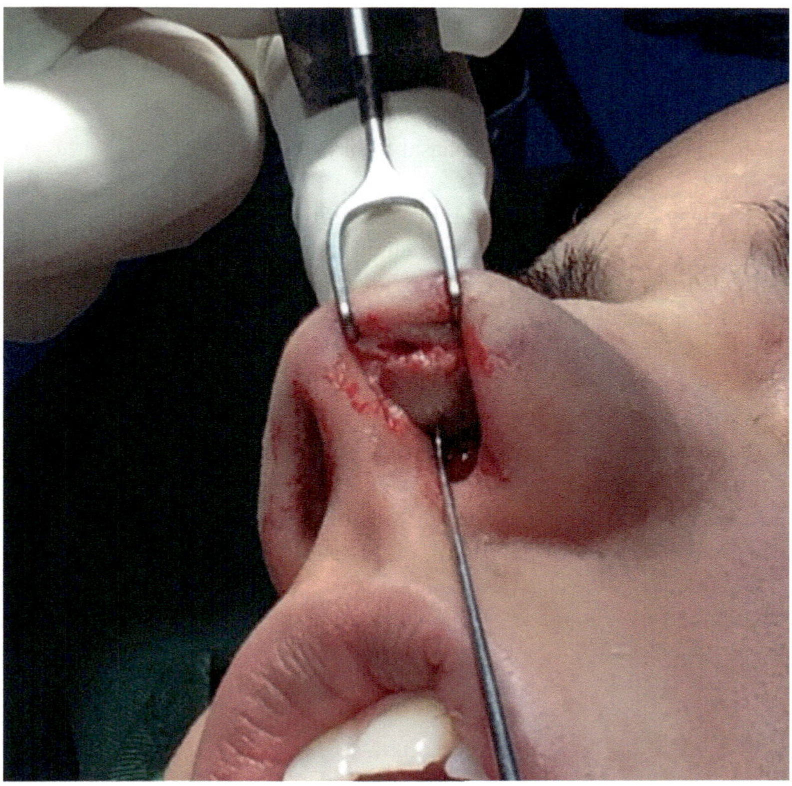

Fig. 21.14 Appearance of the inferior margin of the middle crus

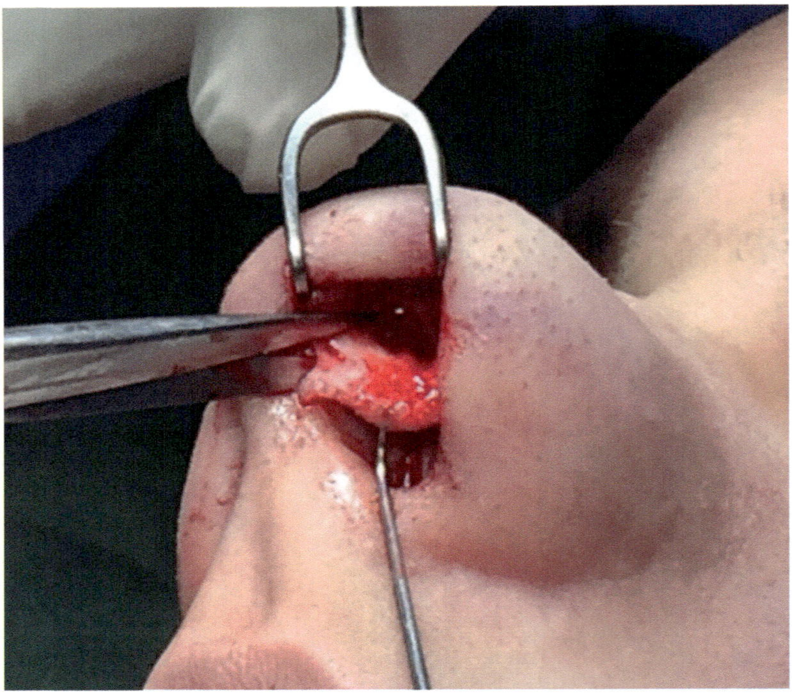

Fig. 21.15 Cutting of the inter-domal band

21.2 Surgery of the Alae Nasi

The alae nasi are two wings like structures that makes the major part of the lateral walls of the nasal aperture tube. They have a major contribution to the aesthetics of the nose. They must be clearly seen at the sides of the nasal front as two beautiful rounded structures.

In many cases especially Middle Eastern and Hispanic noses they are hidden behind a large bulbous front which is made by the large middle and lateral crural bodies.

The solid structure of the alar bodies is essential for maintaining the normal physiology of nasal respiration. Thinning of the alar bodies is to be avoided. Weakening them may severely compromise their ability to maintain a patent airway during inspiration. The rim-sill folds are usually the location of nasal bulk in this area.

Anatomically the alae nasi cannot be dissected or explored as it is made of one solid fibrofatty tissue which does not have any other anatomical components or layers. The alar skin cover is tightly adherent to their bodies both externally and vestibularly.

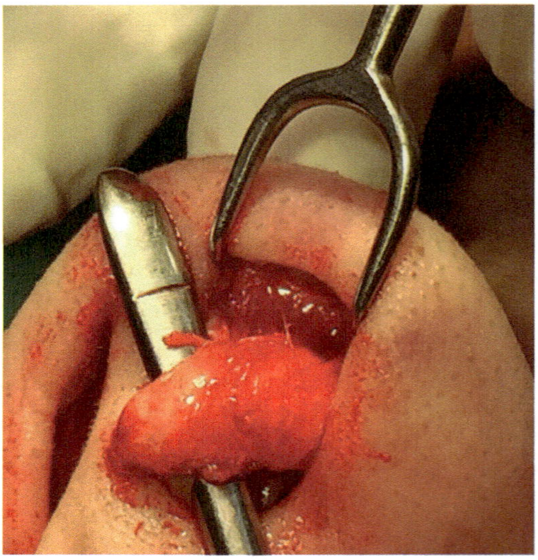

Fig. 21.16 Complete delivery of the lower lateral cartridge like a bucket handle

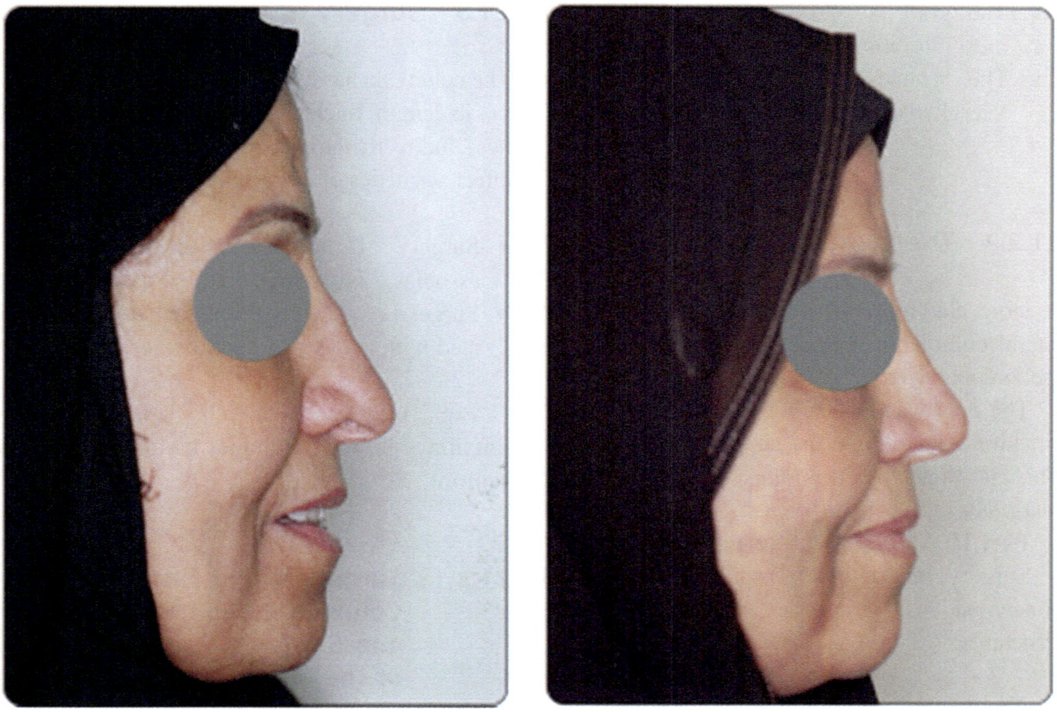

Fig. 21.17 Small Right Ala Nasi

Aesthetically the **size of the alar bodies** plays the most important role. This indirectly affects their shape and location.

21.2.1 Small Ala Nasi

A small size body of the ala nasi is clinically translated to a **high alar margin** in relation to the lateral columellar margin that consequently becomes over-exposed.

Increasing the size of the alar body is not an easy job. These cases are dealt with by **directly supporting the alar margin** using a subcutaneous graft to bring it down.

This needs a fairly **strong and thick graft material**. The most suitable materials are a **thick bony or thick cartilaginous septum**. The thickest part of the quadrilateral cartilage is the most inferior stripe which is embedded into the maxillary groove (Fig. 21.17).

After grafting, the alar margin usually **feels thicker** than the rest of the alar body. Some degree of **resorption** takes place in a few months due to the gradual resorption of the graft material.

Using weak or thin graft material will have a good immediate result but the long-term results are usually disappointing.

In cases of **bilateral high** alar arches, one has to use similar **graft materials for** similar results.

21.2.1.1 Surgical Technique

Many techniques have been described to lower the alar margin. The author only reports his own.

i. Half centimeter incision is made at the inner surface of the alar nasi just posterior to the alar body.
ii. A Dissector, Freer elevator, is introduced gradually and slowly through this incision to create a subcutaneous pocket at the alar margin. The marginal skin stretches gradually and slowly.
iii. A thick part of the septal cartilage or bone is harvested. It is then shaped and cut to the exact length of the high alar arch.

iv. The graft is introduced using a straight mosquito artery forceps.
v. The wound is closed using absorbable Vicryl stitch.

21.2.2 The Large Ala Nasi

A large alar body will exceed the level of the lateral columellar margin resulting in an unaesthetic appearance.

The only way of dealing with this unaesthetic situation is to **reduce the size of the alar body**. This is done by trimming the inferior alar marginal.

Part II: Medial Wall Surgery

Surgery of the medial wall of the nose is concerned with surgeries of the following structures:

1. **The Columella**

The columella has two components:
a. The Firm Anterior Columellar Segment
b. The Soft Posterior Columellar fold

2. **The Medial Crurae**
3. **The Nasal Septum**

Nasal Septal Surgery associated with Rhinoplasty is divided into two clinically different components:
a. The Membranous septum:

The subcutaneous part of the septum that makes the medial wall of the four-walled lower third of the nose.
b. The Osteocartilagenous septum:

The internal part of the septum that makes the medial wall of the three-walled upper two-thirds of the nose.

21.3 Surgery of the Columella

The columella has direct effects on nasal aesthetics via its length, thickness, shape, level and straightness. Indirectly the columella and the medial crurae affect aesthetics of the nasal apertures.

- Surgery of the **firm anterior segment** is associated with surgery of the **medial crurae.**
- Surgery of the **posterior soft fold** is associated with surgery of the **anterior nasal spine.**

Both parts are indirectly affected by the **maxillary crest** and the **caudal vestibular septum.**

21.3.1 Surgery of the Firm Anterior Columellar Segment and Surgery of the Medial Crurae

The inferior borders and parts of the bodies of the medial crurae make the firm segment of the columella (see anatomy section).

Surgery of the firm anterior segment of the columella is in fact surgery of the inferior parts of the medial crurae.

As a subcutaneous structure, the shapes of the medial crurae have a role in nasal aesthetics. In certain situations, they may need direct or indirect surgical intervention.

21.3.1.1 Bifid Ccolumella

The widely separated **inferior margins** and **bodies** of the medial crurae (Fig. 21.18) are to be approximated. The inferior crural margins are explored by direct incisions just next to the inferior columellar margins. The skin is dissected off using the tips of sharp scissors (the inferior margins are readily visualized in the delivery technique of the lower lateral cartilages).

The intercrural loose connective tissue may need to be reduced or removed. The inferior

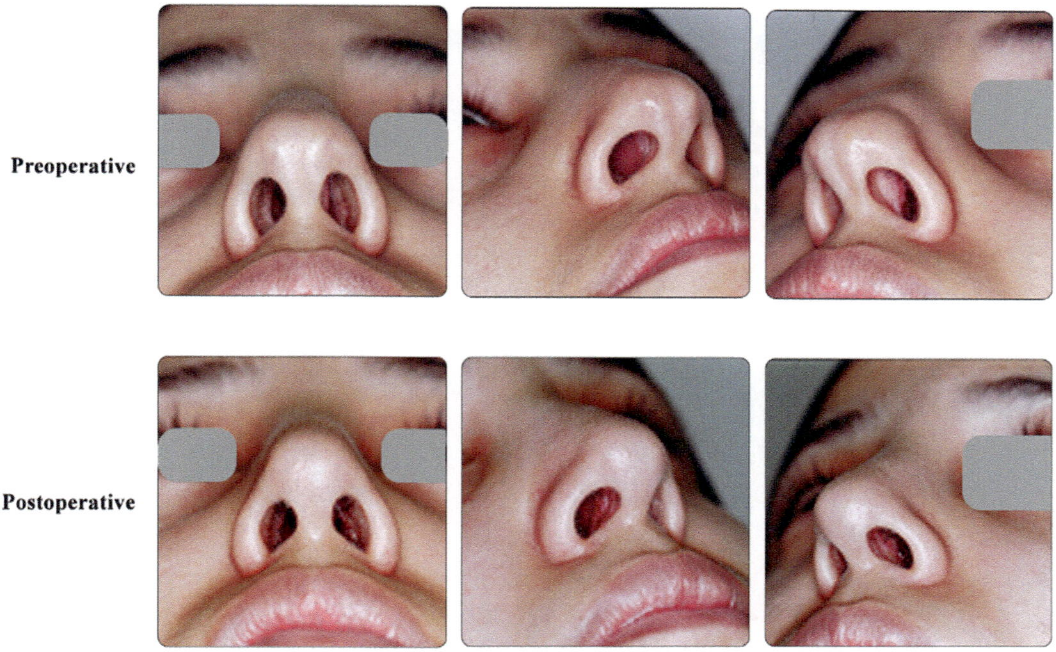

Fig. 21.18 Bifid columella, before and after surgery

margins of both medial crurae are then approximated using Vicryl stitches along the margins.

21.3.1.2 Hanging Columella

This is an unaesthetic deformity caused by the large size of the medial crurae of the lower lateral cartilages. There are downward projection of the bodies of the medial crurae just anterior to soft posterior columellar fold (Figs. 21.19 and 21.22). The crural lower margins and lateral hairy surfaces are relatively large and protrude at a much lower level than the margins of the alae nasi. The medial crurae look like the handles of a ladies bag hence the name is hanging columella.

In these cases, all surrounding structures are within the normal size and position. The only outstanding structures are the oversized medial crurae.

Hanging columella is to be differentiated from:

a. The protruding columella secondary to a long caudal septum or large anterior nasal spine.
b. The small alae nasi exposing the lateral columellar wall with the highly notched alar margin.

Management:

The best and only way of dealing with the hanging columella is by direct surgical reduction of the excess size of the medial crurae.

This is done via a marginal incision as a sole surgery or as part of the overall lower lateral cartilaginous exploration.

21.3.1.3 Overprojecting Medial Crurae

The posterior margins of the medial crurae may be overprojecting and protruding into the cavities of the nasal apertures.

It is important to realize that the **inferior vestibular bands** and the **cartilaginous medial crurae**, both contribute to the overprojection into the aperture space.

Preoperative

Postoperative

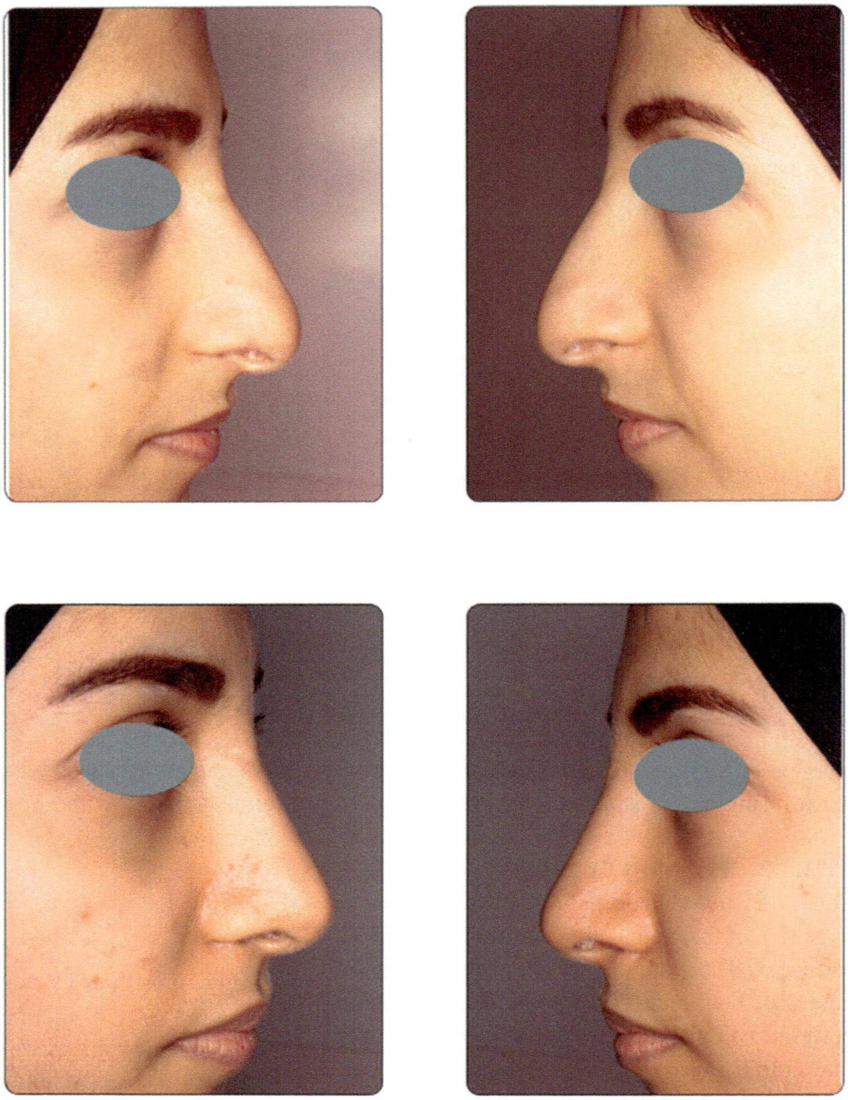

Fig. 21.19 Hanging columella, before and after surgery

In some cases, the projection is predominantly produced by the inferior vestibular bands, while in the others it is the size, shape and relative stiffness of the **cartilage** that plays more important role.

Other factors that may affect the crural projection are the **skin thickness**, the amount of **intercrural tissues** and an extra-long protruding **caudal septum**.

Reducing the overprojecting crurae has an effect on the **size**, **shape** and hence the **aesthetics** of the **nasal apertures**. Medial crural projections may **vary from one nostril to the other** producing **unequal openings** in size and shape.

A normally projecting medial crurae may become too large for the available space after surgically reducing the size of the nasal apertures, e.g., excision of the rim-sill folds.

All factors are to be considered in the procedures of reducing the overprojecting crura, starting from simple **external** approach to a more direct **internal** one as follows:

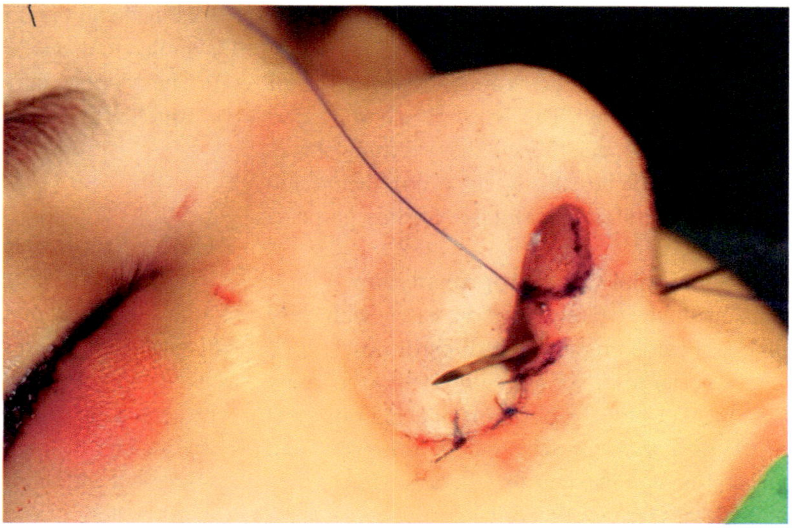

Fig. 21.20 The Transcollumellar Stitch. The transcollumelar stitch going anterior then posterior to the IVB (Inferior Vestibular Band)

External Lintercrural Stitch (Linter-Sill Band)

A **transcolumellar-suture** is used to anchor the **two inferior vestibular bands (IVB)** on both sides of the nose. The crural cartilages are not directly involved in this stitch but rather the two bands are pulled medially by the stitch, which must be **strictly intra-vestibular using prolene** on a **straight needle**. It is taken between **the two medial ends of the nasal sill bands,** i.e., at the **two angles** of the sharp upward turning from their transverse course (Figs. 21.20, 21.21, 21.51, 21.52, 21.53, 21.54, 21.55, 21.56, 21.57, 21.60, 21.61, 21.62, 21.110 and 21.111).

When the two **angles are approximated, they will pull on the posterior free margins of the medial crurae**. This single stitch is usually sufficient.

To further secure the lasting effect of this stitch, a preliminary dissection and **thinning of the subcutaneous tissues between the two crurae is done**. This adds to the thinning of the columellar skin width. The **posterior margins of**

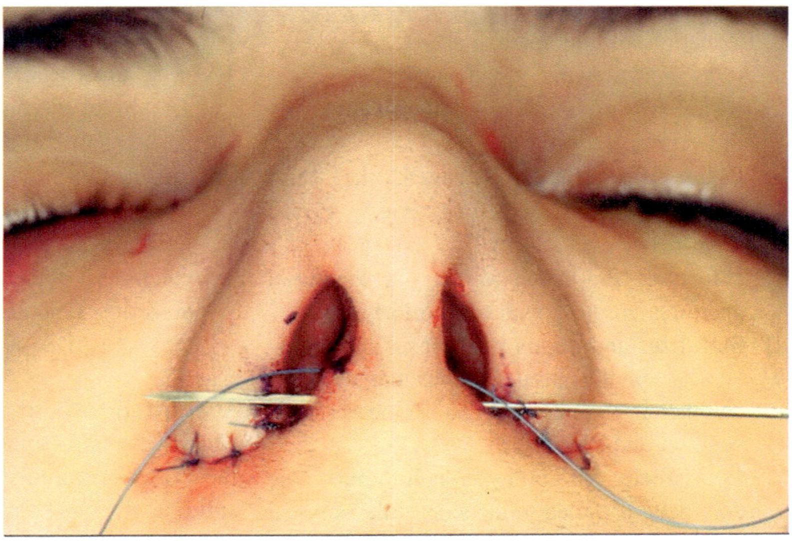

Fig. 21.21 Looking at the transcollumelar stitch from the basal view going anterior and then posterior to the two IVBs on both sides

both crural cartilages may then be anchored by one or more trans-sutures.

The **proline stitches remain in situ for at least two months**. This ensures a strong and lasting fibrosis that keeps the aperture shape. Absorbable stitches, including vycril, dexon and catgut are therefore not suitable for this purpose.

Internal Medial Crural Approximation

This method is rarely used in cases with very diversely wide crurae and stiff cartilages.

It is a more direct and sure method to bring together the bulging posterior and inferior ends of the medial crurae. This can be achieved from the septoplasty incision or otherwise an incision is made at the upper margin of one medial crus. The incision is deepened between the two crurae, to reach their posterior and inferior margins. Some of the intercrural tissues are removed.

A toothed forceps is then introduced from the columellar wound. **The nasal sill band** is picked up just posterior to the **point of maximum crural bulge**. A Bite is taken into the sill band **at the tip of the forceps**. The same is done on the other side. On tying the stitch the two sides are now anchored together pulling the medial crural bulge into midline. An absorbable single stitch is sufficient.

Finally, if the posterior ends of the crural cartilages are very stiff and prominent, they may be **excised** before placing the proline intercrural stitch externally.

Reduction of the medial crural overprojections has the following advantages:

(a) **Equalizes unequal apertures** caused by different crural prominences.
(b) **Better aesthetic appearance**: the nasal apertures become wider posteriorly giving them better oval shapes.
(c) **Improves the nasal airway** as the nasal apertures are now wider posteriorly.
(d) **Stabilizes** and **aligns both nasal sills** transversely on the nasal floor as the alar and columellar wounds may disturb the nasal sill position and stability.
(e) **Centralizes an oblique columella:** The columella is pulled to the side of the surgical knot, i.e., if it is oblique to the left then the knot is made on the right side and the columella is pulled to that side while tightening the knot.
(f) The stitch can be used to **close the columellar incision** on both sides.

21.3.2 Surgery of the Soft Posterior Columellar Fold

This is the **soft fold of skin** that covers the gap between the **upper lip** and the nose which is represented by the **medial crurae**, at the most posterior end of the columella.

<u>**Surgical importance**</u>

The posterior columellar fold derives its surgical importance from two main factors:

(a) It is the only **soft unsupported** part of the columella as it contains loose connective tissue and muscle fibers. The main and only support is gained superiorly from the bony **anterior nasal spine**.
(b) It is located at the **naso-labial** (columella-labial) **angle** which is of great aesthetic value.

21.3.2.1 Factors Affecting the Posterior Columellar Fold

The **size, shape** and **position** of the posterior columellar fold vary according to **age, anatomy** of the surrounding structures and the **contents** as follows:

The Medial Crurae

i. The crural prominence: as the curvatures of the posterior ends of both crurae increase, they depart away from each other producing a **wide fold.**
ii. Position: A superiorly or inferiorly placed columella (hanging columella) moves the posterior columellar fold in one of two directions, i.e., **superiorly** or **inferiorly.**

The Anterior Nasal Spine

This is the most important structure that affects the posterior columellar fold as it is **the only solid** and major support for this critically important soft area.

The nasal spine is part of the palatine process of the maxillary bone. The **size** and **position** of the nasal spine are variable, with consequent effects on the shape and aesthetics of the naso-labial angle, the shape of nasal aperture and indirectly on the supratip areas.

21.3.2.2 Position of the Anterior Nasal Spine

Position of the Anterior Nasal Spine: The sideway deviations of the spine drive the posterior part of the columellar wall of the one side. The caudal septum, the medial crurae and nasal sill bands are also deviated and may encroach upon the nasal aperture space and affect its aesthetics.

21.3.2.3 Size of the Anterior Nasal Spine

Size of the Anterior Nasal Spine: Variations and changes in the size of the anterior nasal spine affects the nose and nasal aesthetics in two main directions and consequently two important areas:

i. **Inferiorly:** affecting the **naso-labial angle** through the **posterior columellar fold**. A large spine produces a protruding columella, while a small spine results in an acute naso-labial angle.
ii. **Anteriorly:** affecting the **height** of the anterior septal angle and hence the **nasal height** at the supratip area indirectly through the **weak triangle**. A parrot beak deformity or supratip depression results as a consequence of a high or low anterior septal angles.

Large Anterior Nasal Spine

A large anterior nasal spine is usually associated with a long caudal septum. There are two clinical presentations of a large anterior nasal spine:

i. Protruding columella:

The columella is lower than the level of the alar margin and the medial vestibular wall is unpleasantly exposed. A large nasal spine will drive the posterior columellar fold, downward protruding and exposing it. The caudal septal cartilage pushes the medial crurae, downward protruding and exposing the rest of the columella.

ii. The Tension Nose:

There are clinical and morphological conditions in which there are special anatomical configuration in the naso-labial area and the surrounding structures that have very significant **aesthetic** and **functional** effects.

Changes may not only affect the nose and the upper lip, but they may also be part of a more **generalized** developmental deformity that affect the growing face. These conditions may therefore be observed both in adults and in children as early as the age of 6–9 years.

There are so many anatomical factors that affect the **soft tissues,** e.g., the zygomaticus, levator labii, depressor septi muscles, the upper lip and the frenulum. The supporting **skeletal tissues** are affected, e.g., the caudal septum the anterior nasal spine, nasal dorsum, maxillary body, alar bone and the mandible.

Clinical Picture:

The basic morphological disorder stems from the fact that the supporting **skeletal** structures are **disproportionately larger** than the overlying **soft tissues**, which become short and tight.

Enlargement of the skeleton may be limited to the anterior **nasal spine** and caudal septum or it may include the **alveolar margin** which may protrude forwards, i.e., pragmatism. Finally, enlargement may include the whole of the **maxilla** and facial skeleton. The clinical picture, therefore, varies according to the increasing degrees of deformities as follows:

i. The "Mobile Tip"

The simplest and earliest feature that may be associated with the tension nose is animation of the nasal tip, i.e., mobile tip due to the overactivity of the depressor septi muscles. The mobile tips may present in an otherwise aesthetically balanced nose.

ii. The "Tethered Lip" or "Tight Lip" Syndrome:

In the more advanced cases, there is gradual obliteration and widening of the **naso-labial angle** by the progressively enlarging anterior nasal spine and the accompanying protruding caudal septum. The upper lip then becomes tethered, shortened and taken up towards the nose.

The frenulum is very short, holding the lip tightly. The lip may become open even at rest exposing the upper incisors. Smiling may show the gums of the upper teeth, i.e., **gummy smile**. These conditions are known as the "**open lip**" or "**Bugs Bunny**" syndrome.

Management of the tension nose:

(a) Children: only conservative measures are needed to improve the nasal airways and relieve the obstruction. **Adenoidectomy** and **submucus diathermy of the inferior turbinates** are sufficient in most children.
(b) **Adults:** depending on the degree of deformity the surgical management is aimed at both the **soft tissue** and the **skeletal structures**.

Although there are so many anatomical deformities that may be involved, yet changes are mainly centered on their aesthetic effects on the **naso-labial angle**, which if released, other deformities seem like secondary ones. In other words, the nasal spine may be the only culprit in these deformities yet it has a significant and central role.

Only deformities that are limited to the nose and naso-labial area are dealt with by the Rhinologists, while more advanced deformities in the face, maxilla and mandible need the cooperation of the Orthodontic and Maxillo-facial surgeons.

Management therefore includes the following:

i. **Bony and cartilaginous skeleton**:

This includes limited and carefully measured reduction of the **anterior nasal spine** and/or caudal cartilaginous septum. **Septoplasty** and, if needed, **rhinoplasty**, to remove the nasal hump are additional measures to improve nasal aesthetics.

ii. **Soft tissue**:

The muscles that may be involved in the tension nose are the depressor septi, the levator labii superioris alaeque nasi and the zygomaticus major and minor.

Preoperative

Postoperative

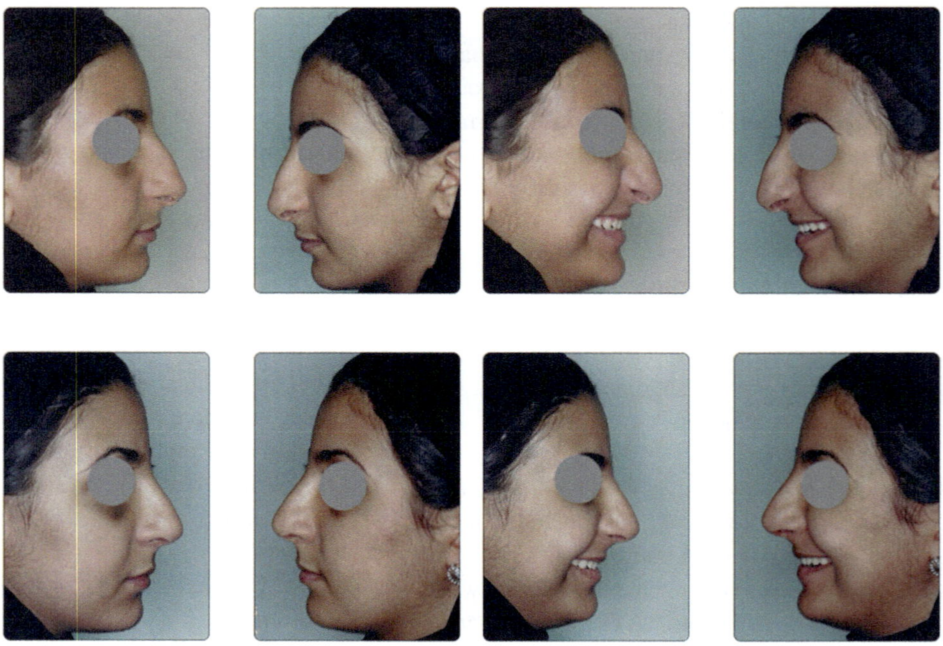

Fig. 21.22 The Plunging Tip

The **depressor septi** muscles contribute the most to the naso-labial tension deformities. They are the **only muscles** that have nearby bony attachments and can either be severed or detached.

Animation is largely abolished after this procedure alone. It may be coupled with cutting the short **frenulum** transversely and stitching the wound longitudinally. The soft tissue work together with the skeletal work on the anterior nasal spine and the caudal septum, **releases the upper lip** which becomes elongated. The naso-labial angle, teeth exposure and the gummy smile are all improved.

Small Anterior Nasal Spine

A small receding nasal spine has two clinical presentations:

i. Retracting columella:

This is caused by the partial or total loss of support of the soft posterior columellar fold by a small anterior nasal spine. It is usually **iatrogenic, i.e.**, caused by over-reduction of the nasal spine during septal surgery or rhinoplasty. Even with well proportioned and aesthetically balanced structures of the lower third of the nose, there may be an **acute naso-labial angle**. Restoring the solid support using bone or cartilage graft is the logical and effective maneuver. The graft is introduced via a labial or vestibular incision.

ii. Plunging Tip:

This term is used to describe a drooping tip that is disproportionally large, coupled with an acute naso-labial angle.

Clinical Picture:

The basic morphological disorder in this condition is that there are large lateral and middle crurae as compared to the relatively small, receding anterior nasal spine and medial crurae (Fig. 21.22).

There may be **other secondary changes** in the region that exaggerate the plunging effect, e.g., long caudal septum especially towards the anterior angle, dorsal hump and overactive depressor septi muscles.

A small anterior nasal spine therefore may not be the only deformity in these conditions. It is rather a part of a much wider morphological changes in the lower third of the nose. In fact the nasal spine may have an acceptable size and position, yet disproportionately small as compared with the large domes and lateral crura.

The final unaesthetic outcome is that of **an acute naso-labial angle** with large **drooping nasal tip**.

Management:

(a) Direct management:

By dealing with the middle and lateral crura, reducing their sizes directly.

(b) Indirect management:

Camouflage surgery, using a tip graft may overcome the deformity. This may be combined with cephalic trim of the lateral crura.

21.4 Surgery of the Nasal Septum

The nasal septum is **one of the four major components** of the surgery of Rhinoplasty. It plays a important role both aesthetically and functionally. These roles must be maintained at all times during surgery.

Clinically, the nasal septum has two segments which are totally different anatomically, aesthetically and physiologically:

1. **The osteocartilagenous septum**: This is a completely intranasal part of the septum and is lined with respiratory mucosa.
2. **The membranous septum:** This is a completely subcutaneous structure that is covered by the vestibular skin. The membranous septum has two components: the loose vestibular skin and the caudal vestibular septum (see Histology).

21.4.1 The Essential Role of the Nasal Septum in Rhinoplasty

The nasal septum is an essential structure that must be considered in every case of Rhinoplasty even if septal surgery is not involved in the procedure. There are fundamental factors that must be understood and maintained in every procedure to ensure successful aesthetic and functional results:

21.4.1.1 Stability and Support

Stability of the three-dimensional structure of the nose is one of the major concerns of Rhinoplasty.

The nasal septum provides a vital support and is a major factor in the overall stability of the nose.

The basic surgical procedures that are performed in Rhinoplasty tend to **weaken** and destabilize the three-dimensional structure of the nose. These procedures are:

- The intercartilagenous incisions;
- Excision of a nasal hump: this includes lateral, medial and superior osteotomies of the bony pyramid;
- Division and separation of the cartilagenous septum from the upper lateral cartilage which is sometimes needed;
- Surgery of the lower lateral cartilages and alar base.

All of these procedures tend to weaken the structure of the lateral walls of the nose, starting from the bony pyramid down to the midvault and the lower lateral cartilages.

Structures on the side walls of the external nose are in a way **disassembled, reshaped** and **repositioned** in better aesthetic locations.

The nasal septum, therefore, must be **preserved as much as possible to maintain nasal stability**. Ideally, the nasal septum should reach from the floor of the nose to the dorsum. If any part of the septum is taken away, e.g., for a graft material, it must not jeopardize the septum's supportive role. A **conservative** attitude must be generally maintained in septal surgery.

Leaving a **10mm strip** of dorsal cartilaginous septum is sufficient to secure the **dorsum**. The strip may be larger or smaller according to the stiffness of the cartilage.

Additionally leaving a caudal strip of cartilage may be necessary to avoid an acute naso-labial angle. The caudal strip is not a necessity in many cases. The anterior nasal spine provides enough support to the naso-labial angle in these cases.

21.4.1.2 Maintaining Dorsal Height

The nasal dorsum starts from the nasion and ends at the anterior septal angle. The nasal septum is a major supportive structure all through from the bony pyramid, midvault and finally the floor of the weak triangle.

A nasal hump is usually osteocartilagenous and is associated with a high bony and cartilaginous septum.

A high **caudal** septum will lead to supratip elevation or parrot beak deformity.

On the contrary, a defective cartilaginous septum and lack of support will lead to a saddle deformity or a supratip depression. Depression and parrot beak deformities are usually iatrogenic, while humps are developmental.

21.4.1.3 Direction of the Nose

A **deviated** septum, especially near the dorsum, may lead to deviation of the nose. An **oblique** septum may lead to, or be associated with, an oblique nose. Deviation and obliquity are associated with cases of bilateral **maxillary asymmetry** (refer to chapter of the Deviated Nose and the Crooked Nose).

21.4.1.4 Source of Graft Material

The nasal septum is the best source of graft material for the following reasons:

- The graft can be conveniently harvested from the nose during surgery without the need for another field of surgery.
- Two varieties of graft materials are available:

i. Cartilage:

  - The cartilaginous septum is usually a good material for the nasal tip and augmentation of the nasal dorsum and sidewalls.
  - The inferior cartilaginous border that is embedded in the maxillary groove is very thick and suitable for augmentation of the alar margin.

ii. Bone: The vomer is an excellent source of bone graft material.

- Septal grafts can be shaped and adapted to the various parts of the nose, e.g., dorsum, sidewalls and tip.
- Rejection of the septal graft is almost unknown.
- Good, long-term results: Compared with other graft materials, septal grafts have a more **predictable** aesthetic outcome in the long term. This is due to **minimal resorption** and the good acceptance of the graft by the body.

21.4.1.5 Nasal Airway

It is imperative that the surgeon must maintain a satisfactory nasal airway. The best aesthetic result will not be appreciated without good nasal airway.

Patients with extreme sinus pathology, e.g., extensive nasal polyps, fungal infection or extensive infection are better treated first before considering any aesthetic surgery.

21.4.2 Nasal Septal Deviation

Nasal septal deviation per se is neither a disease nor is it a pathological diagnosis. Many people have quite severe deviations with very little, if any, symptoms. The only exceptions are the post-traumatic and the severe symptomatizing cases including the localized deviations at the area of the nasal valves.

The nasal septum is not usually strictly midline structure. Very often it has one or more natural curves or deviations. Nasal septal deviation may take place in the bony or cartilaginous parts. The osteocartilagenous junction is another common site for septal deviation.

21.4.2.1 The Bony Deviations

The curves in the bony septum may be mild or quite sharp with a bony spur. Deviations are mostly due to the different sizes of the structures on the both sides of the septum in the lateral nasal walls. The turbinates, the ethmoid and the maxillary sinuses may be larger on one side than the other. The bony septum, which has clear clinical deviation, is in fact exactly in the middle between the two unequal sides. This is clearly seen in the coronal and axial C-T scans of the nose and sinuses.

An S-shaped deviation of the septum may be due to larger inferior turbinate on one side while the middle turbinate and/or ethmoids are larger on the other side.

Severe deviations may reach and even touch the lateral nasal wall. It may be associated with a large and thick bony spur. This usually takes place **at the junction between the vomer and the perpendicular plate of the ethmoid.**

21.4.2.2 The Osteocartilagenous Deviations

The quadrilateral septal cartilage may not have any deviations in its body, but it may be larger than the available space inside the nose. In these cases, the cartilage is forced out of its place in one or more locations within or outside the nose.

i. **Inferiorly:** The cartilage may be dislocated laterally out of the maxillary groove. The posterior septal angle may protrude to one side of the columella, i.e., caudal septal dislocation.
ii. **Anteriorly:** The **anterior septal angle** may appear as a supratip bulge in the weak triangle resulting in a Parrot beak deformity.

iii. **Superiorly:** The long cartilage may angulate at its **junction with the vomer and ethmoid bones** leading to varying degrees of septal deviation.

The osteocatilagenous deviations therefore present in two locations:

- At the meeting with the maxillary crest **inferiorly;**
- At the meeting of the septal cartilage with the vomer and ethmoid bones **superiorly**.

21.4.2.3 The Cartilaginous Deviations

The quadrilateral cartilage of the septum may have quite asymptomatic natural curves or deviations in its body.

Should these deviations be present in the key areas of the **nasal valves**, internal or external, they may strongly affect air entry giving the patient an equally strong sensation of nasal blockage.

21.4.3 General Principles of Septal Surgery in Rhinoplasty

There are common basic recommendations in septal surgery, if it is included in the process of Rhinoplasty:

21.4.3.1 Preservation

Conservative techniques are generally observed, so that dismantling and excisions of the different parts of the nasal septum are reduced to the absolute minimum in order to keep it **firm**, **solid** and **supportive.**

<u>Resection better than Augmentation:</u>

This is an excellent general principle in the surgery of Rhinoplasty.

It is easier to **take** away excess nasal tissues than **adding** them by augmentation and supporting grafts. The lesson to learn here is not to rush into excising tissues.

Adding graft is a fiddling process that takes time and the aesthetic outcome is not always predictable especially in the long term.

21.4.3.2 Intraoperative Timing of Septoplasty

Not only is it important **what** to do in septal surgery but more importantly is **when** to do it. In general, the initial bilateral dissection of the mucoperichondrium, separation of the septal cartilage from the surrounding bones subperichondrially is better made at the beginning of the surgery. Any decision to **resect** parts of the septum is to be **postponed after osteotomies** no matter what the temptations, or despite any clear excess tissues.

21.4.3.3 Maintaining the Integrity of the Septum

It is important to avoid perforating the nasal septum. This will disturb nasal physiology and weaken the dorsal support. Having residual deviation is better than having a perforation.

21.4.4 Technical Details of Septal Surgery

While operating on the nasal septum, the surgeon should have a clear vision of the main targets of the surgery which are

(a) Nasal Stability;
(b) Nasal airway;
(c) Nasal aesthetics.

It is therefore important to have a clear anatomic, physiologic and aesthetic assessment.

21.4.4.1 Subperichondrial Septoplasty

The common use of the term submucus dissection of the nasal septum is a misnomer. The accurate surgical procedure is subperichondrial dissection.

Reaching the subperichondrial layer is the most important step in septoplasty. It is almost true to say that a **successful subperochondrial dissection equals a successful septal surgery.**

Reaching the subperichondrial layer after the initial incision needs:

a. Good **preparation** for a bloodless field;
b. Making the incision in the right place;

c. Going through the different layers one by one till the subperichodrial layer is reached.

Although there is one continuous mucous membrane covering the cartilaginous and the bony septum, yet the **perichondrum** is **not continuous** with the **periostium** of the maxillary crest or vomerine groove. Each has to be dissected separately.

Reaching the subperichondrial and subperiosteal planes is a very meticulous process which needs time and patience. Haste and rush must be avoided at this stage. At the end it pays off, as the rest of the septal surgery becomes much easier and better controlled.

21.4.4.2 Preparation for Septal Surgery

- The upper half of the operating table is elevated or else **reverse Trendelenburg** position, with the head **slightly raised**.
- A suitably sized firm, but not hard, **horseshoe** or a **head ring** is placed under the ball of the head.
- A soft rounded pillow is placed **under the knees** and a small soft pad just **above the heals**.
- Surgery is done under hypotensive general anesthesia.
- Local anesthesia is additionally injected using a one in two hundred thousand (1:200,000) solution of adrenaline with lidocaine 1–2%. Injections are made in the areas of the **membranous septum** and into the **subperichondrial layers on both sides**. The **bevel** of the needle is directed towards the side of the septum. The right level is reached if **blanching of the septal mucosa** spreads as injection proceeds.
- Surgery is delayed for 10–15 min till the full effect of local anesthesia takes place.

21.4.4.3 Instruments

- Good, powerful **head light**. The nasal cavity is a dark deep hole that needs good illumination. Fiber-optic cold light using the true white lighting provides the best condition for surgery.
- Thin-bladed Killian speculae, short and long ones are needed.
- Ordinary metal suction, 3 mm and 5 mm, e.g., Frazier suction tubes.
- A **sharp beveled suction dissection** is usually of great help for a bloodless field, e.g., Haraldsson suction elevator
- A **sharp** and **blunt two ended Freer dissector**
- Double-ended **Cottle's elevator**. The harpoon sharp end of Cottle's elevator helps in dissection of the inferior mucoperiosteal part of the septum while the blunt end helps in disarticulating the osteochondrial junctions.
- **Cottle's columellar forceps** or simple **toothed Adson forceps.**
- Blakesley or Telly Henkle Forceps, 3 mm and 5 mm.
- Janson septum forceps and Janson Middleton through cutting septum forceps.

21.4.4.4 Surgical Steps

The Incision

- The surgery starts by **fully stretching the membranous septum** using Cottle's columellar or simple toothed forceps. Alternatively, a Kelian speculum is used to stretch and directly reach the inferior margin of the caudal cartilagenous septum. This ensures that the skin incision is exactly over the caudal cartilaginous margin at the highest possible level of the membranous septum. This level of the membranous septum is **nearer to the muco-cutaneous junction** where the **vestibular skin is more adherent to the caudal margin**. Dissection at this level is easier and gives more direct access to the perichondrium of the septal cartilage.
- Only with few exceptions, the incision for septoplasty must always be made at the **caudal margin of the cartilaginous septum** which then continues with the intercartilagenous incision for Rhinoplasty. The septal and

intercartilagenous incisions are always **inferior to the anterior angle of the internal valve**.

The incision extends to the whole length of the caudal cartilaginous margin, i.e., from the anterior septal angle to the side of the incisive maxillary crest.

Exposure of the septum must be complete in order to have total control of each and every part of the septum. The **margin** and **angles** of the septal cartilage as well as its bony parts should be explored.

- The incision is gradually deepened through the skin, subcutaneous tissue and then the perichodrium. It is essential to reach the **subperichondrial layer**. It looks pearly white and is quite bloodless.
- Dissecting the mucoperichondrium, using a Freer elevator, becomes then quite easy. Using the suction dissection at this stage is quite helpful for bloodless field.
- It is not infrequent to find it difficult to reach to the subperichondrial layer, especially in post-traumatic cases.

In these cases, it is helpful to use the side of the knife and repeatedly **scratch the perichondrium off** the caudal margin until the white glistening cartilage is seen. The perichondrial margin can then be seen on the side of the scratched area. The subperichondrial layer is entered using the sharp end of Freer dissector.

Septal Exploration before Osteotomies

This step mainly aims at **dissecting the mucoperichondrium off the cartilage** and the **mucoperiostium off the bone**. The **septal cartilage is then separated and freed from its bony attachments**.

- The perichondrium is dissected **anteroposteriory** and then **superiorly**. The anterior and the posterior septal angles are explored. Dissection is then continued **inferiorly** to separate the quadrilateral cartilage from the maxillary groove. If the cartilage was already dislocated from the groove then it is easier to push it further towards the same side of dislocation, i.e., to complete the separation between the cartilage and the maxillary groove.
- The septal cartilage is then dissected off and separated from the vomer inferiorly and the ethmoid plate superiorly. Separation from the latter **must not reach the dorsum** of the nose in order to avoid its collapse and saddling which may take place either immediately or after osteotomies.

At the end of this procedure, the septal cartilage is released from its perichondrial and bony attachments. It becomes almost totally free.

The septal cartilage spontaneously and naturally moves towards the midline. This will have a favorable effect on two anatomical locations:

i. The osteocartilagenous junctional areas, i.e., with the vomer and ethmoid bones. Any **localized bony deviation** is gently pushed and fractured to the midline after minimally trimming its margin.
ii. The nasal valve angle usually widens spontaneously.

It is strongly adviced **not** to **attempt resecting any excess cartilage or bone** at this time and stage of the surgery. All temptations of cutting even the most obvious caudal or inferior cartilaginous excesses or bony spurs must be resisted at all cost. They are postponed until after osteotomies.

Completion of Septoplasty After Osteotomies

Osteotomies, especially if associated with **hump resection**, are usually associated with partial resection of both the cartilaginous and the bony septum anterosuperiorly. The caudal excesses of the septum can now be accommodated inside the nose. It becomes an excellent midline support.

It is only at this time and stage of the operation that any cartilaginous or bony excesses may be accurately resected without jeopardizing the stability of the nose.

Managing the Nasal Septum

The **osteo-cartilaginous septum** and the **membranous septum** are dealt with in different ways because of their anatomic location and aesthetic effects.

The Osteocartilagenous Septum

i. The vomer:

The general attitude concerning the bony part of the septum is **minimal resection** and correction by **manipulation to the midline**, then **fixation.**

The vomer and the lower part of the ethmoid plate are fractured and pushed towards the midline. This is done by the combined use of the long stout blades of a Killian forceps or an equally strong elevator, e.g., Cottle's elevator.

Only minimal trimming may be needed at the osteo-cartilaginous junction from the bony or cartilaginous side or both to correct and release any **severe angulation** at this area.

If a **bony spur** is obstructing the airway, it is either trimmed or very precisely removed. It may be useful to use a strong double action punch (Jansen Middleton's) or scissors (Hayman's or Kaplan's scissors).

Beware of excising large pieces of septal bones, that may weaken the bony pyramid of the nose and jeopardize its stability.

ii. The Incisor Maxillary Crest:

The maxillary crest is a small yet an important part of the bony septum because of its subcutaneous location at the naso-labial angle. It accommodates the posterior angle of the cartilaginous septum.

If the bony crest is deviated, then it should be manipulated to the midline by the stout blades of Killian's speculum or a small chisel.

Breaking it at **one side only**, keeps it partially attached to the floor of the nose with minimal destabilization.

The anterior nasal spine is only trimmed if it is too long.

iii. The Ethmoid Bone:

The highest part of the ethmoid bone is not easy to access, reach or correct both clinically or during septal surgery. If deviated it may not interfere with the nasal airway but it may **obstruct the proper reduction of the side walls of the bony pyramid after osteotomies**. The nose remains **crooked** unless this part of the septum is corrected.

The best and simplest method of correcting this part of the septum is by simple manipulation. It has to be fractured from outside and forced to the midline by **Kassanjian maneuver,** i.e., the sidewalls of the bony pyramid are cross fractured towards the midline.

Kassanjian Maneuver: This is a procedure of cross fracture of the bony pyramid. After osteotomies and medialization of the bony side walls, the deviated bony pyramid is covered by two pieces of dry 4x4 inches gauze swabs. The pyramid is then snappily hammered on the deviated side towards the opposite side. Using both hands, the bony pyramid is then manipulated and centralized more accurately in the midline.

iv. The Internal Cartilagenous Septum:

Excess cartilage is accurately trimmed. Any deviation is corrected or precisely trimmed.

Grafts may be harvested from the septal cartilage. A dorsal stripe of 10mm of cartilage is sufficient to maintain dorsal stability.

21.4.5 The Membranous Septum

This part of the septum is called membranous as it is mostly devoid of firm structures (see anatomy section). The membranous septum is totally vestibular, i.e., covered with vestibular skin. It has two main components, i.e., **loose midline vestibular skin** and the **caudal vestibular septum**. Both play important roles in nasal aesthetics. The caudal vestibular septum has an additional physiological role (see physiology of nasal respiration). The membranous septum has **direct** and **indirect** effects on nasal aesthetics.

A. The **direct effects** are caused by the firm subcutaneous body of the **caudal vestibular septum**.
B. The **indirect effects** are due to the **excessively redundant skin** of the membranous septum with **overactive Depressor Septi muscles**. This results in a condition called **sliding tip**.

21.4.5.1 The Direct Effects of the Membranous Septum

The direct effects of the membranous septum are caused by the firm subcutaneous body of the caudal vestibular septum.

The Caudal Vestibular Septum

The caudal septum is the inferior one fifth segment of the cartilaginous septum, which is free from attachment to the upper lateral cartilage. It is **totally subcutaneous**, i.e., covered by the external skin anteriorly and the vestibular skin internally, being part of the membranous septum. It is also called the **vestibular septum**. The caudal septum is the only **relatively mobile** part of the nasal septum. It is the strongest structure of the lower third of the nose and constitutes a midline stable and robust basis for both nasal aperture tubes.

The caudal septum is of significant **clinical**, **aesthetic** and **physiological** significance.

Clinical Significance

The caudal septum has **a free front** and **fixed base** to the maxillary crest. It is the central support of the lower third of the nose. It forms a firm, strut between the maxillary groove posteriorly and the dorsum of the nose anteriorly.

The **softness** and **mobility of** the membranous septum helps in **absorbing the shock** of frontal **trauma** to the nasal tip.

Powerful frontal trauma may lead to fracture of the caudal septum. The fracture line is at the junction between the **mobile** caudal and **fixed** proximal parts of the cartilaginous septum. It is not an uncommon fracture. Unfortunately, it is often undiagnosed at the time of the accident and is totally neglected. This will lead to **deformity of the nasal tip and disfigurement of the nasal apertures.**

Trauma may take place by direct fall on the nose, hitting a hard object in an accident or by a direct punch.

Fracture of the caudal vestibular septum may not be noticed clinically and is diagnosed on table during the surgery, for the first time.

Aesthetic Significance

Being a subcutaneous structure, the caudal septum directly affects the aesthetic of the nasal tip, supratip area, columella and nasal apertures. These effects are best demonstrated in cases of caudal vestibular septal deviation (Fig. 21.23).

Caudal septal deviation is the dislocation of the caudal septum laterally outside the maxillary groove, under the vestibular skin. Dislocations may be subtle and frequently missed clinically. Clinicians must look for it.

- **The supratip area**

The anterior border and anterior angle of the caudal septum fills the supratip area. Clinically, the supratip area lies above the nasal tip between the domes of the middle crurae. Anatomically this area is known as the weak triangle.

A **high** anterior septal **border** and anterior **angle** will lead to **supratip elevation**. A **low** anterior border and angle will lead to a **supratip depression** (Fig. 21.24).

- **The Nasal Tip**

The anterior margin and the anterior angle of the caudal septum represent the end point of the nasal dorsum. They provide major **support for the nasal tip.**

- A **unilateral bulge** of the middle or lateral crurae is caused by a dislocated caudal septum to one side. Correction of the septum reduces the bulge (Fig. 21.25).

Fig. 21.23 Right caudal septal deviation and dislocation, distorting the anatomy of the right nasal aperture

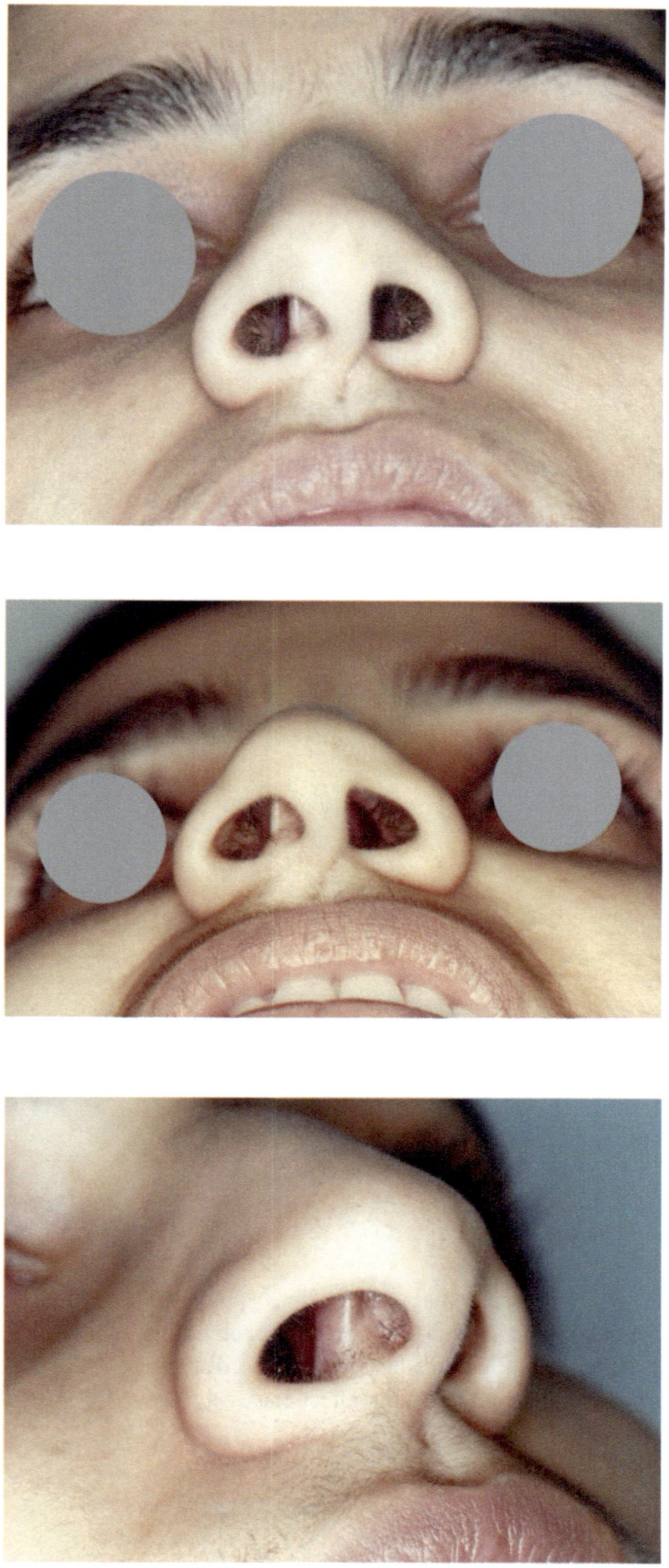

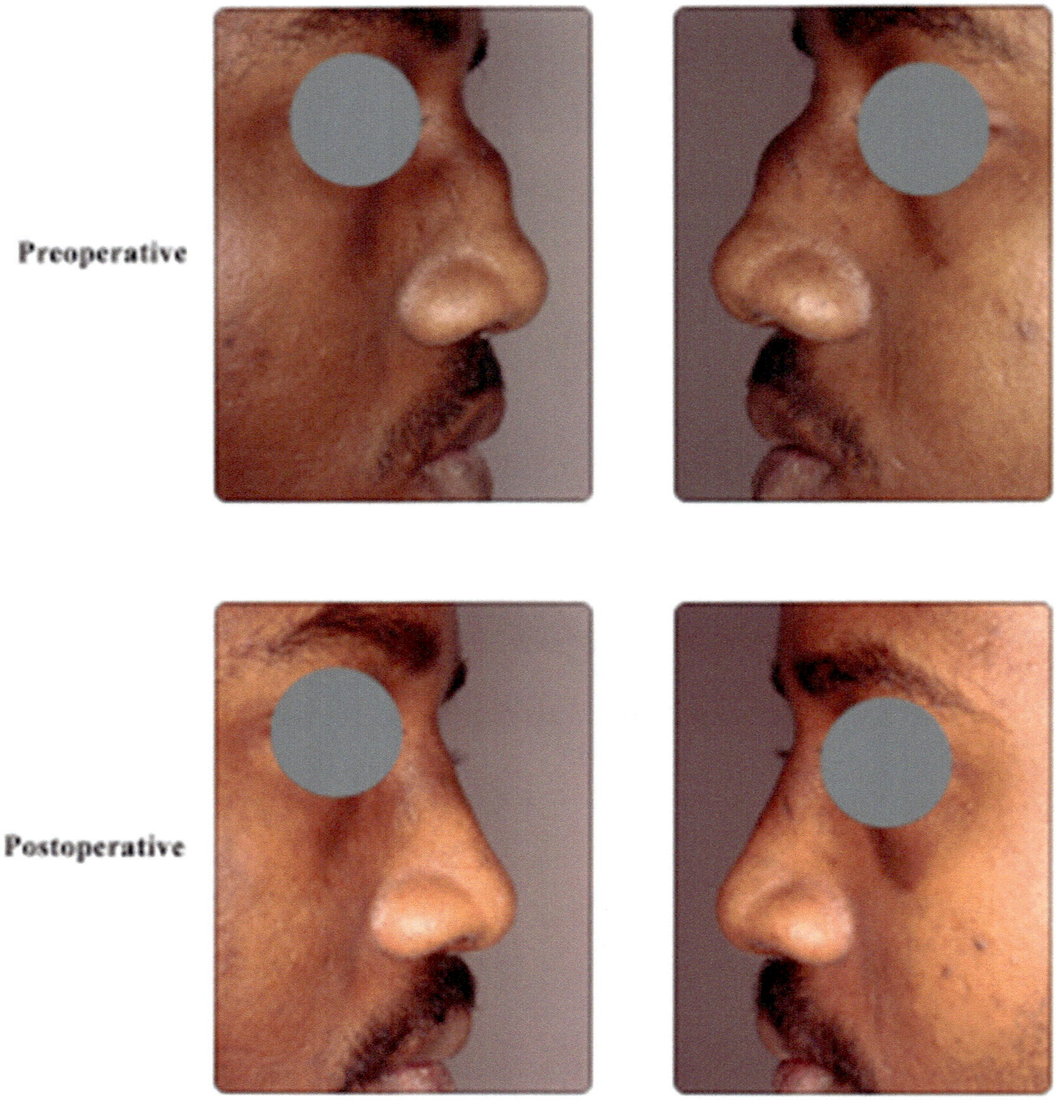

Fig. 21.24 Post traumatic Supratip depression

- **The columella**

A long caudal septal margin may push the medial crurae down leading to a **protruding** columella. The columella may become **oblique or twisted** according to the effect caused by the septum.

- **The Nasal Aperture**

In cases where the caudal septum is dislocated, the caudal margin pushes the **medial crus laterally** and the **nasal sill inferiorly**. Both changes will encroach upon the shape and size of the nasal aperture. The affected side looks apparently smaller and is badly disfigured. One medial crus

Fig. 21.25 Bulge of the left lateral crus by the deviated anterior septal angle. The posterior septal angle is obliquely dislocated to the right side

Preoperative

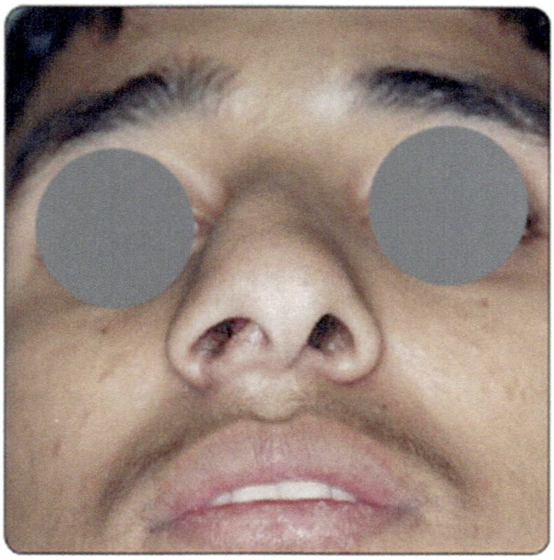

Postoperative

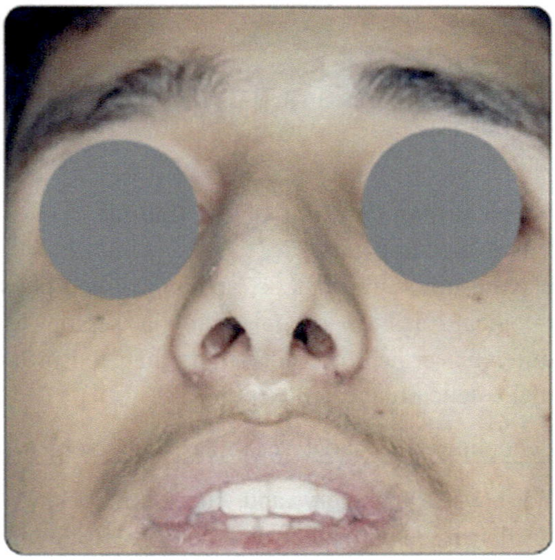

is unpleasantly bulging into the nasal cavity and the nasal sill band is at a lower level than the other side (Fig. 21.26).

- **The Nasolabial Angle**

The posterior angle of the caudal septum is securely embedded in a groove in the maxillary crest. The naso-labial angle increases with the increase of the size of the nasal spine and the protrusion of an elongated posterior angle and vice versa.

Physiological Significance

The caudal septum is the fixed medial wall for the right and left anterior angles of the internal nasal valves (see physiology of nasal respiration).

Preoperative

Postoperative

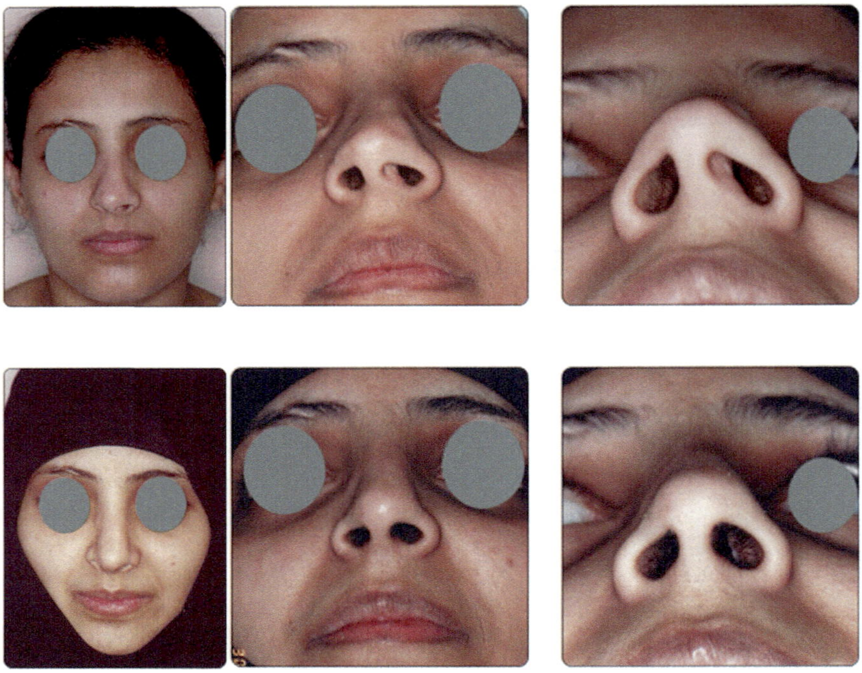

Fig. 21.26 Left caudal septal deviation has led to oblique protruded columella and inferior displacement of the left nasal sill band

Surgical Management of the Caudal Vestibular Septum

Having different aesthetic, anatomical and physiological roles, the caudal vestibular septum has different surgical considerations than the proximal osteocartilagenous septum.

Guidelines for caudal vestibular septal surgery:

To have satisfactory and successful aesthetic results in caudal septal disorders, the following five conditions are observed:

Accurate Height and Length

Accurate height and length: The caudal septum must have the exact **height in the supratip region and length caudally**. The locations of the **anterior** and **posterior septal angles** must be observed successively in each of these locations.

Straight

Straight: The **anterior** and **inferior borders** as well as the **body** of the caudal septum must be straight, or otherwise be straightened, to avoid deviation or crookedness.

Firm

Firm: The caudal vestibular septum has to be firm enough in order to support the supratip weak triangular area.

Midline

Midline: The caudal vestibular septum has to be strictly in the midline to avoid deviation of the lower third and hence the tip of the nose (Fig. 21.27).

Stable

Stable: The caudal vestibular septum has to be securely stable in its position.

Surgical procedures therefore should address these five conditions as follows:

i. **Reduction of Excess Caudal Septum**

(a) Reduction of the **excess height:**

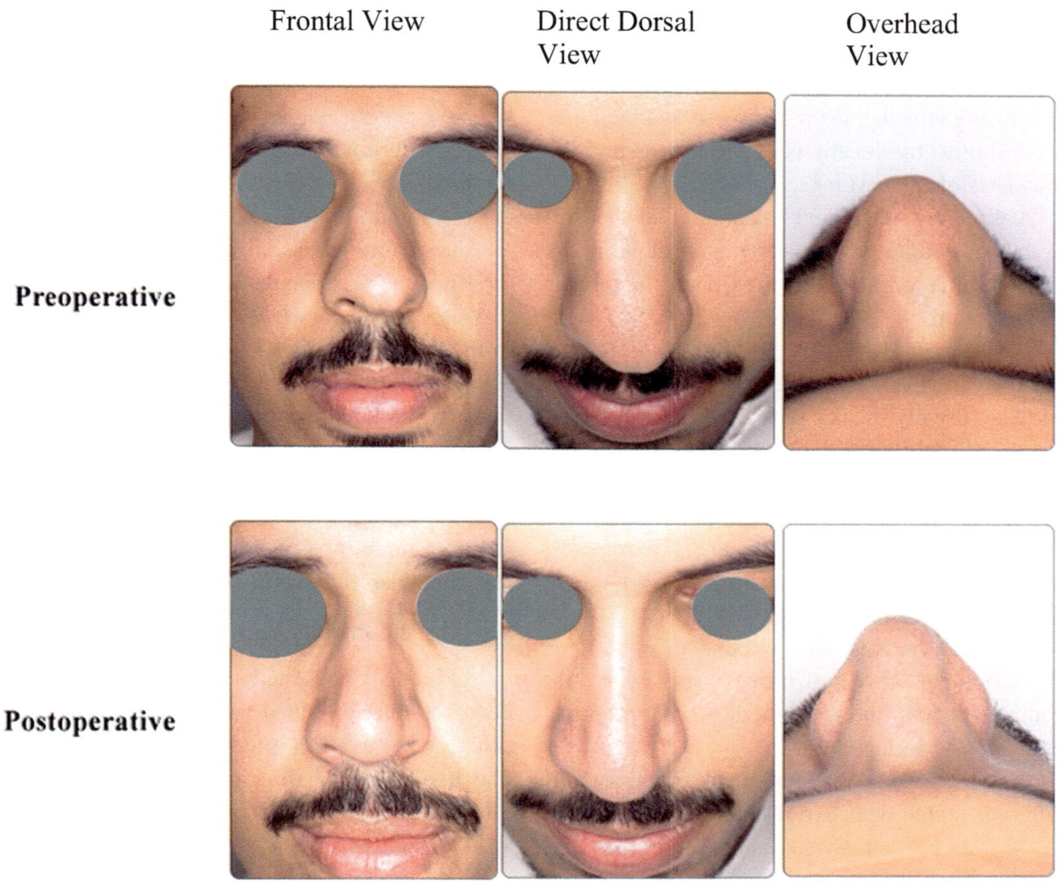

Fig. 21.27 Supratip deviation, due to left caudal septal deviation

The excess caudal vestibular septum is usually at its junction with the maxillary groove. The inferior margin is dissected subperichondrally and then dissected off the maxillary groove. Only the excess cartilage is accurately trimmed using a No 15 bladed knife. Excessive removal will lead to instability and supratip depression.

(b) Reduction of excess caudal length:

The excess length is either at the **anterior angle** or more commonly the **posterior angle** or **both.**

Incision is made at the caudal margin which is dissected subperichondrally. The **anterior nasal spine** may need to be trimmed. The caudal septum is trimmed till the cartilage comes within the maxillary groove.

The anterior valve angle is observed. A small localized deviation of the septum in this area may be **the only part** that needs trimming to improve the valve angle.

ii. **Correction of a Crooked Caudal Septum:**

(a) Curved caudal septum:

The caudal septum may be naturally curved to one side. This curve is dealt with by **scoring** its concave side.

Scoring is made antro-posteriorly parallel to the inferior margin. It has to reach both margins of the septum, anteriorly and posteriorly.

Scoring is made, deep and close to each other according to the locations of the curves and the thickness of the cartilage.

A severely angulated septum is dealt with exactly the same way as a traumatic septum.

(b) Traumatic fracture of the Caudal Vestibular Septum:

In severe trauma to the front of the nose, the septal cartilage usually breaks **at the junction between the distal mobile caudal vestibular part** and **the more fixed proximal part of the quadrilateral cartilage**. The fracture line is usually parallel to the caudal margin and the columella. All or part of the caudal septum is separated partially or totally from the rest of the cartilage.

Trauma disrupts the perichondrium. Perichondrium of the distal broken cartilage is not continuous with the perichondrium of the proximal septal cartilage.

In these cases, they are dealt with as two different septae with two different incisions.

A severely traumatized distal segment may be difficult to dissect or realign with the proximal segment. Should it continue to negatively affect nasal aesthetics or the airway the broken caudal segment may be sacrificed and removed all together. Supratip augmentation is usually needed.

<u>Excess soft tissues:</u>

Excess soft tissues are usually found beside the broken caudal vestibular septum either in the form of a **double cartilage,** or **excess skin** and **fibrous tissues**. They all add to the thickness and the bulk of the septum at the external valve area. Their excision not only improves the nasal airway but also the nasal aesthetics. The columella becomes nicely thin and the naso-labial angle is better adjusted. The excess tissues are usually more on the deviated or dislocated side of the septum, but both sides have to be considered.

iii. A firm, stable and midline caudal vestibular septum:

Having achieved the right height, length and straightness of the caudal vestibular septum, it must be stable, firm and strictly in the midline.

The posterior margin is securely placed in the maxillary groove. The anterior septal angle is centered between the domes of the middle crurae in the supratip region.

Adjustments are also made to the anterior nasal spine and the maxillary crest. A long nasal spine or maxillary bony spur are trimmed. Both are brought to midline, i.e., fractured by the stout blades of a Killian forceps or else by the use of a chisel.

If further stabilization is needed the posterior septal angle is stitched to the anterior nasal spine or the maxillary groove.

If the septum was excessively weakened by the deep scoring or loss of tissues, then extra support may be added by a **strut of cartilage or bone.**

<u>Securing the internal nasal valve</u>

At the end of any caudal vestibular septal surgery, the internal **nasal valve** is inspected especially at the **area of the anterior valve angle**. The **heads of the inferior turbinates** may be trimmed as they may become relatively too large to the available space.

Nasal packing may not be necessary. Two longitudinal **trans-septal stitches** are made superiorly and inferiorly using vycril three zero stitches in a two cm. cutting needle. The **superior stitch** starts high up at, or just above, the osteocartilaginous junction and inferiorly the stitch goes through the septum at the level of the valve angle.

The **inferior stitch** goes as far down to reach as near as possible to the level of the posterior septal angle.

21.4.5.2 The Indirect Effects of the Membranous Septum

The Sliding Tip

In noses where the dorsal height is at a satisfactory level the **two lower lateral cartilages** are at a **lower level**, than the **dorsum,** i.e., **posteriorly displaced** and **depressed,** i.e., sliding backwards (Fig. 21.28).

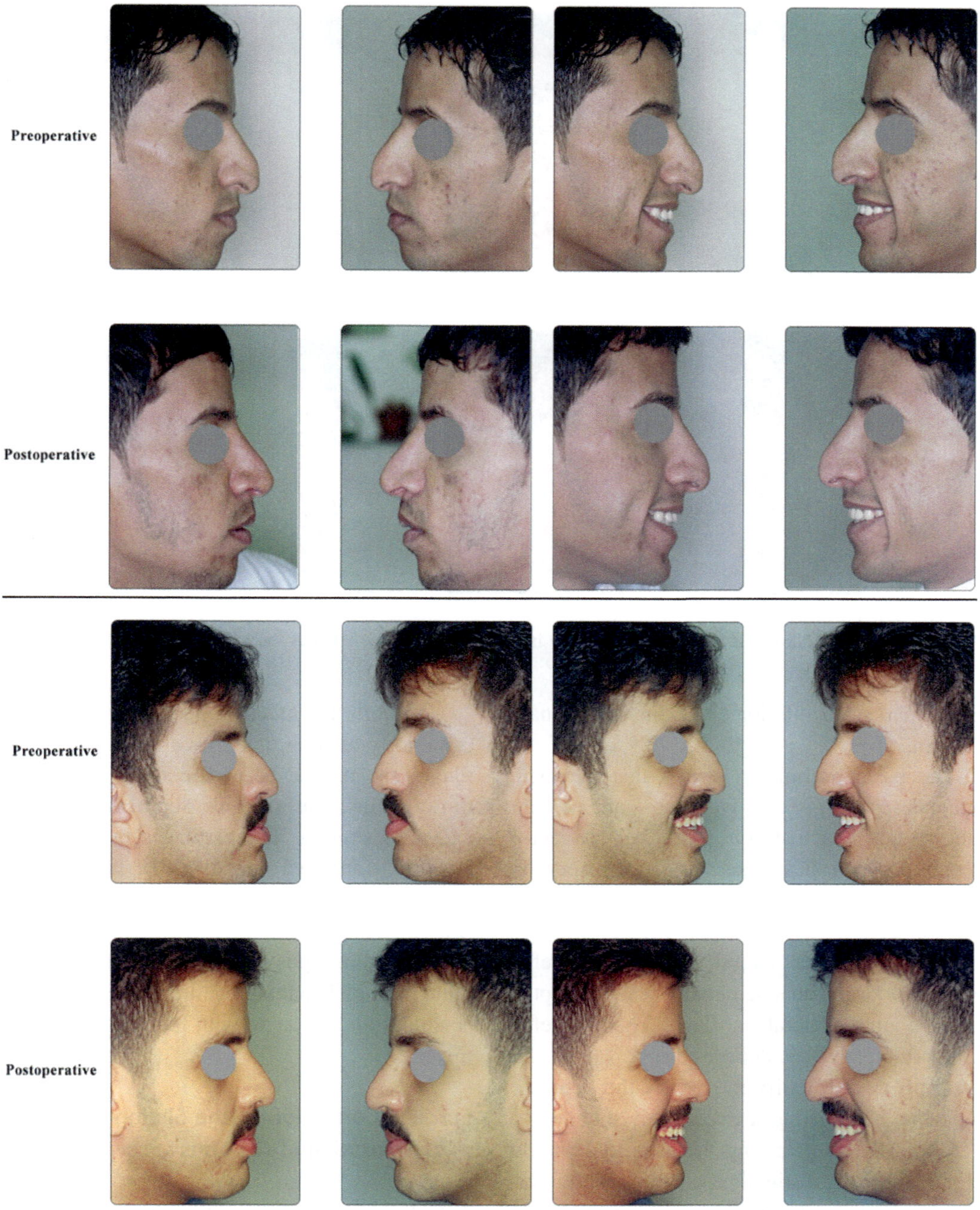

Fig. 21.28 Sliding Nasal Tip , The effect of Smiling. Two cases of sliding tip, i.e. the nasal tip is at a lower level than the anterior septal angle. Sliding exagerated by smiling

Sliding is exaggerated by smiling and by holding the upper lip down by the mouth. There is an overactive Depressor Septi muscle. The main clinical feature of these conditions is the **inferior and posterior movement of the two lower lateral cartilages below the level** of the **anterior septal angle**, i.e., the subcutaneous antro-inferior angle of the cartilagenous septum that can be felt and sometimes seen in the supratip weak triangular area. The anterior septal

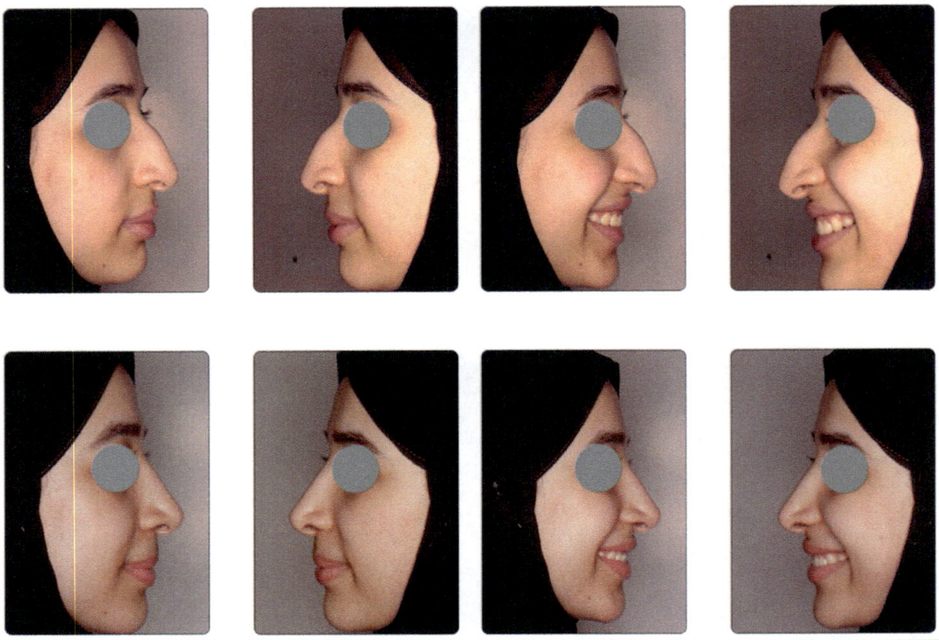

Fig. 21.29 Mobile Nasal Tip. The tip moves only inferiorly at the same level as the anterior septal angle

angle marks the inferior end point of the nasal dorsum.

The basic **pathology** here is that the membranous septum is excessively loose and contains the strongly active or may be overactive depressor septi nasi muscles. The suspensory ligament of the tip is equally loose (if it ever exists).

The two lower lateral cartilages therefore become loosely attached to the caudal septum and the upper lateral cartilage. They therefore slide posteriorly, i.e., depressed (Fig. 21.28). The nasal tip can be easily moved by the depressor septi muscles making it excessively mobile.

Clinically on palpating the nose, the anterior septal angle is distinctly palpable, while both lower lateral cartilages are easily maneuverable around the caudal septum. They can be replaced back to their appropriate position by gently pushing the tip of the nose upwards, i.e., sliding back or disliding the nasal tip.

This is frequently rehearsed by the patients at home. They very swiftly demonstrate it to their doctors as they are very well trained to do it.

A **mobile tip** may not necessarily be sliding posteriorly as long as the two lower lateral cartilages are maintained **at the same level of the dorsum, i.e., the anterior septal angle** before and after smiling. The cartilages in these cases are firmly attached to the rest of the nose particularly to the caudal septum and septal angle (Fig. 21.29).

The sliding tip is to be differentiated from the plunging tip. The main feature in the latter is the acute naso-labial angle with long drooping nasal tip.

Surgical Correction of the Sliding Tip

(a) **Exploration of the anterior septal angle**:

This can be achieved by the meeting of the two **intercartilaginous incisions** on both sides with the **complete transfixing columellar incision,** i.e., exploring the whole length of the inferior septal margin. The incision must be **strictly on the inferior septal margin** after fully stretching the membranous septum. From the two incisions **the skin is undermined over the nasal dorsum**

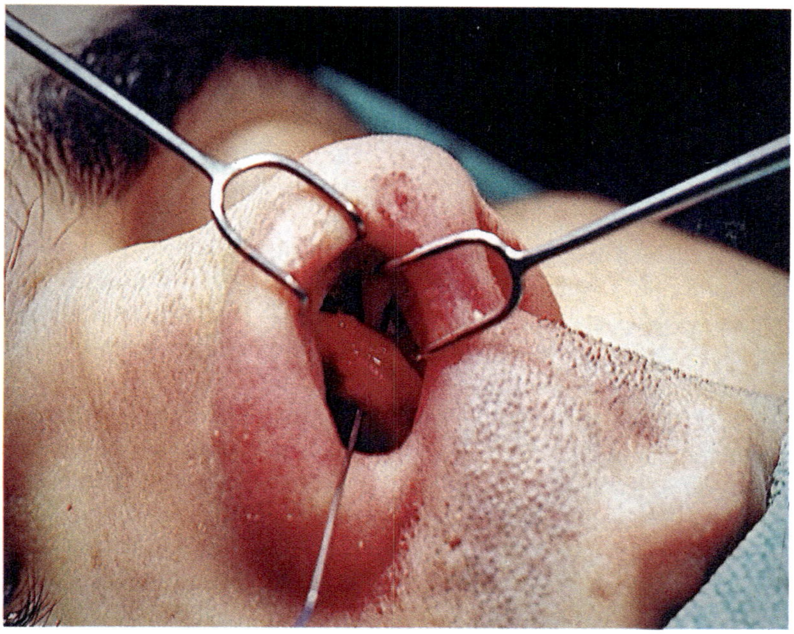

Fig. 21.30 Exploration of the anterior septal angle. Trans Septal stitch, after excision of the membranous septum

and **around the septal angle** anteriorly and inferiorly. This divides the aponeurotic-like tissue that connects the two middle crurae to the anterior septal angle and acts as a suspensory ligament of the tip of the nose. Division of the lateral perichondial attachment of the lower end of upper lateral cartilage may be necessary for the further exploration.

The **anterior septal angle,** together with its caudal margin, becomes now free and clearly prominent into the surgical field. The two lower lateral cartilages with their covering skin are **freely mobile around the septal angle**. In other words, the caudal septum and the two lower lateral cartilages are fully and freely **separated from each other.**

(b) Excision of the membranous septum and elevating the Sliding Tip:

The loose skin of the **membranous septum** is **completely excised** including the Depressor Septi muscles, the membranous part of the inferior vestibular bands and all the loose skin and subcutaneous tissues, so that the **cartilaginous septum** superiorly and the upper margins of the **medial crurae** inferiorly are **clearly seen.**

A judgment strip of caudal septum may need to be excised with its covering skin depending on the degree of nasal projection.

A straight needle on nylon stitch (prolin) is passed transversely through, the anterior septal angle (Fig. 21.30). The free **nasal tip** is now **rotated superiorly** to the appropriate position. The needle is then passed back, transfixing, both medial crurae and the stitch is tied down. **The septal and the medial crural cartilages are now in direct contact with each other**. A second supporting stitch is similarly taken more posteriorly.

(c) Detaching the Depressor Septi muscles:

The previously excised Depressor Septi muscles must now be **detached from their maxillary origin** via the nose or the buccal sulcus. This secures the post-operative immobility of the nasal tip and avoids animation. There are three methods of cutting the Depressor Septi muscles:

i. **Transbuccal Approach**

- Buccal Stab wounds

This is the easiest and simplest method of detaching the Depressor Septi muscles. The upper lip is elevated using a sharp pronged alar retractor. The sharp pointed harpoon end of Cottle's elevator is introduced into the buccal sulcus. The mucosa is stabbed by the tip of the harpoon on both sides of the frenulum. The elevator sharp harpoon head is then introduced further deeply and the Depressor Septi muscles are meticulously scraped off their maxillary attachments. Grating sound of the bone is heard. Avoid going to the inferior bony margin of the nasal aperture (Fig. 21.31).

No need to cut the frenulum. Only if there is tight upper lip, the frenulum is divided transversely and stitched longitudinally.

- Buccal incisional wound

The upper lip is elevated by a sharp pronged alar retractor. The frenulum is cut just above the central incisors by a **transverse incision**. The incision is then deepened to the nasal spine and extended laterally on both sides. The Depressor Septi muscles are scraped off their bony maxillary attachments on both sides of the nasal spine using a periosteal elevator. The wound is then closed **longitudinally** by Vicryl stitches (Fig. 21.32).

While scraping the periostium, avoid scraping the midline, especially the anterior nasal spine with its attachment to the posterior septal angle. This area, if disturbed might affect the stability of the supratip area and lead to a **supratip depression.**

ii. Transnasal Approach

From the posterior end of the columellar wound, a periosteal elevator is introduced. It is then directed towards the anterior surface of the maxillary fossa, inferior and lateral to the anterior nasal spine. The muscle fibers of the Depressor Septae are scraped off their bony insertion, until the grating sounds of metal on bone are heard (Fig. 21.33).

Part III: Surgery of the Bony Pyramid

The bony pyramid is the solid foundation for the distal soft tissue structures of the nose. It is the most important source of stability to its three-dimensional structure.

The base of the nasal bony pyramid is provided by the strongest facial bones, i.e., the **two maxillae** that contribute to their frontal processes, and **the frontal bones**, that contribute to their nasal parts. Both are quite compact and firm bones. On top of them articulate the much weaker **nasal bones**.

From this solid foundation the rest of the nasal structures take their basic attachment to build its cartilaginous, membranous and fibrofatty three-dimensional structures. The **undersurface** of the **nasal bones** provides firm attachments for the **upper lateral cartilage** which in turn articulates with the **undersurface of the** lateral crurae of lower lateral cartilage. The alae nasi are directly attached to the upper lip and lateral nasal wall.

21.5 Nasal Stability and Rhinoplasty

In Rhinoplasty, one major concern of the surgeon is **the stability of the nasal structure** during the whole course of the procedure.

As a three-dimensional structure, the nose stands out in air as firm stable organ that is maintained by its accurately integrated parts. Breaking the structural integrity will lead to the fall and **collapse** of part or the whole of the upper two-thirds of the nose.

In this concept, the nose is like a strong nice looking building that keeps its firm shape through the well integrated and accurately designed columns and walls. The collapse of one or more of these walls and columns may lead to the collapse of part or the whole building.

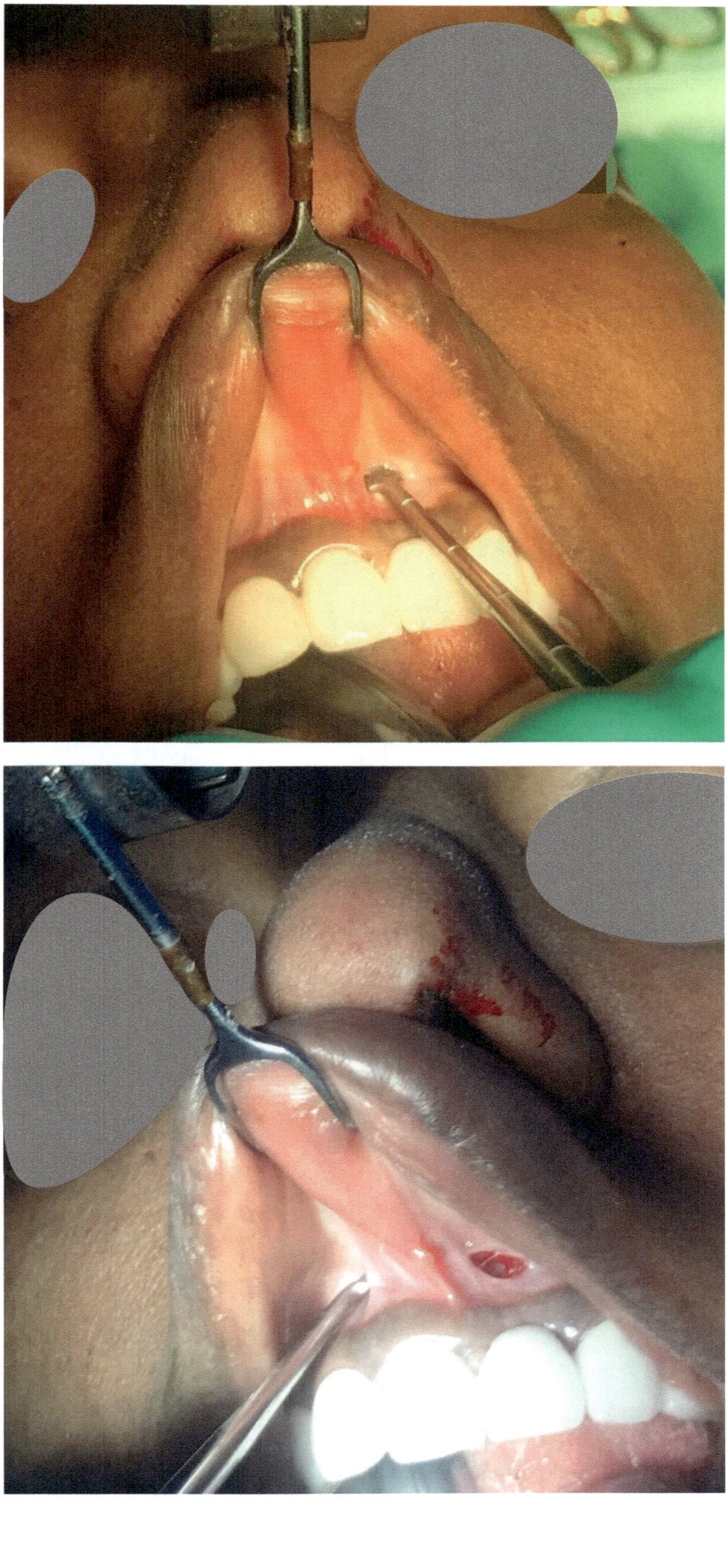

Fig. 21.31 Transbuccal stab. Buccal stab by the harpoon end of Cottle's elevator, to scrape the Depressor Septi Muscles

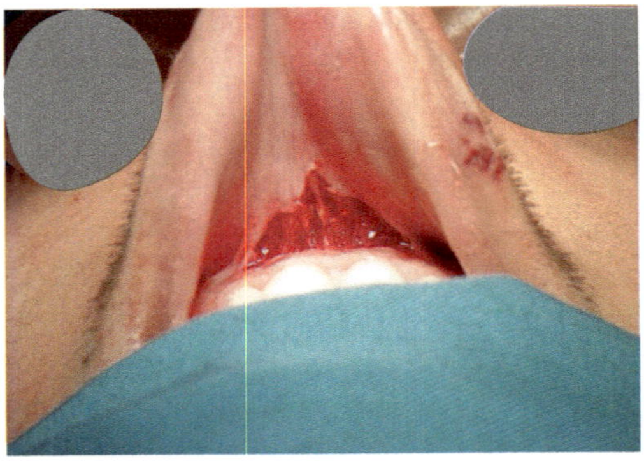

Incision at the vestibular margin cutting the frenulum and extending from the second right to the second left upper incisors.

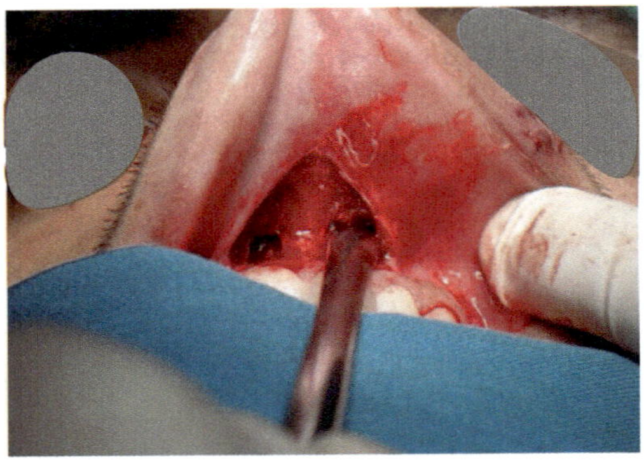

Separating the right and left Depressor Septi muscles by scraping them off the anterior maxillary wall using a periosteal elevator.

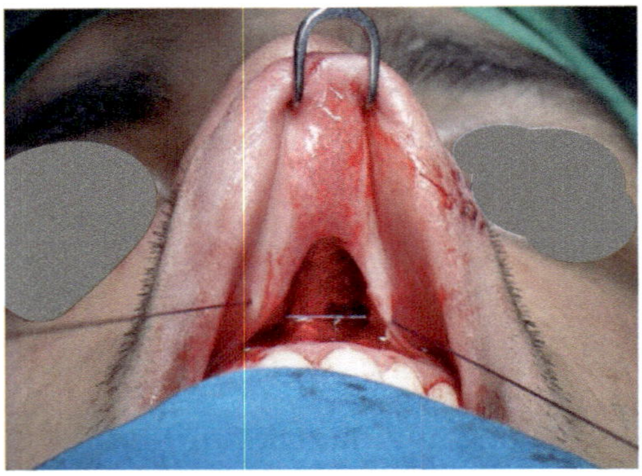

The wound is closed longitudinally using 2-0 Vicryl stitch on a large rounded needle. (Fig. 15)

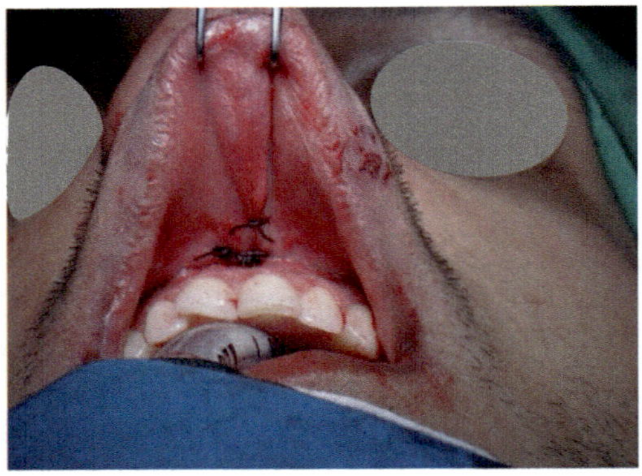

Stitching is completed.

Fig. 21.32 Tranbuccal Devision of the Depressor Septi muscles

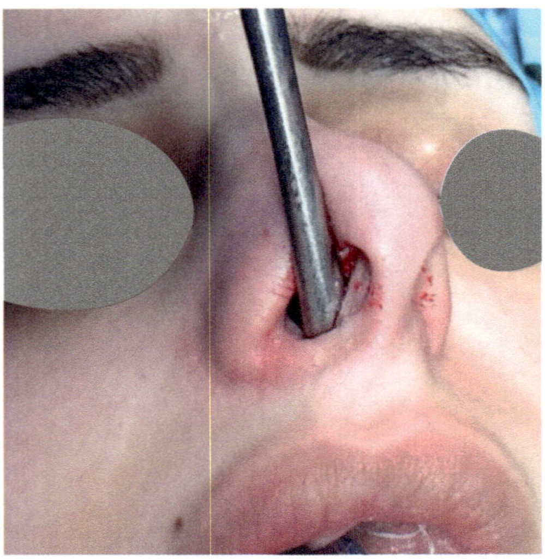

Scrapping of the depressor Septi Muscles off the interior maxillary wall using the Periosteal elevator.

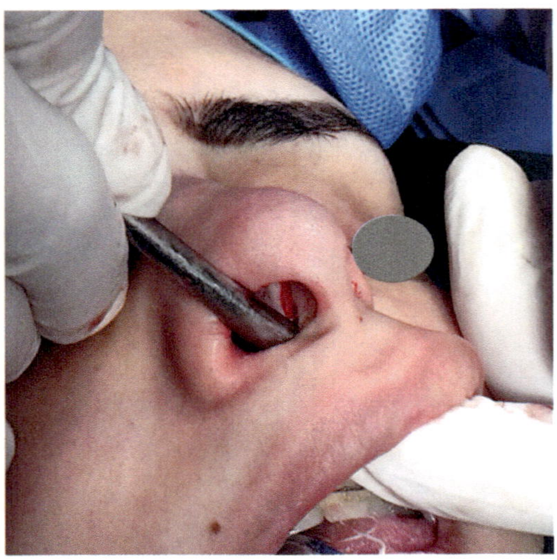

Palpating the anterior maxillary wall as the elevator scrapes the depressor Septi Muscle

Fig. 21.33 Transnasal Division of the Depressor Septi Muscles

By far the most important stabilizing structures in the nose are the walls of the **bony pyramid** and the **nasal septum, bony and cartilaginous**. The lateral cartilages and the alae nasi are more of an aesthetic and physiologic structure.

21.6 Aesthetic Assessment of the Bony Pyramid

Correct assessment of the aesthetics of the bony pyramid is fundamental for the final outcome of Rhinoplasty.

A **wide bony base** is consequently followed by **wide, soft tissue sidewalls**, including the alar base. A **high bony hump** is usually, but not always, followed by a high cartilaginous dorsum. A nasal hump has therefore an osteocartilagenous component.

The following questions are necessary in order to help the decision of surgically reducing the width, and/or altering the height of the bony pyramid.

- Is the bony pyramid of a **good size**?
- Is it **wider** than aesthetically acceptable compared to the rest of the nose?
- Is the cartilaginous dorsum of acceptable height?
- Is the **width of the bony base** suitable for the final aesthetics of the lower nasal soft tissues so that the sidewalls and the alar base are of reasonable width?
- Is the bony pyramid **deviated, crooked or irregular?**

The Aesthetics of the Nasal Sidewalls:

The bony sidewalls begin from the root of the nose, at its narrowest, curving gradually downwards and laterally till their inferior margins which are attached to the tough membranous floors of the muscular triangles and consequently to the alae nasi. The **lateral position of the bony walls therefore dictates the lateralization of soft tissue lateral walls** including the alar base.

Diagnostic assessment of the bony sidewalls is made both **clinically** and **photographically**. Looking at the nose in the **frontal** and **direct dorsal views**, the bony sidewalls look wider than the middle of the nose, just above the level of the upper lateral cartilage.

The nasal sidewalls together with the eyebrows make a **C-shaped and an inverted C-shaped course**. Any bulge of the bony sidewall inside the C-shape curve is looked upon as an indication of a wide base or irregularity in the bony sidewall that may need correction (see Photography Section).

The aesthetics of the **eyes** are directly related to aesthetics of the bony sidewalls. The eyes are the two most attractive organs of the face. They are like a beautiful picture that has a four-sided frame, viz., the eyebrows superiorly, cheeks laterally and inferiorly and finally the nasal bony sidewalls medially. If the latter are irregular or bulging, the beauty of the central picture is negatively affected.

There is a definite improvement in the aesthetics of the eyes after reduction of bulging or irregular bony sidewalls. They look wider and nicer. Irregularities of the bony sidewalls no longer distract the attention.

21.7 Indications for Osteotomies

Osteotomies in Rhinoplasty are useful and important procedure. In this procedure, each side of the bony pyramid is surgically divided and separated so that they can be manipulated to aesthetically better location. In most cases, they are pushed and moved medially to reduce the width of the bony base.

The procedure of osteotomy has quite a fundamental necessity in many situations in aesthetic rhinoplasty. These situations are:

21.7.1 Wide Bony Base

In these cases, the nose is broad and may be large. Osteotomies alone simply reduce the width and the size of the nose. Medialization of the bony side walls will lead to elevation of the dorsum of the upper two-thirds of the nose.

21.7.2 Bony Hump

Excision of a bony hump is usually associated with an **open roof deformity**. As the nose becomes smaller, the base of the pyramid is now relatively wide. Osteotomies are necessary to close the deformity and reduce the base.

With preservation push down and pull down techniques there is no open roof, nevertheless the size and height of the bony pyramid are reduced.

21.7.3 Facial Asymmetry and Oblique Pyramid

Cases of facial assymetry usually have a wide bony base and an osteocartilagenous hump. The bony pyramid is deviated to the larger side. Osteotomies is mandatory to centralize the bony pyramid.

21.7.4 Traumatic Fracture of the Nose

The bony pyramid is usually wide, irregular, crooked or deviated. Osteotomies are needed as part of correcting the deformities.

21.7.5 Wide Alar Base

The bony pyramid, with its sidewalls, makes a **stout basis of a series of attachments** of the soft tissue structures distally on both sides of the nose. These series begin with the attachment of the superior border of the **upper lateral cartilage** to the undersurfaces of the **two nasal bones**. The inferior border of the upper lateral cartilage in turn is attached to the lateral crurae.

At the base of the bony pyramid, i.e., further posteriorly, there are the attachments of the **tough fibrous membrane** between **frontal process of the maxillae** and the **lateral crurae** of the lower lateral cartilages.

The position of these soft structures is determined by the bony sidewalls. The **wide-based sidewalls** of the bony pyramid take with them the rest of **the soft structures farther away laterally**.

A **wide alar base** therefore is almost always associated with **wide bony base.**

Reduction of a wide alar base will never be completed before the reduction of the bony basal attachment. After osteotomies and medicalization of the nasal sidewalls, the shape of the nasal openings will be transformed from rounded with transverse axes to a vertically oblong shaped openings with longitudinal axes. The bony and cartilaginous dorsum will be better projecting forwards.

21.8 Osteotomy Techniques

The goal of osteotomies is to separate the two sides of the bony pyramid in order to be able to manipulate each side into its new medialized position. Each side has to be cut **laterally, medially** and **superiorly**.

Although the osteotomy procedure is one of the first basic techniques taught in Rhinoplasty, yet many of the causes of disappointing results are due to faulty technique or because it was totally omitted. Studying the details of this technique, its diversities and pitfalls is necessary.

Osteotomies are either **external** or **internal**. Each surgeon better continue with the technique that he can do best. Nevertheless, he should be acquainted with the other technique. One technique of osteotomy may either fail or become difficult to command or complete despite the experience. Another technique becomes handy in these situations.

21.8.1 The Lateral Osteotomies

21.8.1.1 Internal Lateral Osteotomies

The advantage of the internal lateral osteotomy is that it has no external scar. The question of hematoma in general depends on the experience, speed and patient's response. It is important to press on the side of the wound for 2–3 min after osteotomy is completed. Ice is used externally during this period. This avoids a lot swelling.

An incision is made just anterior to the head of the inferior turbinates, at, or just inside the muco-cutaneous junction. The incision is deepened till the inferior margin of the frontal process of the maxilla is reached. A thin **freer elevator** is used to raise the periosteum. **Two or three millimeter chisel** is introduced at the incision site. It may be better to use a **guarded chisel,** e.g., Converse or Masing curved chisel. The lateral protrusion of the guard can be felt subcutaneously during the whole process of osteotomy.

As the chisel is held tightly with one hand, the hammer is used by the other hand to tap on the head of the chisel.

Alternatively, the chisel is held by one hand and the index finger of the other hand is used to palpate the guarded chisel subcutaneously, while the assistant is snapping the head of the chisel repeatedly. The chisel is directed upward and medially along the sidewall of the bony pyramid till it reaches the level of the lacrimal tubercle, just inside the medial canthus of the eye.

Lateral osteotomy must be law, i.e., flush to the face, to avoid step deformity.

21.8.1.2 External Lateral Osteotomies

Using a **two mm. chisel, a mark** is made on the external skin at the junction between the body of the maxillary bone and its frontal process, i.e., tie at the origin of the frontal process (Fig. 21.34).

With a no.15 blade **a stab** is made at the mark. The chisel is again placed inside the stab wound, and the **periostium is cut** at his point by a single snap on the head of the chisel using a hammer.

The author's preference is 4–5 oz weight hammer with one plastic and one metal side. The plastic side is used for the lateral and superior osteotomies, while the metal side is used for the medial osteotomies.

The periostium is then continued to be marked and cut along the line of osteotomy at the base of the bony pyramid, i.e., from this point upwards till the lacrimal tubercle, just inside the medial canthus of the eye (an external indicator to the lacrimal sac which is inside the orbit) and then downwards to the free margins of the frontal process of the maxilla.

The osteotomy line must be low, i.e., flush with the facial surface of the maxillary bone to avoid stepping of the sidewall.

The bone is then pierced at three or four places along these lines by stronger snaps on the chisel head. The **first** piercing osteotomy point is made at maximum convexity of the frontal process, halfway between the lacrimal tubercle and the inferior free margin. This is the **thickest** part of the frontal process of the maxilla. From this point superiorly and inferiorly the frontal process is quite thin and easily pierced by the chisel or osteotome.

The chisel must be sharp and held firmly against the bone, to avoid slipping. The chisel is sharpened each time by a blade sharpener and better replaced if the edge becomes irregular or dull.

The osteotomy line starts from the free margin of the frontal process inferiorly, till the lacrimal tubercle (see anatomy of bony pyramid).

21.8.2 Superior Osteotomies

Using the index finger, two important landmarks are palpated at the upper end of the lateral bony wall of the nose which are

i. The lacrimal tubercle, just next to the inner canthus of the eye.
ii. The nasofrontal suture at the junction between the two bones, i.e., the nasal bone and the nasal process of the frontal bone. It is situated at a slightly higher level than the lacrimal tubercle.

The superior osteotomy is made at, the level of the inner canthus of the eye (Fig. 21.35).

A **mark** and **a stab** are made in the external skin at this level using a two mm chisel and a no. 15 blade. The periostium is cut and marked by the chisel.

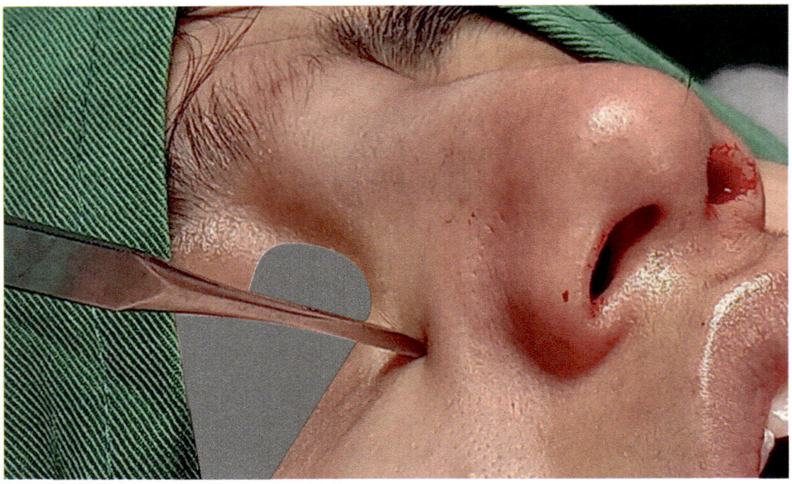

Fig. 21.34 Right external lateral osteotom

Osteotomy is then pursued at two or more points. The chisel is held **firmly** and **obliquely from above downwards** against the osteotomy line, so that the hammering force is directed safely **downwards and medially**. This avoids going through the harder nasal process of the frontal bone as well as the inadvertent slipping into the higher part of the nasal cavity.

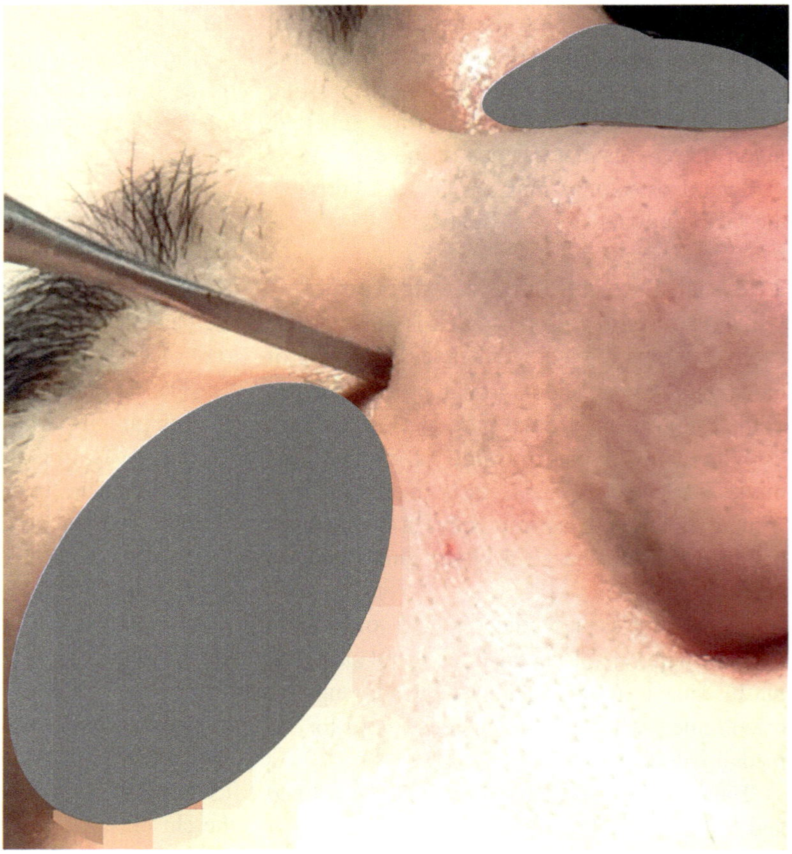

Fig. 21.35 Superior external osteotomy

P.S. A controlled superior osteotomy dictates the line of superior bony separation. This is better than the blind technique of green stick fracture which may take place at two different, and perhaps unwanted, low levels on both sides of the nose.

21.8.3 Medial Osteotomies

To complete the full separation of both sides of the bony pyramids, medial osteotomies have to be secured.

The nasal bones are cut on both sides from their medial attachment to each and separated from the posterior attachment to the perpendicular plate of the ethmoid bone. Most of this separation may already be achieved if a large bony hump is removed.

Using the metal side of the hammer, the sound of hammering suddenly changes to a dull sound as the solid frontal bone is reached.

21.8.3.1 The Technique of Medial Osteotomies

A sharp thin 14–16 mm wide osteom, e.g., Robin's, is used, depending on the size and the height of the nose. The use of a thick heavy osteotome may have more damaging effect.

The osteotome is introduced from the nasal opening abutting the nasal septum. It is pushed gently upwards and forward.

Just before reaching the lower margin of the nasal bone, the anterior angle of the osteotome is forced further forwards to pierce and cut through the upper lateral cartilage. The anterior angle of the osteotome will be both seen and felt under the dorsal skin.

The most important rule at this stage of medial osteotomy is that the **anterior angle of the osteotome must be at a higher level than the bony dorsum**. The edge of the osteotome must be **felt and seen subcutaneously at all times** while it is proceeding antrosuperiorly. This avoids the inadvertent superior slipping of the osteotome intracranially. The loose undermined skin during the skeletonizing exposure makes this job quite easy.

Medial osteotomy proceeds superiorly till the level of the medial cantus of the eye at the rhinion.

21.9 Infracture

After completion of the osteotomies, now the two sides of the bony pyramid are free to be mobilized.

The bridge of the nose is covered by one or two 4x4 inches gauze. With the flat of the two thumbs, the two sides of the bony pyramid are pushed and displaced medially.

If successful the pyramid will immediately look thinner. Now, with the tip of each thumb, we can feel the cut edges of the bony base as well as the gaps created between them and the newly infractured sidewalls.

This is the sign of successful osteotomies and infracture of the bony pyramidal walls.

The height of the cut edges is palpated in order to make sure that it is almost flush to the face and not too high. The whole length of the bony base must be included in the cut line.

The extent of infracture, or medicalization, of each side may be controlled and varies, should one side is more lateralized than the other, as in cases of bilateral maxillary asymmetry.

21.10 Pitfall of Osteotomies and Infracture

The osteotomy procedure may apparently fail to achieve its goals. For one or more of the following reasons:

21.10.1 Failure of Infracture

Failure of infracture or medialization of one or the two bony walls may take place. It is usually caused by **incomplete lateral osteotomies** especially in the external technique in a hard thick sidewall bones. **Osteotomy is revised** on the affected side. The use of a slightly bigger chisel, 3mm, might be necessary.

If infracture continues to be difficult, despite securing good osteotomies, then **outfracturing** of this side will completely dislodge it and makes it more free to medialize.

21.10.1.1 Technique of Outfracture of Bony Sidewall

The thin 14–16 mm osteotome is introduced abutting the septum up to the hard nasofrontal angle and then swayed laterally with the lateral bony wall, till it is completely out fractured.

Finally if the surgeon fails in completing the fracture by the external technique he has to revert to the **internal osteotomy technique** or vice versa, i.e., **from internal** to **external** technique.

21.10.2 Oblique Bony Pyramid

The bony pyramid becomes oblique if its two sides are unequal. This may be caused by one or both of the following factors:

i. One bony side is originally longer than the other, e.g., in cases of bilateral maxillary asymmetry and cases of accidental or surgical traumas.
ii. Osteotomy is inadvertently height on one side than the other. A high step is felt on the affected side. Revision low osteotomy is done on the affected side will balance the pyramid. The chisel is introduced from the same wound and the stump of the nose is chiseled down.

21.10.3 Deviated Bony Septum

Deviation bony pyramid that only appears after osteotomies and infracture is mostly caused by a **high deviation of the bony septum**. Deviation may be an original anatomical, developmental or post-traumatic. This problem is dealt with by one of the following procedures:

i. Out fracture of one or both sides of the pyramid.
ii. **Kassanjian** maneuver, i.e., cross fracture of both sides of the bony pyramid (fig).

21.10.4 Defective Area

After osteotomy one side may look smaller and defective than the other. This defect may hardly be noticed preoperatively and even before osteotomies and infracture.

Retrospectively it appears as a subtle difference between the two sides in the **pre-operative photographs**.

The defect most frequently is present **over one side of the upper lateral cartilage**. Rarely over one side of the **bony pyramid**. An accurately measured **cartilaginous septal graft** is used to fill the defect over the upper lateral cartilage and **bony graft** over the bony pyramid.

21.10.5 Step Deformity

A step may appear on one on both sides of the bony walls. The commonest cause is **high lateral osteotomy**. A low osteotomy, i.e., flushes to the face gives better aesthetic result and corrects the step deformity.

21.11 The Nasal Dorsal Hump

A prominent dorsal hump is an aesthetic challenge that always comes in the way of any surgeon who decided to perform rhinoplasty. It seems like an excellent chance for the beginners. The simple disappearance of the hump perse is a great psychological boost to both the patient and the surgeon alike.

The surgeon has a sense of achievement and satisfaction especially at the beginning of his career in his early experience in rhinoplasty.

As he becomes more experienced, he realizes that **there are more in each nose that can be achieved** to add to its aesthetics than just removing the hump. Not only that his technique and ability to judge the exact amount to be removed but also his sense of balancing that with the aesthetics of other areas of the nose gradually improves.

There are many factors that have to be considered in the surgical procedure of hump removal:

21.11.1 The Normal Anatomy

The nasal bones are anatomically and naturally convex forwards in their lower half. This convexity may need to be flattened and treated as if it is a hump in certain situations, e.g., as part of the overall reduction of the size of the nose.

21.11.2 Anatomy of the Dorsal Hump

The dorsal hump is made of **bony** and **cartilaginous** components. They vary in size and proportion according to the proportionate anatomical variations and to the size of the hump. The bony dorsum may be quite small anatomically while the cartilaginous hump is larger and vice versa.

21.11.3 The Large Nose

In a large nose, removal of a nasal hump is **only part** of the overall reduction in the size of the nose. Reduction may include wide alar base, skin thickness, the nasal tip and the midvault. The nose may remain high and long even after removal of the hump. Further reduction of the dorsal height from the root of the nose to the anterior septal angle is necessary to successfully reduce the size of the nose. It is easy to blame the hump alone for the high and long nose.

21.11.4 Associated Deformities

Overlooking associated unaesthetic deformities while removing the hump may end up with unpleasant or even disappointing result. These deformities may be one or more of the following:

21.11.4.1 Deviated and/or Oblique Bony Pyramid

Deviated and/or oblique bony pyramid, as in cases of maxillary asymmetry or post-traumatic.

21.11.4.2 Flat Naso-frontal Angle

Nothing worse than having the hump removal and end up with a solid straight nose. The hump was creating a false nasofrontal angle above it.

The nasofrontal angle must be re-established after the removal of the hump for better results. A special curved nasofrontal rasp is used.

21.11.4.3 Areas of Defects

After removal of the hump and osteotomies, a depressed area may become apparent that was not clear before the surgery.

These are usually on one side of the upper lateral cartilage, or the bony pyramid.

21.11.4.4 The Trumpet Deformity

The lower third of the nose may appear disproportionately large if only the large-sized bony pyramid is reduced, omitting the large wide alae nasi and/or large frontolateral walls. The outcome is a nose that has a long narrow root and large wide distal end and looks like a trumpet.

21.11.4.5 Post-traumatic Bony Pyramid

In some patients there is a clear history of trauma from an accident, assault or sports followed by bleeding and deformity of the nose. In many others, trauma may be quite presumptuous, especially in the cases of bony pyramidal deviation. There is no clear history of trauma. These cases might be a forgotten childhood trauma or bilateral maxillary asymmetry in which trauma is assumed to be the cause.

Class 1 Nasal Fracture "Chevallet"

In these cases, fracture may only involve the **cartilaginous septum between its two fixed points**, i.e., the **nasal bones** and the **maxillary spine**. The **caudal vestibular segment** is usually involved.

The thin tip of the nasal bone may be broken leading to a ski-slope deformity (fig).

This type of fracture may not be noticed at the time of injury due to support of the underlying upper lateral cartilage. It is only apparent if the broken end is impacted under the proximal part of the bone.

Class 2 Nasal Fracture

The **frontal process of the maxilla** is broken and depressed on one side with clear C-shaped deformity. The opposite side is prominently pushed in the opposite direction.

This fracture is usually associated with another C-shaped fracture of the nasal septum "Jarjavay fracture". This involves the quadrilateral cartilage and the perpendicular plate of ethmoid bone. It is quite impacted by the overlapping segments of fracture. This segment must be excised to release the tension off the nasal bone at **the time of injury**. The **late treatment** of these cases especially in the course of Rhinopalsty a more **conservative approach is pursued**. Areas of excision are to be weighed against the stability of the bony pyramid in the process of rhinoplasty.

Traumatic Saddle Deformity

Traumatic saddle deformity may involve the bony, cartilaginous or both parts of the nasal dorsum. The degree of saddling is variable according to the severity and cause of trauma. Surgical and non-surgical traumas, septal hematoma and chronic infections are the commonest causes (fig).

Comminuted Bony Trauma

In these cases, the bony pyramid is made up by irregular pieces of broken bones, i.e., comminuted fracture. Externally sharp edges of broken bones are seen and felt subcutaneously, giving the bony pyramid quite an irregular appearance. This may be due to multi-injuries, failed reduction or trauma by hard objects.

Childhood and Forgotten Trauma

Injuries that take place in life may delay the growth of the affected part of the bony pyramid. Growth may become squinted or crooked (Persig and Lehmann, 1975).

21.11.5 Techniques of Hump Removal

There are different techniques for removing the hump. The surgeon should stick to the technique that he can do best, but he should be familiar with other techniques as well.

21.11.5.1 Preservation Pushdown and Let Down Technique

Preservation reduction of the osteocartilagenous hump is made by preserving the keystone area. Sequential septal stripes are resected. Lateral trimming of the nasal process of the maxilla may be needed in large humps. Mobilization is then made of the bony pyramid which is pushed down or let down according to its size and height. Details of this technique are seeked (Preservation Rhinoplasty ISBN 978-605-68971-1-5, 2020 Septum publisher)

21.11.5.2 The Osteotomy Technique

Using a sharp osteotomy the exact size of the osteocartilagenous hump is cut from below upwards. The osteotome is introduced into the intercartilagenous incision, placed at the lower end of the cartilaginous hump. A cut is made by the sharp end of the osteotome, or by using a knife. The osteotome is then driven through the hump using the hammer. Avoid the tendency for the head of the osteotomes to move deeper leading to over reduction. The osteocartilagenous hump comes out all as one piece.

P.S. The osteotome must be thin and sharp.

- Fractured nose: The use of osteotome in these conditions carries the risk of shattering the broken pieces of bones and collapse of the bony pyramid.

21.11.5.3 The Saw Technique

It is an old technique that Tony Bull tried to modernize by using a thin saw that has one raw of sharp teeth. Unfortunately, the manufacturing companies have modified the saw to a much thicker double row of teeth that are probably stronger and more effective, yet quite harsh and unsuitable for this delicate task (personal contact).

The saw has a bayonet double angle shape and a good gripping handle. It is introduced via the intercartilagenous incision. Contrary to the osteotome sawing from the bony down to the cartilaginous segments of the hump. It all comes out as one piece with a part of the septum attached to the inner surface.

21.11.5.4 The Rasping Technique

In this method, the bony pyramid is rasped down using a crisscross card-bite rasp to avoid avulsing trauma to the upper lateral cartilage. Rasping better be in an oblique fashion. The bony hump is rasped completely down until it becomes almost at the same level of the nasion.

The natural convex curve of the lower half of the nasal bones is also flattened. The dust of the bone that results from rasping is flushed with saline and sucked away.

The rasp is reversed so that the teeth are facing the dermis of the skin. It is then used to sweep away out the bone dust that might stick to the surface of the skin (Tony Bull personal contact)

The cartilaginous hump is cut away in a reverse manner from above downwards (JackSheen). A No.2 blade is used after breaking the tip away to avoid piercing the external skin. No.2 blade has the advantage of having a straight long edge that cuts the hump evenly and equal on both sides.

The knife is introduced from the intercartilaginous wound to superior end of the cartilaginous hump. With a sawing movement the hump is shaved down at the same level of the rasped bony dorsum.

21.12 Surgery of the Upper Lateral Cartilage

The upper lateral cartilage is the site of surgical interest in Rhinoplasty in certain situations:

21.12.1 Cartilagenous Hump Excision

The upper lateral cartilage usually has the major share in the formation of the nasal hump. It has to be removed for the completion of the procedure of hump excision.

21.12.2 Unequal Sides of Upper Lateral Crurae

Developmental or post-traumatic defect is on one side of the upper lateral cartilage. Diagnosis is made clinically or photographically before surgery. Sometimes the condition is only seen intraoperatively after osteotomies.

Cartilagenous graft is excellent in balancing the two sides of the nose. The thickness of the graft needs certain judgment. It is usually thicker than a single layer of lateral crural cephalic trimming cartilage. Either two layers of these or thicker layer or crushed septal cartilage graft.

21.12.3 Broad Middle Third

Having finished surgeries to the bony pyramid and nasal tip, the nose may be found to be broad in its middle third at the area of the upper lateral cartilage.

Using No. 15 blade or straight pair of scissors used to cut its medial attachment to the cartilaginous septum longitudinally helps to break the wide curve of the upper cartilage and narrow the area.

The medial cut of the upper lateral cartilage, better be short of cutting the anterior angle of the nasal valve, i.e., its most inferior end, knife therefore is a better tool for its purpose.

21.12.4 The Subdermal Fat

The lower end of the upper lateral cartilage near the weak triangle is covered by a layer of loose fibrofatty tissues which continuous naturally and anatomically with the soft pad of fibrofatty layer that fills the weak triangle.

This layer may need to be removed in certain cases as part of overall reduction of the nasal size.

Care must be taken to avoid supratip depression.

Part IV: Surgery of the Inferior Wall

The inferior wall of the nose is made is the **vestibular floor** and the **flat triangle** also known as the soft triangle. Surgery of the inferior nasal wall therefore includes

A. **Alar Base Surgery**
B. **Surgery of the Flat Triangle**.

21.13 Alar Base Surgery

The **alar base** is defined as the area of contact between the soft lower third of the nose, i.e., the alae nasi and the upper lip (see anatomy).

The meeting between the **alae nasi** and the **upper lip** is of particular surgical interest. The firm structural bodies of the **alae nasi** are attached to the **Orbicularis Oris muscle** and its overlying adherent skin (see anatomy section).

Only the **upper two-thirds** of the **posterior alar border** is attached to the **upper lip**. The **lower third** is separated from the lip by a gap that is filled by the **rim-sill** soft fold of skin (the superior segment).

Alar base surgery, therefore, focuses on the **size,** the **bulk** and the **aesthetics** of the junction between the ala nasi and the lip in which the rim-sill fold plays an important role. It is noteworthy that the **rim-sill fold** has two components, the superior wedge behind the alar body, i.e., the **posterior segment** and the inferior round fold at the vestibular floor, i.e., the **inferior segment** (see anatomy section)

<u>Types of Alar Base Surgeries:</u>

I. Alar Base Enlargement Surgery
II. Alar Base Aesthetic Enhancement Surgery
III. Alar Base Reduction Surgery

21.13.1 Alar Base Enlargement Surgery

Widening of the nasal or alar base is not usually an aesthetic demand, but it might be necessary in two situations:

21.13.1.1 Lateral Angulation and Alar Flattening

Overzealous resection of the **adherent vestibular** skin cover of the ala nasi leads to **collapse of the lateral alar wall** and **lateral angulation** of the nasal opening, i.e., **posterior vestibular stenosis**.

(a) <u>Lateral Angulation</u>

Overzealous excision of the inferior segment of the **rim-sill fold** as well as the **adherent vestibular skin** over the lower third of the ala nasi. This will lead to lateral angulation of the external nasal opening with flattening of the alar groove (Fig. 21.36).

(b) <u>Collapse of Lateral Alar Wall</u>

Overzelous excision of the adherent vestibular skin of the upper two-thirds of the ala nasi will lead to its collapse. The alar body loses its nice rounded contour and both alar grooves become shallow and flattened.

This condition is treated by adding **free skin graft** to replace the lost skin in the lateral alar wall and vestibular floor. The lateral wall will regain both its **freedom,** i.e., the natural physiological movement as well as **its natural external rounded** body and a natural curve with the nasal sill (Fig. 21.37).

The skin graft is either taken from the external alar skin or a larger size may be taken from the post-auricular skin. It is better to have a generous size of skin as the graft usually **shrinks** when harvested and **contracts** after healing, i.e., almost double the size of the defective area is better harvested.

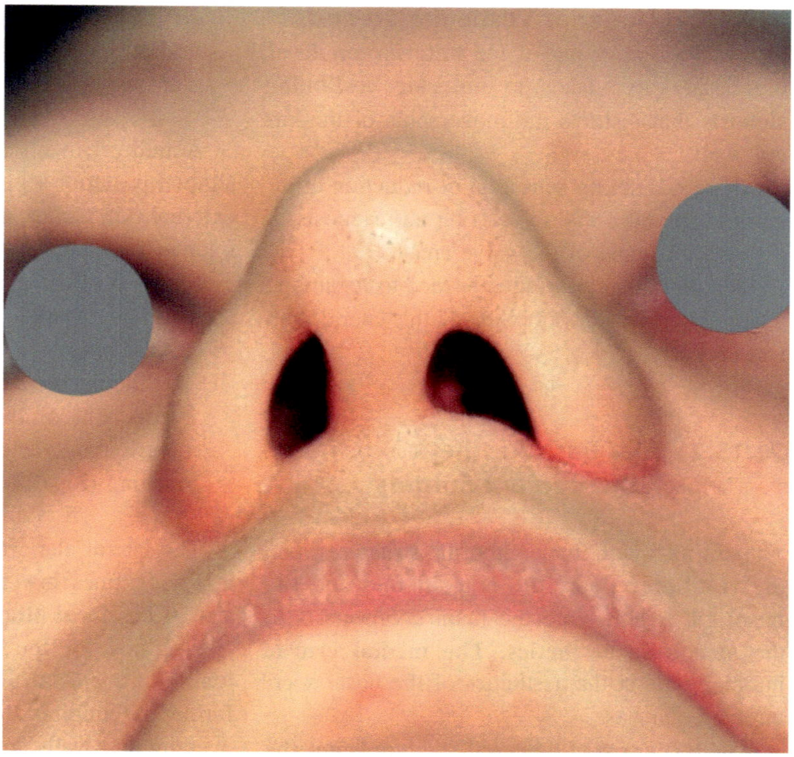

Fig. 21.36 Lateral angulation of left ala nasi

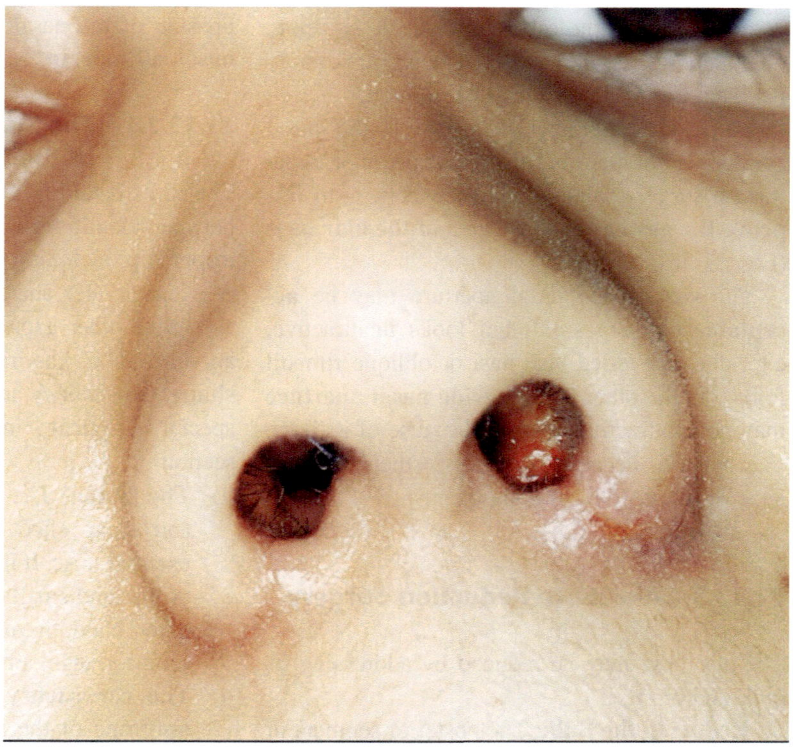

Fig. 21.37 Surgical treatment of Alar Collapse. Left vestibular free skin graft for left alar collapse

21.13.1.2 Anterior Vestibular Stenosis

Overzealous resection of the **anterior angle** of the nasal valve leads to **anterior vestibular stenosis** that restricts the movements of the lateral wall.

There is a strong sensation of reduction of air entry to the nose due to scarring and stenosis of the anterior angle of the valve area.

Generous skin grafting is needed to regain the anatomy, hence the mobility of the lateral wall and air entry.

21.13.2 Alar Base Aesthetic Enhancement Surgery

The **ala nasi** with its neighboring structures, i.e., the **vestibular floor**, **the rim-sill fold** and **the nasal sill** together are the main contributors to the **alar base aesthetics**. **The medial crurae** indirectly affect the aesthetics of the nasal aperture and alar base.

The large size of the nasal aperture **is not the only cause of** its unpleasant appearance. **Unaesthetic relations** between the anatomical components of the alar base may be quite unattractive and gives negative facial impression, i.e., snarling or angry facial expression.

In many conditions the size of the nasal aperture is not therefore the real concern or target for the surgery, but the main concern is to **improve the aesthetics** of the area **of the alar base** (Fig. 21.38).

The **size** of the nasal aperture may be **acceptable** or even **small** but looks unattractive, e.g., due to everted alae nasi or oblique rim-sill folds. On the other hand, a **wide nasal aperture** may be unattractive not only because of its large size but also because of the unaesthetic appearance of its anatomical components.

21.13.3 Alar Base Reduction Surgery

The alar base may be reduced by addressing its bulk and/or size.

i. **Reducing the Bulk**: The posterior segment of the **rim-sill fold is a major contributing structure to a bulky alar base.** Bulky alar bodies may also contribute to the bulk of the alar base (Fig. 21.39).

A bulky rim-sill fold usually has a **wedge-shaped** posterior segment which has much wider external skin surface as compared to the narrower internal vestibular surface.

Excision of the posterior segment of the rim-sill fold has a marked effect on reducing the bulk of the alar base.

ii. **Reducing the size**: The **inferior** rounded component of the rim-sill fold is a major contributing factor to the **size** of the nasal opening (Fig. 21.40).

The lateral alar wall needs to be **medialized** and sometimes **lowered** in order to reduce the **size** of the **areal attachment to the upper lip**.

The **size** of the **vestibular floor** and the **length** of the **nasal sill** may need to be reduced if further reduction in the size of the nasal aperture opening and walls are needed.

The alae nasi, in its new **medial** and **lower** location, has to be well and firmly stitched to the lip side of the nasal base, i.e., in line with the **nasal sill margin**.

21.13.3.1 The Surgical Significance of the Rim-Sill Fold

The rim-sill fold is a **transitional soft skin area** between the **ala nasi**, **the nasal sill band** and the **upper lip** including its underlying Orbicularis oris muscle (see anatomy section).

Unlike other gaps and soft areas in the nasal aperture tube, the rim-sill fold has a unique **shape, consistency** and **location** that makes it of special surgical importance (see anatomy section).

(a) **The shape**: The rim-sill fold has its direct and clear effect on the aesthetics of the external nose. It might be too bulky and large or thin and small (posterior segment). On the other hand, it might be too long or short (inferior segment).

(b) **The consistency**: The rim-sill fold is **the only** one of the soft skin gaps in the nasal aperture tube that is both **soft** and

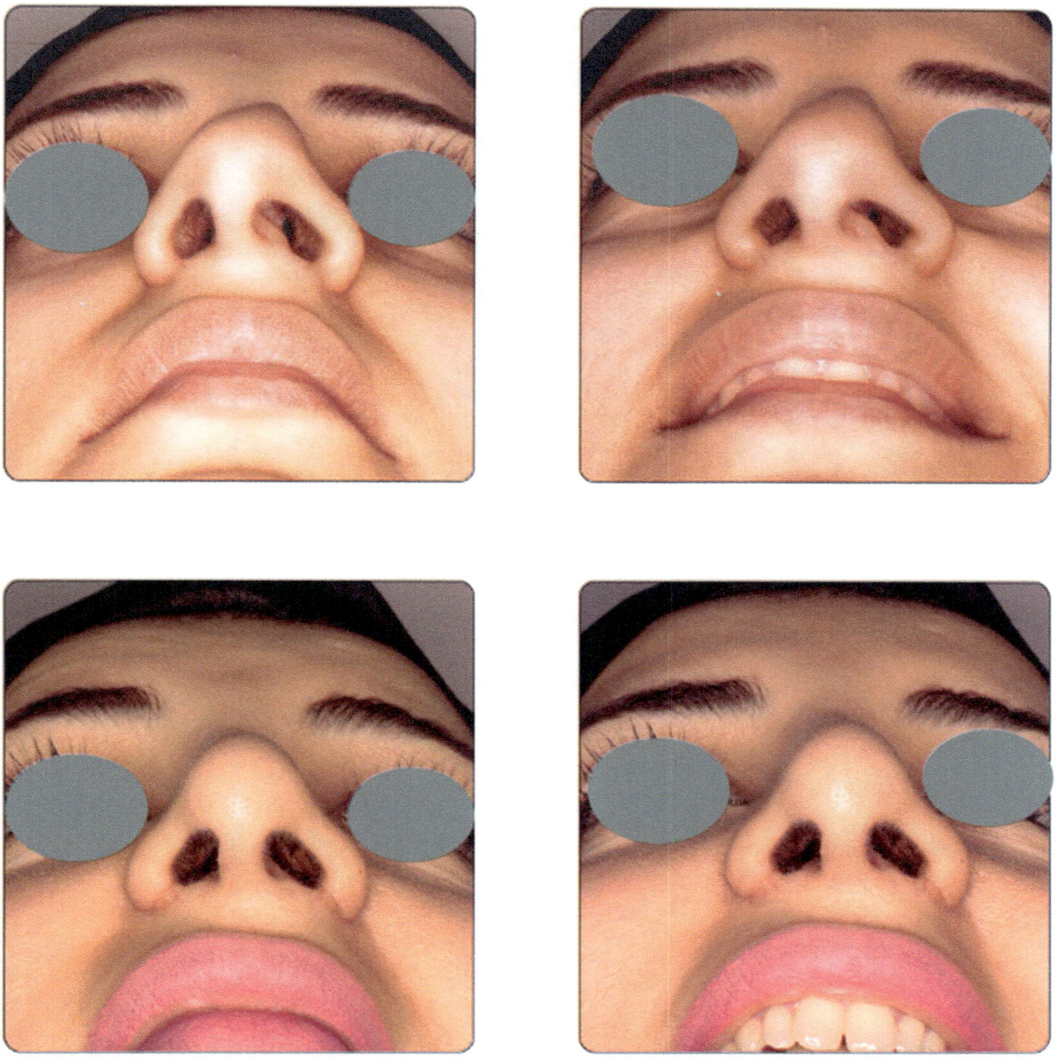

Fig. 21.38 Improved size and aesthetics of the nasal aperture after rim-sill excision

stretchable (refer to anatomy). Smiling elongates the lips transversely taking both alae nasi laterally which in turn stretches the skin of both rim-sill folds and the whole of the vestibular floor.

This type of skin gives the rim-sill folds two major advantages:

- **Surgical incision** in this type of skin heals nicely with minimal, unsightly scaring.
- **Surgical excision** of part or all of the rim-sill folds reduces, **size, bulk** and abolishes the expansion of the nasal apertures on **smiling**. They all are greatly wished aesthetic demand.

(c) **The location**: The rim-sill fold is located at the **most inferior** and **posterior** end of the nose. This location has two great surgical advantages:

(i) It shares in the formation of the **posterior alar groove**, which is a perfect place for a **well hidden, out of sight scar**. Not only this, but also it is a favorable site to **create an attractive alar groove** in a nose which

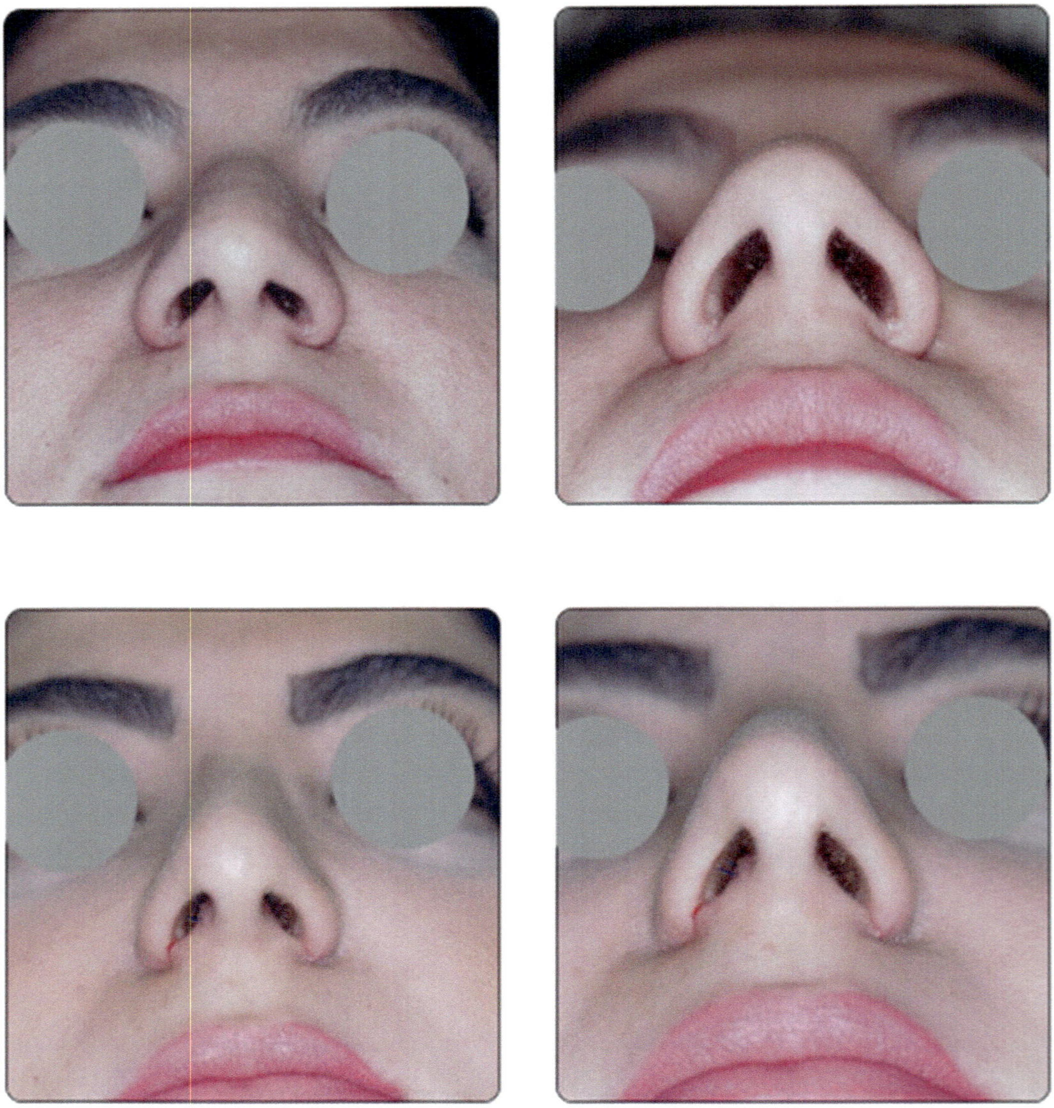

Fig. 21.39 Reduction of the bulk of the nasal apertures after excision of the rim-sill folds

has a less favorable shallow groove, as in the Asian noses.

(ii) The rim-sill fold is at the junction between the **freely mobile lateral alar wall** and the **relatively fixed vestibular floor**.

Incision in the rim-sill fold not only makes the lateral alar wall **more free** but it also gives free access to the vestibular walls and cavity.

The rim-sill fold, therefore, is the gateway to the nasal aperture tube, i.e., the vestibular cavity. It is the only anatomical location where the **vestibular cavity may be entered** without jeopardizing the aesthetics of the external nose.

Once the vestibular cavity is entered, **many surgical procedures** may then be carried out, e.g., excising part or all of the rim-sill fold, repositioning of the lateral alar wall, adding or excising parts of the vestibular wall.

In conclusion, the **location** and the **consistency** of the rim-sill folds help in making a

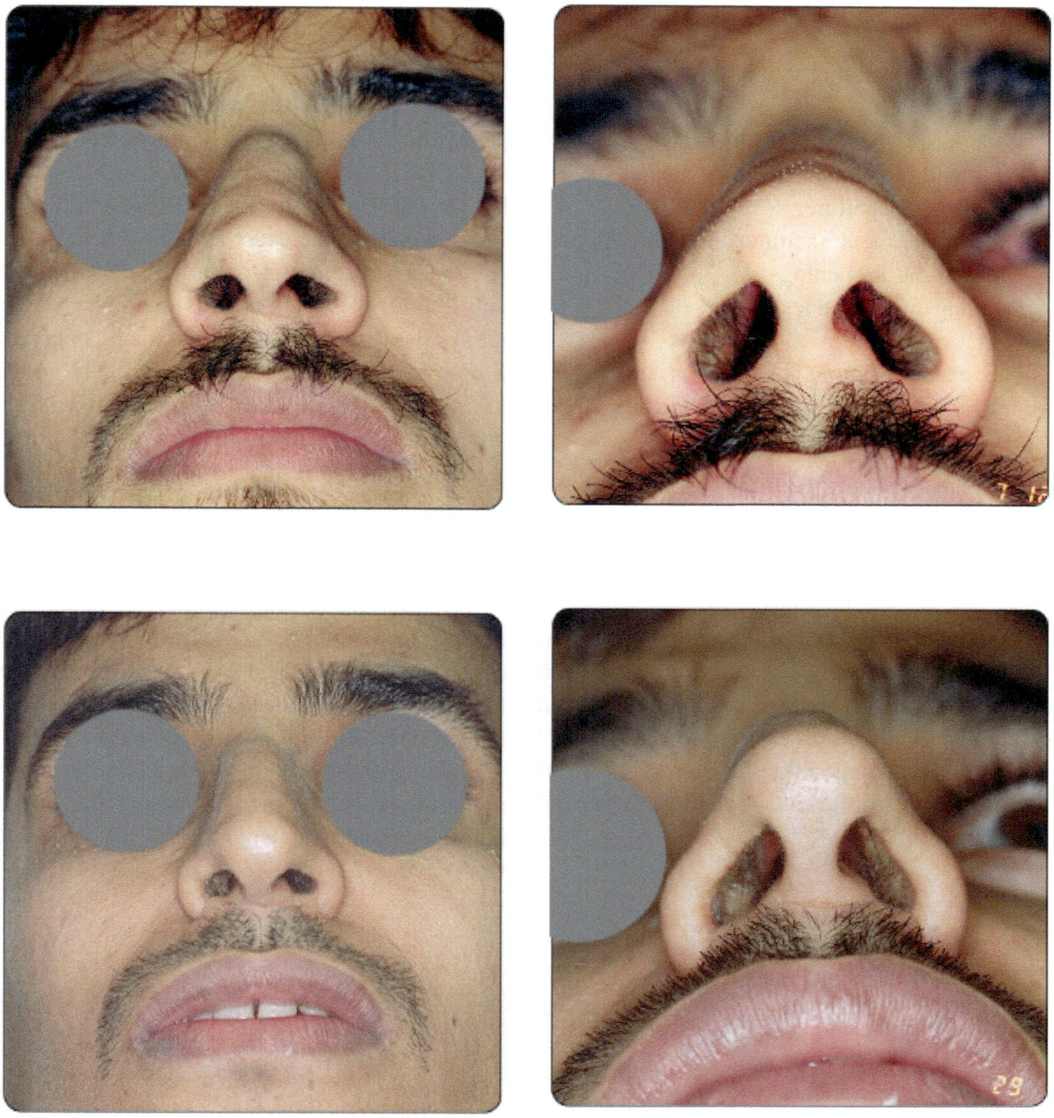

Fig. 21.40 Reduction of the size of the nasal apertures after excision of the rim-sill folds

surgical incision both **well hidden** and heals with minimal scarring.

21.13.3.2 Defining the Location of the Rim-Sill Fold

The location of the rim-sill folds must be defined clinically, photographically and intra-operatively.

The exact meeting lines of the folds with the **nasal sill, alar rim** and **upper lip** are seen and marked.

The rim-sill test clearly defines these lines. This test can be repeatedly made clinically and in the operating theater under anesthesia.

Only occasionally these lines are quite evident without the need of the rim-sill test.

21.13.3.3 Surgery of the Rim-sill Fold

Rim-sill surgery essentially is based upon **accurate anatomical planning**. Planning is made in two steps:

1. Diagnosis

This means defining the aesthetic problem:

- Wide nasal aperture;
- Wide and large nasal aperture tube;
- Bulky nasal aperture;
- Unaesthetic nasal aperture;
- Unequal nasal openings.
- Defining Incision lines

The exact locations of incision lines must accurately be defined, mostly with the help of the Rim-sill test.

Planning for the Incisions

Incision sites are a mainstay of successful alar base surgery, i.e., naturally beautiful nasal apertures with well-camouflaged scar.

There is **no standard or stereotyped incision** used routinely in nasal aperture surgery. Each incision is planned and tailored to the surgical anatomical findings in each individual nostril even in the very same nose. Incision in the **right nostril** may be **different** from the **left nostril** (Fig. 21.41).

Marking

The Sill Line

The **lateral end of the nasal sill** is located, by performing the rim-sill test on the operating table (Fig. 21.75) and a mark is made, i.e., a single dot by the marking pen (Figs. 21.65 and 21.76). Using a caliper, the exact length of the nasal sill is measured **from the columella** to its **lateral end** (Fig. 21.42). Both nostrils should have equal nasal sills. If shortening of a nasal sill is planned, a new mark is made more medial. The longer nasal sill is shortened to be equalized with the other side.

Measurement of the nasal sill length starts from **the columella** medially and not from medial crural prominence which is variable from one nostril to the other (Fig. 21.43).

Unequal nasal sills are not an uncommon finding in normal individuals who never had surgery before. This is usually discovered for the first time on table during surgery. It is easily missed clinically and photographically.

Starting from the sill mark, a line is drawn **posteriorly,** i.e., **inwards,** crossing the margin into the nasal vestibule, and stops just inside the margin (Fig. 21.47).

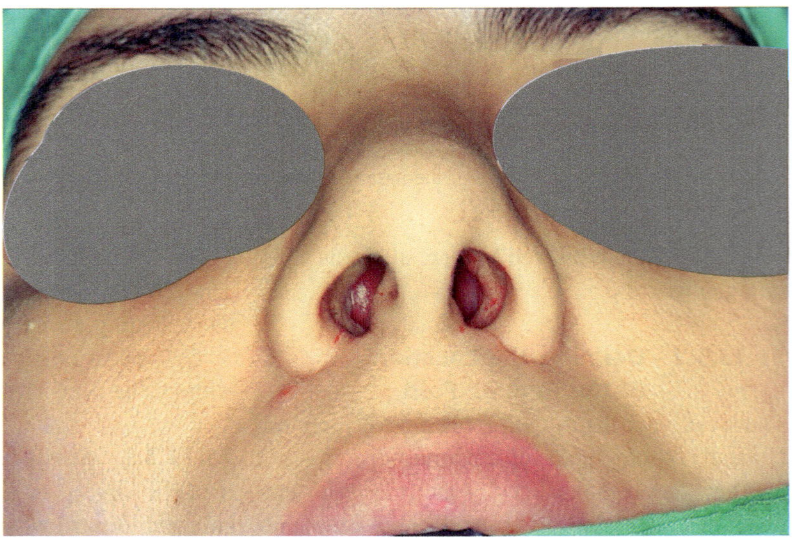

Fig. 21.41 Pre-operative basal view. Note the right posterior lateral crural prominence

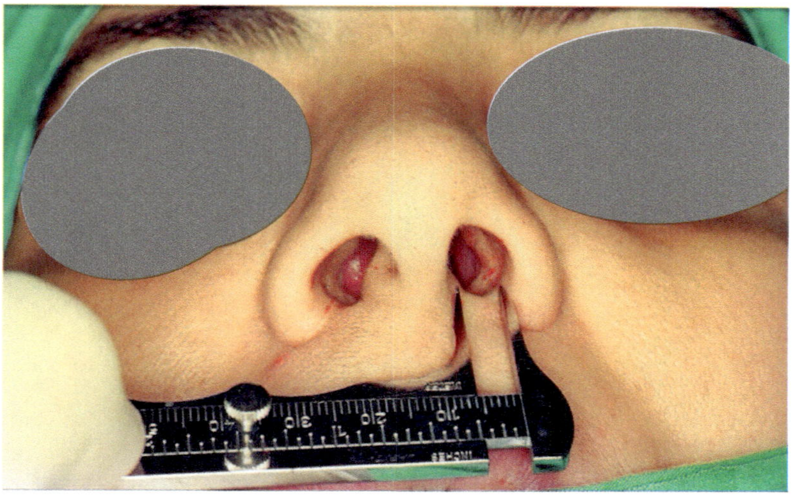

Fig. 21.42 Measuring the width of the left nasal aperture

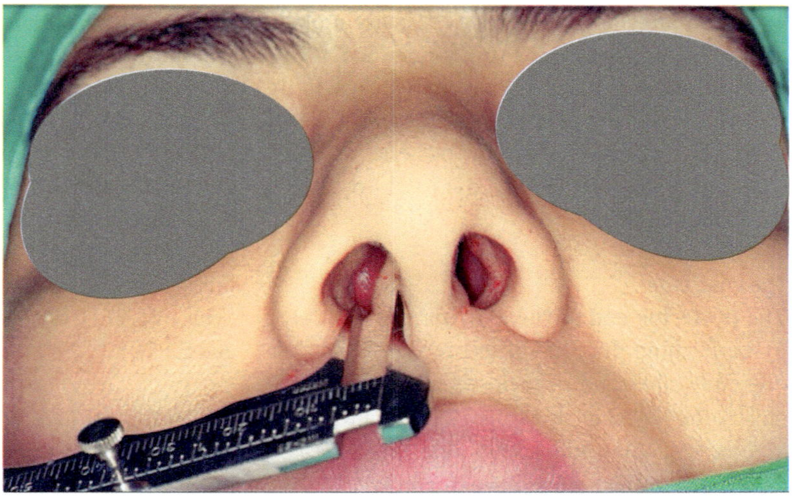

Fig. 21.43 Measuring the width of the right nasal aperture. Measuring starts from the columellar margin avoiding the lateral crural prominence

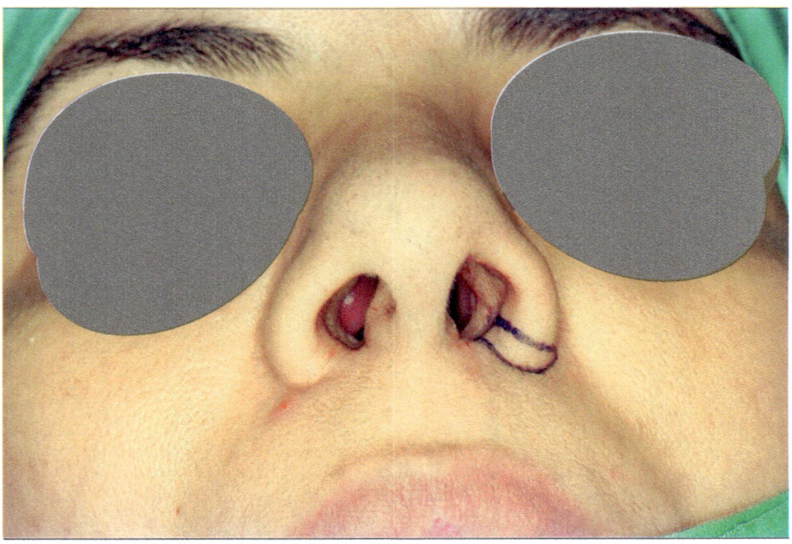

Fig. 21.44 The left sill line and alar line

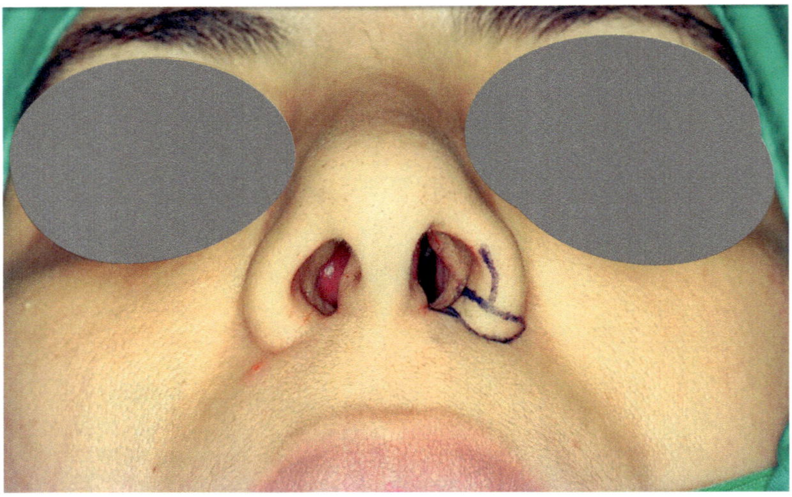

Fig. 21.45 The Marginal Lines. The left marginal lines at inferior alar margin and anterior surface of the sill band (correspond to the lines of light reflexes)

Externally the line crosses the margin **anteriorly** till it reaches the naso-labial junction.

From this point, the line continues **strictly into the posterior alar groove**, for one-third of its length, i.e., the length of the posterior segment of the rim-sill fold (Figs. 21.45, 21.46, 21.47, 21.66 and 21.67).

The Alar Line

The **posterior end of the alar margin** is located by performing the rim-sill test repeatedly on the operating table, and a **mark** is made, i.e., a single dot by the marking pen (Figs. 21.65 and 21.76).

From the **alar mark,** the **alar line** starts by crossing the alar margin **externally**. It then follows the **posterior margin of the ala nasi**, for one-third of its length until it meets the **sill line** (Figs. 21.44, 21.45, 21.46, 21.47, 21.66, 21.67, 21.77, 21.78, 21.79 and 21.88).

The posterior margin of the ala nasi is clearly seen by the repeated rim-sill test intraoperatively.

Going **inwards** from the alar mark the alar line crosses the alar margin into the nasal vestibule and stops just inside the margin (Figs. 21.47, 21.66, 21.67, 21.68, 21.69, 21.77 and 21.79).

The Vestibular Line

At this point inside the nasal vestibule the two lines, alar and sill lines, are joined by a transverse

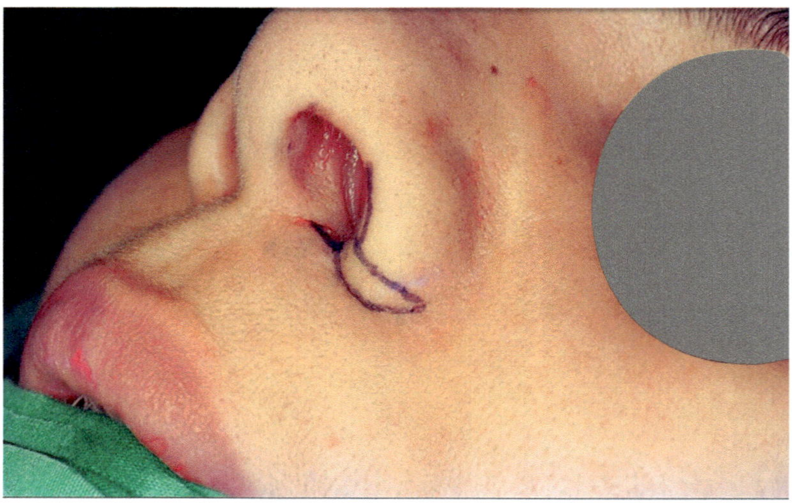

Fig. 21.46 The sill and alar lines meet at the superior end of the posterior segment of the rim-sill fold

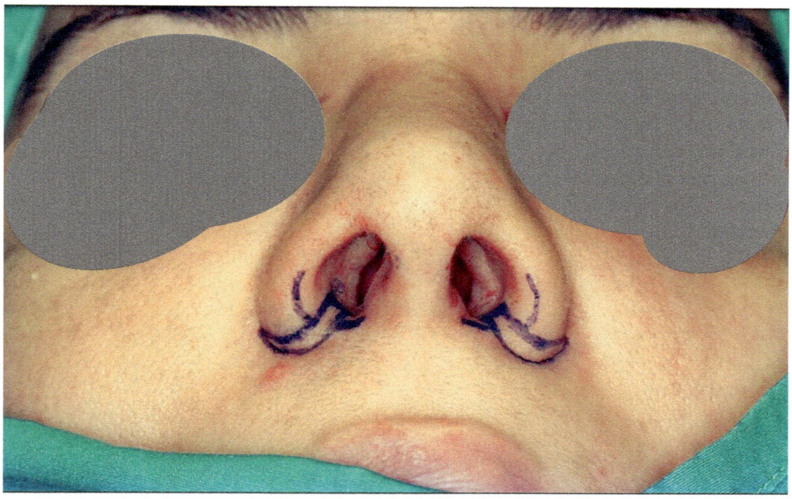

Fig. 21.47 The Sill, Alar, Vestibular and Marginal Lines. Complete marking of the rim-sill folds, after adding the vestibular lines

line, the **vestibular line** (Figs. 21.47, 21.68, 21.77 and 21.78).

No dog's ear deformity is formed by joining the two margins together as the vestibular skin is quite loose with abundant subcutaneous tissue.

As the vestibular skin is closely adherent to the body of the ala nasi, the posterior alar margin is easily recognized at the **junction between the loose skin at the vestibular floor and the adherent alar skin**. Care must be taken to avoid encroaching upon the adherent skin.

It is noteworthy that only **the lower third** of the posterior alar margin can be explored externally as the external nasal wound cannot go higher than the soft rim-sill wedge of skin. Higher medialization of the alar base, and hence the posterior alar groove can be achieved from inside the nose without the need for extending the external scar.

N.B. Crossing the **aperture margins** aims at reducing the **aperture size** while external wedge resection of the alae nasi aims at **reducing the alar flare** and alar **bulk**.

The Marginal Lines

These are lines which are marked over the **lines of light reflexes** on the **inferior alar margin** and the **anterior surface of the nasal sill band** (Figs. 21.45, 21.46, 21.47, 21.48, 21.58, 21.59, 21.60, 21.61, 21.62, 21.67, 21.78, 21.79, 21.80, 21.81 and 21.82).

The line starts from the sill mark onto the **nasal sill band** medially and from the alar mark onto the **alar margin** laterally. The two lines are interrupted by the area to be resected between them, i.e., the inferior segment of the rim-sill fold (Fig. 21.48).

These two lines join each other after surgical resection of the inferior segment of the rim-sill fold to become **one continuous circular line** (Figs. 21.48, 21.49, 21.59, 21.81 and 21.82). They are an excellent guide for the surgeon in rejoining the margins of the alae nasi and nasal sill bands and in keeping the **natural curve** of the nasal aperture (Figs. 21.49, 21.50, 21.51, 21.52, 21.53 and 21.54). Marginal lines also help avoiding excessive **rotation** of the alar margin internally or externally.

Surgical Excision of the Rim-Sill Folds

A sharp pronged alar retractor is used to elevate the ala nasi (Fig. 21.66). Local anesthesia 2% lidocaine with adrenaline is injected in the rim-sill folds from within its vestibular side. A No.11 blade is better used as it has a straight sharp blade that corresponds with lines of cutting at the alar base (Figs. 21.69, 21.70, 21.71 and 21.72).

The **first cut** starts across the nasal sill at the **sill mark,** i. e. at the lateral end of the nasal sill band, down to the vestibular floor internally and the naso-labial crease externally (Fig. 21.69). Cutting then follow the sill line **strictly into the posterior alar groove** (Fig. 21.70).

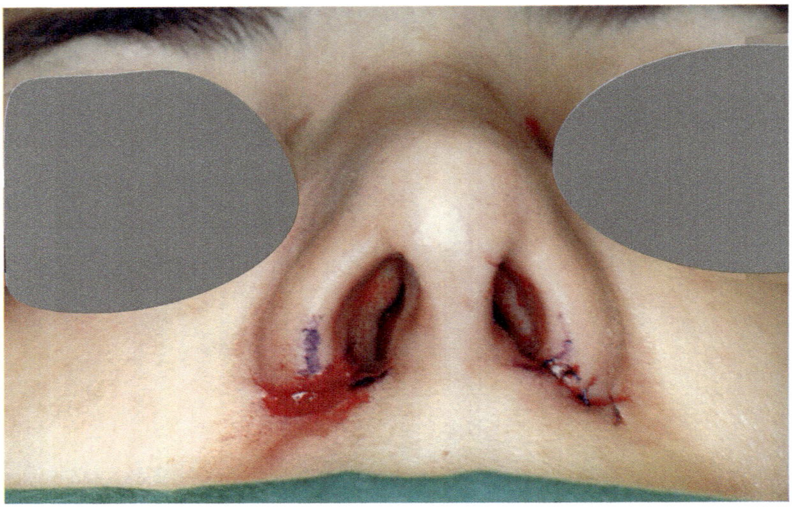

Fig. 21.48 Rim- Sill fold excision and stitching. Excision of the inferior and posterior segments of the right rim-sill fold. The wound is closed on the left side. The left alar and sill lines join each other to become one continuous line

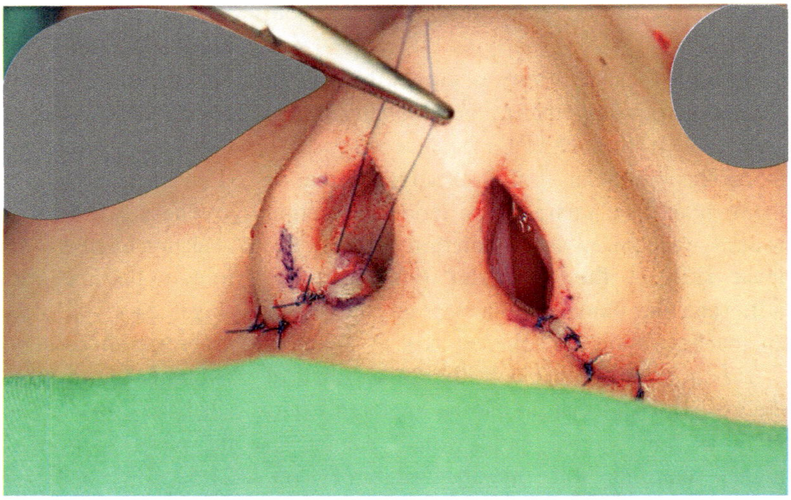

Fig. 21.49 The three marginal skin stitches. The rim and sill lines become one continuous line

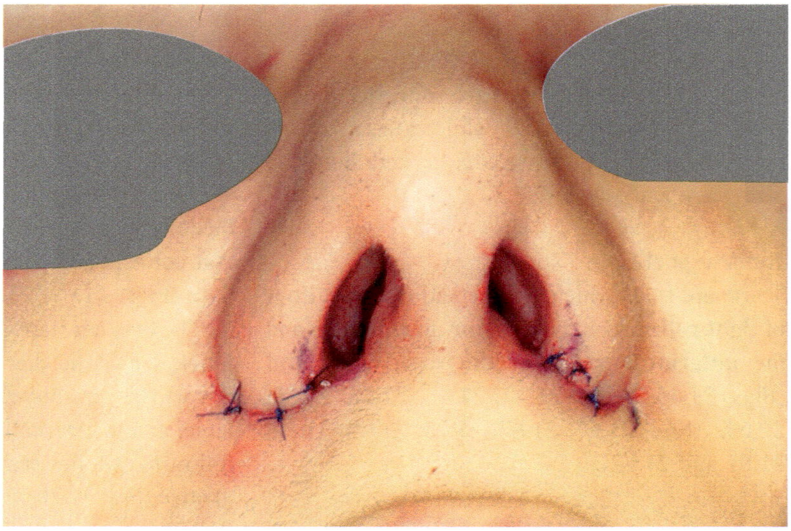

Fig. 21.50 Unequal nasal openings due to larger right lateral crural prominence than the left

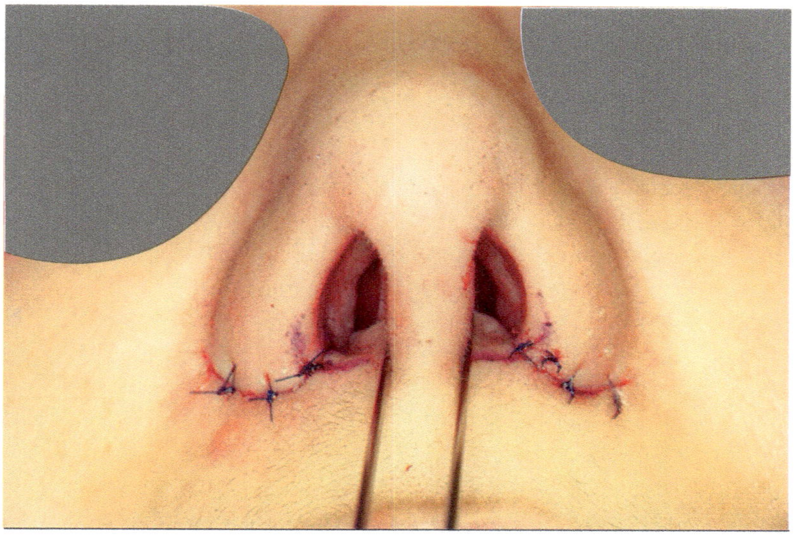

Fig. 21.51 Abolishing the effect of the lateral crural prominences using a thin forceps

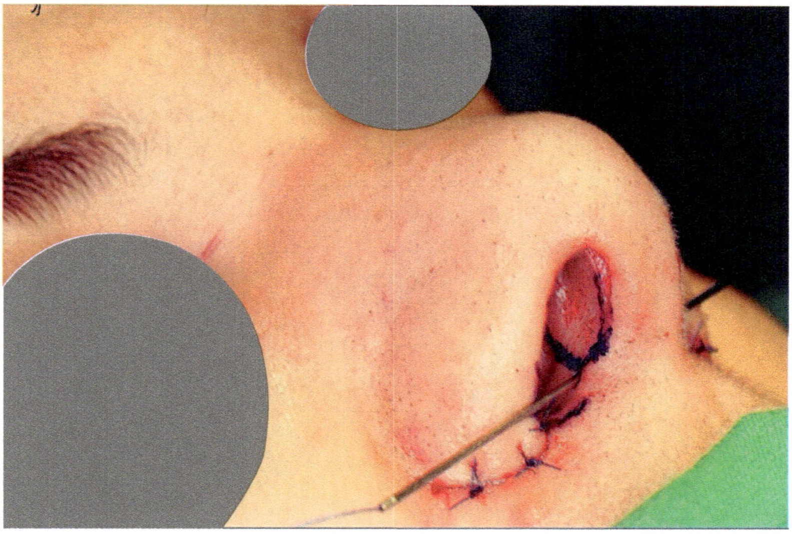

Fig. 21.52 Transcollumelar stitch going anterior to the IVB (Inferior Vestibular Band)

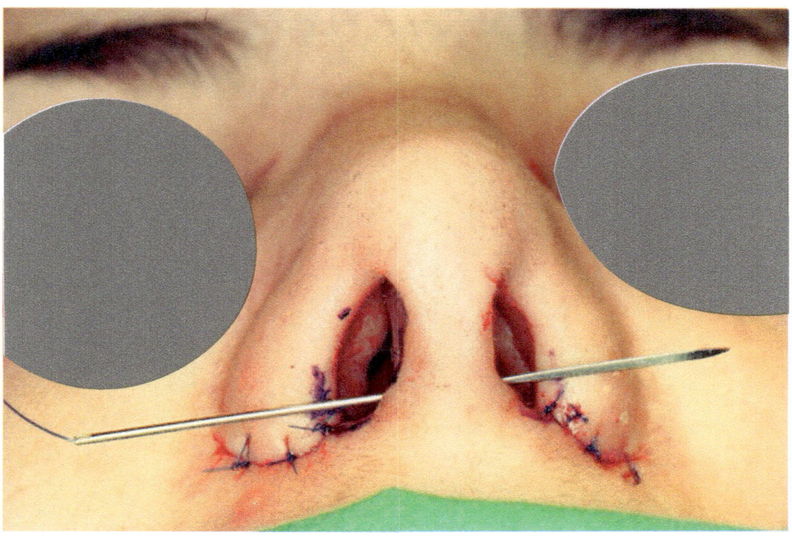

Fig. 21.53 Looking at the transcollumelar stitch from the basal view

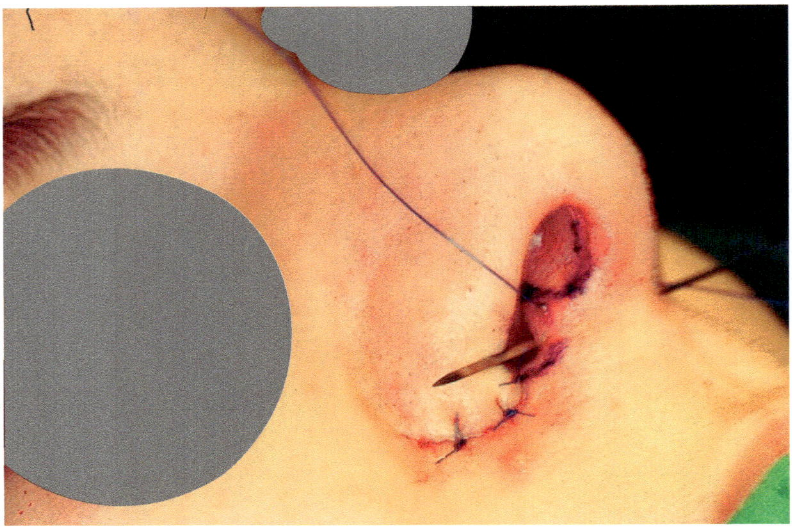

Fig. 21.54 The transcollumelar needle coming back posterior to the IVB (Inferior Vestibular Band)

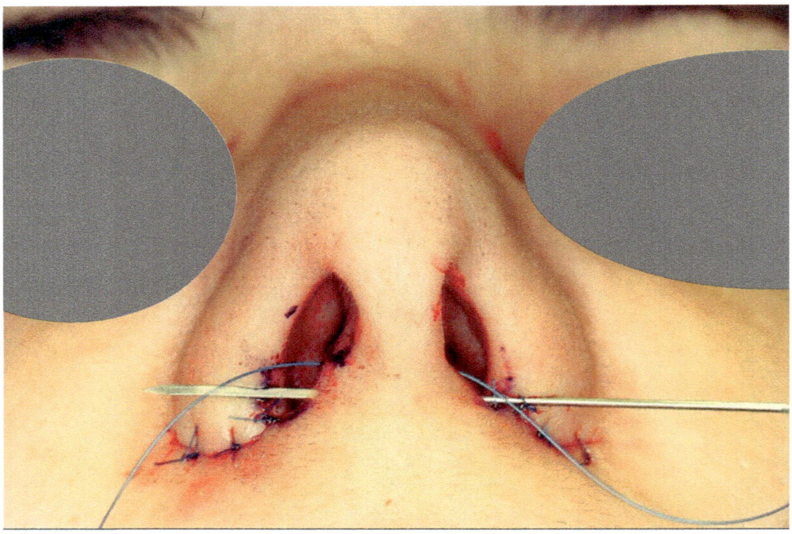

Fig. 21.55 The transcolumellar stitch going anterior, then posterior to the two IVBs (The inferior vestibular band) on both sides

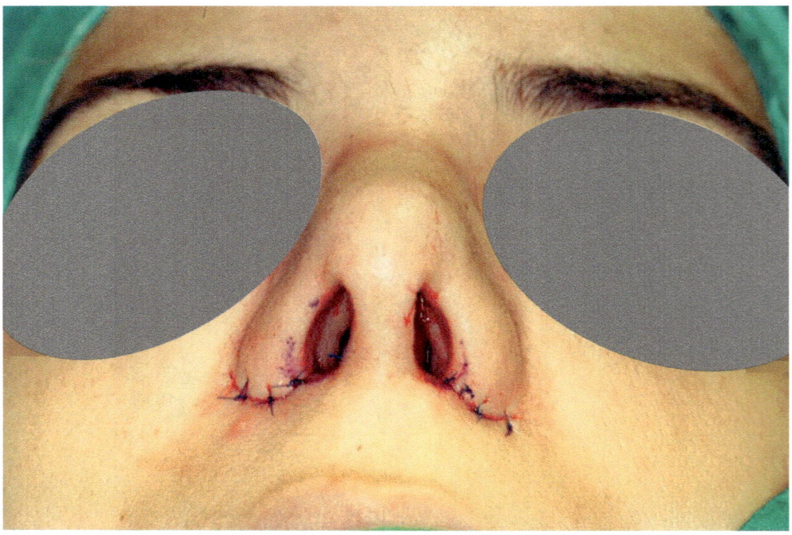

Fig. 21.56 Equal nasal apertures after transcollumelar stitch

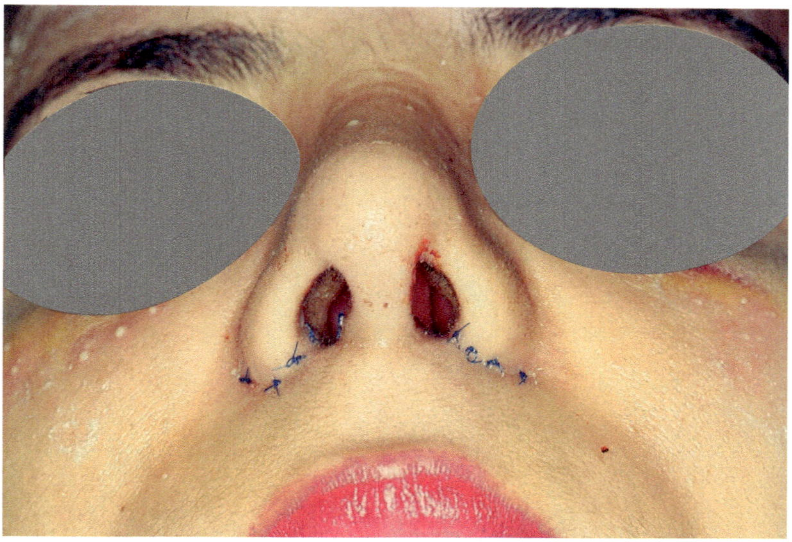

Fig. 21.57 Post Operative Appearance on the seventh day

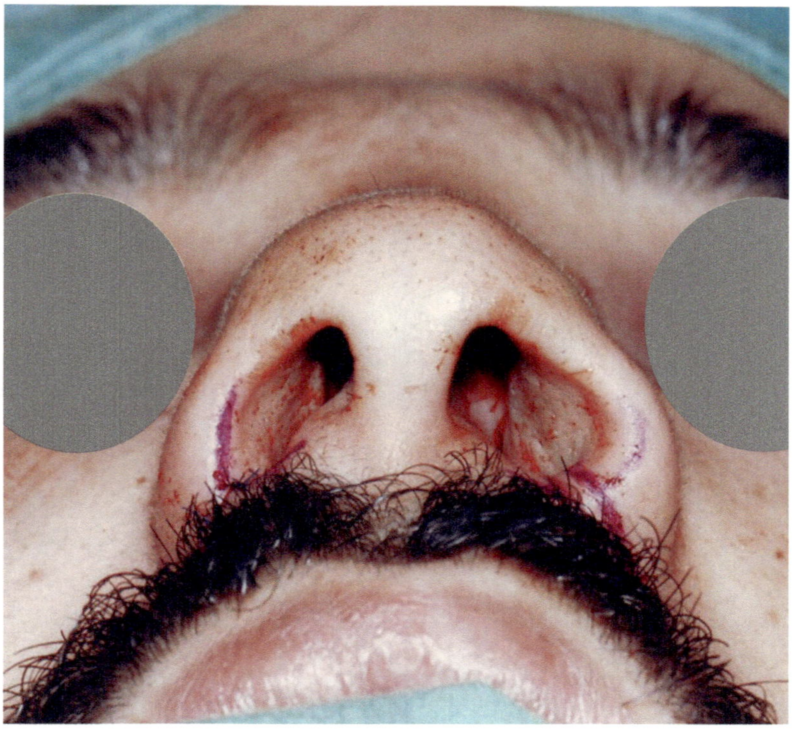

Fig. 21.58 Unequal nasal apertures after initial rim-sill excision

The **second cut** starts at the **alar mark,** i. e. at the lower margin of the ala nasi. Cutting goes across the alar margin **just inside the nasal vestibule**. **Externally** cutting continues **posteriorly** along the junction between the **firm posterior alar margin** and the **soft skin** of the posterior segment of the rim-sill fold, till it meets with the upper end of the posterior groove incision (Figs. 21.71 and 21.72).

Cuts are then deepened, while the rim-sill fold is held by the toothed forceps and the lateral alar wall is counter elevated by the alar retractor, till the whole fold is completely excised (Figs. 21.72, 21.73 and 21.75).

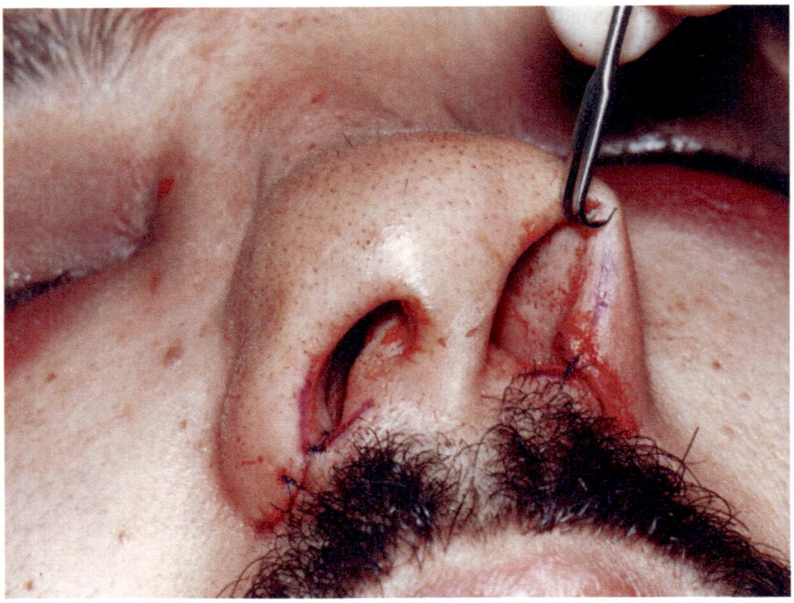

Fig. 21.59 Further alar ressection while the marginal stitch in stu

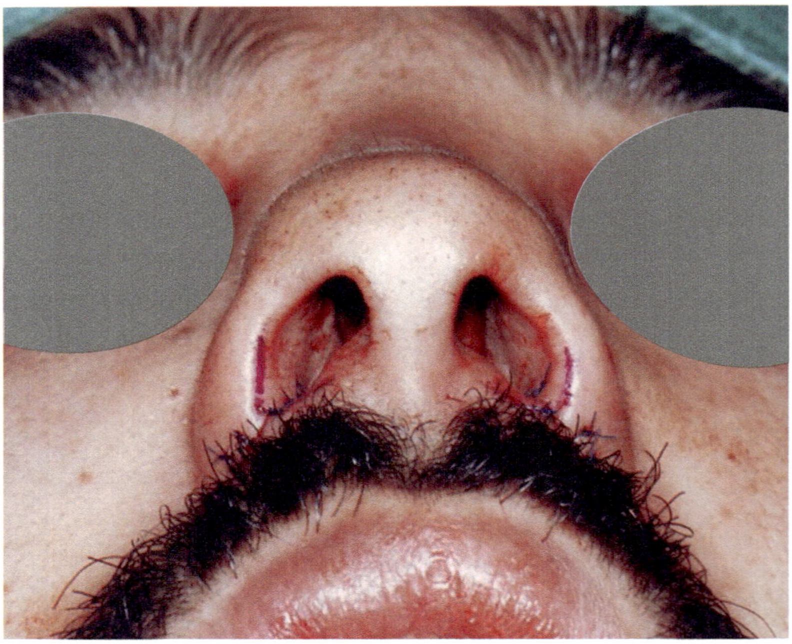

Fig. 21.60 Equal nasal apertures but disturbed by unequal lateral crural prominences on both sides

Practical Guidelines:

i. It is better to cut off the rim-sill folds on **both sides**, right and left, **simultaneously** before deciding to reconstruct the rim-sill wounds.

ii. Only parts, and not all, of the rim-sill folds may be excised. Each case is judged according to the aesthetic requirements of either reducing the size, the bulk or both.

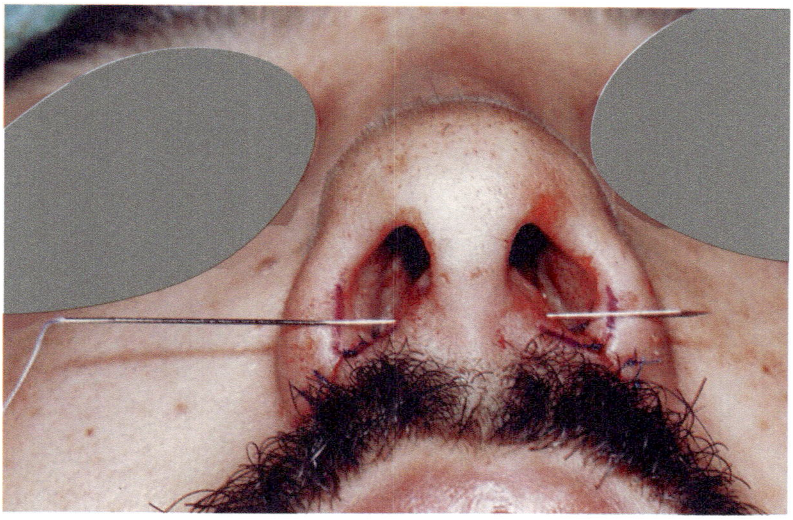

Fig. 21.61 Transcollumelar Stitch

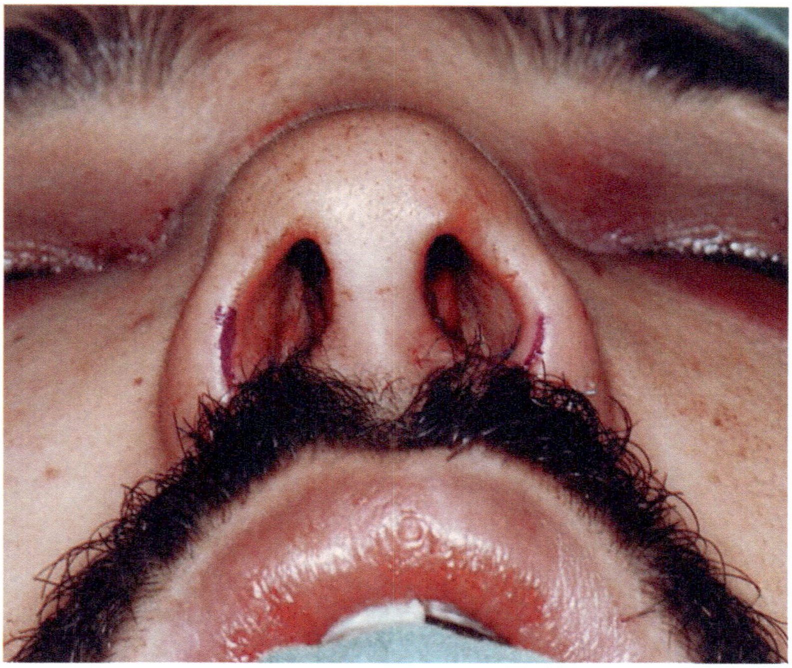

Fig. 21.62 Completely equal nasal apertures after abolishing the The effects of the medial pr prominences

iii. It is wise to **resect less skin** than believed necessary. Further reduction is possible, but **not** the opposite.

iv. The general assessment is made by looking at both apertures from a distance after placing the preliminary subcutaneous stay sutures.

v. Similar apertures not only mean that they are as close as possible in size and shape, both also both alar grooves are close to each other in their depth and position.

vi. Should one side is seen to be larger than the other after primary resection, then further resection is made while stitches are in place. Usually,
1–2 mm is all that needed medial crural prominence (Figs. 21.58, 21.59 and 21.60).

vii. The two nasal openings sometimes have completely different **shapes** that might be

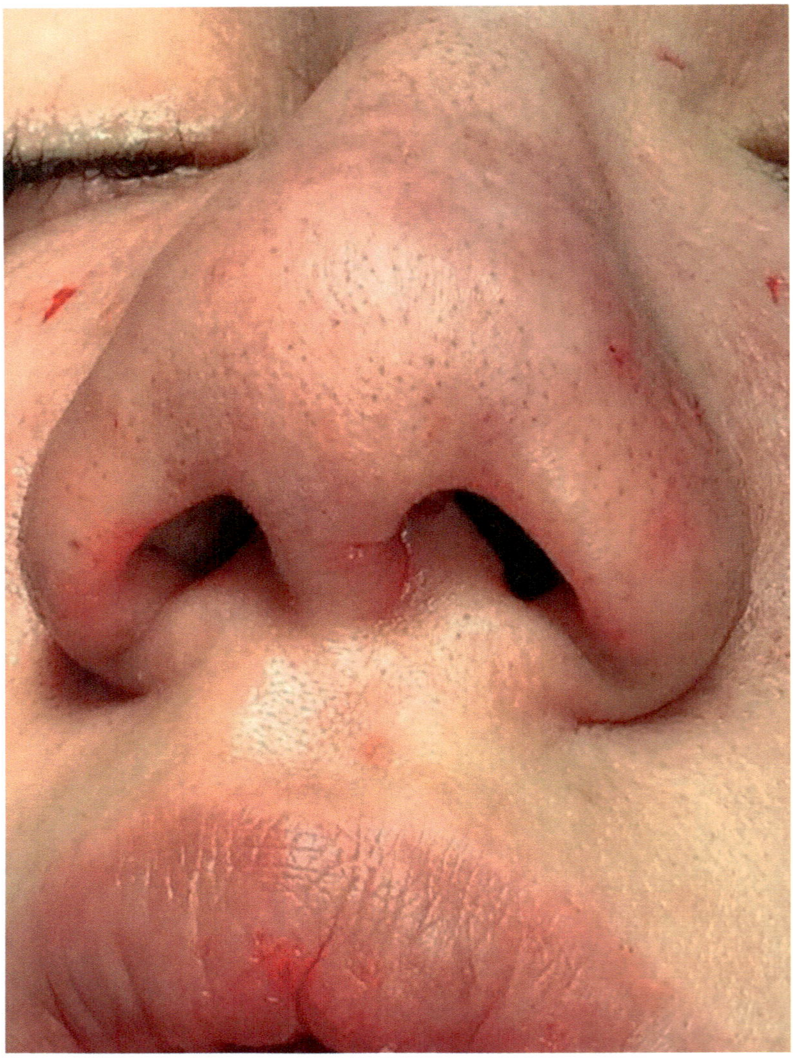

Fig. 21.63 Extremely thick skin alar base. The posterior segment rests on the upper lip like a flat tire

difficult to change for matching with each other. In these cases having two openings that are equal in **sizes** regardless of the shapes procedure is the best aesthetic result.

Type of Rim-Sill Aesthetic Surgeries

The rim-sill fold may be long, thick or both. This leads to a wide, thick nasal aperture or both. It is important to remember that each rim-sill fold has two anatomical segments. Each segment has its own aesthetic effects. The **inferior segment** is between the nasal sill and the inferior alar margin and mainly contributes to the **width** of the nasal openings (Figs. 21.75, 21.76, 21.77, 21.78, 21.79, 21.80, 21.81, 21.82, 21.83, 21.84, 21.85, 21.86 and 21.87). The **posterior segment** extends behind the alar margin and its main contribution is to the **bulk** of the nasal aperture (Figs. 21.63, 21.64, 21.65, 21.66, 21.67, 21.68, 21.69, 21.70, 21.71, 21.72, 21.73, 21.88, 21.89, 21.90, 21.91 and 21.92).

Rim-Sill surgery aims at improving the aesthetic of the alar base. It is no longer restricted to the mere reduction of the width of the alar base (Fig. 21.88).

According to the aesthetic needs, there are many goals that may be achieved.

(a) **Posterior segment** excision is mainly concerned with reduction of the **bulk** of the alar base.

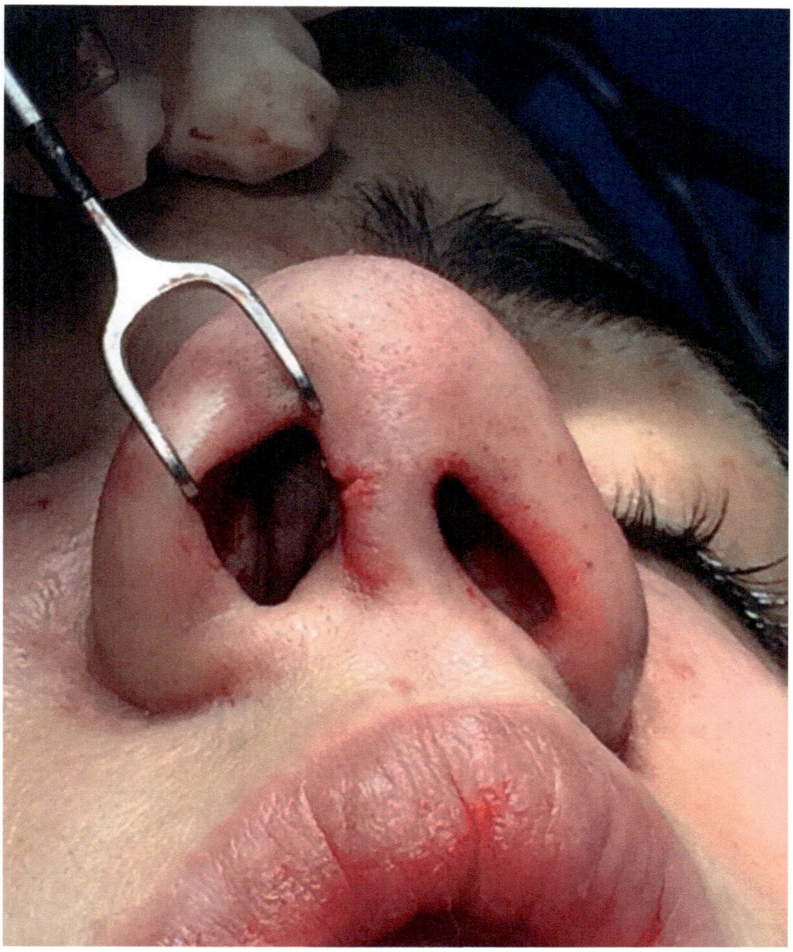

Fig. 21.64 Stretching the rim-sill fold using an alar retractor

(b) **Inferior segment** excision is mainly concerned with reduction of the **size** of the nasal aperture.

(c) Reducing the size of **the whole length of the nasal aperture tube**: This is required in very wide nasal aperture coupled with wide and sizable lower third of the nose, i.e., wide nasal aperture tubes. In these cases, reduction in the size of nasal aperture walls is required.

In these cases cutting continues through the vestibular floor along the alar and sill lines till they reach the mucocutenous junction at the superior limit of the nasal aperture tube, i.e., the posterior vestibular margin (Figs. 21.106, 21.107 and 21.108).

Care is taken to avoid encroaching upon the adherent skin over the inner surface of the alae nasi to avoid lateral angulation of the nasal aperture.

(d) **Aesthetic enhancement** of the alar-sill relationship, e.g.,

i. Everted alae nasi gives a snarling impression
ii. Thin rim-sill folds produce visual interruption of the inferior nasal margin
iii. Oblique rim-sill segment is unsightly and sometimes exposes the columellar wall.

Rim-Sill Post-excision Reconstruction

Excising the rim-sill fold leaves the nose with an open wound that has **two cut ends**, the **alar margin** and nasal **sill margin**.

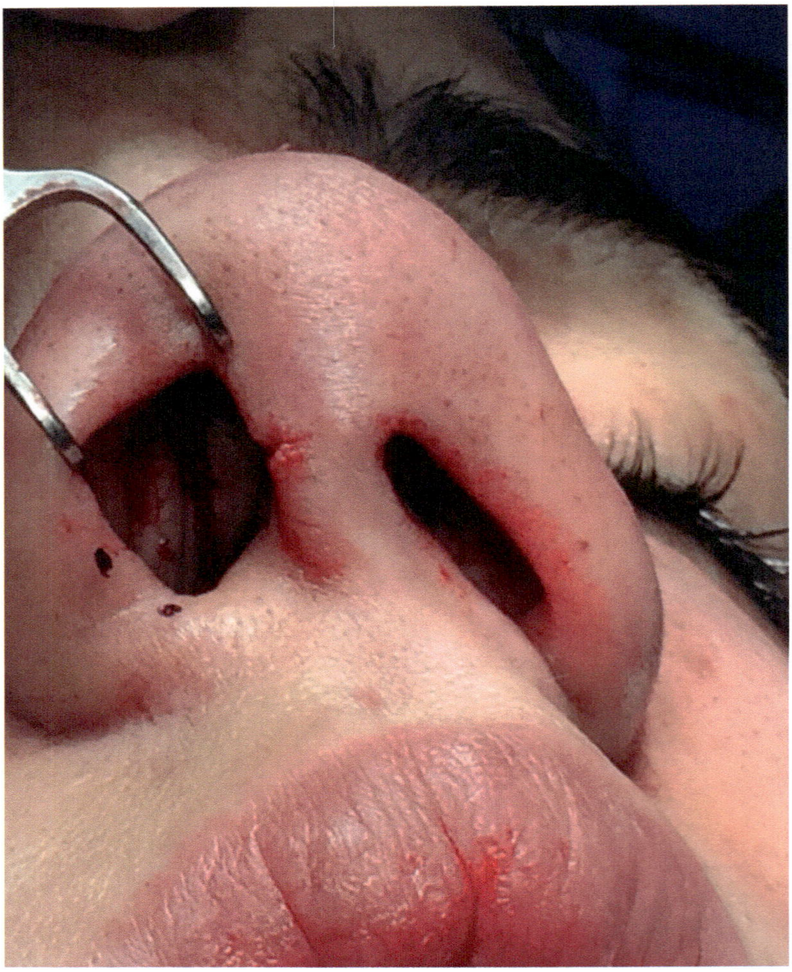

Fig. 21.65 Marking the posterior alar margin and the lateral end of the nasal sill

These are **two firm structures**. Each cut end has a **rounded margin**, and is made of **thin skin** which is **adherent** to the underlying firm fibrous tissues (Fig. 21.89).

The gap between these two structures has to be reduced subcutaneously to approximate and align the two firm margins before finally closing the skin (Figs. 21.90, 21.91 and 21.92).

The Submarginal Approximation

Using a No. 4 or 5 absorbable vycril stitches, a **submarginal stitch** is taken 1–2 mm. away from the rounded margin of each side. Both stitches have to be at the same distance from the margin. The knot must be neatly square, so that the two curved skin surfaces match when they join each other and make one naturally curved margin without stepping (Figs. 21.93, 21.94, 21.95, 21.102 and 21.103).

Skin Closure

This is the final important step following the previous preparations, starting from clinical examination to photography, planning, drawing, cutting and then subcutaneous stitching.

The final appearance of the nasal aperture in most cases usually becomes apparent after the submarginal stitch (Figs. 21.95 and 10.9).

The Three Marginal Skin Stitches

The purpose of these stitches is to accurately match together the two rounded semicircular cut edges of the alar and sill wounds. The submarginal stitch is an excellent preparatory base that brings the two margins close to each other

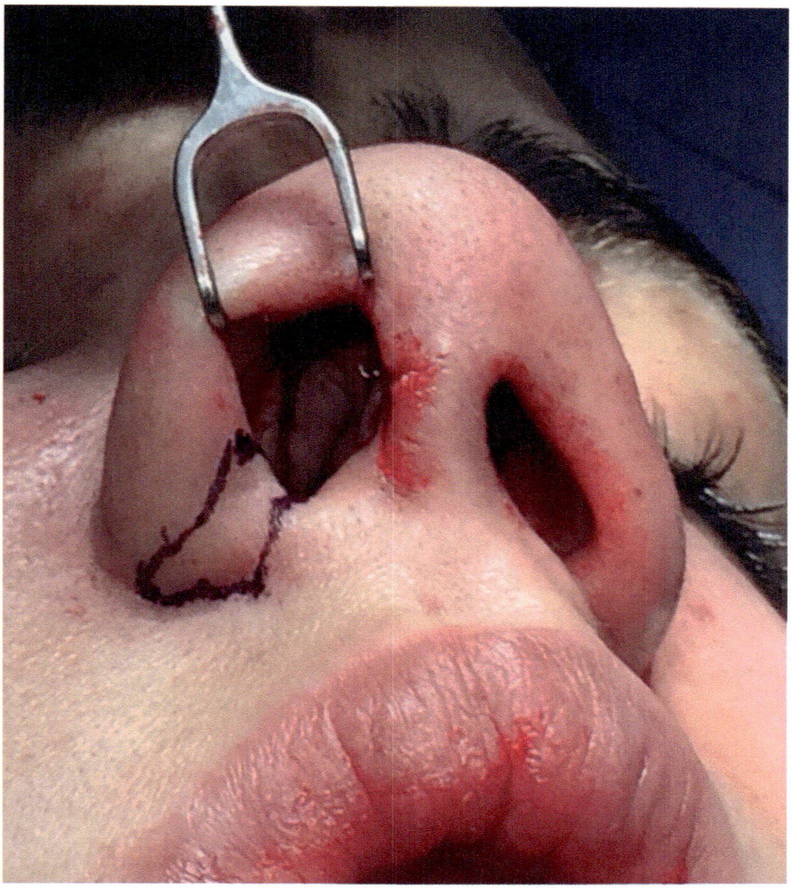

Fig. 21.66 The sill and alar lines crossing the sill and alar margins. The two lines meet at the superior end of the posterior segment of the rim-sill fold

(Figs. 21.92, 21.93, 21.94, 21.95 and Figs. 10.9, 21.103 and 21.104).

There are **three** important key stitches which are quite necessary in order to round up the curved margins and have complete control over them, so that when healing is completed the two margins will unite smoothly and uniformly with each other in such a way that they continue as a naturally curved margin.

A five or six zero **fine nylon** (proline) in a ½ cm cutting needle is used. Each of these stitches must be **deep square** one that includes the two layers of the thin skin and its underlying firm fibrous tissue on both sides. These three stitches are: (Figs. 21.49, 21.50, 21.81 and 21.82)

(1) **The middle or marginal stitch**: As the name implies this stitch is in the middle between the external lip and internal vestibular stitches. It is taken exactly at the rim and sill **marginal lines**. The two lines now join each other to become one continuous marginal line (Figs. 21.49 and 21.81).
(2) **The External lip stitch**: This stitch is at the **outermost** side of the curved margins, i.e., at the junction between the two margins, alar and sill, with the upper lip (Figs. 21.49 and 21.81).
(3) **The Internal vestibular stitch**: This stitch is at the **innermost** side of the curved margins, i.e., at the junction between the two margins with the vestibular floor (Figs. 21.49 and 21.81).

Ideally, we should start by the marginal stitch, followed by the other two stitches. The order of stitching may vary from one case to another.

The rest of the alar skin wound can now be easily closed, using the same fine nylon stitches,

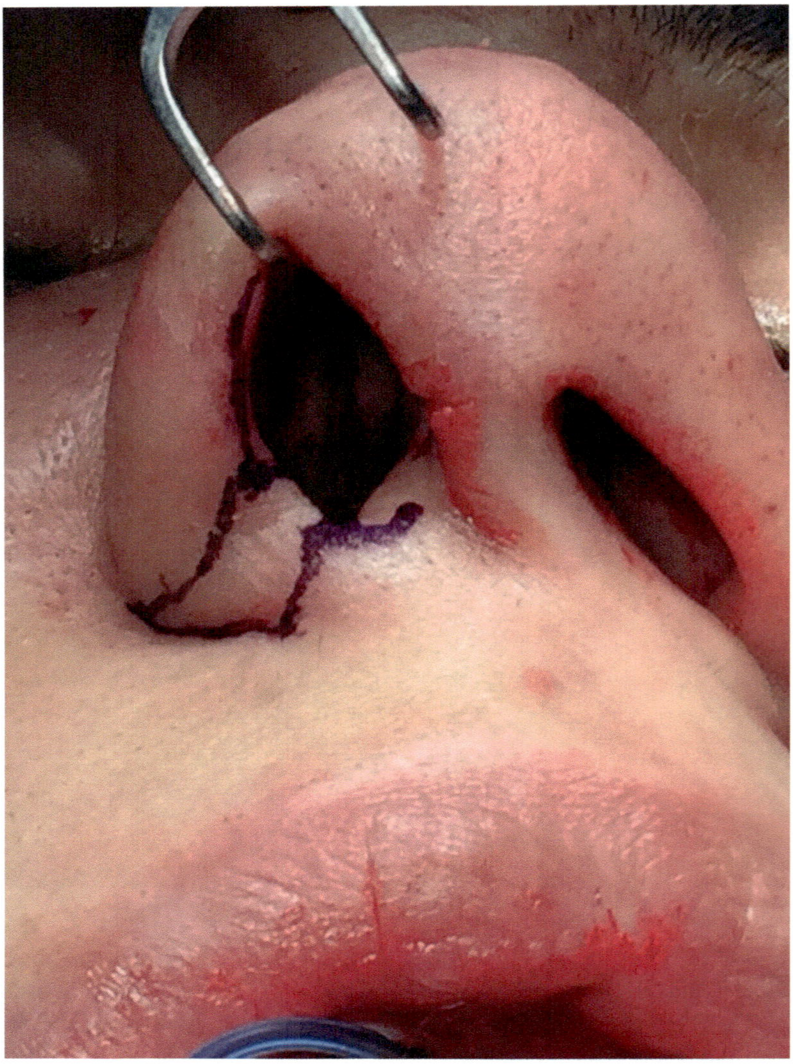

Fig. 21.67 The two marginal lines, the inferior alar and the anterior nasal sill margins

both inside the **nasal vestibule** and outside at the **posterior alar groove**.

Management of the Wide Nasal Aperture Tube

In cases of very wide nasal aperture tube, the size of the vestibular floor needs to be reduced as part of reduction of the size of the nasal aperture.

In these cases, the alar line and the sill line do not stop just above the aperture margin. They rather continue inside the vestibular floor for a variable distance, depending on the amount and the level of reduction in the size of the nasal aperture tube.

Both lines, and hence the vestibular line, may reach as high as the **muco-cutaneous line,** i.e., the upper limit of the aperture tube, In these cases, the whole length of the aperture tube is reduced in size.

The **alar line**, inside the nasal vestibule, must accurately follow the posterior alar margin. Care must be taken not to encroach upon the adherent vestibular skin of the inner surface of the alar nasi to avoid lateral angulation (Figs. 21.107 and 21.108).

Closure of a Wide Aperture Wound

Excision of a large and bulky rim-sill fold leaves a **wide gap** between the **ala nasi** and the **nasal**

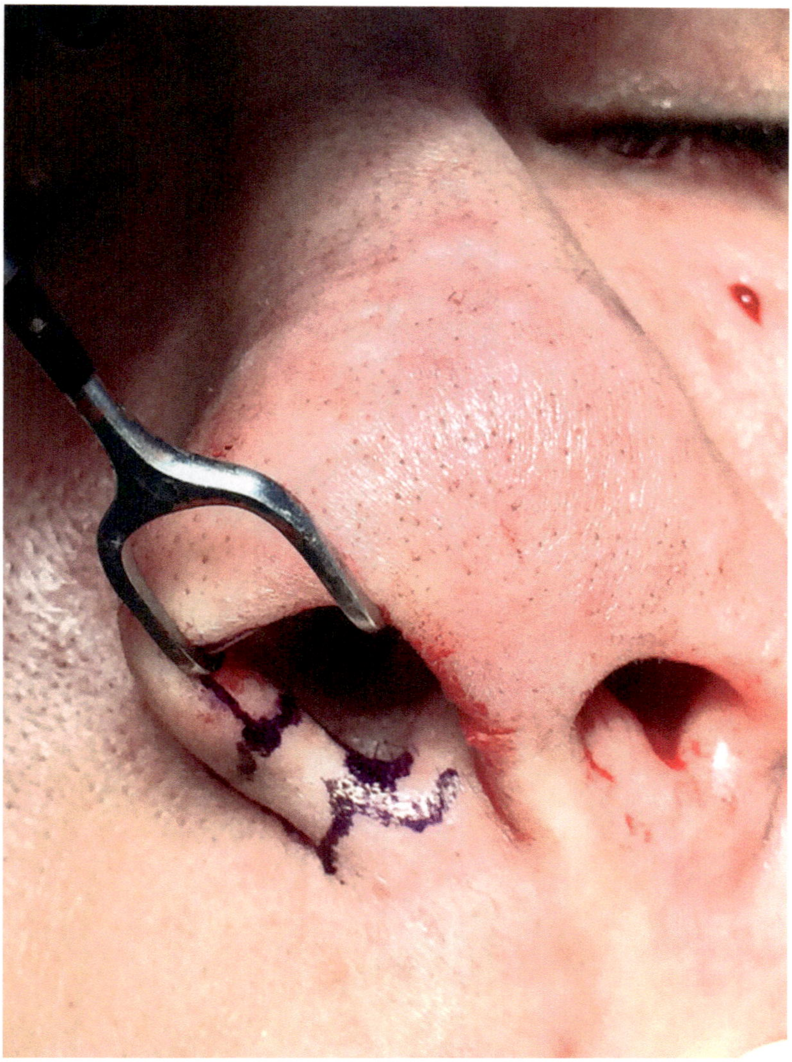

Fig. 21.68 The inferior segment of the rim-sill fold is stretched and the vestibular line, just inside it

sill band. **Four wound surfaces** are now present. **Firstly** is the nasal **sill margin** which is usually small as it is made of the stump of the sill band semicircular cut edge. **Secondly** is the **posterior alar margin** which is relatively long after excising the high posterior segment of rim-sill fold. **Thirdly** is the wide **raw surface in between the alar and sill margins**. This area lies over the orbicularis oris muscle. **Fourthly**, should part of the **vestibular floor** be excised, the resultant surface will be continuous with the previous raw surface (Figs. 21.89 and 21.96).

The wide gap between the **rim** and **sill** cut margins must be reduced so that the **submarginal stitch** can ultimately be taken accurately.

Reducing the Alar-Sill Gap

One or more stitches may be needed to approximate the **alar margin** to the **nasal sill band**. Using an absorbable 3 or 4 zero vycril, stitch that has ½ cm needle is used to approximate between the **posterior margin of the ala nasi** and the **medial end of the nasal sill band,** i.e., to bring about the two tough structures near to each other. This stitch has two sides of attachments:

(a) **The lateral side:**

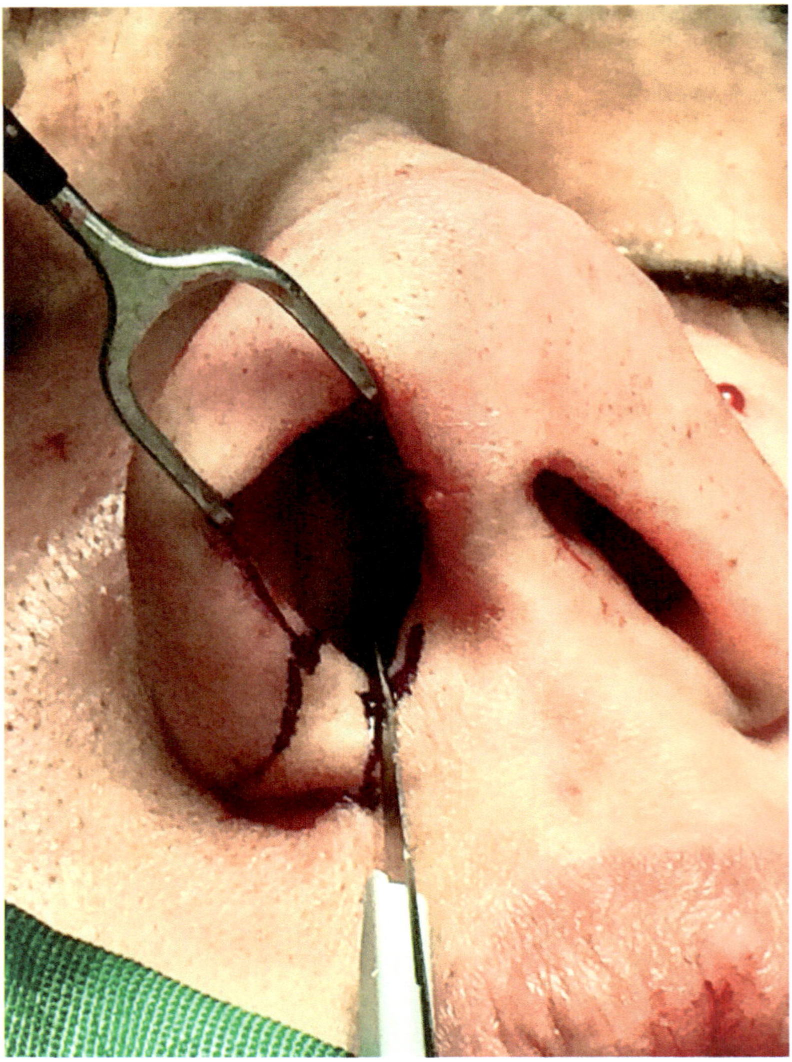

Fig. 21.69 Cutting through the sill line, down to the upper lip

A deep bite is taken through the tough body of the **posterior alar margin**, as it is exposed in the wound, at its junction with the soft connective tissue floor over the lip (Figs. 21.90 and 21.98).

(b) **The medial side:**

A second deep bite is taken by the needle through the **soft connective tissue floor** medially. The needle then comes out **just close** to, but not through, the **cut edge of the nasal sill band** (Figs. 21.91, 21.99 and 21.100).

Tightening of this stitch will move the **body of the ala nasi** both **medially** and **inferiorly**. This consequently will have the following effects:

i. The nasal or **alar base** is **reduced in size**.
ii. The **posterior alar groove moves medially** and the **superior groove** moves **inferiorly**. The **depth** of both grooves either maintained or deepened.
iii. The semicircular **cut margins** of the **ala nasi** and **nasal sill** become closer to each other and ready for the **submarginal stitch** (Figs. 21.92 , 21.93 , 21.100 and 21.101).

Now the **two tough structures** of the lateral **alar** and inferior **sill** walls are brought together to

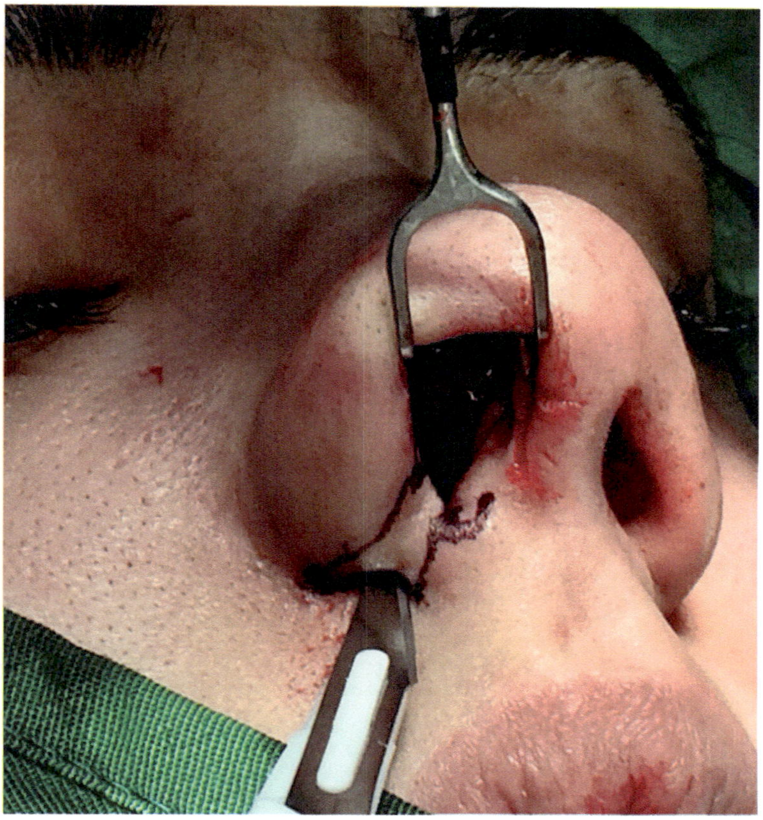

Fig. 21.70 Cutting into the posterior alar groove, through the sill line

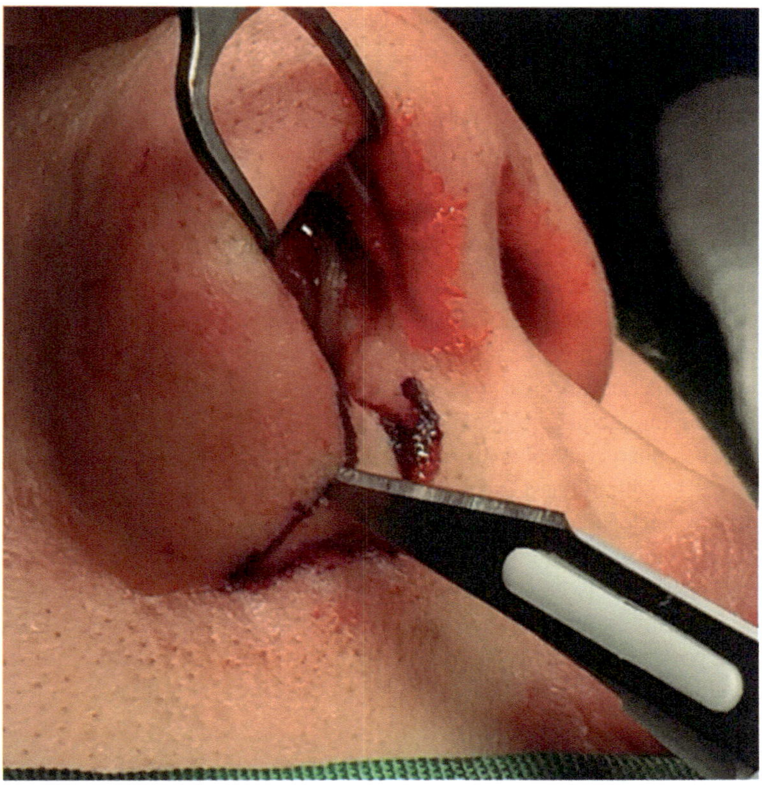

Fig. 21.71 Cutting through the alar line at the junction between posterior alar margin and the posterior segment of the rim-sill fold

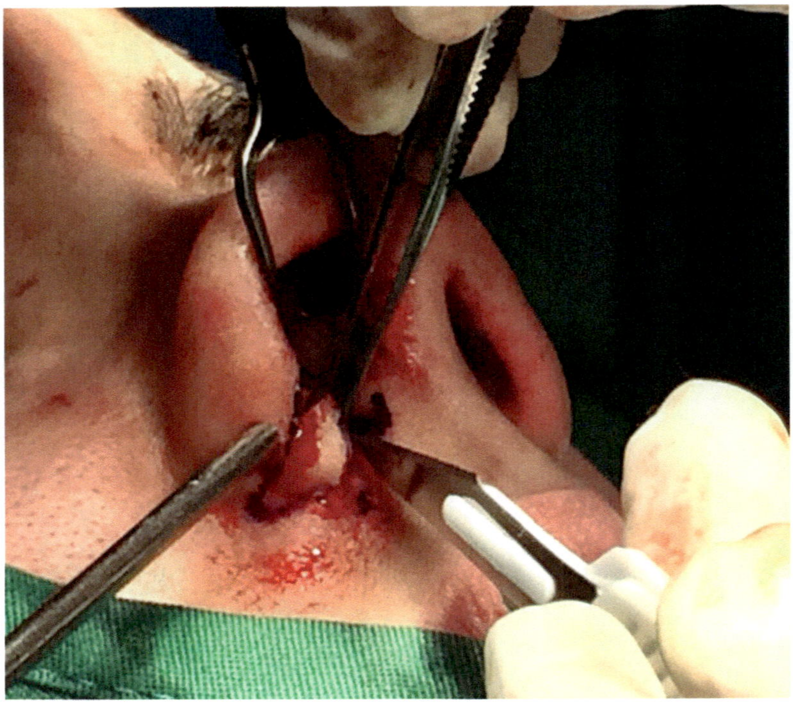

Fig. 21.72 Connecting the two incisions inside the nasal aperture margin, through to the vestibular line

make a new **smaller**, **aesthetically** pleasing and **firmly** structured nasal aperture.

Closure of the Vestibular Floor Wound

Absorbable vycril four zero stitches in a cutting ½–1 cm needle are preferred to close the vestibular skin wounds. Nylon stitches are difficult to remove post-operatively. Direct **deep square stitches are taken to evert** the vestibular skin margins.

Medialization of a Lateralized Ala Nasi

A **laterally placed ala nasi** may present in a naturally large nose or it may be iatrogenic following unequal surgical reduction of alar base. It may be unilateral or bilateral (Fig. 21.105).

The **posterior alar groove** has to move medially with ala nasi to reduce the overall basal attachment of the nose.

Medialization should take place from within the nasal cavity, via the rim-sill exploration, without any further external wounds. The inferior and posterior segments of the rim sill fold are accurately marked and excised after measuring an equal length of the nasal sill with the opposite side.

A judgement segment of the loose vestibular skin parallel to the inner side of the posterior alar margin is marked and excised (Figs. 21.106 and 21.107).

The posterior margin of the ala nasi is clearly seen through the lateral side of the wound (Fig. 21.107). A lateral bite is taken, by a cutting one cm vycril needle, close to or may include the posterior alar margin. The medial bite goes deep into the vestibular subcutaneous connective tissue, before it finally comes out at the medial cut wound edge of the vestibular floor (Fig. 21.108 and 21.109).

Finalization of the Alar Wounds

The external alar skin wound is closed using five or six zero proline stitches. The distance between the stitches should be close enough so that the alar wounds finally look neat and clean without any blood ooze. Opsite spray is useful to reduce the disturbing post-operative crustation and infection (Figs. 21.110 and 21.111).

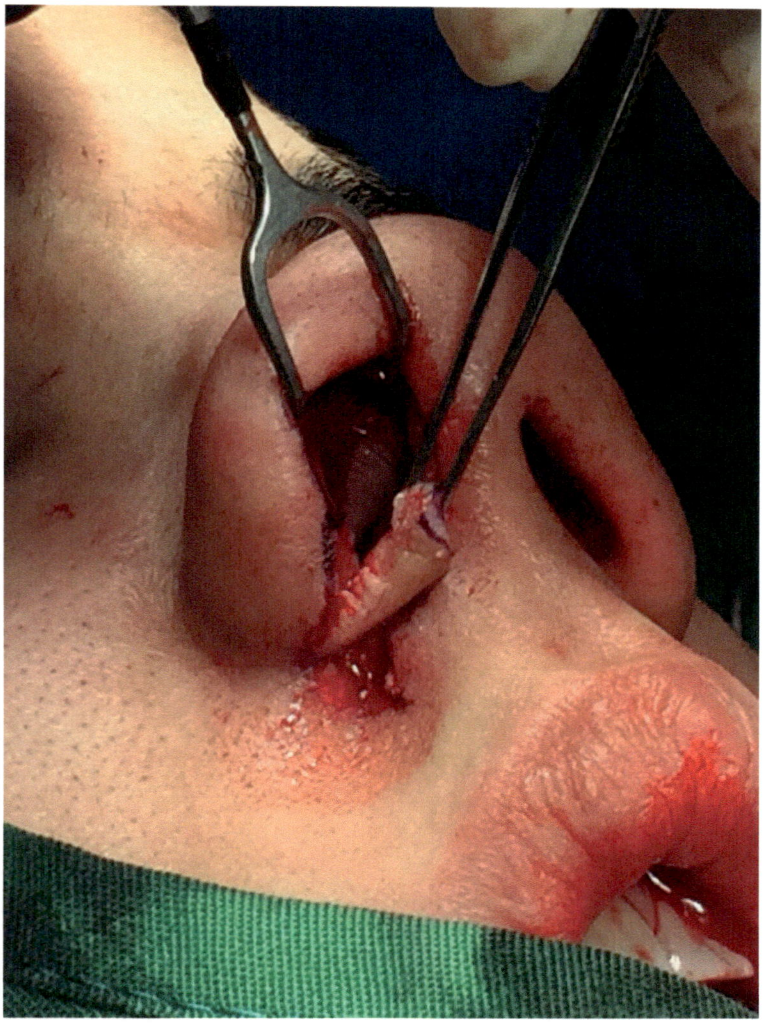

Fig. 21.73 Excising the posterior and inferior segments of the rim-sill fold en bloc

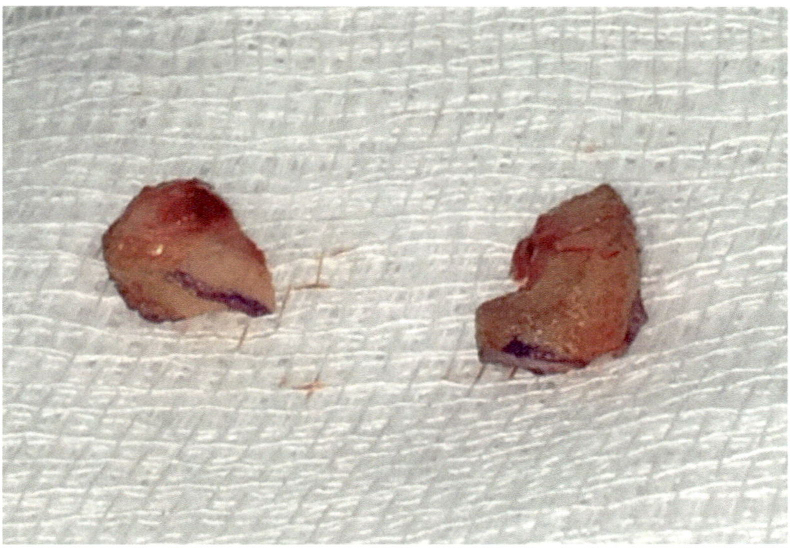

Fig. 21.74 The two rim-sill folds after excision

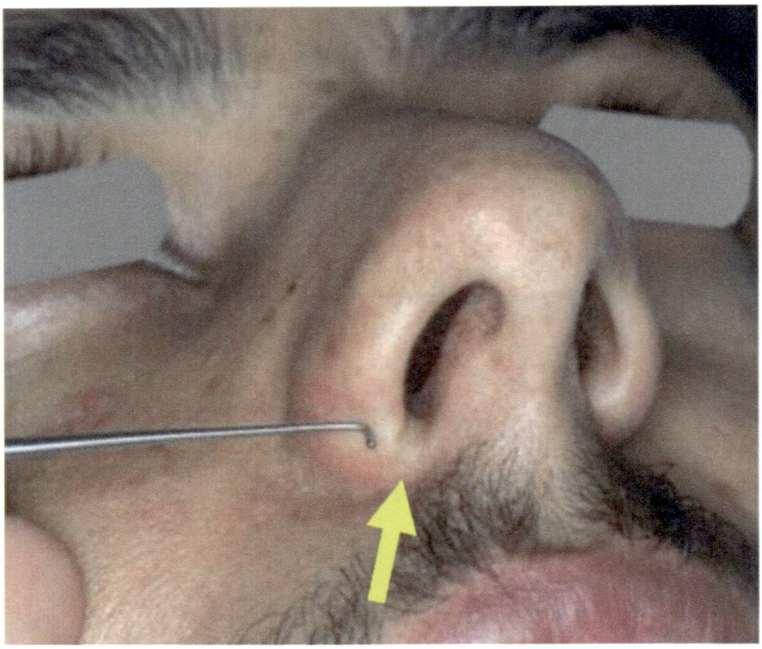

Fig. 21.75 Performing the Rim-Sill test. The soft inferior Rim-Sill segment (yellow arrow) is shown between the two creases: the inferior alar margin laterally and the nasal Sill Band medially

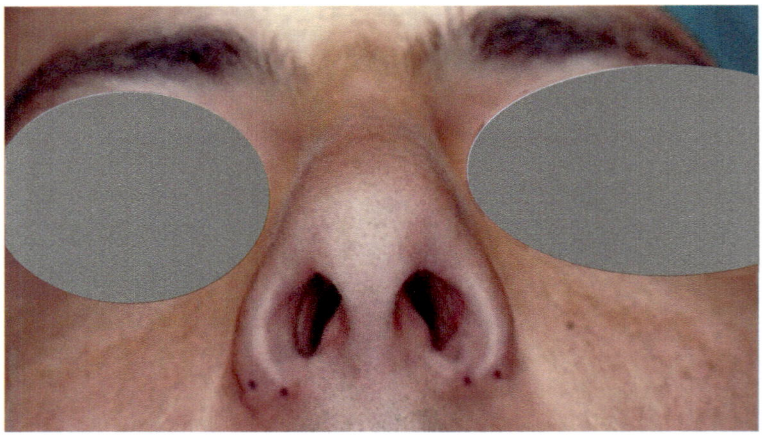

Fig. 21.76 Two dots are added. The lateral dot at the posterior margin of the alar rim and the medial dot is at the lateral end of the nasal Sill Band

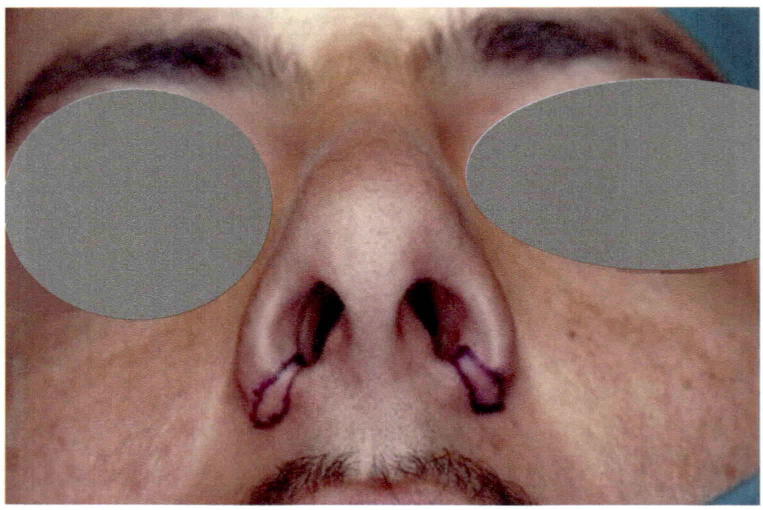

Fig. 21.77 Marking the inferior segment of the Rim-Sill Folds by the sill line medially and alar line laterally

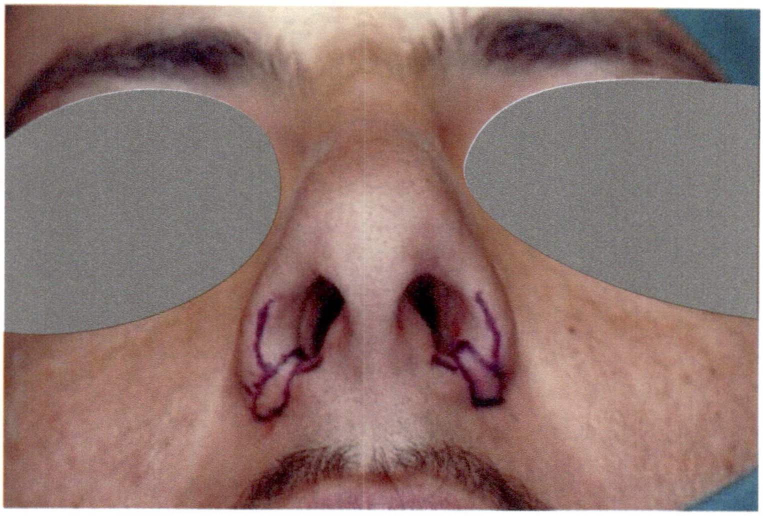

Fig. 21.78 The marginal lines (corresponded to the light reflex) and the Vestibular lines are placed

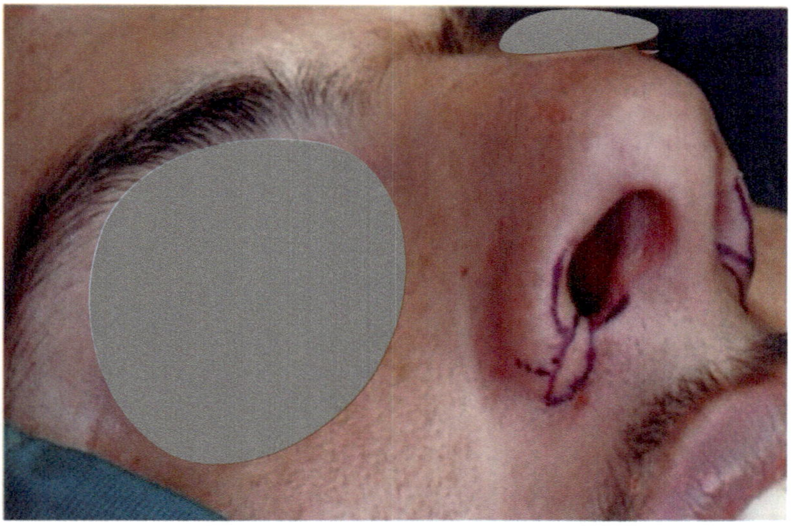

Fig. 21.79 The posterior segment of the Rim-Sill fold is marked with a dotted line

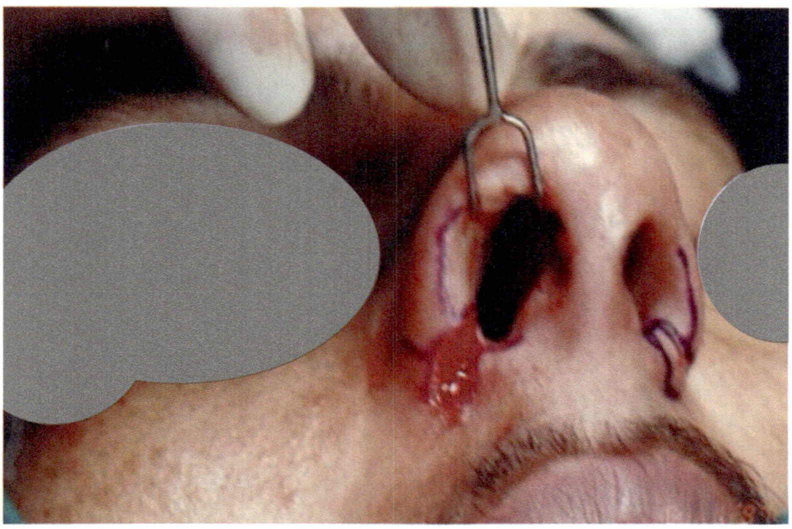

Fig. 21.80 The inferior segment of the Rim-Sill fold is excised

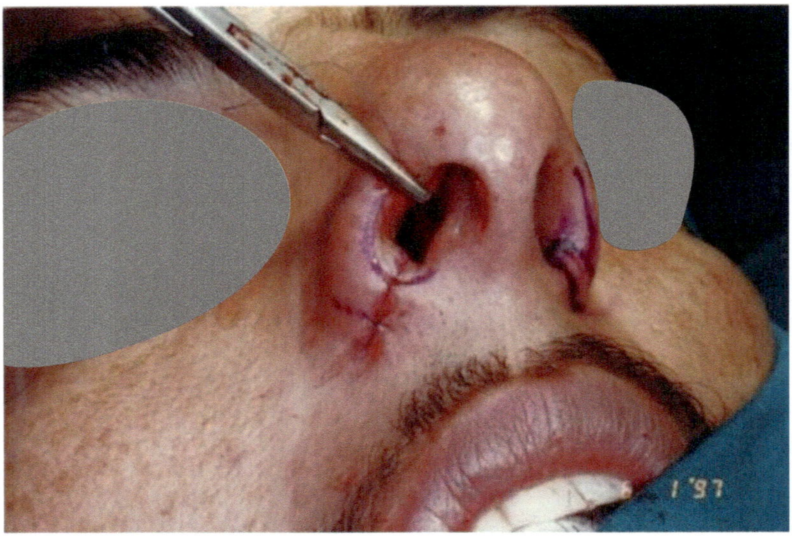

Fig. 21.81 The three-stitch technique. The rim and sill lines become one continuous line

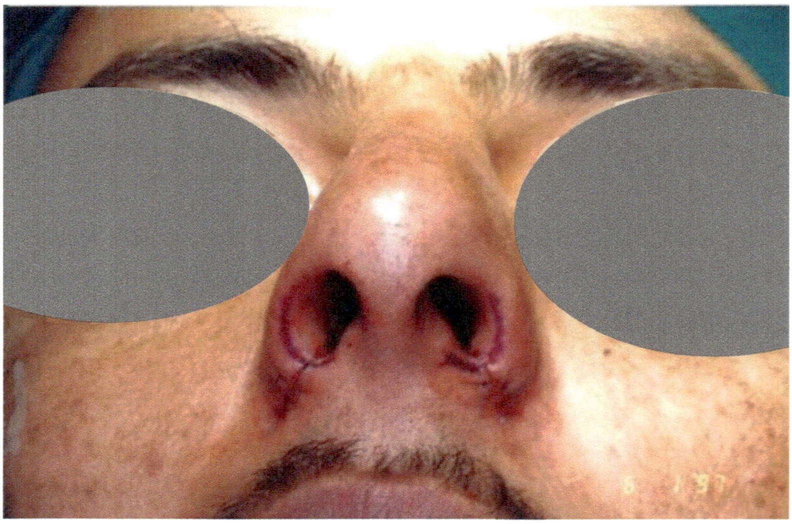

Fig. 21.82 The two inferior segments of the Rim-Sill folds are excised. There is a natural continuation between the inferior alar margin and the prominence of the nasal Sill Band

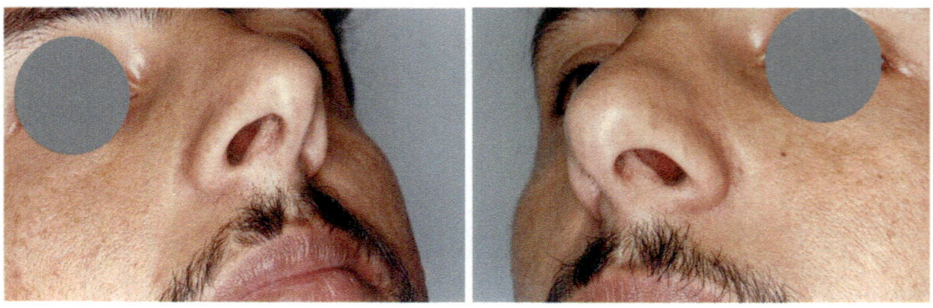

Fig. 21.83 Pre operative right nasal aperture view

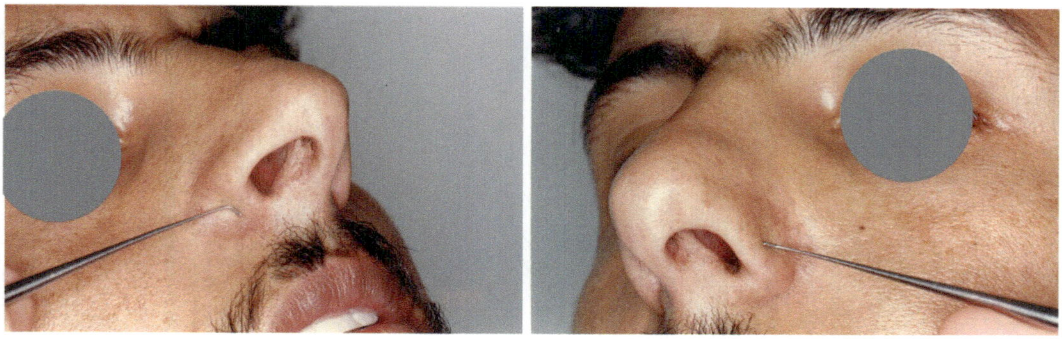

Fig. 21.84 The left rim-sill test demonstrates the inferior segment while the right rim-sill test demonstrates the posterior and inferior segments

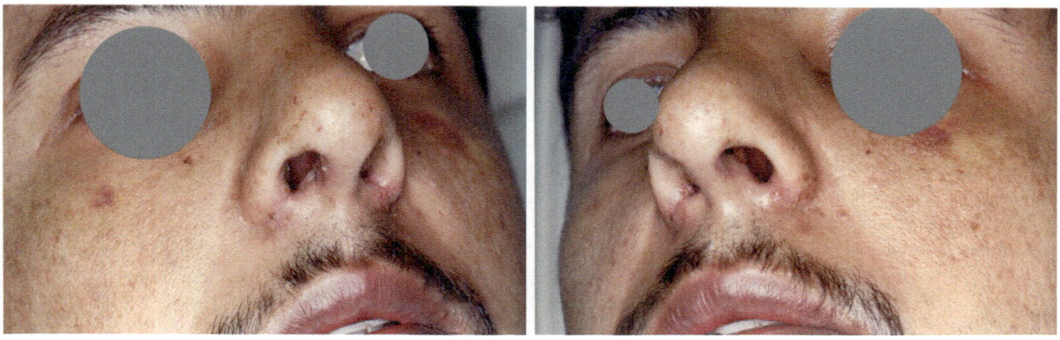

Fig. 21.85 One-week post-surgery, immediately after removing the stitches

Fig. 21.86 Preoperative basal view

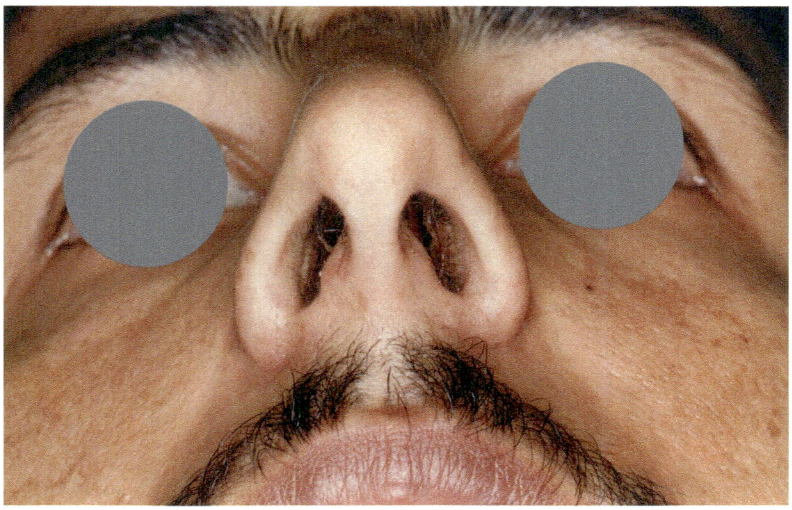

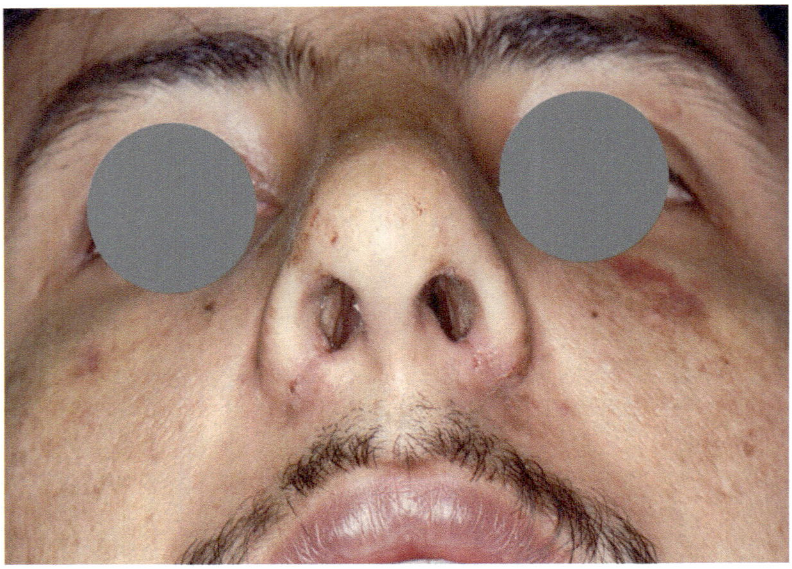

Fig. 21.87 Basal view one week after surgery. The photograph taken for the patient demonstrated in (Figs. 21.75, 21.76, 21.77, 21.78, 21.79, 21.80, 21.81 and 21.82) before, during and after surgery

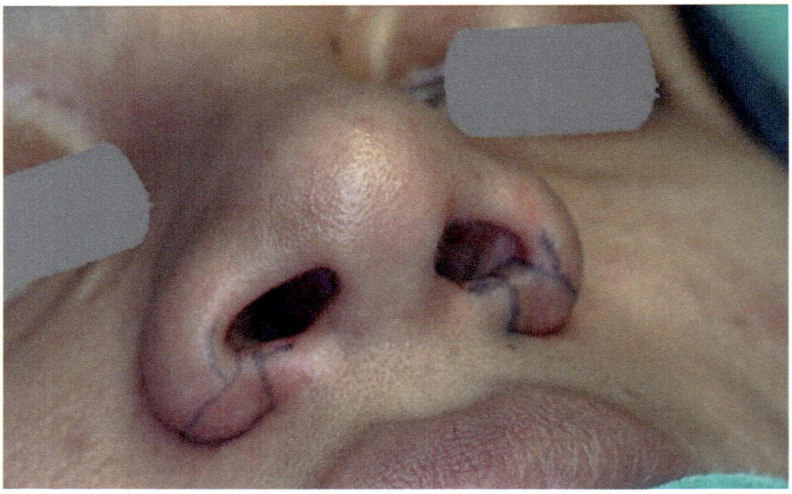

Fig. 21.88 Complete marking of the rim-sill folds. Sill line, alar line, marginal lines and vestibular line

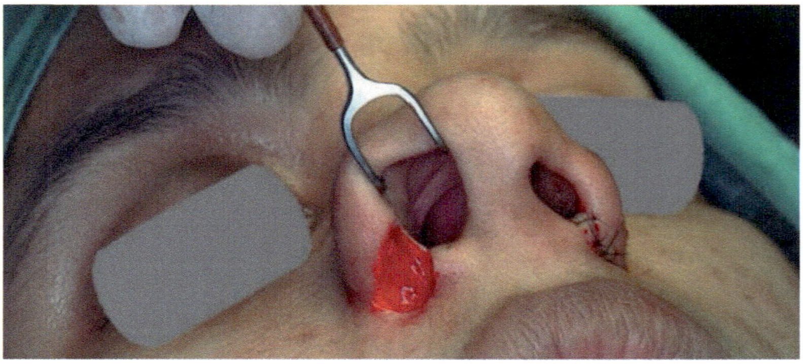

Fig. 21.89 Wide gap after excision of the two segments of the right rim-sill fold

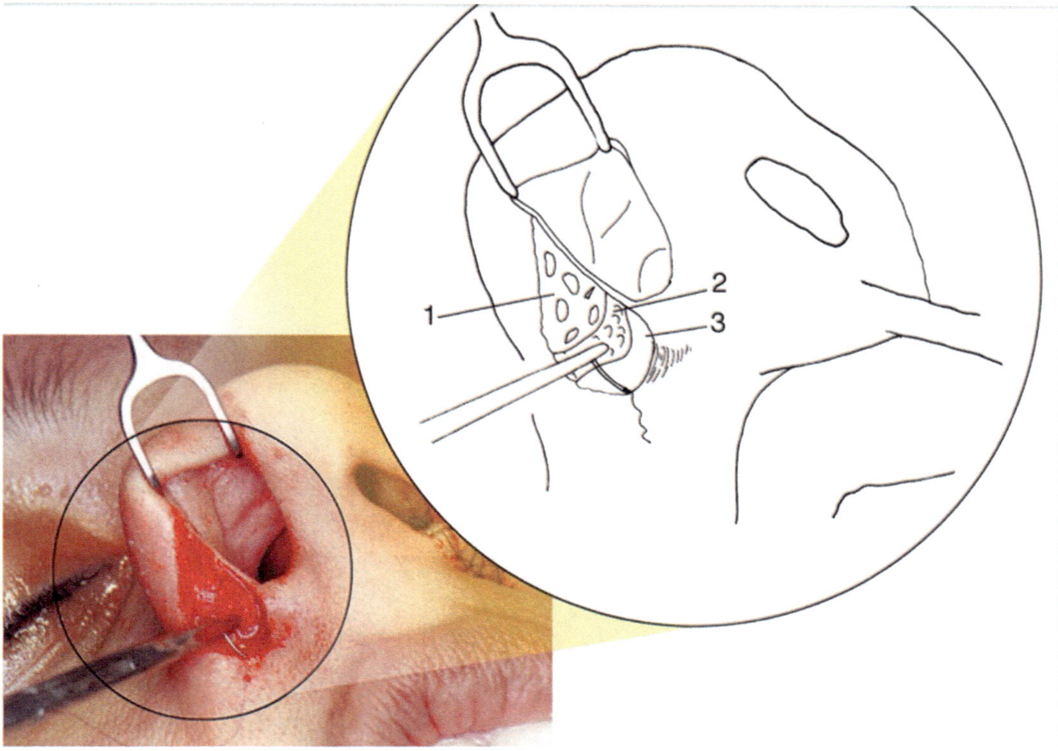

Fig. 21.90 Reducing the wide Alar-Sill gap. The subdermal stitch is taken from the floor of the wound near the cut edge of sill band to the posterior alar margin. 1. Posterior Alar Margin. 2. The floor of the rim-sill wound. 3. The lateral cut edge of the nasal sill band

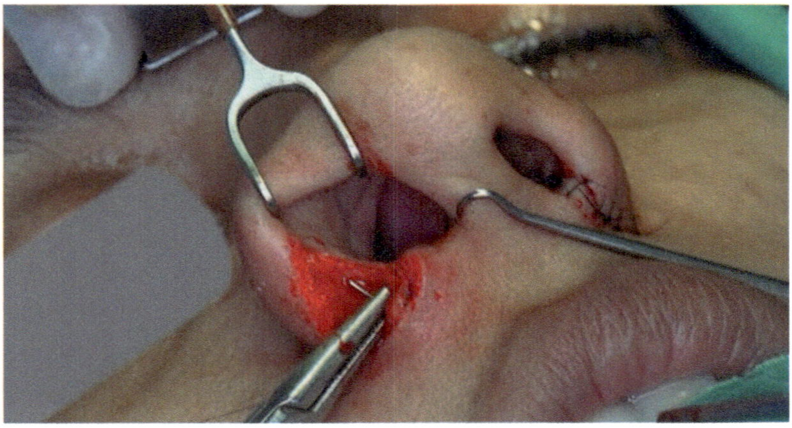

Fig. 21.91 The medial stitch, from the floor of the rim-sill wound to the area close to the nasal sill band

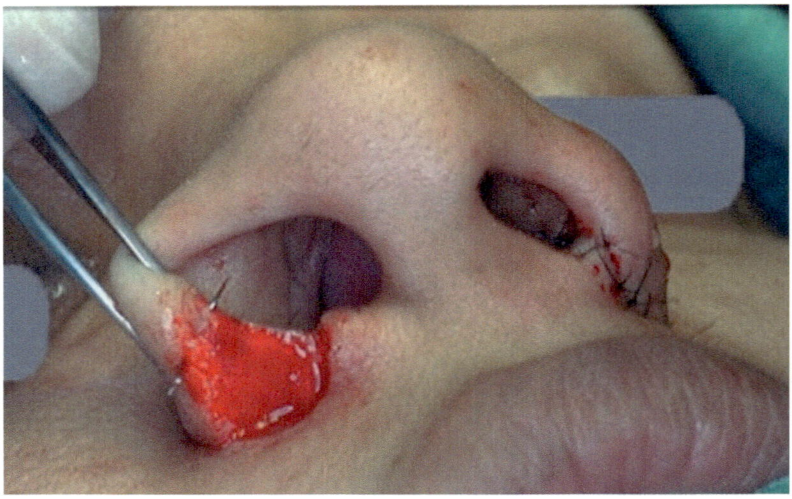

Fig. 21.92 The alar submarginal stitch. The rim-sill gap has been narrowed down

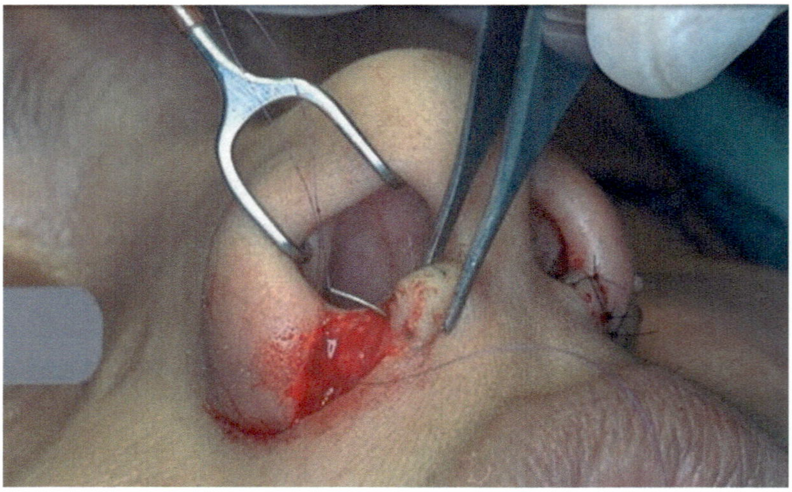

Fig. 21.93 The sill submarginal stitch

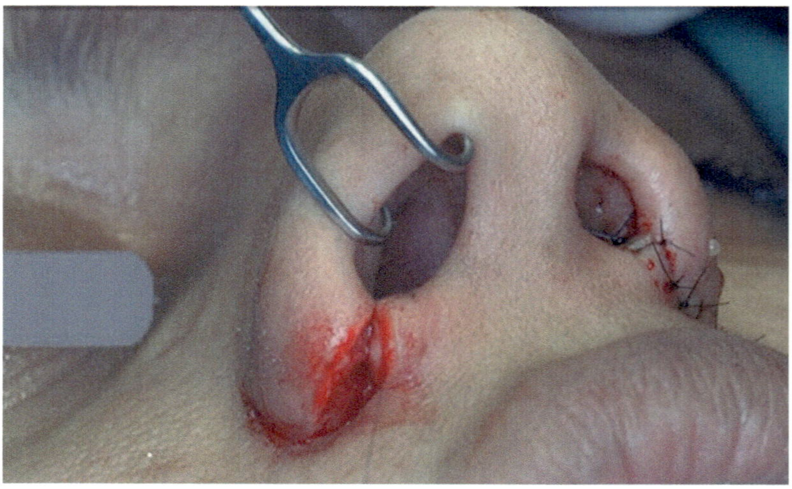

Fig. 21.94 Closure of the submarginal stitches together

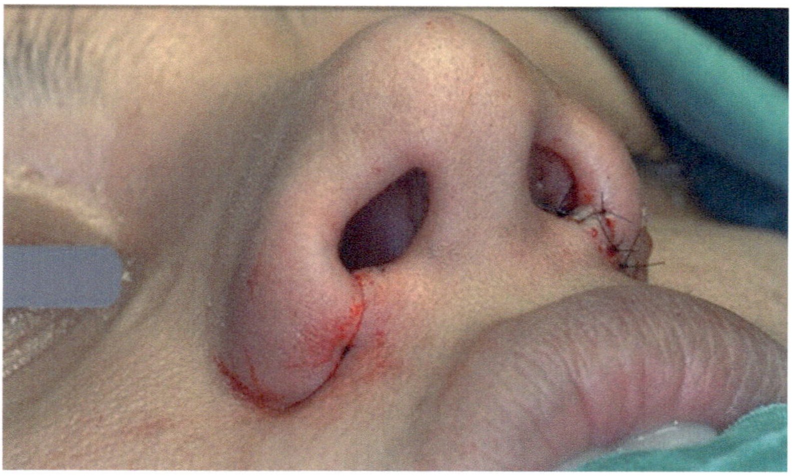

Fig. 21.95 The natural appearance of the aperture margin. The posterior alar groove angle is wider

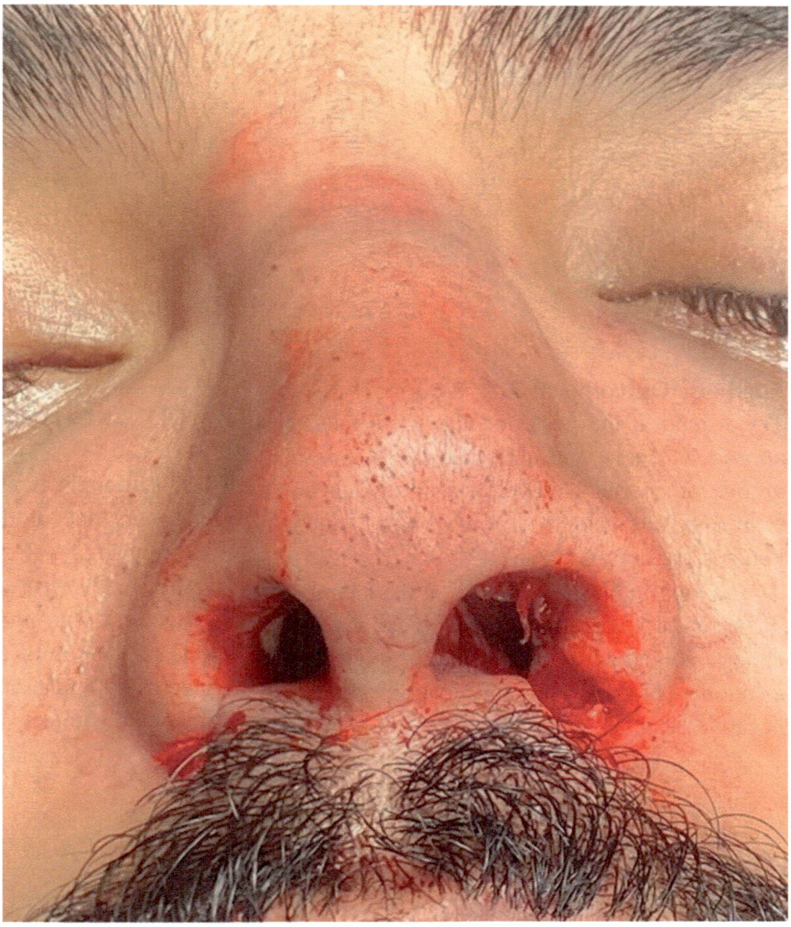

Fig. 21.96 Reducing a wide Alar-Sill gap in a small nose. Wide gap after excision of a large left inferior rim-sill segment

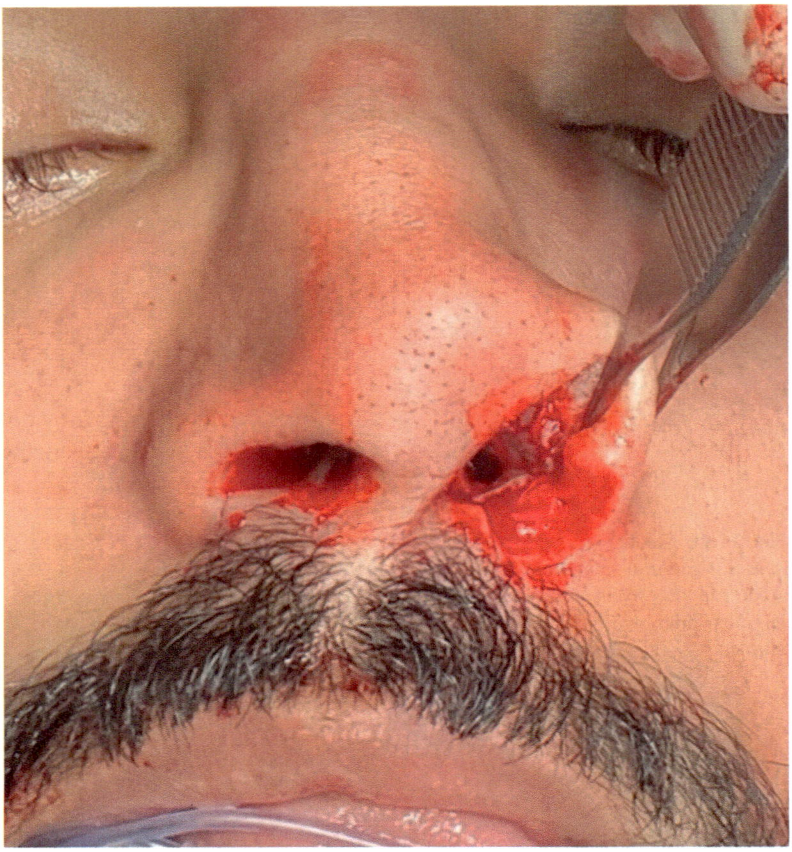

Fig. 21.97 Pulling the ala nasi laterally demonstrates the width of the gap

Aesthetic Outcome of Alar Wounds

The wound at the posterior alar groove usually appears as a new and quite natural looking alar groove or crease. It never appears as a wound right from the moment of removing the stitches. Patients are quite satisfied.

The longitudinal cut wounds at the lateral end of the nasal sill appear as two linear scars that almost, totally disappear in 2–3 months. Its location is hidden away and does not have any negative aesthetic effect.

21.14 Surgery of the Flat Triangle

The flat triangle is a two-layered soft skin area that covers one of the nasal gaps at the nasal floor.

Any inadvertent injury that may lead to damage and scarring of the skin and subdermal connective tissue of this triangle will lead to an aesthetically unpleasant notching that looks ugly. The notching defect is seen anteriorly in the nasal front.

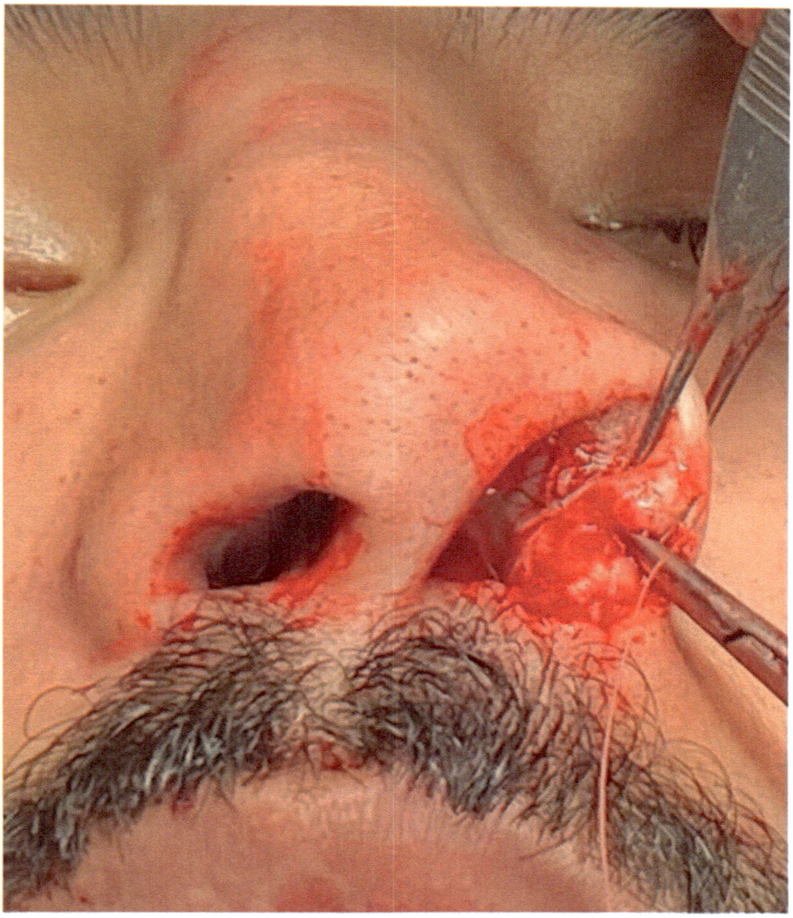

Fig. 21.98 The lateral subdermal stitch

The commonest cause of damage to this triangle is a long-standing nasogastric tube that usually slides anteriorly against the flat triangle causing trauma, infection and scarring.

The fibrosed notched triangle is quite an unpleasant difficult surgical challenge.

21.14.1 Acute Injury of the Flat Triangle

If the fold of the flat triangle was inadvertently cut or damaged during surgery, this must be recognized and dealt with immediately by primary repair.

The skin fold has to be stitched in two separate layers, the vestibular skin and the external skin, using six zero Vicryl or nylon stitches. It is preferable to use absorbable Vicryl rapid for the vestibular skin, because it would be quite a difficult task to remove the nylon stitches amid the vestibular hair (Figs. 21.112 and 21.113).

The connective tissue layer must be kept free. Stitches of each skin layer must only include one layer at a time and avoid transfixing or anchoring the other layer.

This avoids scaring of the subdermal connective tissue layer and hence late notching or depression of the flat triangle.

21.14.2 Chronic Damage of the Flat Triangle

Delayed unrecognized damage to the flat triangle will lead to fibrosis and contraction of the

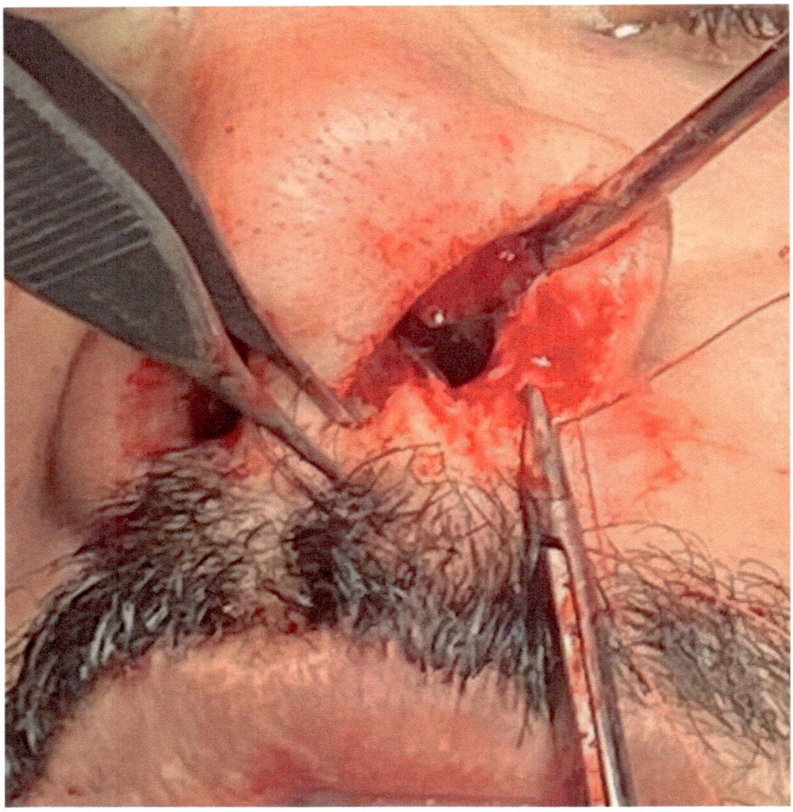

Fig. 21.99 The medial subdermal stitch

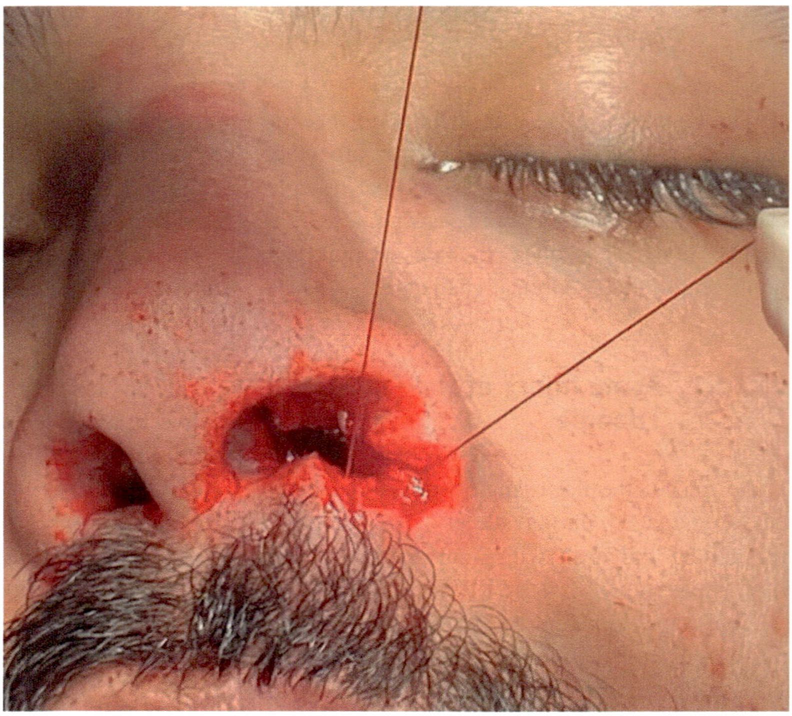

Fig. 21.100 Pulling on the two sides of the stitch, demonstrating the gap to be closed

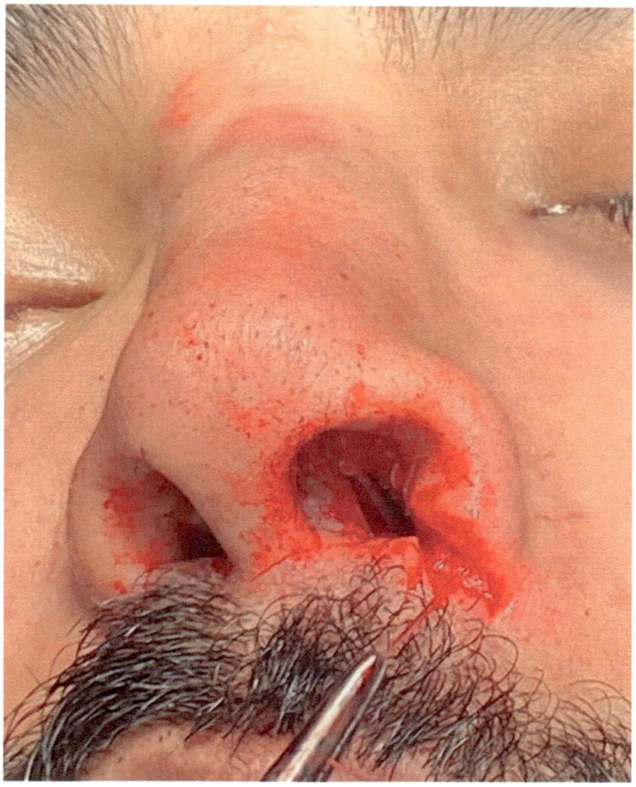

Fig. 21.101 Reduction of the gap, after tightening the subdermal stitches

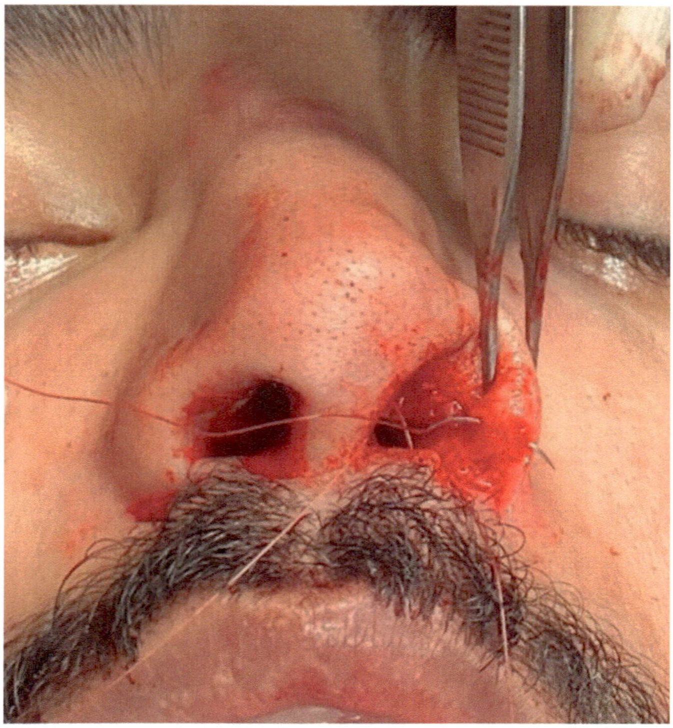

Fig. 21.102 The alar submarginal stitch

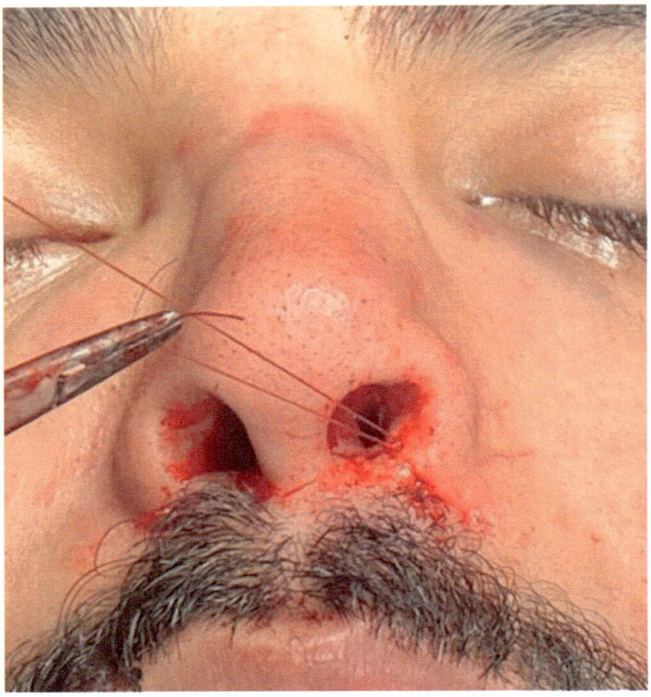

Fig. 21.103 Closure of the submarginal stitches resulting in a naturally rounded margin. Note the continuous line of light that reflects from the inferior alar margin and the anterior margin of the nasal sill

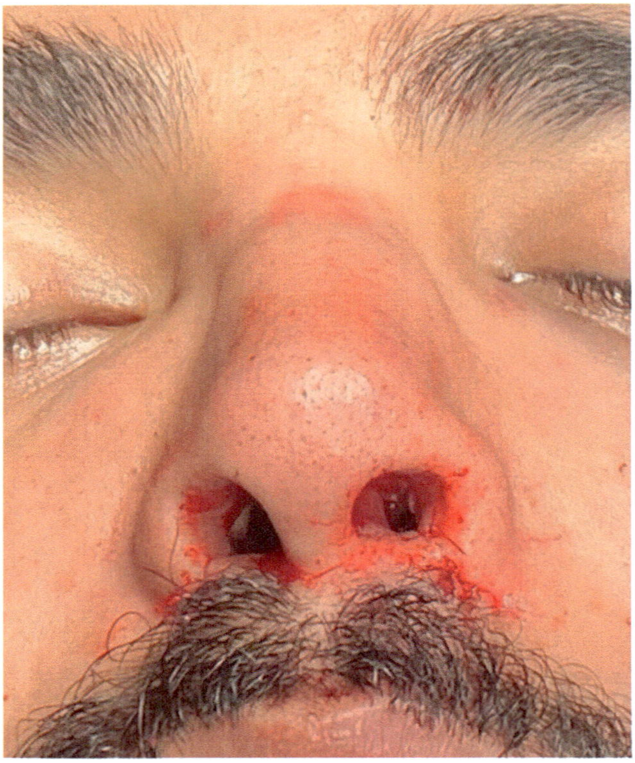

Fig. 21.104 Nasal aperture looks naturally round with invisible wound. Note the continuous line of light reflex

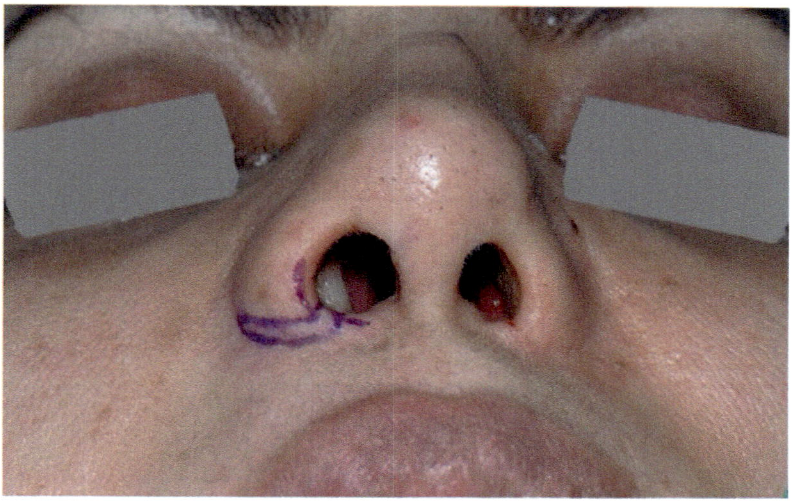

Fig. 21.105 Medialization of a secondary lateralised right ala nasi

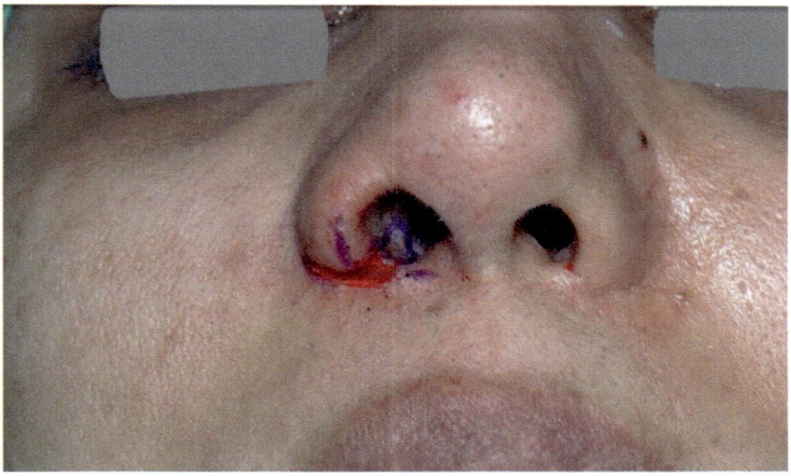

Fig. 21.106 The posterior and inferior segments of the rim-sill fold are excised. Note, the marking of the planned segment to be excision from the vestibular floor

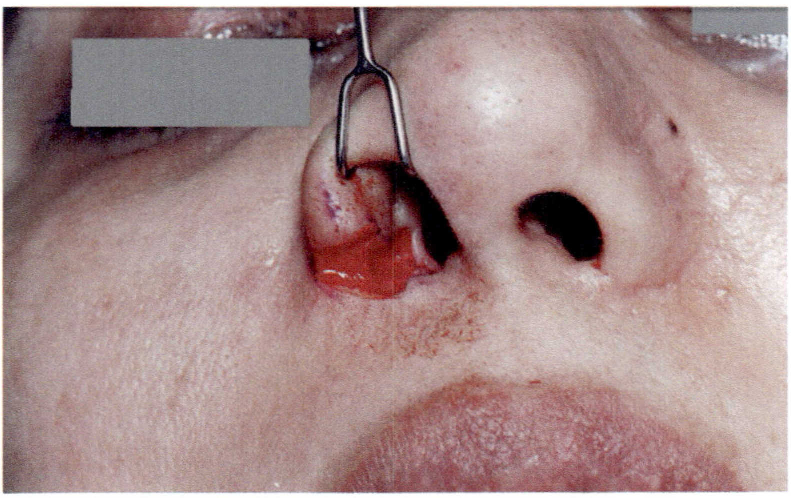

Fig. 21.107 Segment excision of the vestibular floor up to the muco-cutaneous junction, just medial to the posterior margin of the right ala nasi

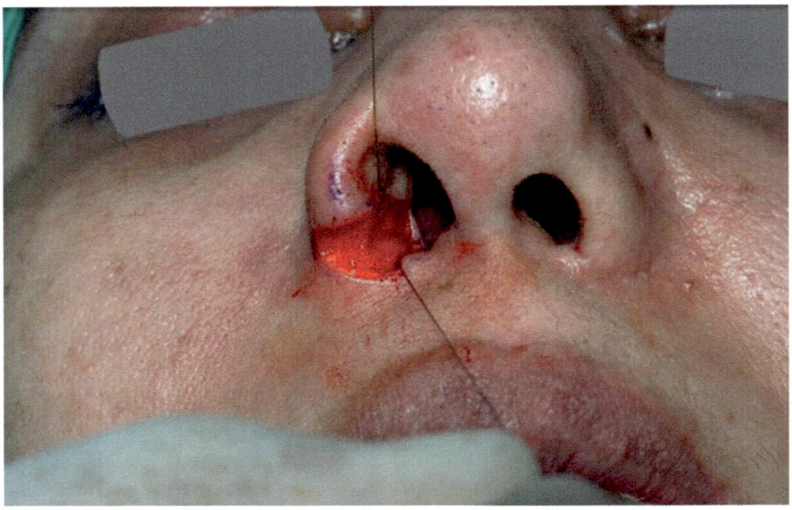

Fig. 21.108 Stitch between the posterior alar margin to the most medial deep end of the wound

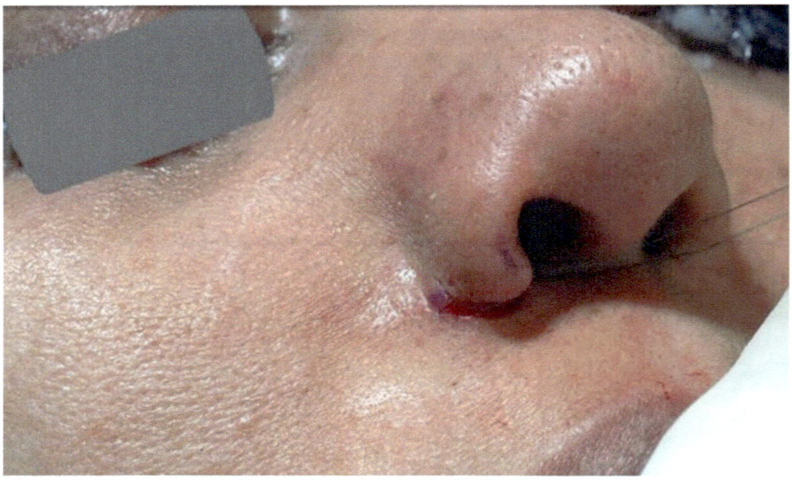

Fig. 21.109 Medialization of the ala nasi, on tightening the vestibular stitch

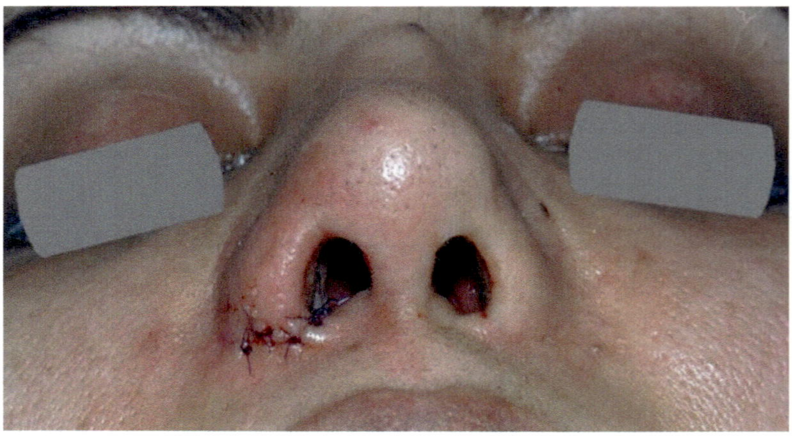

Fig. 21.110 Final appearance with equal nasal apertures. Minimal lateral crural prominencies are noted

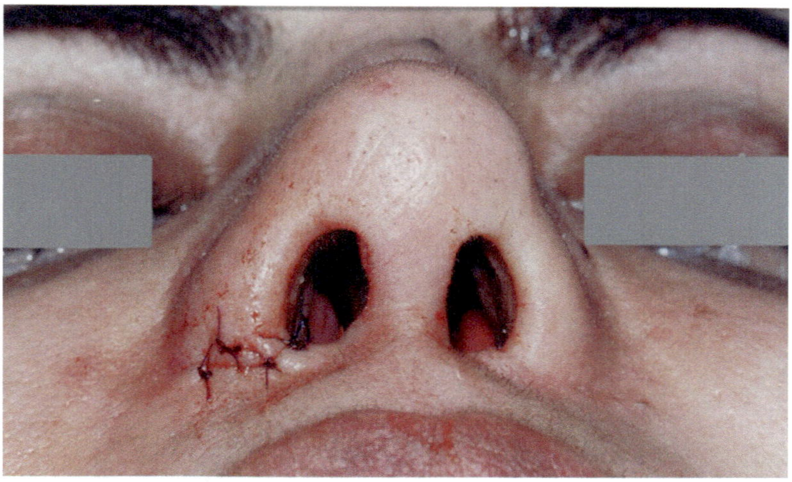

Fig. 21.111 The lateral crural prominencies are abolished by a transcolumellar stitch. Swelling of the posterior alar groove settles in a few weeks time

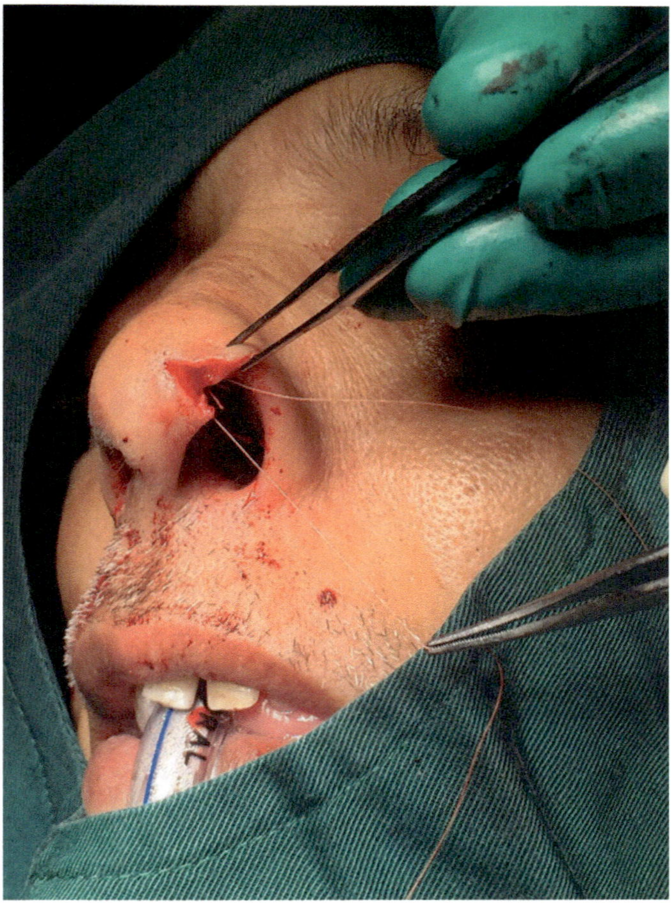

Fig. 21.112 Surgery of acute injury of the flat triangle. Stitching the vestibular skin layer of the left flat acute triangular wound

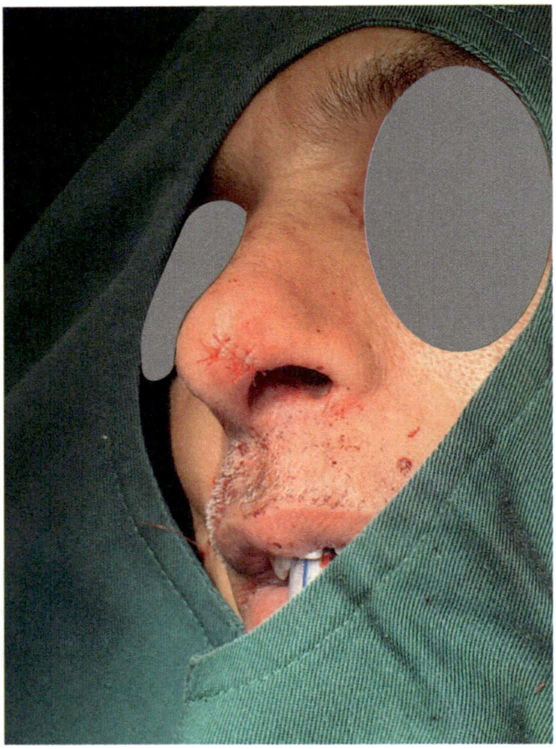

Fig. 21.113 The stitching of the external skin layer of the left flat acute triangular wound

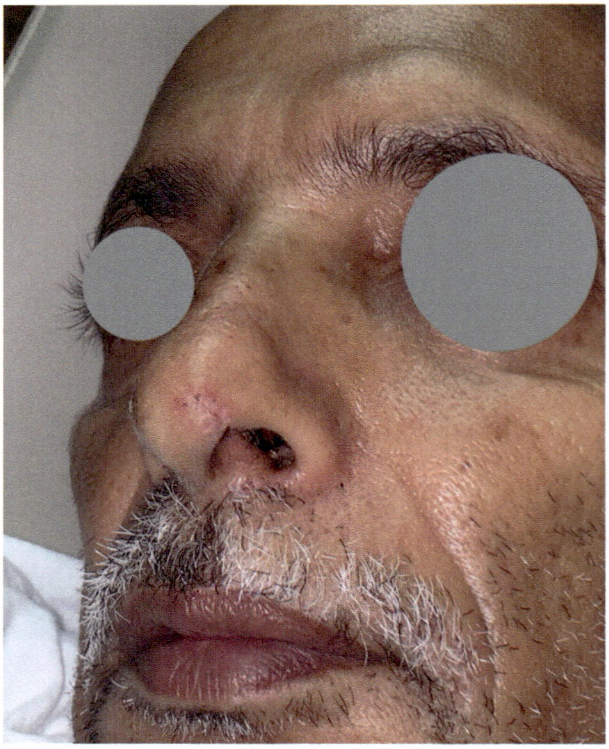

Fig. 21.114 The appearance of the wound one week after surgery. Note there is slight notching at the alar margin

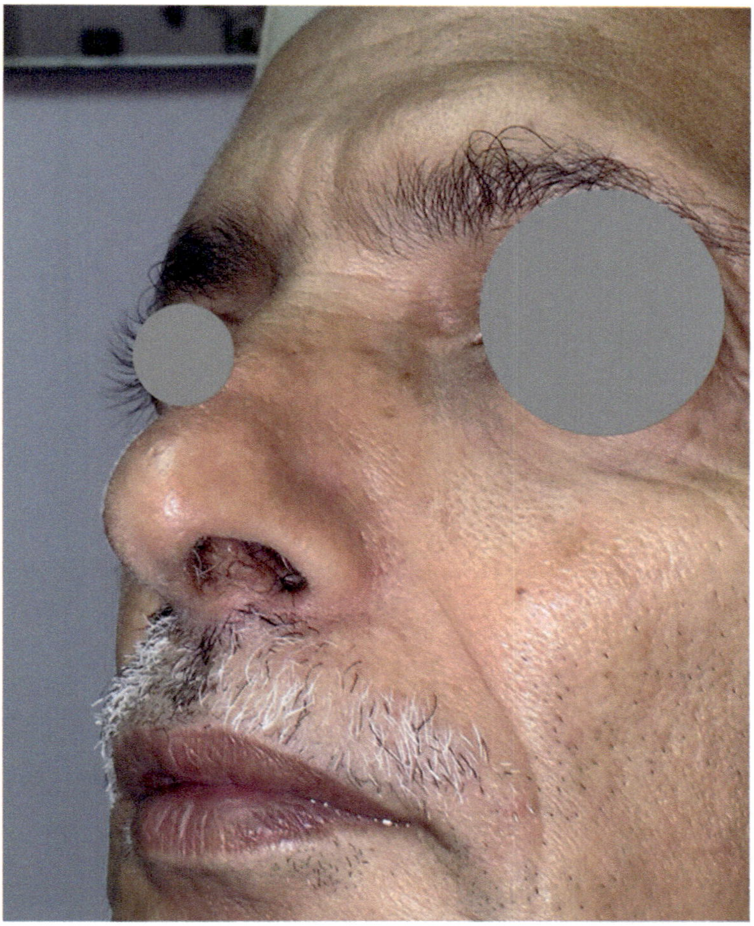

Fig. 21.115 Six weeks after surgery. The external surface and alar margins are naturally smooth

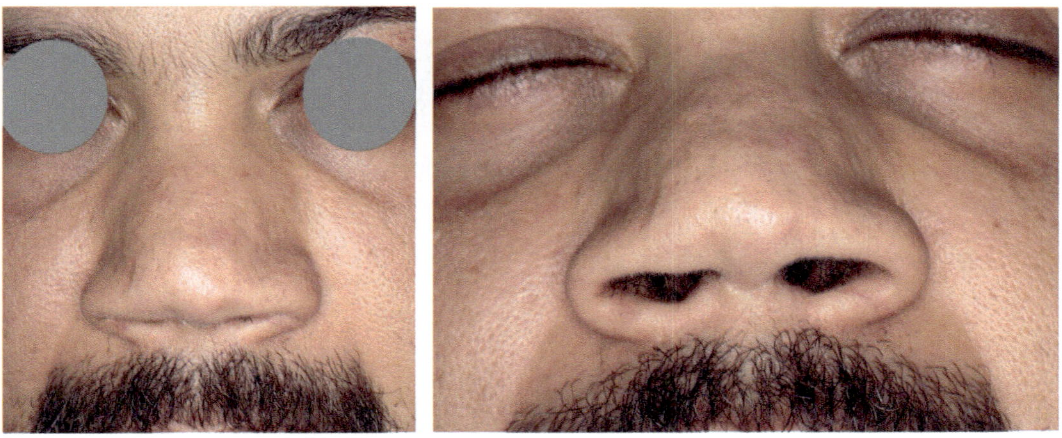

Fig. 21.116 Chronic depressed scarring of the right flat triangle. Preoperative frontal and backward tiling views. Scarring and depression of the right flat triangle

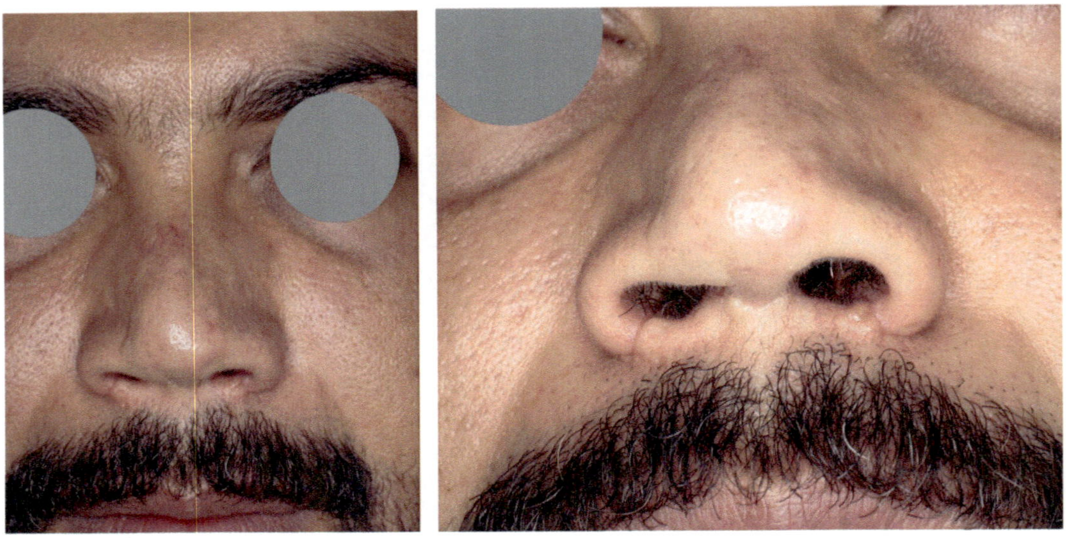

Fig. 21.117 The use of bone graft in filling the severely scarred flat triangle. The right flat triangle regained its contour post-operatively

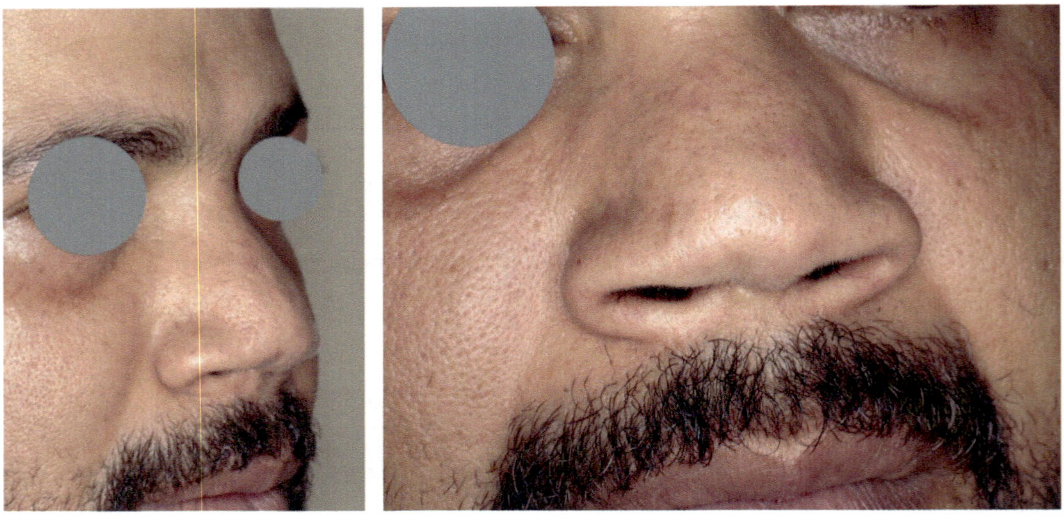

Fig. 21.118 Oblique views demonstrating depressed scarred right left triangle

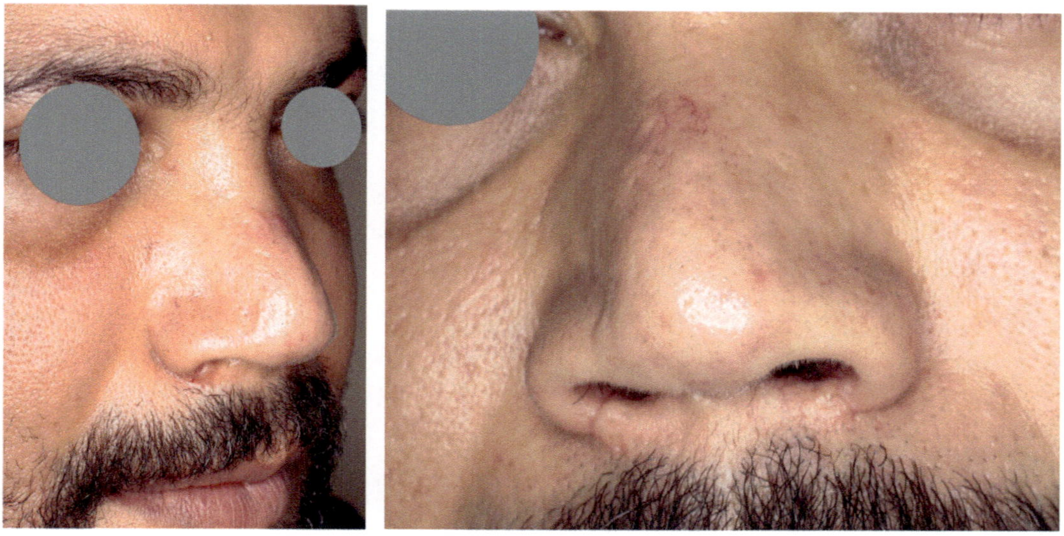

Fig. 21.119 Another post operative views. The right flat triangle regained its contour post-operatively

subdermal connective tissue layer. This consequently makes the triangle lose its nice, smooth, soft and flat surface. Instead, it appears as an ugly **depression** (Figs. 21.116 and 21.118) or a **notch** on the frontal surface of the nose.

Causes of Chronic damage are:

i. A misplaced and neglected nasogastric tube. Constant pressure and accumulation of secretions will lead to infection and gradual erosion of the skin fold of the flat triangle.
ii. Neglected injury leads to infection and scarring.
iii. Undue manipulations and injuries that affect the flat triangle during surgery of the middle and lateral crurae.

21.14.2.1 Management

There is no way to regain the lost connective tissue layer. The only way to deal with this situation is to **fill the** potential space between the two skin layers of the **triangle** with **a piece of thick bony septal graft**. The crushed cartilages do not give enough support and it will resorb and fibrose in the long term (Fig. 21.119).

22 Clinical Varieties of Rhinoplasty

Abstract

There are wide varieties of clinical conditions that may present for Rhinoplasty. One predominant feature me be the most prominent anesthetic part of the nose. A person may present predominantly because of his large nose, bulky nose, deviated nose, oblique nose, crooked nose or fractured nose. People from different ethnic backgrounds may ask for Rhinoplasty. Pediatric and secondary Rhinoplasty are is another group which may seek Rhinoplasty. Finesse Rhinoplasty. These are individuals who have noses that we see every day as normal or even attractive. Many of them do not seek surgery, and if they ask then they may be helped. These noses have no apparent deformities, injuries or defects, yet they present for Rhinoplasty.

Keywords

Finesse rhinoplasty · The large nose · The bulky nose · Defatting · The deviated nose · The crooked nose · Bilateral maxillary asymmetry · Rhinoplasty of the fractured nose · Fracture of the cartilaginous septum · Fracture of the nasal bones · Fracture of the frontal process of maxilla · Secondary rhinoplasty · Clinical varieties of secondary rhinoplasty

22.1 Part I: Finesse Rhinoplasty

These are individuals who have noses that we see every day as normal or even attractive. Many of them do not seek surgery, and if they ask then they may be helped. These noses have no apparent deformities, injuries or defects, yet they present for rhinoplasty in one of the following clinical presentations:

(1) A patient may have quite an **attractive-looking nose**, yet seeks further improvement in the appearance of the nose.
(2) A patient may have an **attractive nose**, yet there are **one or more** areas that are **not in harmony** with the rest of the nose, e.g. protruding columella, wide alar base, broad bony pyramid or the presence of certain defect or protrusion.
(3) A nose that is generally **acceptable**, yet not quite attractive. Only minimal changes in one or more areas are necessary to transform this nose into an attractive nose.

In all types of rhinoplasty, the patient has to be prepared psychologically and physically.

All four areas are examined clinically.

22.1.1 The Frontolateral Walls

Despite being attractive the frontolateral walls may be slightly large, overshadowing the alae

M. H. A. Shafy, *Innovations in Rhinoplasty*,
https://doi.org/10.1007/978-3-030-94573-2_22

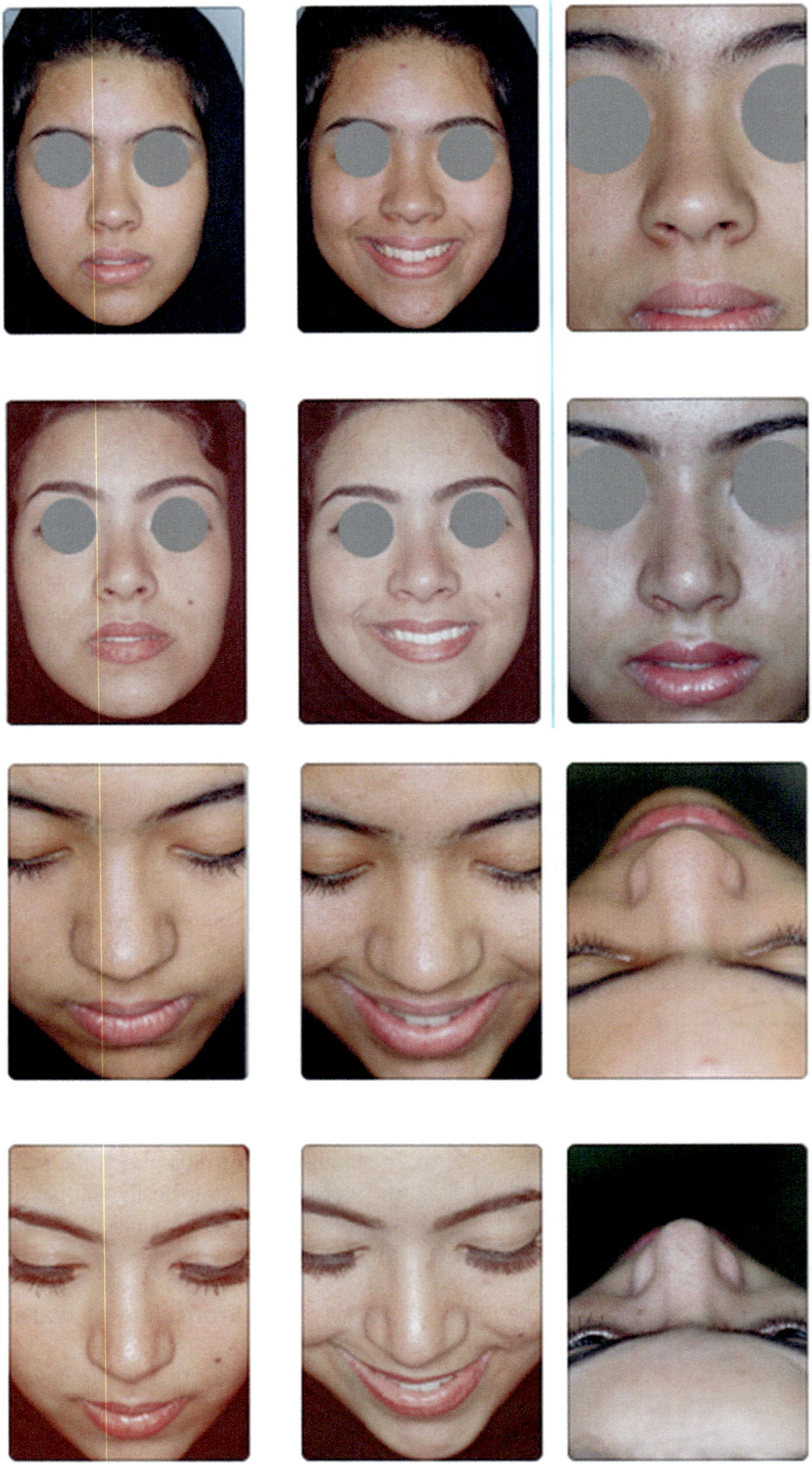

Fig. 22.1 Predominant Frontolateral Wall Surgery

nasi. The latter does not have their fair share in nasal aesthetics.

Simple defatting of the frontolateral walls coupled with medialization of the bony pyramid sidewalls usually has a positive aesthetic enhancement to the nose and the face (Fig. 22.1).

22.1.2 The Medial Wall

A protruding or hanging columella, mobile tip, animation or sliding tip, all could have negative effects on an attractive nose. Each condition is simple to overcome (Fig. 22.2).

22.1.3 The Bony Pyramid

Irregularities on the dorsum, wide base, unequal sides or slight deviation. All these may not affect the overall attraction of a nose, but if corrected the nose looks more attractive (Fig. 22.3).

22.1.4 The Nasal Base

Nasal apertures may look unaesthetic, wide, unequal or undue exposure of one side or both sides of the columella (Fig. 22.4).

22.1.5 Combinations

An attractive nose may have a combination of minor factors in the different areas of the nose that if diagnosed and addressed delicately the outcome is quite stunning (Figs. 22.5 and 22.6).

Examples for finesse rhinoplasty are endless and demonstrated in the atlas for rhinoplasty.

22.2 Part II: The Large Nose and the Bulky Nose: Differences and Surgical Management

The large nose is a very different condition from the bulky nose. Clinical recognition and diagnosis of each type must be clearly made as each has a totally different surgical management.

A **large nose** is mainly the result of an increase in the **sizes** of the nasal structures while a **bulky nose** is the result of an increase in the nasal **soft tissue mass**.

The increase in **size** may affect **some** or **all the structures of the nose** while the increase in **bulk** only affects the **lower third** of the nose.

The **large** nose and the **bulky** nose are two major surgical problems that all rhinoplasty surgeons have to face. They are a real surgical challenge that demands detailed anatomical knowledge and **all the skills and techniques** of the surgeon.

Bulky noses are much more common in Africans, Middle Easterns, Hispanics and Asians. Should we need to reduce the size of Anglo Saxon noses, the lower third has to be proportionately reduced in size and bulk at the same time in order to have a proportionately sized nose.

Big noses, therefore, are mainly due to the increase in their **size**, **bulk** or **both**.

22.2.1 Nasal Size

The increase in the **size** of some or all of the **nasal walls** and their **communicating folds** may be the result of one or more of the following:

a. A wide-based and large **bony pyramid** with or without a large nasal **hump**. This is usually associated with a large and sometimes high upper lateral cartilage.
b. A large lower third of the nose with a **wide alar base** and wide nasal openings.

The overall outcome is a **large nose** with a wide-based and sometimes high **bony pyramid** and/or wide **alar base** and hence wide nasal openings.

22.2.2 Nasal Bulk

A large bulk means an **increase in** the **nasal soft tissue mass. A nose may be small in size but bulky** looking due to the excess in its soft tissue

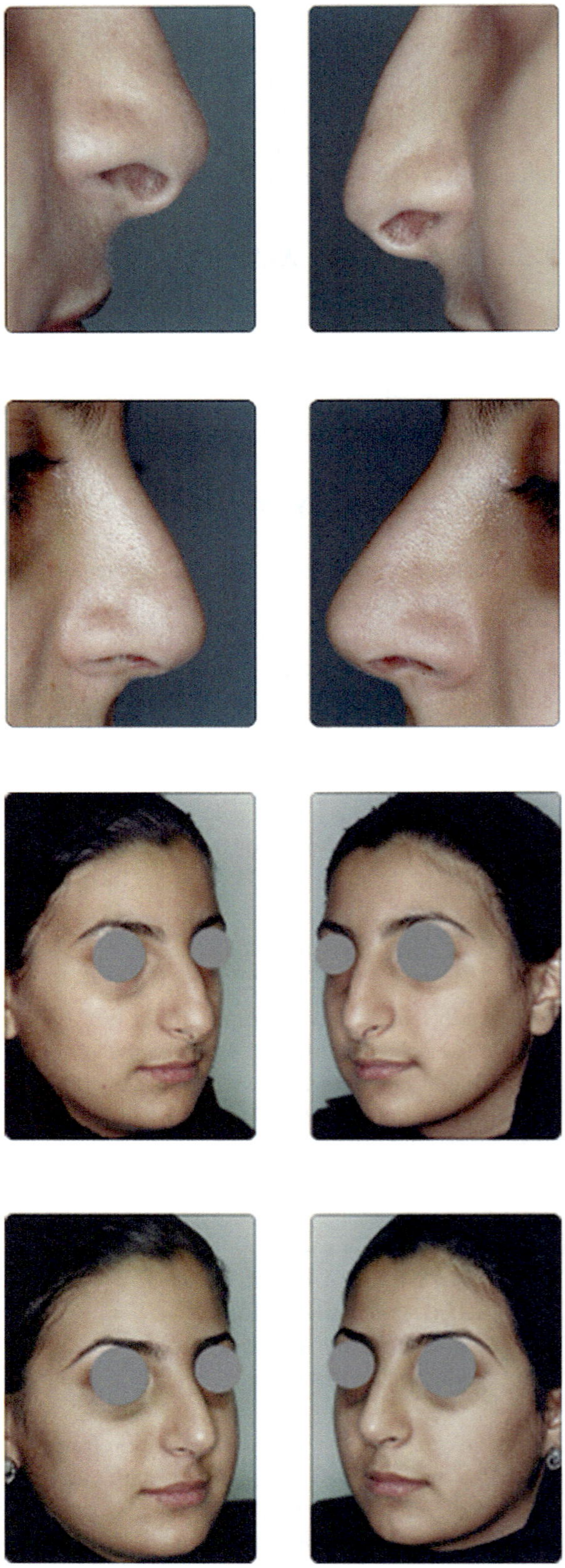

Fig. 22.2 Predominant Medial Wall Surgery : Surgery of the Medial Crurae

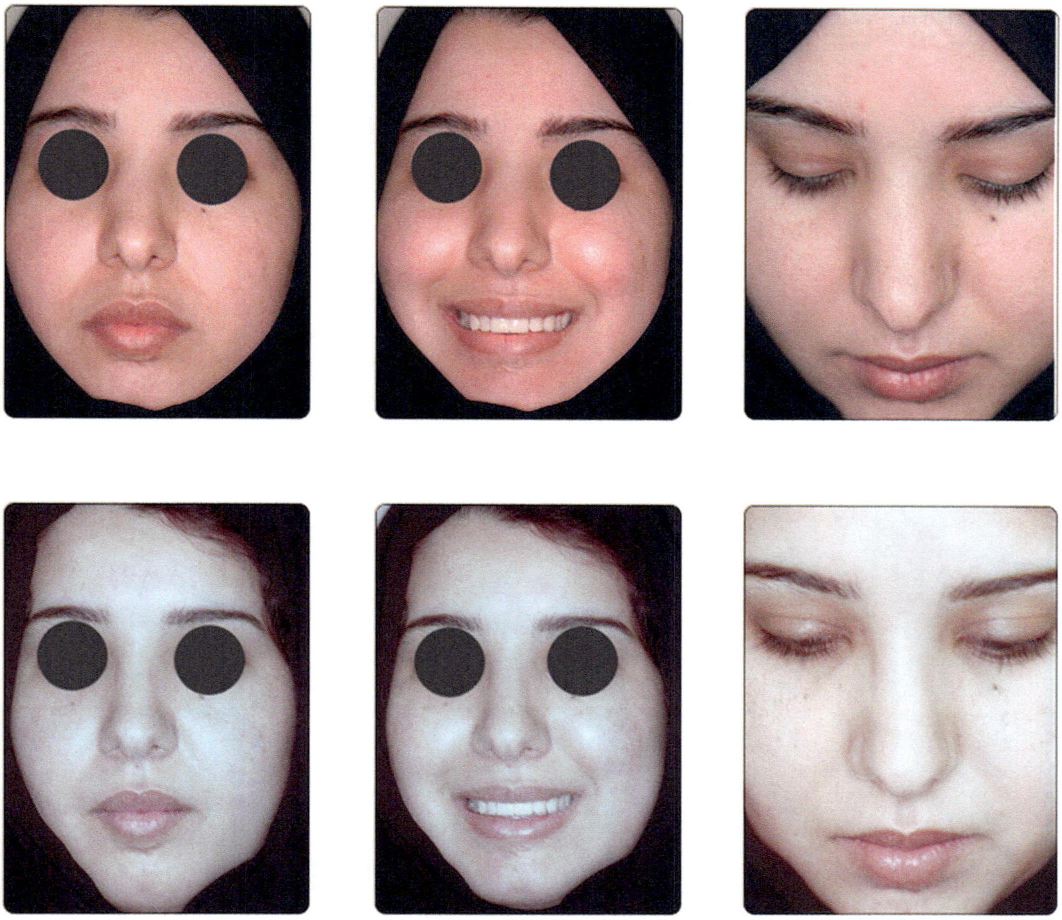

Fig. 22.3 Predominant Surgery for the Bony Pyramids

content. The overall outcome is a **thick, bulky** and **heavy-**looking nose.

The mass of the soft tissue is mainly contributed by **the skin** with its thick dermal and/or **subdermal fibrofatty layers** which are only present in the skin of the **lower third of the nose.** In this part of the nose, the skin is tightly adherent to the underlying lower lateral cartilages and the fibrofatty wings of the alae nasi.

The skin in the upper two-thirds is thin and loosely sliding over the nasal bones and the upper lateral cartilage.

The main **contributors** to the **bulk** of the lower third of the nose are:

i. The skin of the **frontolateral walls**, i.e. the middle and lateral crurae.
ii. The **rim-sill folds** of skin.
iii. The **alae nasi** with their bulky fibrofatty bodies.

In the **African noses**, the main contributor to the nasal **bulk** is the large, bulky **rim-sill folds** rather than the **frontolateral walls**. The **Asian** noses tend to have the main bulk in the **alae nasi**. For the **Middle Eastern** and **Hispanics,** the main bulk is in the **crural skin of the frontolateral walls**.

In conclusion, the **large nose** is due to the increased **size** of the **bony and cartilaginous** skeleton as well as the **soft communicating folds of skin** while the **bulky nose** is due to an increase in the **soft tissue mass** in the lower third of the nose.

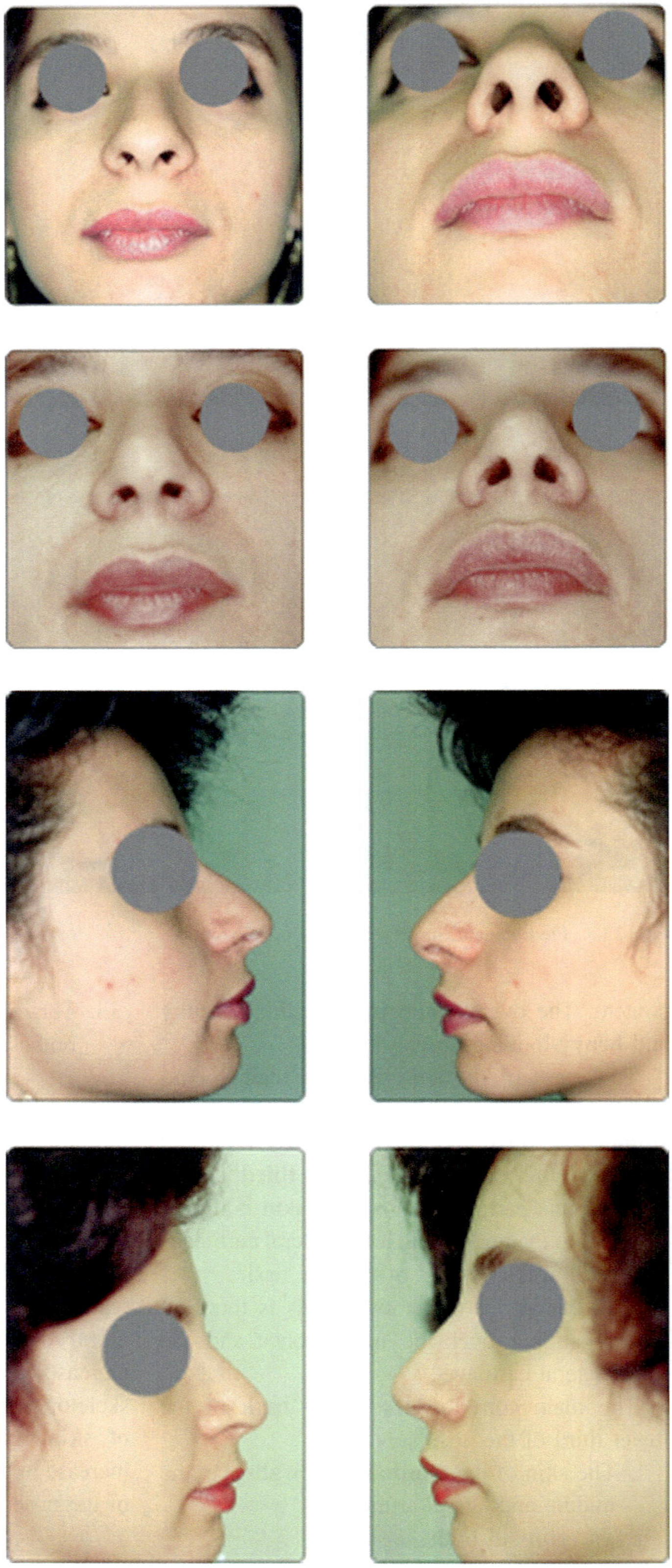

Fig. 22.4 Predominant Alar Base Surgery

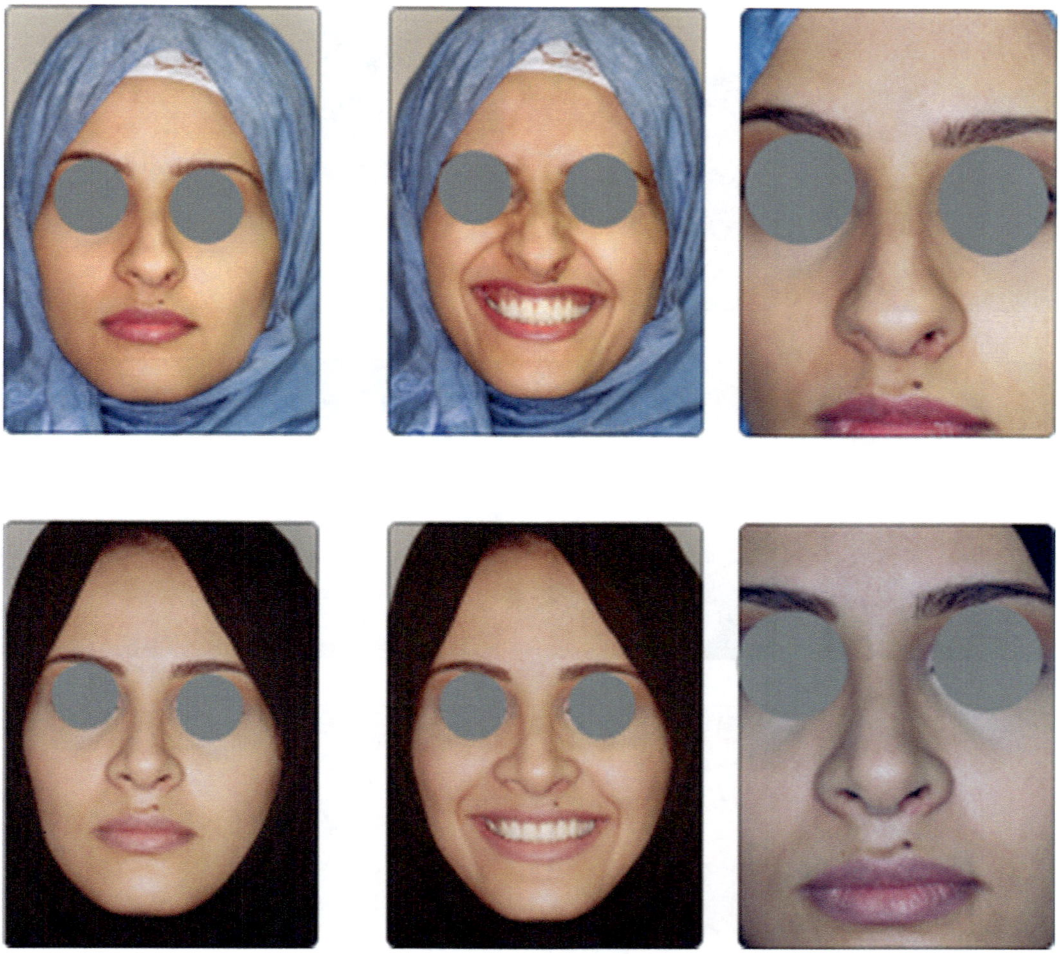

Fig. 22.5 Combined Surgery to the Nasal Tip, Septum and Bony Pyramid

22.2.3 Causes of the Large Nose and the Bulky Nose

Factors that affect the **size** and the **bulk** of the nose may intermingle with each other. Therefore the size and bulk are discussed together as their management is through a series of integrated surgical procedures.

22.2.3.1 Large Bony Pyramid

A large bony pyramid **directly** increases the **size** of the upper two-thirds and **indirectly** increases the **size** of the lower third of the nose (Fig. 22.7).

A **wide-based** bony pyramid drives the lateral walls of the soft nasal aperture tube further away from the midline. The **alar base** becomes wider with nasal openings that have a transverse rather than antero-posterior long axis.

22.2.3.2 Large Upper Lateral Cartilage

The size of the midvault or the upper lateral cartilage either matches the size of the bony pyramid or is disproportionately larger in size (Fig. 22.7).

22.2.3.3 Large and/or Bulky Lower Lateral Cartilages

The lower lateral cartilages are the main structure that makes **the shape** of the frontolateral walls of the lower third of the nose. They are therefore the main contributors to **the size** of these walls (Fig. 22.8).

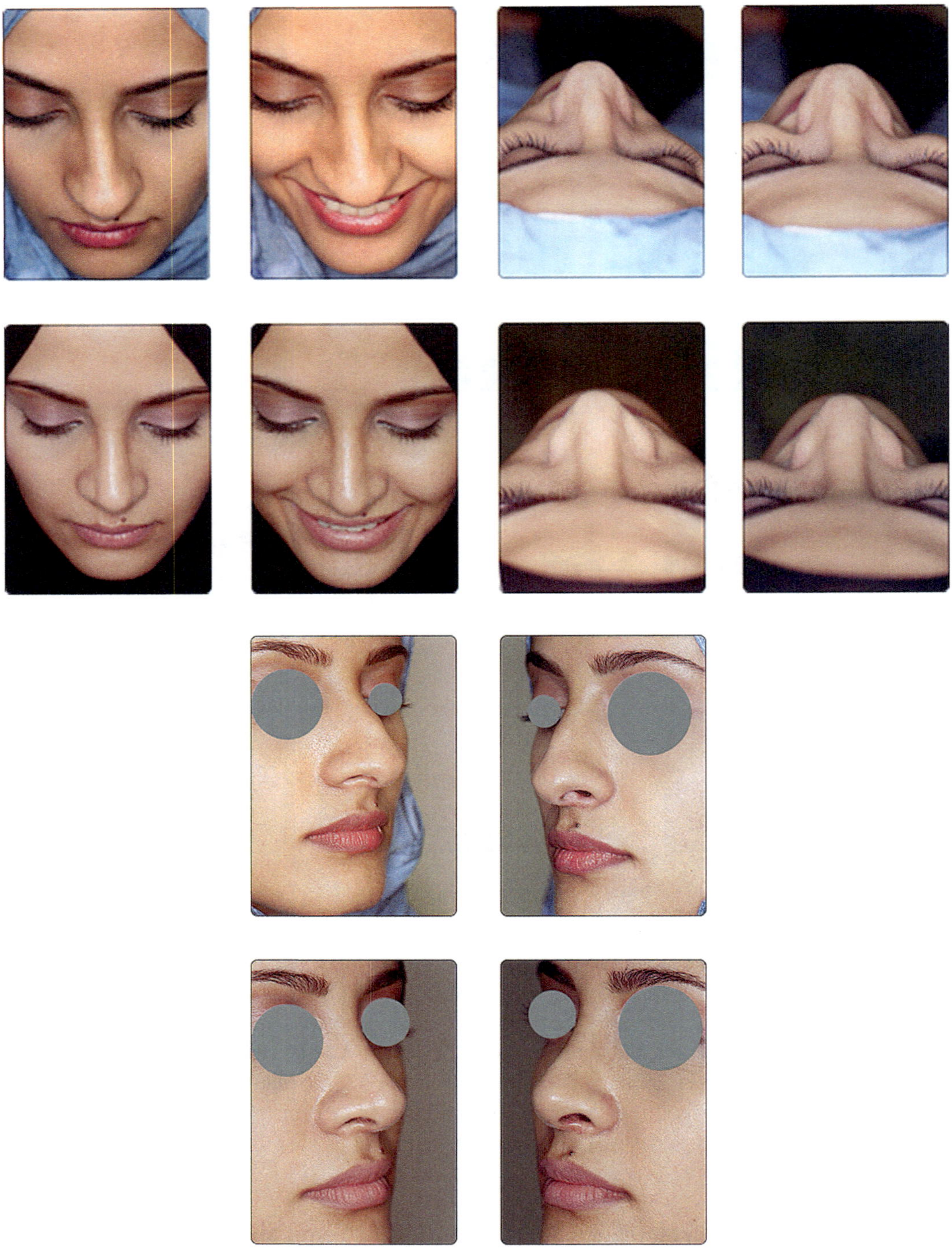

Fig. 22.6 Combination of unaesthetic areas of the boney pyramid, medial wall and alar base

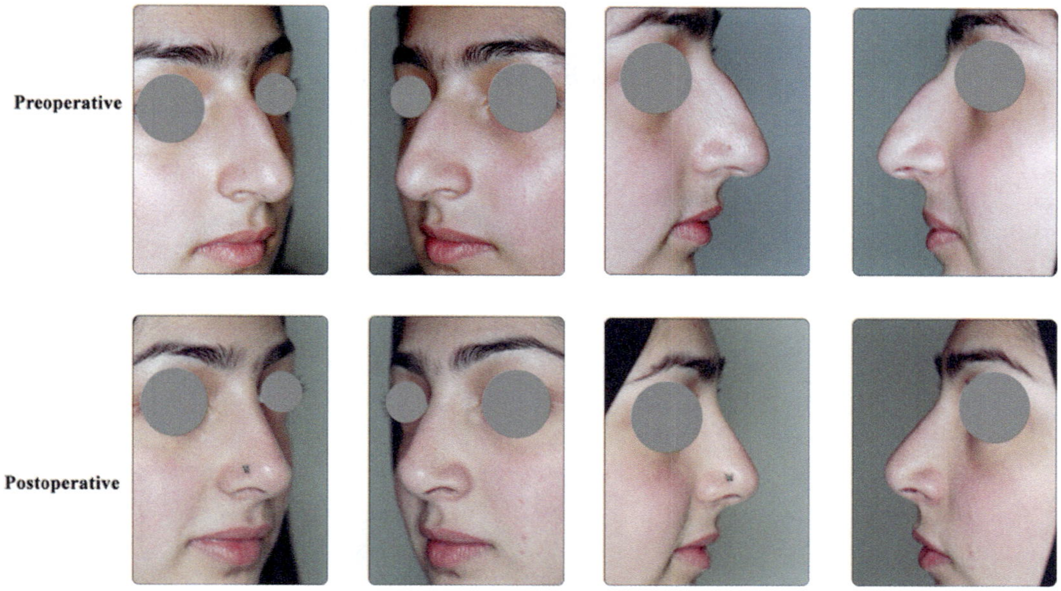

Fig. 22.7 Large osteocartilaginous hump and large lateral crurae

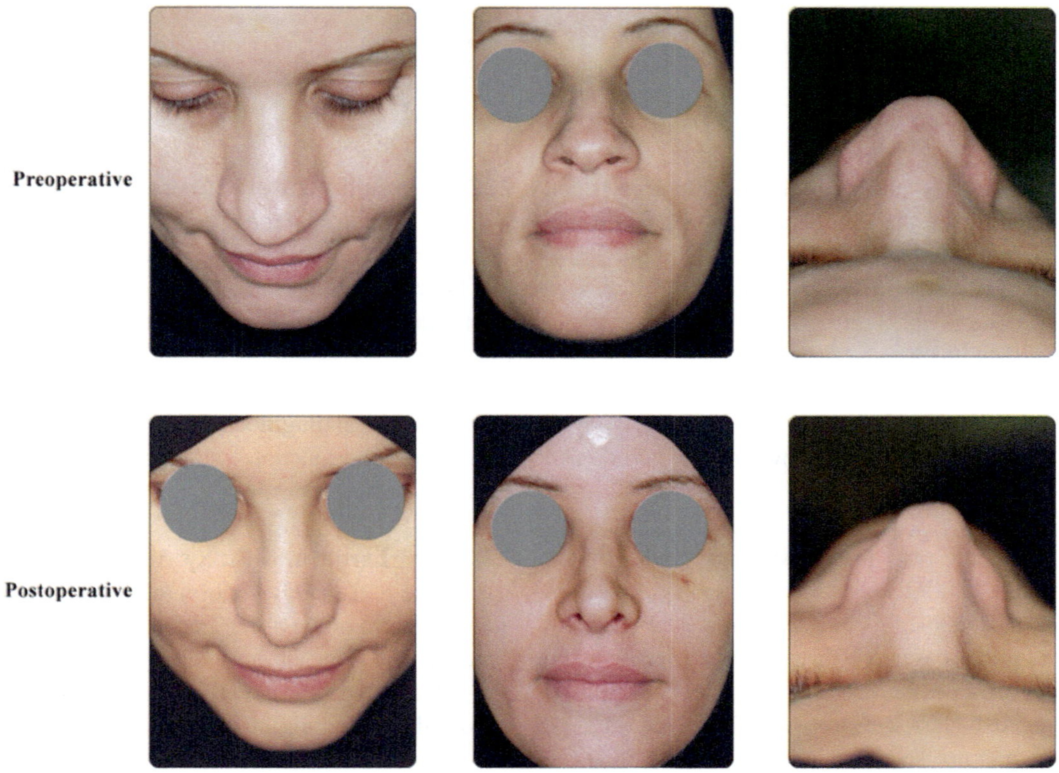

Fig. 22.8 Large and bulky middle and lateral crurae

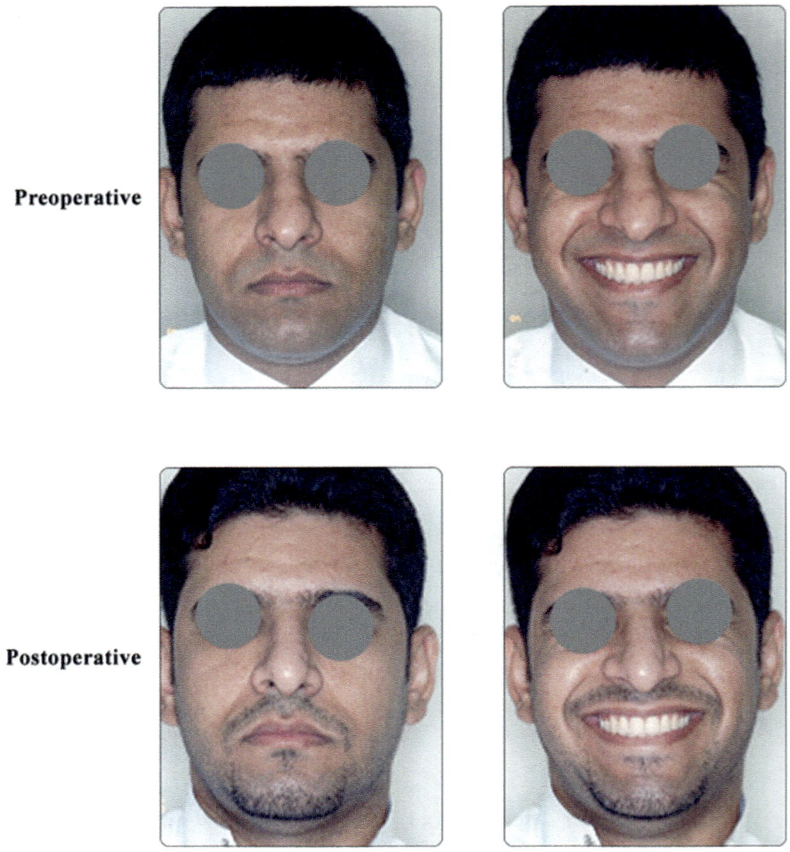

Fig. 22.9 Bulky crural overlap (scroll area)

A bulk is added to the middle and lateral crurae by the thick and heavy three layers of the external skin:

i. The thick greasy epidermis;
ii. The thick fibrous dermis;
iii. The thick two layers of fat;
 - A hypodermal loculated panniculus adiposus;
 - The capsule of fat covering the middle and lateral crurae.

The increase in the **size** and **bulk** of the **middle** and **lateral** crurae may enlarge the front and sidewalls of the nose. The resultant is a large and bulky nasal tip which may **overshadow the alae nasi** on the lateral walls. The characteristic curved bodies and grooves of the alae nasi are lost and not seen as they are hidden behind the Large and bulky crurae.

22.2.3.4 Bulky Lateral Crural Overlap (Scroll Area)

The **overlap** of the **lateral crurae** over the **upper lateral cartilage** may become very **prominent and bulky**. It is both unsightly and adds to **the bulk** of the nose (Fig. 22.9).

This is usually caused by the excess in the **overlapping cartilaginous folds of the lateral crurae** at their junction with the upper lateral cartilage on both sides.

22.2.3.5 Large and Bulky Alae Nasi

Large alae nasi mainly contribute to the **bulk** of the lower third of the nose. This is more common in **Asian** and **African** noses (Fig. 22.10).

Although the skin cover is slightly thick and greasy, the main bulk of the alae nasi is in their **fibrofatty bodies**.

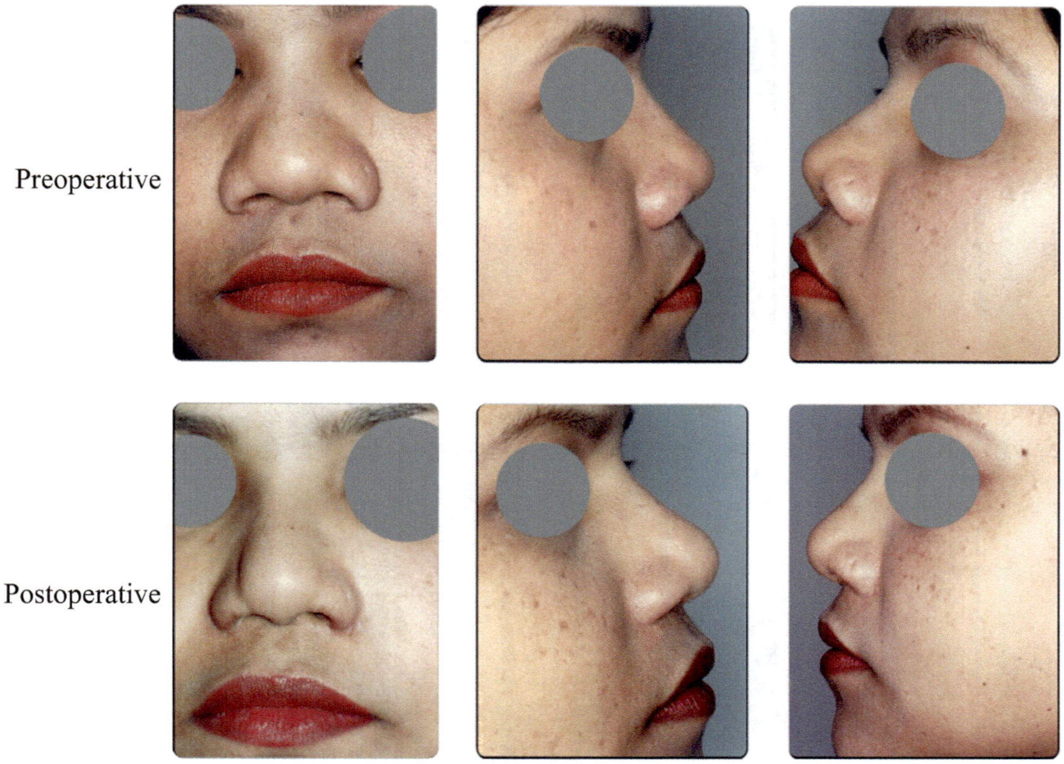

Fig. 22.10 Large and bulky alae nasi before and after surgical reduction

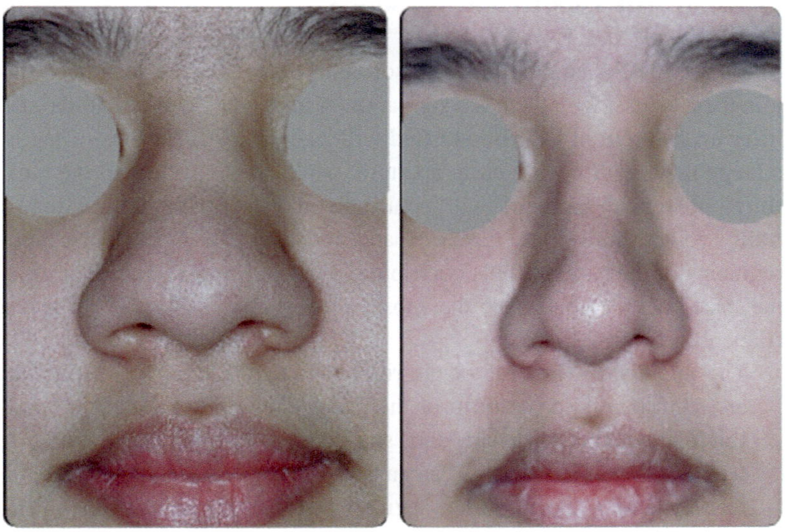

Fig. 22.11 Bulky lower third of the nose before and after defatting of the frontolaterl walls and the excision of the rim-sill folds

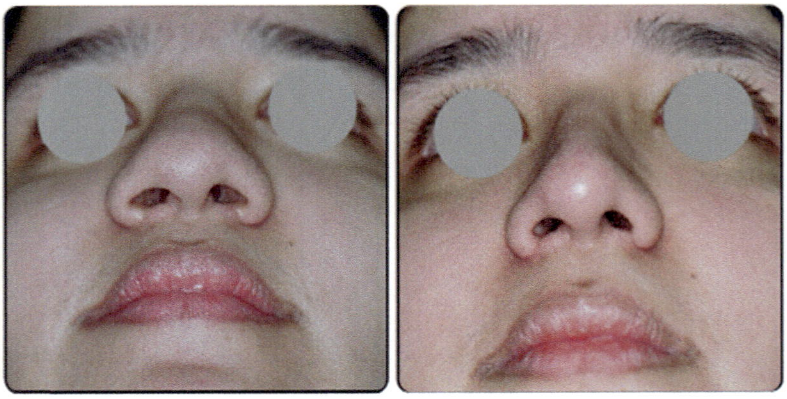

Fig. 22.12 Backward tilting view showing the nasal dorsum, tip and alar base before and after surgery

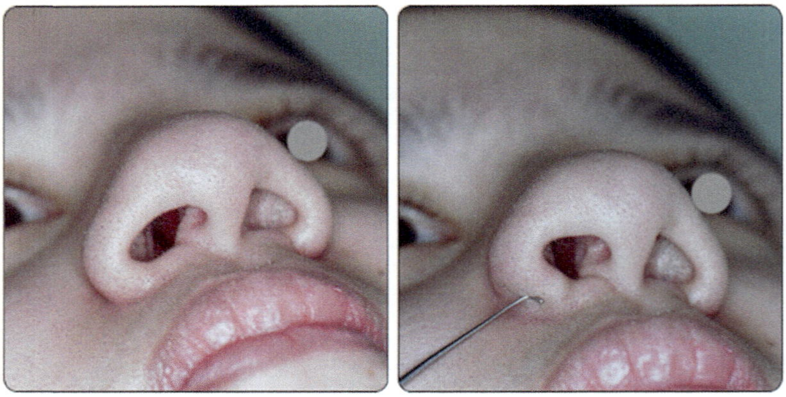

Fig. 22.13 Right nasal aperture view. Rim-sill test demonstrating the rim-sill folds

22.2.3.6 The Length and Thickness of the Rim-Sill Folds

These are the transitional areas of soft skin that join the alae nasi with the nasal sill bands. A **long inferior segment of the rim-sill fold** will lead to a **large nose** with a wide nasal aperture, while a **thick posterior segment** will contribute to a **bulky** lower third. The posterior and inferior segments of the rim-sill folds contribute to either the size or the bulk of the nose or both (Figs. 22.11 and 22.12).

a. The **posterior segments** of the rim-sill folds are contributors to the **bulk** of the nose. The **thick-skinned** folds take the shape of a **wedge** having a **narrow** segment **intranasally** and a much **wider** segment **externally**. This gives the nose a very heavy and thick appearance (Fig. 22.13).
   The excess thick skin rests flatly on the upper lip on both sides like a flat tire of a car. This is aesthetically unpleasant because of the acute angles with the lip as well as the heavy bulk of the skin.
b. The length of the **inferior segments of the rim-sill folds** affects the **width** of the nasal apertures. They may also be **bulky** and contribute to the bulk of the nose. These inferior segments extend on the floor of the nose in direct continuation with the nasal sill bands taking their exact shapes and contours (Figs. 22.14 and 22.15).

22.2.3.7 Bulky External Skin

Thick skin is the most important factor that adds to the **nasal bulk**. Also, the **rim-sill folds,** the other main contributing area to the nasal bulk, are the **skin cover of the middle and lateral crural cartilages**. The one major contributing factor to its thickness is the two **fibrofatty layers** that spread between the perichondrium of the crural cartilages and the smooth fibrous inner surface of

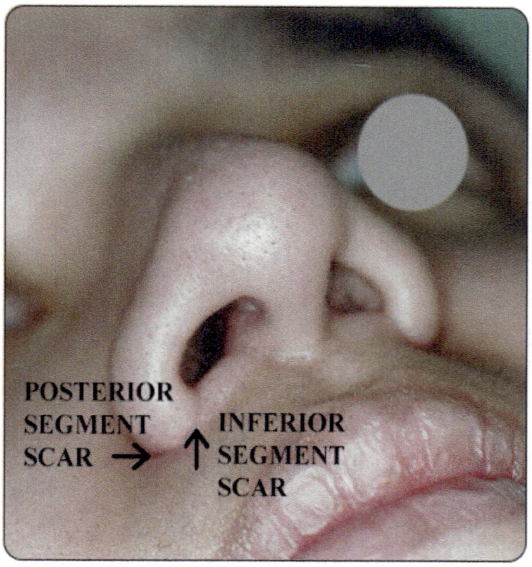

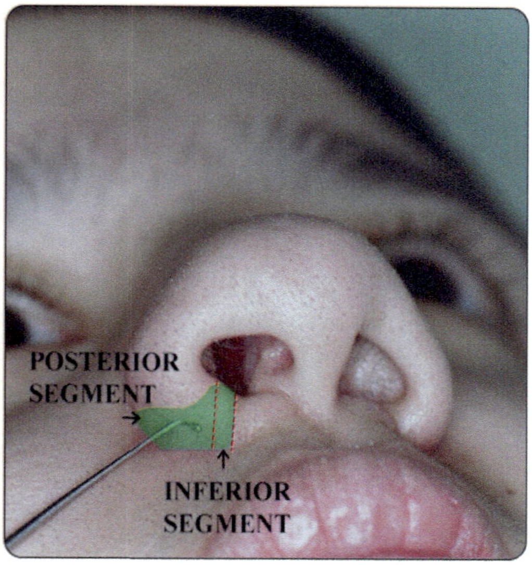

Fig. 22.14 The inferior and posterior segments of the rim-sill fold before and after surgical excision

the fibrous dermal skin (see Chapter on Nasal Skin).

The more fat in these layers, the thicker the external skin and vice versa. The fat that covers the weak triangle further adds to the thickness of this area.

The **skin cover of the alae nasi is thick, greasy and adherent**. There are no subdermal layers. The fibrofatty layers are the contributors to the bulk and/or size of the alae nasi.

22.2.4 Surgical Reduction of the Size and the Bulk of the Nose

Surgery for large and bulky noses is a classic example of the integral and inseparable approach to the whole of the nose, bony, cartilaginous and soft tissue.

The reduction of the size and the bulk of the nose has to be **anatomical**, **natural** and **proportionate** so that the nose does not lose its characteristic shape and look.

The nose of each individual has its **very own characteristics**, almost exactly **like a fingerprint**. It is meant to specifically suit each individual's face in order to keep his own nasal configuration that he is familiar with. We can almost say that every face has its own **nasal print**. The idea of rhinoplasty is to **enhance the beauty of these characteristics without losing their personal individuality**. This can be achieved by the following:

(a) The **upper two-thirds** are mainly concerned with nasal **size** while the **lower third** is concerned with nasal **bulk**. The size of the upper two-thirds indirectly affects the size of the lower third.
(b) Accurate **anatomical diagnosis** of the exact location of the bulky or sizable part of the nose.
(c) The proportionate **size and shape** as well as **relations** of all structures of the nose have to be considered **together as one unit**. They are all integrated into the construction of the external shape of the nose.
(d) Reducing the bulk of fat of the frontolateral walls without directly interfering with the original shape and sizes of the upper lateral cartilage will result in preserving the original shape of the person's own nasal print.

22.2.4.1 Reduction of the Size of the Bony Pyramid

A wide base of the bony pyramid, with or without an osteocartilaginous hump, is reduced

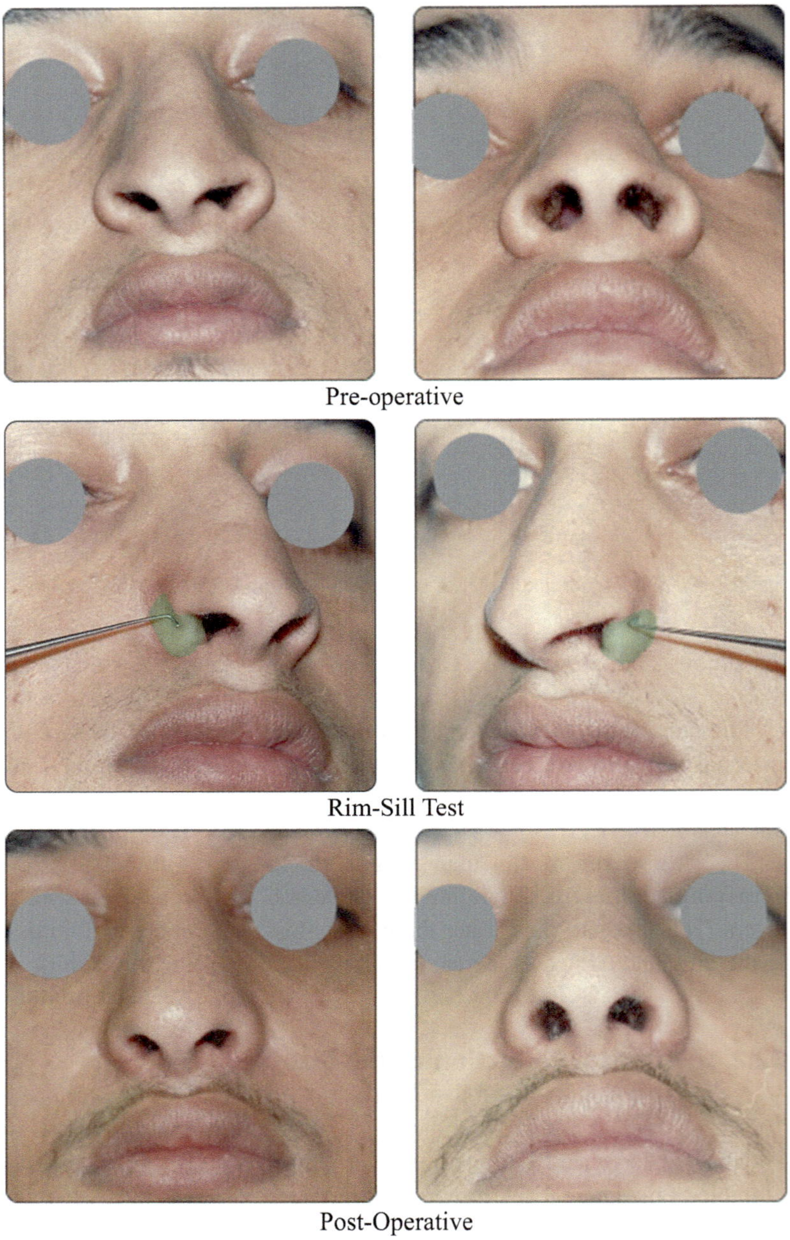

Fig. 22.15 Long and oblique rim-sill folds. The rim-sill folds are making a fourth nasal aperture wall. The two segments are integrated in making one large fold

in size by removal of the hump, osteotomies and medialization of the bony sidewalls.

The push-down and pull-down techniques have the same effect.

A large nose may have **wide rounded** nasal apertures. Following the reduction in **the size** and **the bulk** of a nose, it becomes **smaller** and **slimmer**, yet the nasal openings may remain unaesthetically **rounded** in shape.

In these cases, reduction in the aperture size is better coupled with **osteotomies** and **medialization** of the bony sidewalls. This will drive the lateral aperture walls medially, thus transforming the openings of the nose from a **transversally rounded** shape to a more aesthetic **longitudinally oval** shape.

Osteotomies may be the only work needed for the bony pyramid. No further aesthetic modification such as soft tissue work to the nasal tip or alar base is needed.

22.2.4.2 Reduction of the Size and Bulk of the Alae Nasi

Defatting of the lower lateral cartilages and excision of the rim-sill segments reduces the size and the bulk of the lower third of the nose. Further reduction of the nasal size and/or bulk rarely requires direct surgery to the bodies of the alae nasi.

Extreme large sizes of the alae nasi may be seen in **Asian** and **African** noses (Fig. 22.10).

22.2.4.3 Reduction of the Length and/or Thickness of the Rim-Sill Folds

A **thick posterior segment** of the rim-sill fold usually contributes to the nasal **bulk** while a **long inferior segment** contributes to the **large size** and wide nasal openings (see Chapter on Anatomical Variations). **Both may be the site for a bulky nose.**

Each or both segments may be surgically excised for the purpose of reducing the bulk and/or the size of the alar base and the nose in general.

22.2.4.4 Reduction in the Size and Bulk of the Lower Lateral Cartilages

The Size of the Medial Crurae

The size of medial crurae: Large medial crurae are seen in the **hanging columella**. Direct reduction of the crural sizes is necessary to reduce the overall size of the nose.

The Middle Crural Domes

The domes may increase **the size** of the anterior nasal wall due to the **wide curvatures and/or** their large sizes which produces a **broad and/or large nasal tip.**

Reduction of curvature and/or size of the domes is made directly or indirectly.

i. Directly: This can be achieved by weakening the external surface of the domes using cross-hatching cuts. Only rarely that the size of the domes needs to be reduced.
   Direct square stitch across the tip between the anterior end of the medial crus and the beginning of the lateral crus. This increases the angle of the dome and makes it more prominent. Both domes can then be stitched together.
ii. Indirectly: By the use of a tip or a shield's grafts.
iii. Two-step defatting: The new innovative two-step technique of defatting the fronto-lateral walls of the nose reduces the size as well as the bulk of the middle and lateral crurae. There is no need for the use of direct stitching of the domes. The nose keeps its own nasal print at a smaller scale and thinner skin.

The Lateral Crurae

There are three ways of reducing the **size** and the **bulk** of the lateral crus:

i. **The cephalic trim**: As the middle crus ends at the lateral genu there is a cephalic increase in the size of the cartilage. It is usually the cephalic part that is trimmed away in this type of surgery.
ii. **The bulky scroll area of overlap**: Direct trim of the thick or long folded overlapping lateral crus via the intercartilaginous exploratory incision. This reduces **the bulk** of the scroll area and has an excellent aesthetic outcome.
iii. **Two-step defatting** of the frontolateral walls. Removal of the two layers of fat of the middle and lateral crurae reduces the size and bulk of both structures. The skin is thinner.

Defatting: The Two-Step Reduction of Crural Bulk and Size

Based on the anatomical knowledge of the hypodermal fatty layers, this procedure aims at defatting the crural hypodermal layer of panniculus adeposus.

Thinning of the nasal skin is the main target in this surgical procedure and is addressed to the frontolateral walls of the lower third of the nose. Removal of the two subdermal layers of fat will clear away their two-step enlargement effects on the crurae which in turn regain their original small sizes, i.e. there is a two-step reduction in crural sizes. The small crurae are now covered directly by the thinned out dermal and epidermal layers of skin. The outcome is thin skin covers small crurae that have their exact original shapes, i.e. the nose print is maintained.

The following procedures of defatting and reducing the thickness of dermal skin can only be achieved in **closed rhinoplasty.** The blood supply of the nasal tip is not compromised as the two **columellar arteries** are not severed as in the open technique.

Defatting of frontolateral walls of the nose means **cutting, sucking** and **scraping** the **two fibrofatty layers** that lie between the **anterolateral nasal skin walls** and the **lower lateral** and **medial crural cartilages**. In order to reach these layers, **complete delivery of both lower lateral cartilages** must first be done. The fibrofatty layers under the anterior and lateral walls are now explored and thoroughly removed in **three clear steps**:

Division of the Fibrous Bands

A three-step incision is made for the delivery of the three crurae (see Chapter on Surgery of the Frontolateral Walls). After making the initial inferior marginal incisions of the lateral, medial then middle crurae, a right-angled epidural hook is used to pull on the proximal margin of the vestibular wounds. The fibrous bands are seen stretched between the dermis and the crural capsular layer (Figs. 22.16, 22.17 and 22.18) The bands are cut using a Joseph scissor (Fig. 22.19). The marginal incisions thus are deepened until it communicates with the intercartilaginous incision. The lower lateral cartilage is delivered like a bucket handle (Fig. 22.20).

Removal of the Crural Fibrofatty Capsule

The **fibrofatty layer that envelops the outer surfaces of the domes and lateral crurae** of the lower cartilages is removed. This fatty layer can be picked up and cut off the cartilages by a pair of toothed forceps and curved scissors. Sometimes it is easier to cut the capsule using the tip of a No. 15 bladed knife. The capsular fatty layer is then excised. As the **lateral crurae** have large bodies, they naturally **have thicker** and **more abundant fat** on their external surfaces than the domes. Residual fatty tissues over the cartilages may be scraped by a No. 15 bladed knife (Figs. 22.20, 22.21 and 22.22).

Removal of the Hypodermal Fat

The lower lateral cartilage is pulled down away from the field by a right-angled epidural hook. A blunt pronged alar retractor is used to elevate the alar margin, while the tip of the ring or middle finger counter pushes the anterior and lateral skin walls inwards (Figs. 22.23 and 22.24).

The fibrofatty layer is now seen and **cut** using a pair of curved Joseph's scissors (Fig. 22.25). At the same time, the assistant **sucks** the cut-off fatty tissues with a 3 mm straight suction.

The suction may be used to **draw** the fat out by the assistant. The surgeon then cuts it away (Fig. 22.24).

The suction is then swept all around the inner surface against the external pressure of the ring or middle finger to **scrape** and suck away any loose and residual fatty tissue. Any residual fat is thoroughly and neatly **shaved away** by the No. 15 bladed knife (Fig. 22.26). Rarely a **small curette** is needed especially in cases of secondary rhinoplasty with extremely tough fibrofatty tissues.

All fat over the lateral crurae is removed. Their extreme lateral ends are carefully reached and defatted.

Defatting is completed when the smooth pearly white dermal layer is seen (Fig. 22.27).

Defatting the Weak Triangle

The fibrofatty layer of the weak triangle and the lowermost part of the upper lateral cartilage is now clearly seen via the same previous exploration. Removing their fat cover may only be done if the supratip area is wide, thick and high that needs to be reduced in width, thickness and height. Unwise removal of this layer in a thin nose that has a normal height will lead to depression in the supratip area. Fat can be easily picked up by a pair of Addison's forceps and cut away. The whole of the weak triangle and the

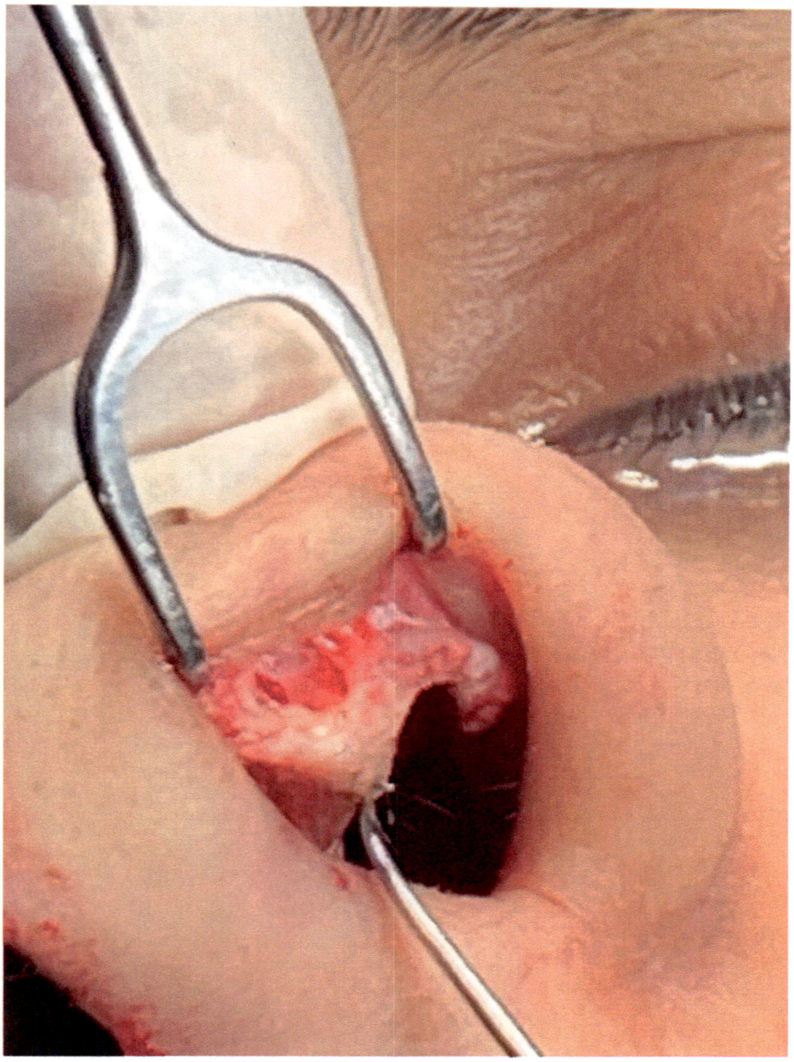

Fig. 22.16 Exploring the fibrous bands between the dermis and the middle cus

lower part of the upper lateral cartilage is clearly seen shining after the complete removal of the fat.

There is a **prominent** ridge **or step of fibro-fatty tissue** which is usually seen on the inner skin surface **at the junction between the skin that covers** the **upper and** the **lower lateral cartilages**. This ridge must be picked up by Addison's forceps, cut and removed in order to reduce the external crease of demarcation or sometimes a step between the skin of the lower and upper lateral cartilages.

At the end of the procedure, both the dermis and the cartilaginous surfaces of **the lateral crus** and **the lower end of the upper lateral cartilage** must be seen to be **evenly smooth, white and shining**. Any extra irregular fibrofatty tissues must be carefully and smoothly **scraped away by a knife**. A No. 15 blade is usually a suitable size for this task. These tissues if left may later grow into small lumps that appear as unaesthetic irregularities on the external surface.

The **routine scraping** of the **excess tissues off** both cartilaginous and skin surfaces, after fat

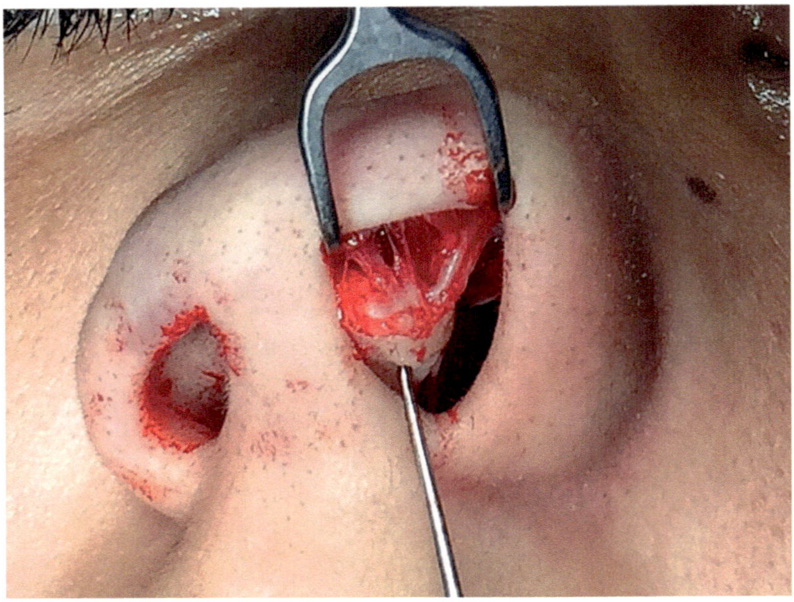

Fig. 22.17 Fibrous bands connecting the dermis to the fatty capsular layer covering the left middle crus

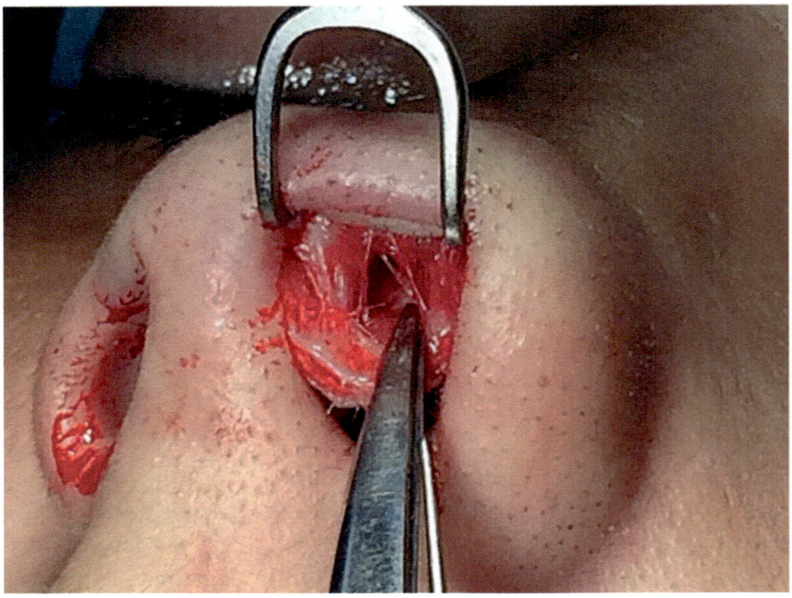

Fig. 22.18 Fibrous bands connecting the dermis to the fatty capsule covering the left lateral crus

removal, ensures uniformly smooth surfaces and has better results.

A 3 mm suction is finally used to scrape and suck away any excess fat that may not otherwise be seen.

Having finished **cutting**, **sucking** and **scraping** the fibrofatty layer, the **lower lateral cartilages** are now **replaced** in their original position.

Special Defatting Conditions

Some noses may have different anatomical changes that may affect the judgment and the management of fat removal.

Revision Rhinoplasty

In **revision rhinoplasty,** the anatomical distinction between the two layers of fat is lost. They are mostly replaced by tough fibrous tissues

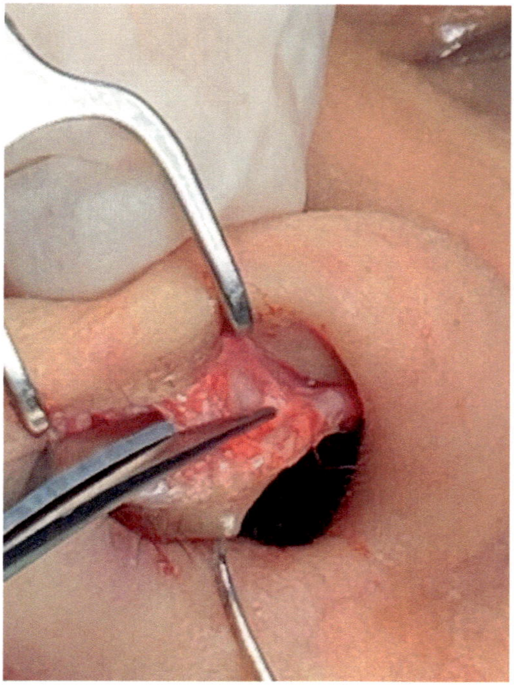

Fig. 22.19 Cutting the fibrous bands

that are **more adherent** to the underlying perichondrium of the lower lateral cartilage as well as over the smooth inner dermal surface.

The only way to remove this layer is to **scrape** it off using the side of a No. 15 bladed **knife**. Cutting it with scissors or using suction is both difficult and ineffective.

A curved **rasp** may sometimes be necessary to remove away an exceptionally thick and tough fibrofatty layer.

Post-traumatic Cases

In a **post-traumatic** nose, the affected side has a tough, thick, fibrofatty layer over the lateral crus. Clinically, it looks larger than the opposite side and, therefore, hides the wing of the ala nasi behind it. This thick tough layer is removed in the same way as in revision rhinoplasty.

Thick Dermal Layer

Occasionally after accurate and complete defatting, the dermal fibrous layer may be seen to be **regularly** or **irregularly thick**. One side may look higher or thicker than the other. Thickness reduction is achieved by gently and **gradually rasping the thicker side** using a small curved rasp. Care must be taken not to overthin the dermal layer. The surgeon must gradually rasp and regularly check for the blood supply and the thickness of the skin.

Defatting Small Noses and Thin-Skinned Noses

In small or thin-skinned noses, their lower third usually has very little fat, however, defatting of such noses **enhances the beauty of the nasal front** and **proportionately reduces the size of the nose**.

Adding Grafts in a Defatted Nose

Removing the fat leaves excess external skin and wide loose space underneath. Adding grafts in the supratip area or over the upper lateral cartilage **needs to be fixed by a transcutaneous stitch**, as the grafts are slippery and may become slippery and easily displaced.

In certain situations, the nasal tip may be augmented by small pieces of diced cartilages to produce more projection or to balance an uneven tip.

Reducing the Size and Bulk of a Child's Nose

Reducing the size and the bulk of the nose is possible starting from the growing ages of 12–16 years.

The **rim-sill folds** and the subdermal **fibrofatty layers** may change in size and shape with age but their excision at an early age **will not directly affect the growing process of the nose**.

The sites of **osteotomies** at the root of the nasal processes of the maxillae and the midline **do not affect the growing nasal bones** or maxillae.

Procedures such as **rim-sill resection, defatting** of the anterior and lateral walls, **osteotomies** and **cross-hatching of the middle crural domes** may have a profound positive effect on the appearance and psychology of a child **without jeopardizing the growth** of the child's nose and face.

The early resection of the fibrofatty layer, as well as the rim-sill segment, greatly reduces their future increase in size and bulk as well as the change in their shape.

They are **soft structures** that are present **in between** and **communicate** the growing stronger

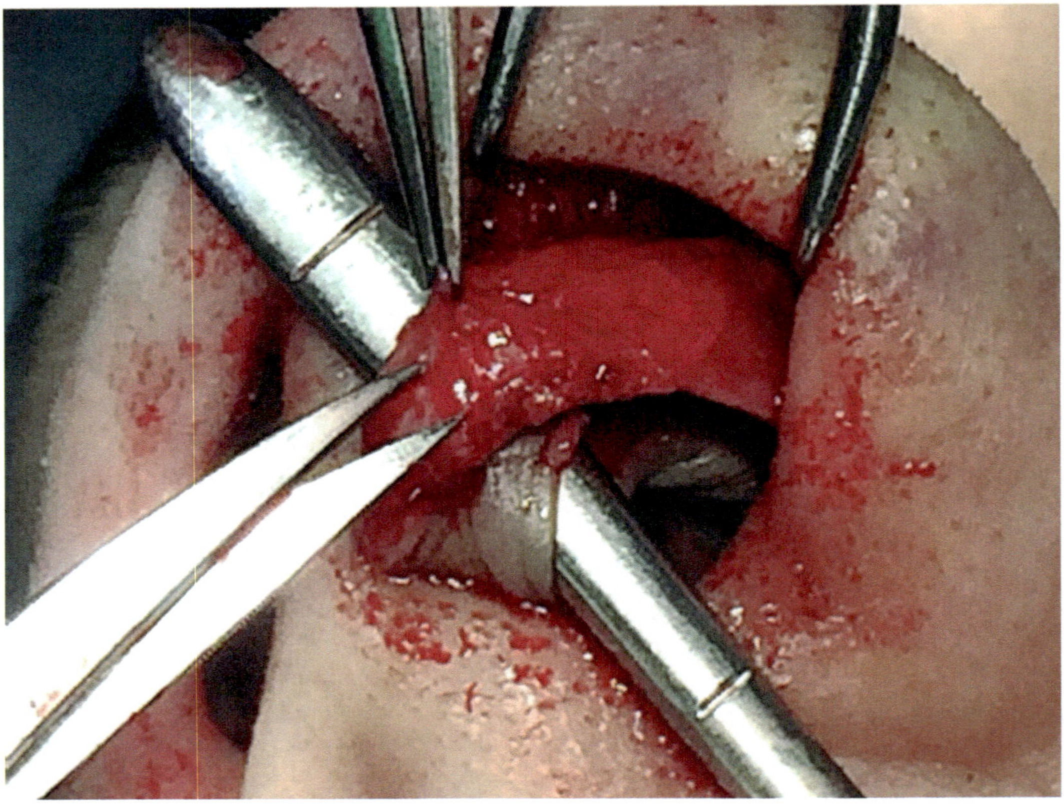

Fig. 22.20 Identifying the fibrofatty capsule covering the left middle crus

and **tough structures** of the alae nasi, alar cartilages and nasal sills.

Future rhinoplasty may possibly be needed for other areas in the nose.

Anatomical Effects of Defatting

If the **adherent hypodermal fibrofatty layer is surgically excised**, the remaining thickness of the external skin will only have its **dermal** and **epidermal layers**.

On the other hand, should the **capsule of fat** be taken off the **lower lateral cartilages**, then they become amenable for surgical reforming to the desired **shape and position** if needed.

The new **unpadded skin** is capable of being directly molded and shaped over the lower lateral cartilages, as it is now **thinner** and **pliable**. The skin can easily take the shapes of the lower lateral cartilages.

Camouflage surgery in the form of cartilaginous **tip grafts is** direct tip stitching and strut grafts are not needed.

The great gain and the major advantage of defatting is that the **tip projection** is beautifully achieved by **the patient's own domes** of the lower lateral cartilages. Each person will keep **his own characteristic nasal appearance**. Noses will no longer appear **uniformly the same**.

It is important to note that the cartilages will **not** be **over projected**, blanching or **seen through** the skin. Unlike tip grafts, the **natural curves of the domes do not** have **sharp edges** and the overlying skin keeps its **full thickness of the dermal layer** as well.

The **surgical excision** of the two layers of fat overlying the crurae, not only **debulks** the anterior and lateral walls but also **shrinks their sizes** by the contraction of the fibrous tissue layer that follows surgery.

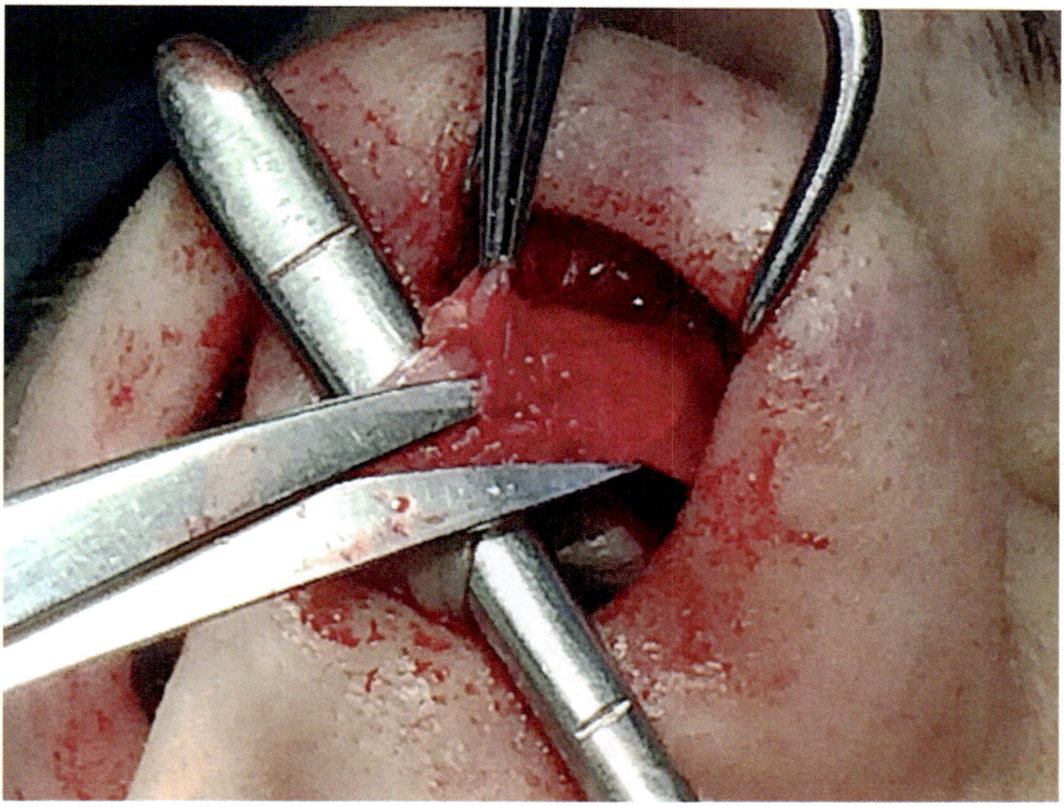

Fig. 22.21 Entering the fibrofatty capsule covering the left middle crus

Removing fat layers leaves a relatively thin layer of skin that takes the shapes of the underlying lower lateral cartilages.

The consequent **reduction in size is uniformly equal** and **natural** so that the tip of the nose does not lose its **characteristic** nasal print.

The Eight Aesthetic Benefits of Defatting

There is a **definite immediate** smooth and **uniform reduction in the bulk**, and consequently the size of the front and sidewalls of the lower third of the nose.

The Nasal Openings

Defatting of the antero-lateral walls has an indirect effect on the size and the shape of the nasal openings. They become **smaller in size** and assume **oval shapes** rather than rounded ones. Alar base surgeries are avoided in many cases.

Defatting reduces the height difference between the thick skin cover of the lateral crurae and the thin skin cover of the upper lateral cartilage.

In some noses, the skin cover of the middle and lateral crurae is prominently thicker and higher than the skin cover of the upper lateral cartilage. Sometimes there is a crease or a step between the two areas so that the tip and sidewalls are prominently bulbous and appear semidetached from the middle third of the nose.

After defatting, the skin of the frontolateral walls becomes thinner, softer and continues smoothly with the upper lateral skin. The semidetached appearance of the lower third of the nose disappears as it becomes continuously smooth with the middle third.

The general size of the lower third is consequently reduced as a result of reducing the bulk.

The nose keeps its original nasal print image. It becomes proportionately smaller, smoother and the skin looks thinner. The irregularities of

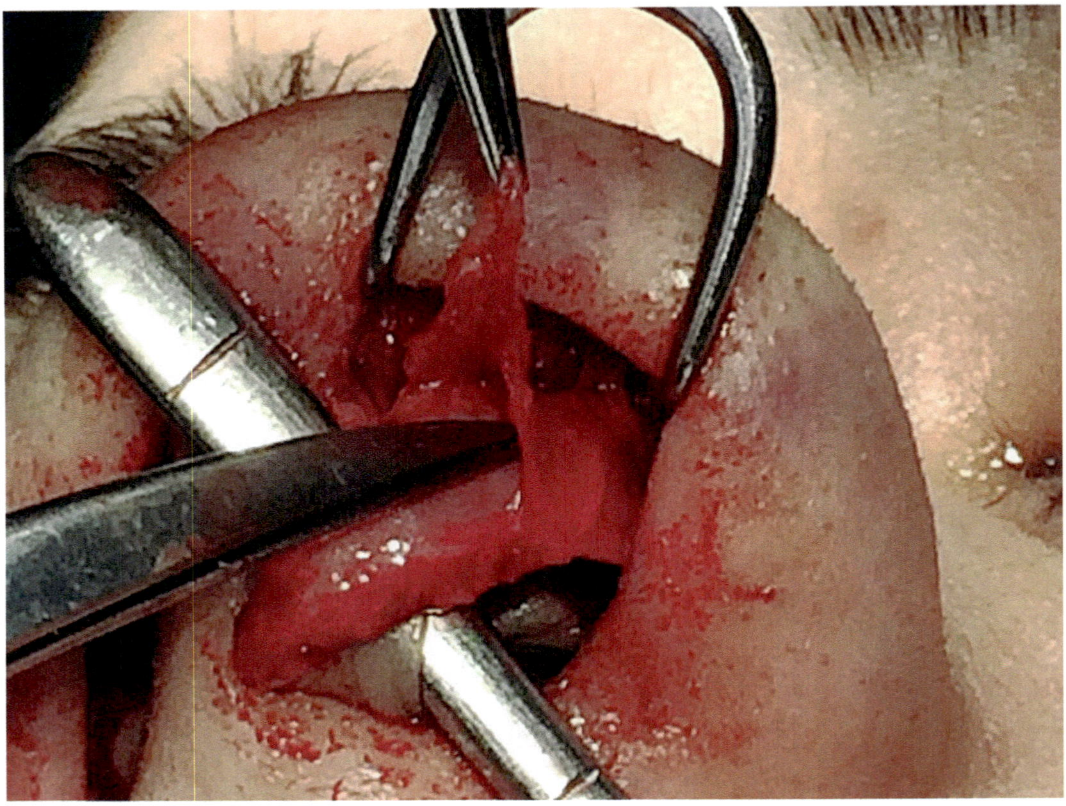

Fig. 22.22 Dissecting the fibrofatty capsule covering the left lateral crus

bulky skin over the lower lateral cartilages disappear as the shape becomes more uniform.

The patient is therefore quite happy as she or he does not lose the original identity but maintains their own nasal and facial image. The nose looks quite natural and not surgically enhanced.

Time is in favor of this type of surgery. The more the time passes, the better is the look of the nose. It continues to look naturally smoother, softer and smaller. Noses continue to improve up to two years after surgery. Some cases were followed for as long as five years, they continue to look better. Pregnancy and aging processes do not enlarge the size of the nose. The loss of fat plus the fibrotic fixation of the telescopic overlaps of the lower lateral over the upper lateral cartilages keep the size of the nose and prevent its enlargement.

Defatting **does not affect the thickness of dermal** or **epidermal skin layers**. Cartilages of the domes and lateral crurae will **not** be **visible, or show through the skin**, as the true skin is not any thinner than before; it is only defatted. Blanching effects of tip grafts are largely avoided.

Defatting leaves the skin of the **bulky African, Middle Eastern and Asian noses**, quite **thin** and **pliable**. Procedures of **cephalic trim of the lateral crurae** and **cross-hatching of the domes** are now more effective in changing the overall **shape** and **size** of the nasal front. The nose gains the **triple effect** of reducing the **size** and the **bulk** and improving the **aesthetics**.

There is **less need for procedures** to reduce the size of the nasal tip, e.g. Goldman's procedure or transdomal stitching, in an attempt to

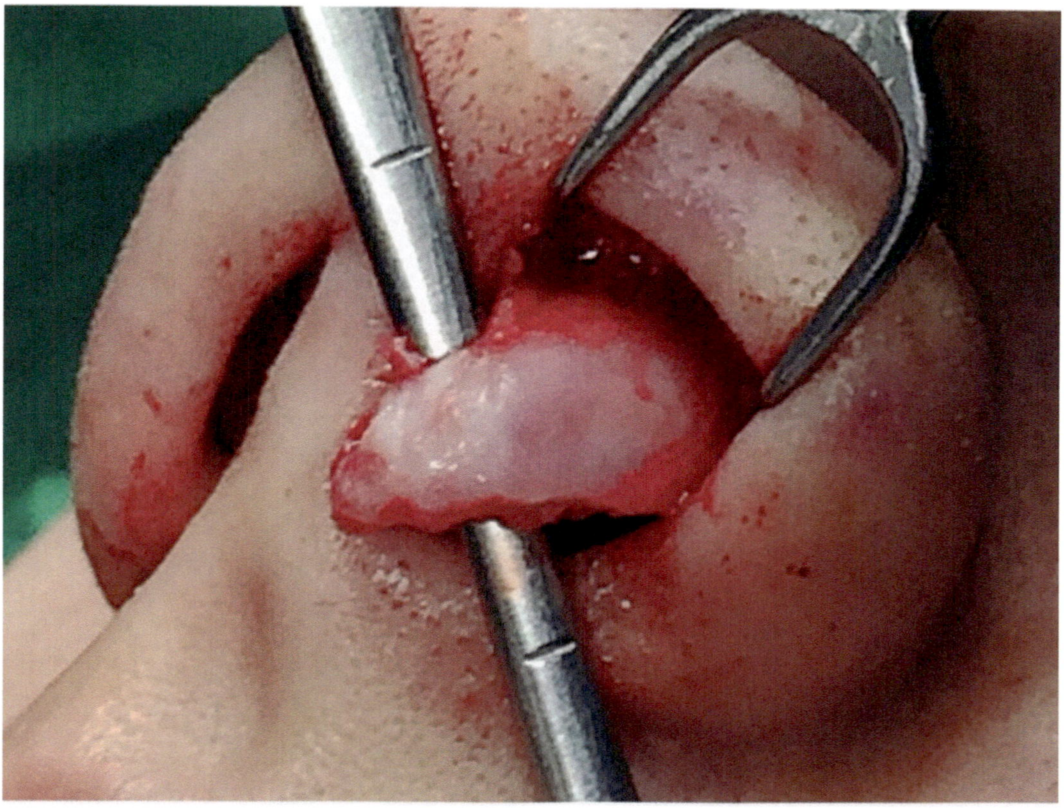

Fig. 22.23 The glistening white surface of the left crural cartilage after complete removal of its covering fibrofatty capsule

narrow the tip. These techniques **only reduce the size of** the nasal front and **not the bulk** of the nasal soft tissues.

Following **hump reduction**, especially, if it was predominantly cartilaginous, the whole of the **upper two-thirds** of the nose is **reduced in size**. The **lower third becomes disproportionately large** and the nose looks like a trumpet. This may affect the thick-skinned, the regular skinned or even the thin-skinned noses. **Defatting** is the **best single procedure** that can proportionately reduce the size and the bulk of the lower third of the nose and regain its natural-looking balance.

In this sense a **new aesthetic concept** is introduced, i.e. **reduction of a nasal hump means the reduction of the whole size of the nose**. As well as the routine hump reduction, **defatting is** now **mandatory for a better aesthetic result**. Alar base resection may be needed.

22.3 Part III: The Deviated Nose and the Crooked Nose: Differences and Surgical Management

Under normal anatomical conditions, the nose is made of paired structures that meet to make a single midline organ which is well balanced by the near equal bilateral subunits, i.e. the frontal processes of maxillae, nasal bones, two sides of upper lateral cartilage and the lower lateral cartilages. The nose looks deviated or crooked if the bilateral differences in size are wide enough to have an obvious unaesthetic external visual effect. One must differentiate between a deviated nose and the crooked nose.

The **deviated nose** is a condition where the whole of the patient's nose including the bony pyramid, the lower two-thirds and the nasal

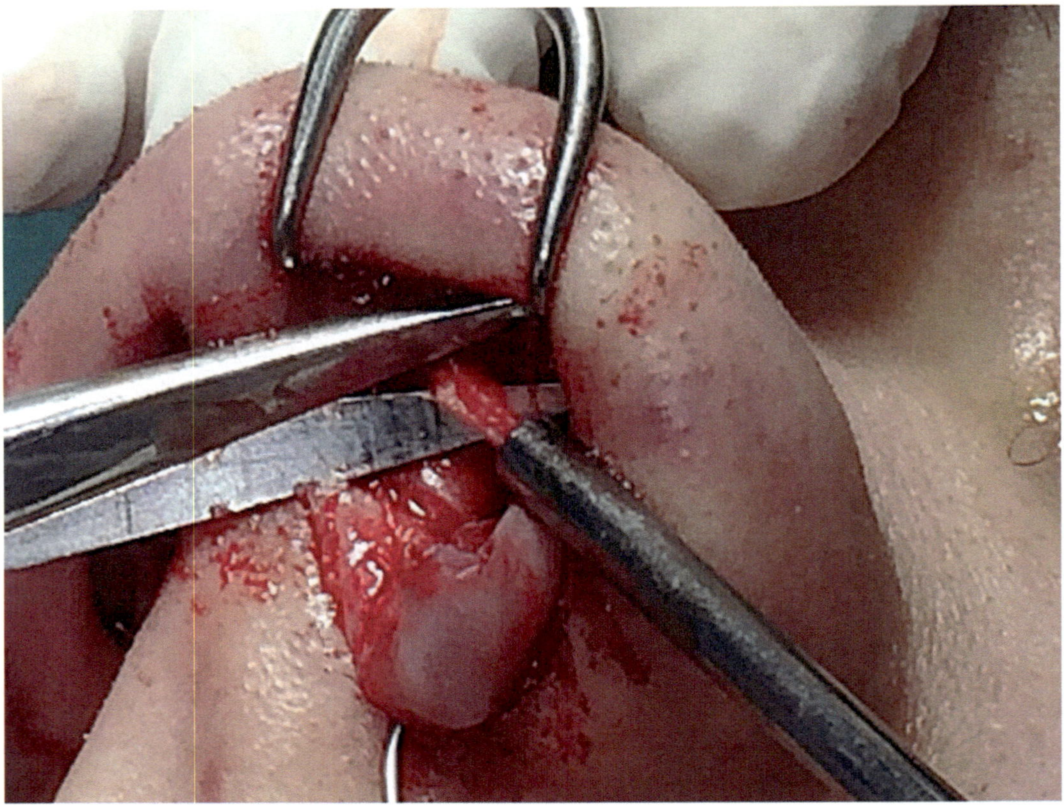

Fig. 22.24 Sucking the fat of the hypodermal layer and cutting it with scissors

septum are all obliquely deviated in the same direction.

A **crooked nose** is a condition in which the nose may take an S-shaped, C-shaped or totally irregular external appearance. The bony pyramid, the midvault and the lower third of the nose are in different directions from each other.

The **bony pyramid** is the main culprit and contributor to the deviation and the crookedness of the nose.

The lower two-thirds of the nose either **follow the same direction** of the pyramidal deviation resulting in the overall **deviation, of the nose**, or **each third may go in a different direction** resulting in **crookedness of the nose.**

Deviation and crookedness of the nose may be natural **developmental** or acquired **post-traumatic**. The latter is either surgical or accidental trauma.

The **developmental** cases usually have **smooth external surfaces**, despite the obvious deformity and the nasal walls are **regularly shaped** while the post-traumatic cases usually have **ragged external surfaces** and **irregularly shaped** walls.

22.3.1 The Deviated Nose

Deviated noses mostly have **smooth** external surfaces with **regular** changes in their structural walls. Therefore most, if not all conditions, of nasal **deviations** are of developmental origin, while **crooked** noses are more commonly **acquired**, post-traumatic cases.

22.3.1.1 Bilateral Maxillary Asymmetry

Bilateral differences in **sizes** and **shapes** of maxillae are almost the rule in normal

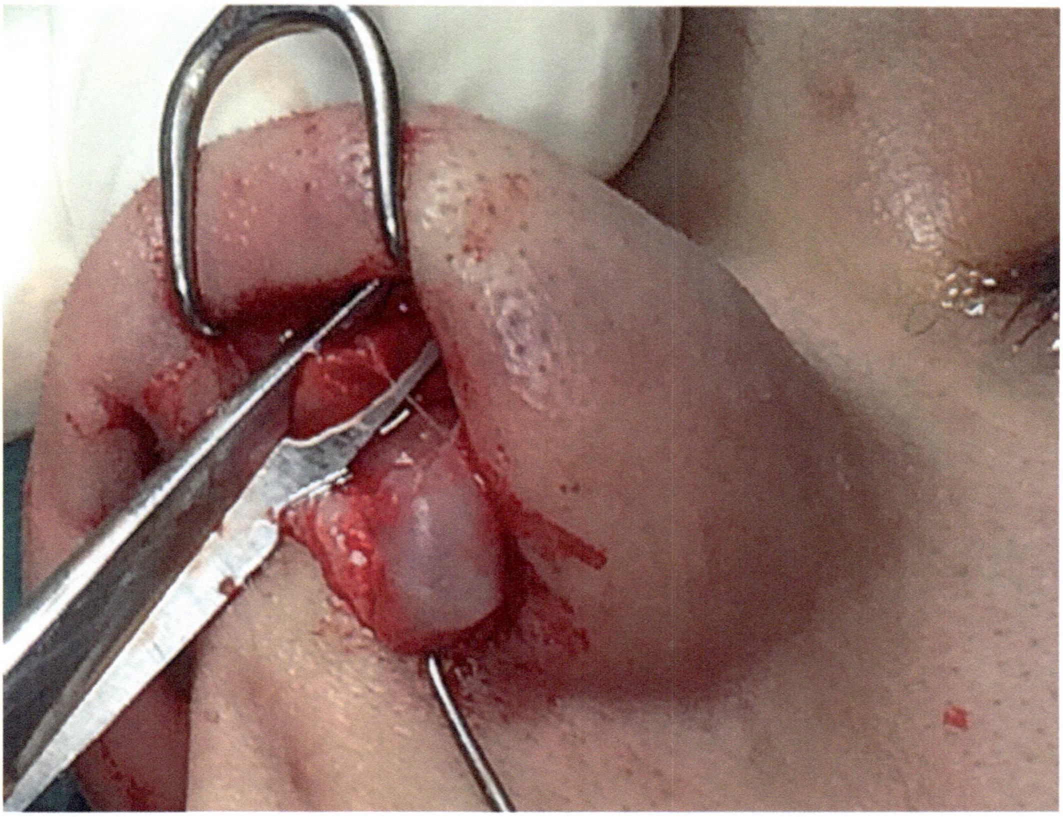

Fig. 22.25 External pressure by the tip of the middle finger allows direct cutting of the hypodermal fat by the scissors

individuals. Subtle differences between the two sides of the face are usually unnoticed and have a negligible effect on nasal aesthetics.

Considerably wide bilateral differences become apparently clear as the structures meet in the midline to make the nose. The nose may become deviated or crooked.

The frontal processes of the maxillae on both sides of the face are the main contributors to the bony pyramid of the nose. The two nasal bones are only two small curved flat bones that cap the pyramid.

The obliquely deviated bony pyramid, in most of these conditions, is a natural result of varying degrees of bilateral facial asymmetry. The facial bones, including zygamas, are larger in size on one side of the face than the other. Consequently, one side has a larger contribution of the frontal process to the nasal bony pyramid.

The degree of nasal obliquity and deviation increases proportionately with the degree of bilateral variations.

The meeting of the two asymmetrical sides drifts the nose away from the midline, resulting in varying degrees of unaesthetic outcomes. The larger frontal process drives the smaller process to the opposite side in two directions:

i. **Horizontal** direction in the **axial plane** leads to an **oblique** bony pyramid as compared to its horizontal base.
ii. **Vertical** direction in the **sagittal plane** leads to **deviation** of the bony pyramid off the vertical midline.

The outcome of these two effects on the bony pyramid is that it becomes both **oblique** and **deviated**.

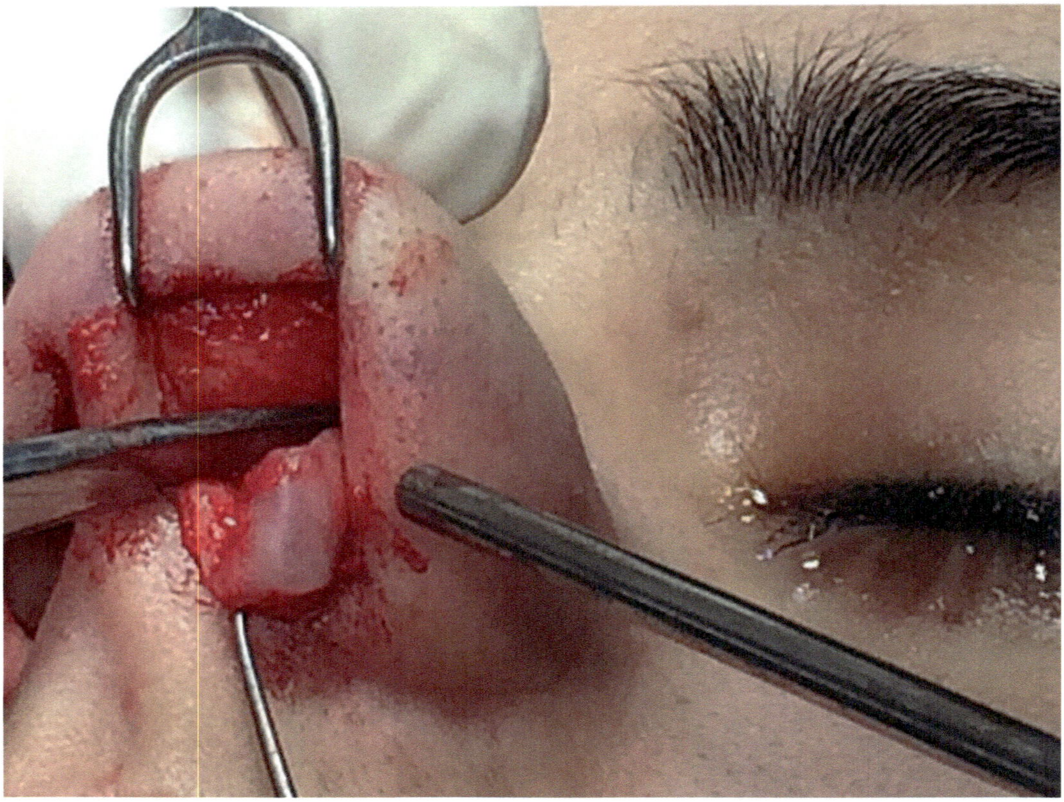

Fig. 22.26 Scraping the residual hypodermal fat using the side of the No. 15 blade

The **smaller side** usually has a **narrower** and **higher cheek**, i.e. Zygomac body with **smaller narrower basal attachment**, of its frontal process. The **larger side** has a wider and **lower cheek** with a **larger and wider basal attachment** of the frontal process.

This arrangement tends to naturally reduce the size differences between the two sides and hence improve the overall aesthetic appearance.

22.3.1.2 The Unaesthetic Outcomes of Maxillary Asymmetry

As the two unequal zygomas meet via their frontal processes, in the midline to make the nose, there are some unaesthetic outcomes that may result:

Oblique and Deviated Bony Pyramid

The oblique and deviated bony pyramid results in oblique and deviation of all supportive structures of the nose, i.e. the bony pyramid, midvault and the nasal septum (Fig. 22.28).

Osteocartilagenous Hump

Because of the deviated and oblique bony pyramid the hump predominates and drifts toward the smaller side. **Photographically** the hump is more apparent in the **oblique views,** especially if taken from the angle of the **larger side**. Patients are usually aware of this and try always to avoid photographs from these angles. The **lateral views** also show the hump but without any difference between the two sides regarding the size of the hump (Fig. 22.29).

Asymmetrical Maxillary Bodies and Cheeks

The **smaller side** has a **high narrow cheek** with a **smaller**, **closer** and **more vertical** side of the **bony pyramid** while the **larger side** has a **wide, lower cheek** with a **larger** and **wider** attachment

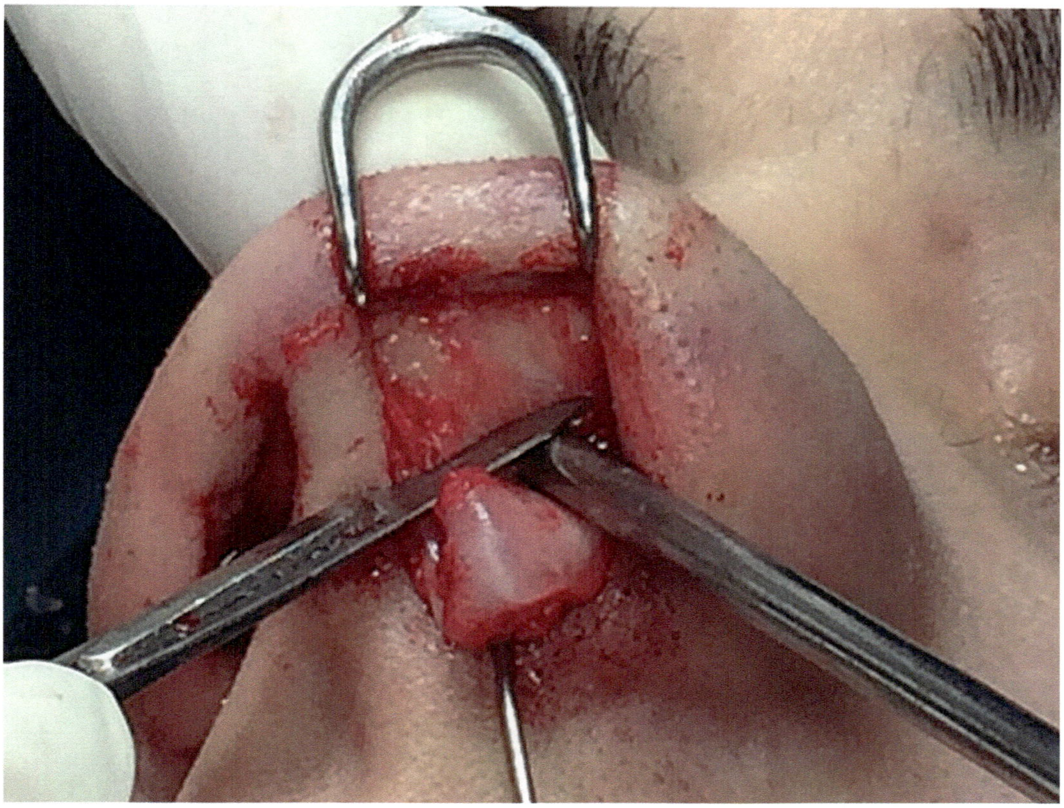

Fig. 22.27 The shining white surface of the dermis is the indication of the end of the defatting process

base of the bony pyramid. This is better seen in the **backward tilting** and **basal** views as well as other views, e.g. frontal overhead and direct dorsal views.

22.3.2 The Crooked Nose

The crooked nose, contrary to the deviated nose, does not look straight in its external appearance. There may be an obvious bend, angulation, protrusion, depression or other types of irregularities.

The **three components of the nose,** i.e. the bony pyramid, the midvault and the lower third, are **in different directions from each other** so that the nose may become **S-shaped**, **C-shaped** or **irregularly irregular**.

Each component may be irregular, e.g. depressed, protruded, smooth or ragged.

The crooked nose may be natural developmental or acquired post-traumatic.

22.3.2.1 The Developmental Crooked Nose

The nose may look quite deformed with obvious angulation, bend, hump, caudal dislocation of the septum and unequal nasal openings, yet the following are observed:

(a) There is no history of accidental or surgical trauma.
(b) The external surfaces of the bony pyramid, midvault and lower cartilaginous third are smooth and regular.

There are no irregularities, sharp edges of broken bones or ragged surfaces.

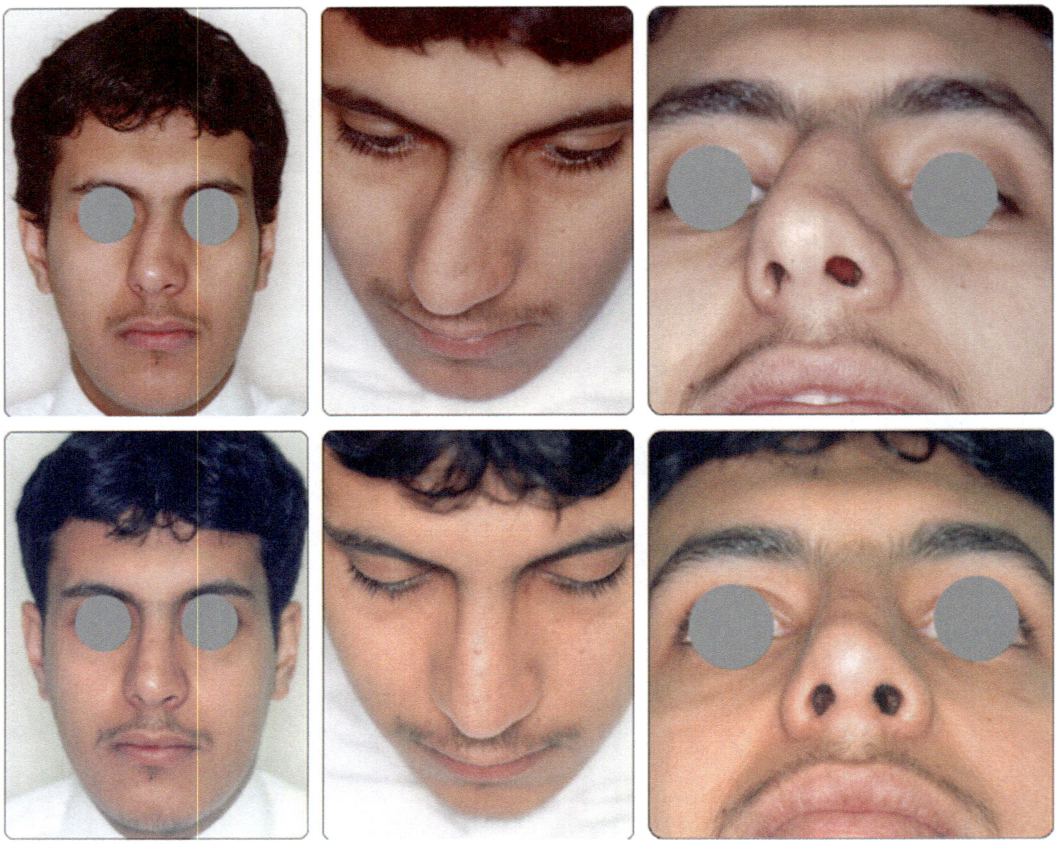

Fig. 22.28 Oblique and deviated bony pyramid secondary to bilateral maxillary asymmetry. Before and after surgery

(c) Bilateral Maxillary Asymmetry

Asymmetry of both sides of the face is clearly seen if the bony pyramid and the cheeks are examined in isolation from the rest of the nose. The small side has a **narrow** and **high** cheek, while the **bony side of the pyramid** is **smaller, closer** and **more vertical,** and vice versa. The large side has a wider and lower cheek with a larger and wider attachment to the sidewall of the bony pyramid.

The midvault and lower third of the nose are in different directions from the bony pyramid (Fig. 22.30).

22.3.2.2 The Post-Traumatic Crooked Nose

Accidental or surgical trauma may result in various types of nasal disfigurements and crookedness (Fig. 22.31).

The classic appearance of a depressed fracture of the bony pyramid following lateral trauma, e.g. a sport trauma as in boxing will lead to an obvious deviation of the bony pyramid of the midline and in the opposite direction from the midvault and the lower third of the nose.

Other types of trauma to the midvault and lower third are discussed in the section on Post-traumatic Rhinoplasty.

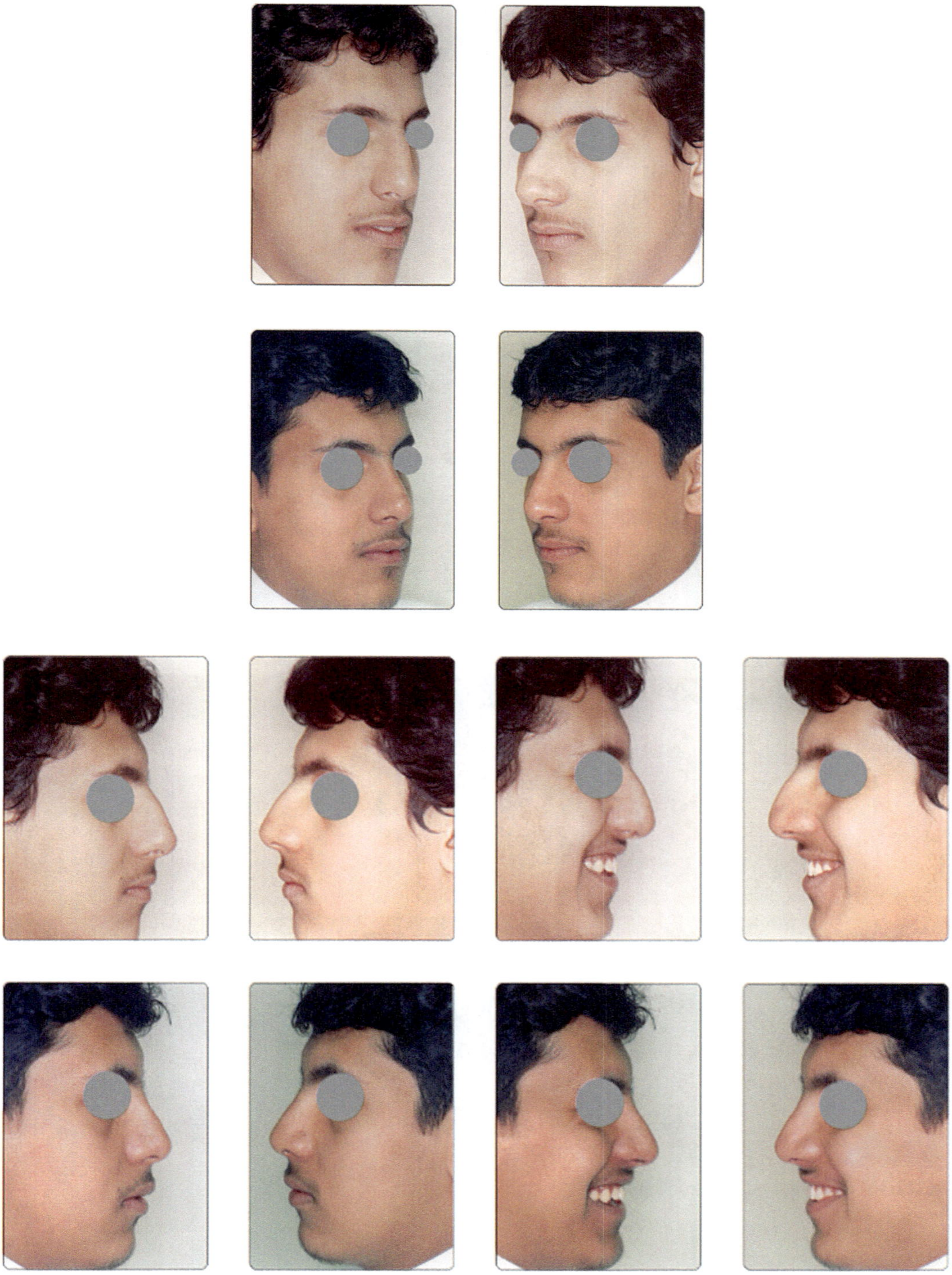

Fig. 22.29 Osteocartilagenous hump in bilateral maxillary asymmetry, before and after surgery

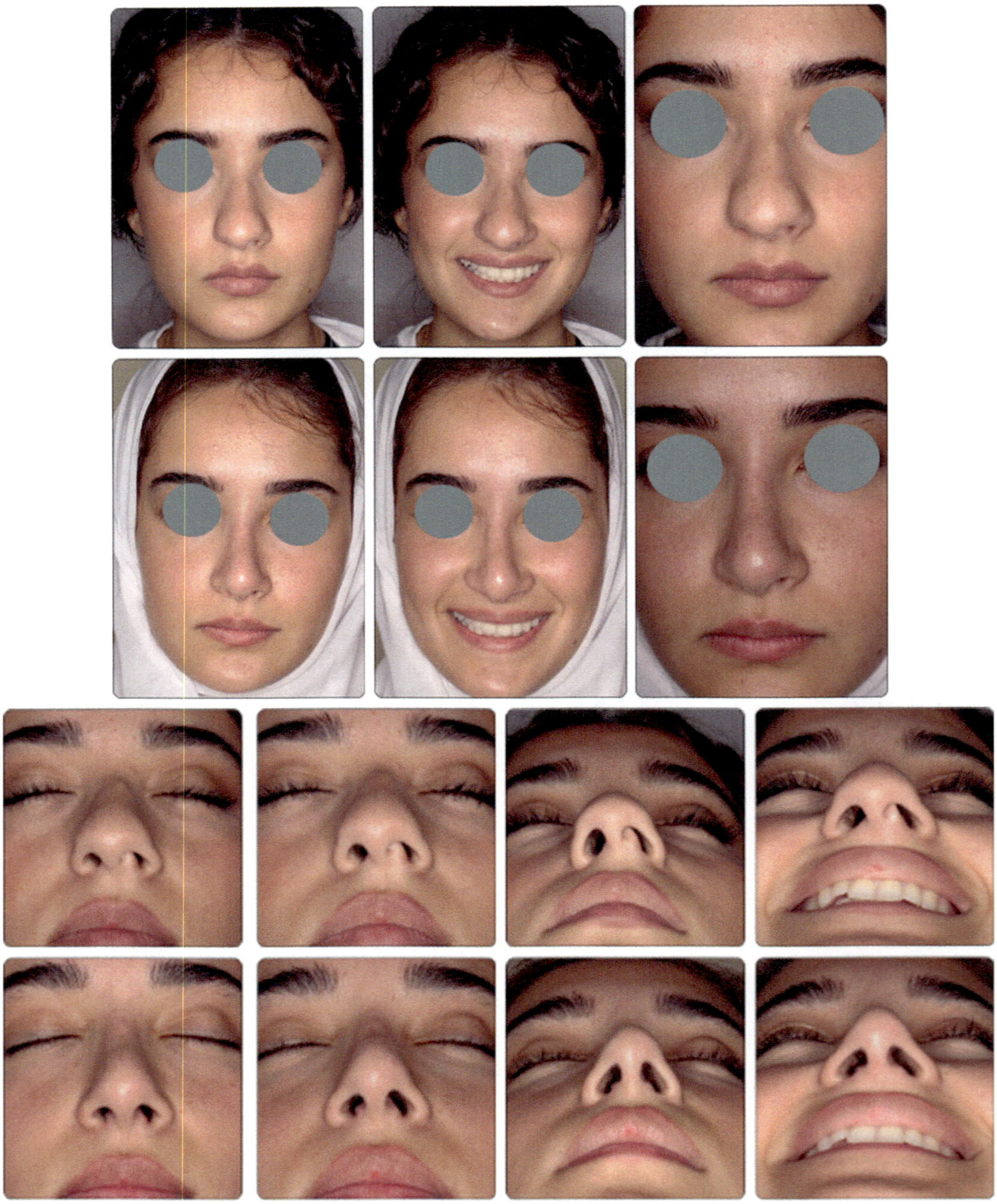

Fig. 22.30 Developmentally Crooked Nose

In contradistinction from the developmental crooked nose, there is a clear **history of trauma**, the nose is **irregularly irregular**, with ragged, rough unsmooth surfaces. There may be protrusion of bony spicules. No other features of bilateral facial asymmetry.

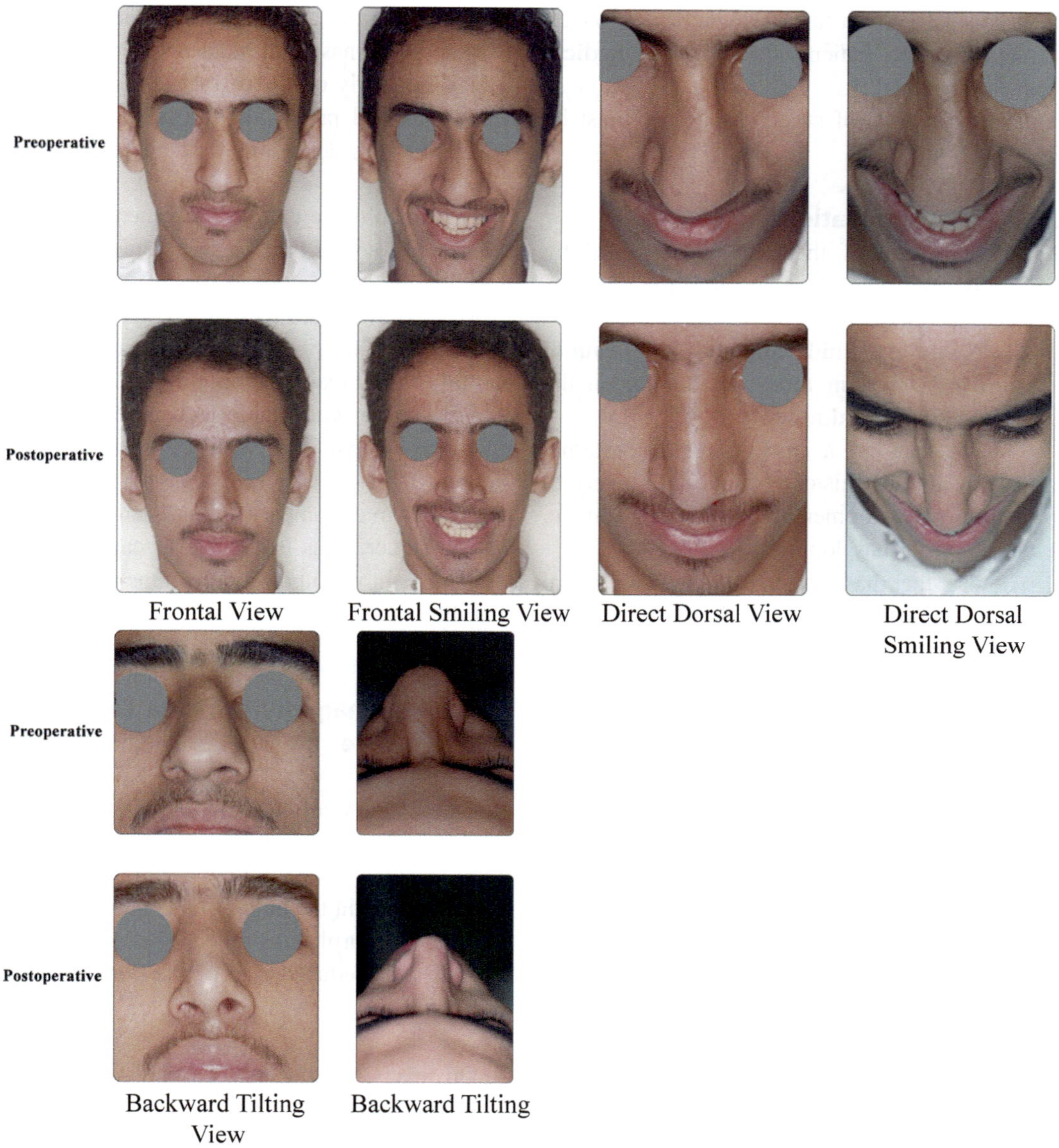

Fig. 22.31 Post- Traumatic Crooked Nose

22.3.3 Clinical Assessment of the Deviated and the Crooked Nose

Both conditions of nasal deviation or crookedness are assessed by carefully going through the history, examination by inspection and palpation and finally photographic studies.

22.3.3.1 History

A history of previous surgical or accidental trauma to the nose. Trauma that causes any deformity in the bony pyramid or dislocation of the caudal septum must be a **considerable unforgotten** one with severe **bruising**, **swelling** and **bleeding** at the time of the accident or injury.

It is usually a bad fall, accident, strong punch or sports injury. Patients usually **seek medical** help in a hospital.

The exact time of surgery or injury must be known.

22.3.3.2 Examination

Each component of the nose is examined by inspection and palpitation for any irregularities, defects and sharp edges.

The **bony pyramid, midvault** and **caudal septum** are the main focus of attention in the deviated and crooked nose.

A nose that has a smooth, regular external wall with no clear history of trauma is likely to be naturally developmental rather than traumatic, even though it may look quite crooked.

A nose that has irregular, ragged or sharp edges over the nasal dorsum, bony pyramid or caudal septum is likely to be traumatic.

22.3.3.3 Photographic Diagnosis

All views of photography are useful in diagnosing and seeing the different parts of the nose in both conditions of deviation and crookedness, yet depending on the location, some views are better in demonstrating a specific deformity than others.

- The **degree** of nasal deviation and crookedness is better appreciated in the **direct dorsal**, the **over head** and the **frontal** views.
- The osteocartilaginous **humps** and the bony pyramids are better seen in the **oblique** and **lateral views.**
- **Maxillary asymmetries** are better demonstrated in the **backward tilting and basal** views. The height and width of both cheeks as well as the bony pyramid are well demonstrated, with a direct comparison between the two sides. Other views may also help in appreciating the bony pyramid and the location of its **origin from the face,** e.g. the **overhead**, **direct dorsal** and **frontal** views.
- **Caudal septal dislocation** and **deformities** are best seen in the **basal** and **nasal aperture** views. The caudal margin may be seen protruding out of the nasal aperture. The two nasal openings are falsely different in size and shape. The nasal sill band is pushed laterally and inferiorly on the dislocated side.
- Defects and protrusions are seen in the different views depending on their location.

Photographs are the best documents that give the surgeon ample time to study the deformities in each area of the nose in detail.

Many of these are seen and diagnosed for the first time in the photographs, despite previous careful clinical examination.

More time is available to be spent with the photographs than that with the patients. **Both sides** of the nose and face are seen **simultaneously** for direct comparison and study.

The camera lens is capable of capturing certain angles in various magnifications and lighting that the human eyes may miss.

22.3.4 Management of the Deviated Nose

Deviated noses are usually large in size that needs overall reduction. Mainly the bony pyramid includes the humps and the nasal tip. Reduction in the bulk of fat contents and size of the lateral cartilages of the nasal tip is required to match the reduced size of the bony pyramid and midvault.

- On excising the osteocartilaginous hump, more bone is reduced from the larger side.
- After osteotomies, the nose may continue to have deviated. Cross fracture of the bony pyramid is needed to adjust it to the midline, i.e. **Kassanjean maneuver**.
  - Two pieces of 4 × 4 inches gauze swab are placed across the bridge of the bony pyramid. The side of the bridge is briskly hammered from the deviated side across to the midline. A crack is heard and the bony pyramid is now centralized. Further adjustment is secured by using the flat of the two thumbs.
- The deviated nose is almost always associated with **deviation of the nasal septum,**

especially in its caudal end. This needs correction by a **conservative septoplasty**.

22.3.5 Management of the Crooked Nose

(a) The developmental crooked nose is dealt with in exactly the same way as the deviated nose.
(b) The post-traumatic crooked nose is dealt with as described in the chapters of secondary rhinoplasty and fractured nose rhinoplasty.

22.4 Part IV: Rhinoplasty of the Fractured Nose: Types and Surgical Management

There are various types and degrees of facial and nasal fractures. In rhinoplasty, we are only concerned with the simple uncomplicated **types of nasal fractures** which are classified as **class 1** and **class 2** types of nasal fractures. In the order of frequency and according to their **weaknesses** and **vulnerabilities,** the most **common nasal fractures** that are met with in rhinoplasty are:

1. **Fractured cartilaginous septum** caused by direct **frontal trauma;**
2. **Fractured nasal bones** caused by **fronto-lateral trauma;**
3. **Fractured frontal process of maxilla** caused **lateral trauma.**

The common causes of nasal trauma are:

- **Frontal trauma**: As in boxing, walking into a glass door, or a direct fall on the nose;
- **Lateral trauma**: Accidents, assault, fighting and group sports, e.g., football, squash, wrestling, karate and rugby.

22.4.1 Fracture of the Nasal Septum

Fracture of the nasal septum may take place in isolation, or in association with fracture of the bony pyramid as in class 1 nasal fracture. There are two types of septal fracture that affect its cartilaginous and bony components:

22.4.1.1 Fracture of the Cartilaginous Septum

Also known as the **vertical fracture of Chevallet**. This, by far, is the most common nasal fracture which on many occasions is usually **missed and not treated, at the time of injury,** as the deformity may not be apparent externally and hence not diagnosed. It is caused by a moderate **direct frontal trauma**, classically seen in boxers. The cartilaginous septum is the most prominent, firm and breakable cartilage of the nose.

The quadrilateral cartilage is broken vertically between its two fixed points, i.e. the **anterior nasal spine of the maxilla** and the **nasal bones**.

Depending on the severity of the trauma, the fracture line may go for a certain distance **down** from the nasal bones or **up** from the anterior nasal spine. In severe trauma, the fracture line goes all the way to connect these two points.

Cartilaginous fracture of the septum usually takes place **in isolation** without any damage to the bony pyramid despite the considerable force of the trauma, i.e. frontal punch or walking into a door.

By far the most common line of cartilaginous fracture is at the junction between the relatively mobile caudal vestibular septum with the fixed internal respiratory cartilaginous septum.

Occasionally, the **distal thin tip of the nasal bone** is involved in the trauma leading to a **ski-slope deformity** of the nose. This is especially true if trauma took place in the childhood period.

Aesthetic Effects of the Vertical Fracture

The vertical fracture of the cartilaginous septum results in the **separation of a distal**

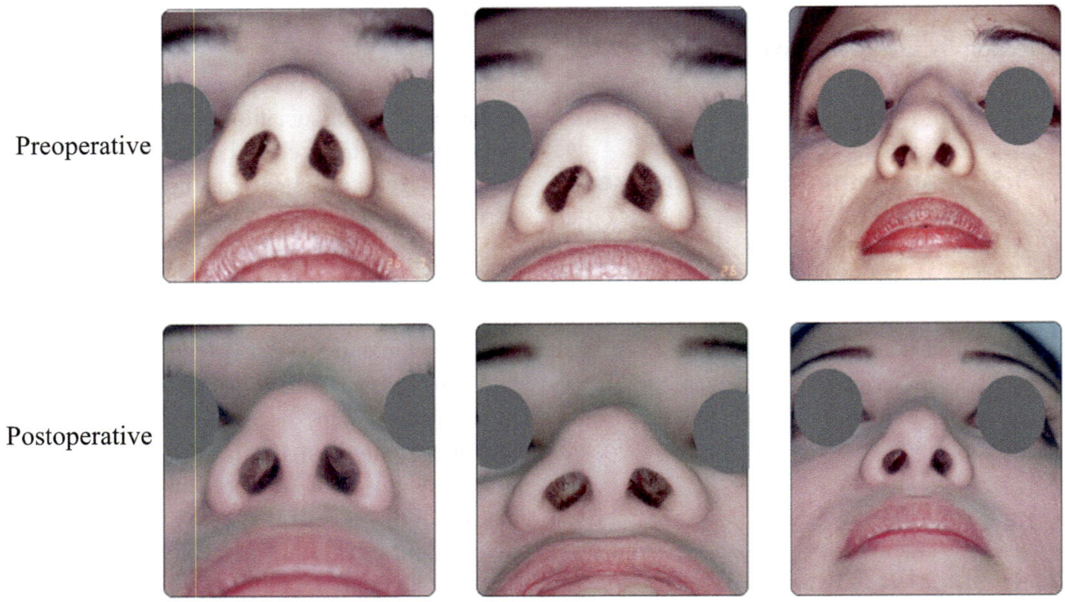

Fig. 22.32 Fracture of Caudal Cartilaginous Septum: Dislocated to the Right

subcutaneous segment which is usually **displaced laterally to one side**.

It is derailed off the maxillary groove, although a piece of cartilage is always present inside the groove. The displacement of the distal segment has the following aesthetic effects:

Unequal Nasal Openings

The displaced inferior border produces unequal nasal openings both in **size** and **shape** (Fig. 22.32).

The **medial crus** is pushed **laterally** and the **nasal sill band inferiorly**, considerably disfiguring the nasal aperture and narrowing the airway.

The caudal cartilaginous margin of the septum may be hidden behind these structures, or in severe conditions, it is seen freely in the nasal opening.

Unilateral Domal Bulge

The anterior border and anterior angle of the broken displaces caudal septum, pushes the **dome** of the middle crus and **forwards laterally,** resulting in an unpleasant **unilateral bulge** and broadening of the nasal tip (Fig. 22.33).

Duplication of the Septal Cartilage

Duplication is secondary to the separation of the perichondrium as a result of the trauma.

The **distal segment is now made of two parts**, viz., the **laterally displaced** segment and the newly formed segment. The latter is usually not uniformly made with some irregularly thin and thick areas of cartilages and fibrous tissues.

The duplicate cartilaginous septum adds to the disfigurement of the nasal aperture.

Saddling

This is not an uncommon complication that may follow accidental or surgical trauma to the cartilaginous septum. The saddle deformity may be immediate or delayed.

Immediate Saddling

Saddling may follow an accidental trauma, but more commonly it inadvertently happens during septal surgery. Destabilization of the supportive

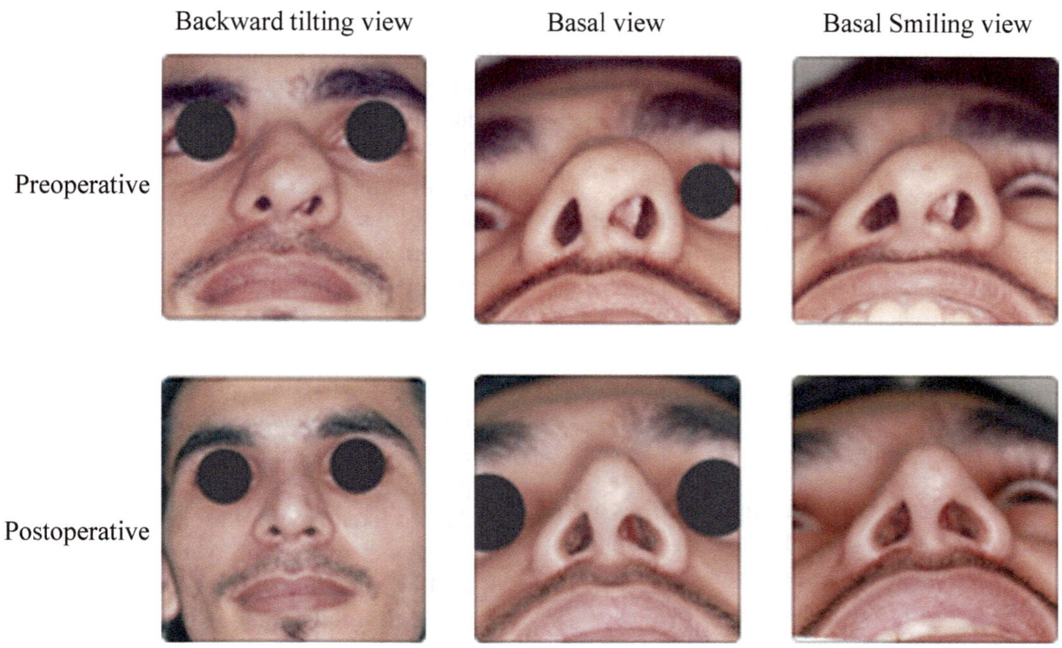

Fig. 22.33 Fracture of Caudal Cartilaginous Septum: Dislocated to the Left

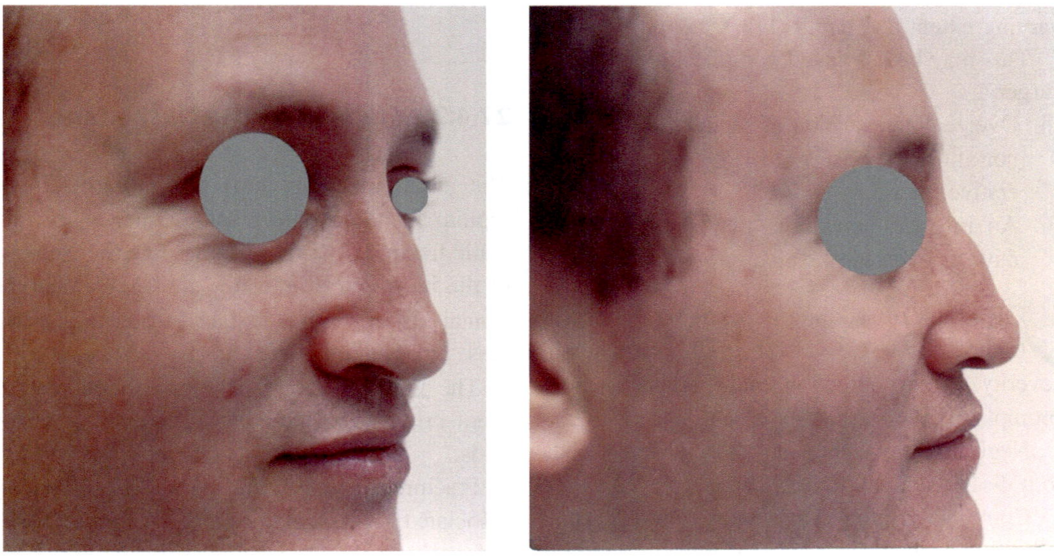

Fig. 22.34 Mild delayed saddling, five years after overzealous septoplasty

mechanism of the septum to the dorsum **at the two fixing points** is the most common cause of the immediate saddling:

- The High Saddle

This results from **too high dissection of the cartilaginous septum.** If the cartilage is inadvertently separated from the ethmoid plate, at the level of the fixing point of the nasal bone, a drop of the nasal dorsum takes place and immediate saddling appears externally.

- The Low Saddle:

This takes place **in the supratip area** at the level of the anterior nasal spine. Disarticulation of the cartilaginous septum from the maxillary groove and/or uncalculated excessive removal of the cartilage and/or bones will lead to an immediate drop of the dorsum at the supratip region.

Delayed Saddling

Anatomically delayed saddling is located between the nasal bones and the nasal tip with varying extent and depth (Fig. 22.34).

This may be a delayed complication of septal surgery.

i. Overzealous excision of septal cartilage may not affect the nose in the immediate postoperative period.
ii. An infected hematoma may present a few days or even weeks after surgery.

The extent of saddling depends on the extent of trauma, tissue loss, size of the hematoma, severity of the infection and finally on how prompt was the surgical intervention.

Neglected septal hematoma or abscess leads to a disastrous disfiguring saddle (Fig. 22.35).

Complete healing and maturation of septal scar tissue may take **12–18 months**. Dorsal depression and saddling may not be apparent and complete before that time.

22.4.1.2 Fracture of the Bony Septum

This is also known as the **C-shaped fracture of Jarjavay**. This is an uncommonly seen fracture that involves both the **bony** and **cartilaginous** septum. It is associated with a **fracture of** the **nasal bones** and the **frontal process of the maxilla**. A stronger frontolateral trauma is necessary to produce it.

The C-shape of the septal fracture starts from the **quadrilateral cartilage** under the nasal bone, posteriorly through the **perpendicular plate of the ethmoid** bone, then curves down before it comes **forward through these two structures again** near the level of the vomerine bone.

i. In a **recently broken nose,** it is important to disimpact the broken bony septum by immediate submucus resection in order to secure a stable reduction of the broken bony pyramid.
ii. An **old fixed fracture** of the bony septum is dealt with more conservatively, with **minimal or no submucus resection in order to avoid destabilization of the nose**. It is preferred that the deviate bony parts of the septum are possibly fractured and **pushed to the midline**, using Killian speculum or a strong elevator. Only minimal resection might be needed.

22.4.2 Fracture of the Nasal Bones

The nasal bones are next to the cartilaginous septum in its weakness and frequency in traumatic fracture. The **nasal bones are the weakest of the bony pyramid**. They are weaker than the frontal processes of maxillae and the nasal processes of frontal bones.

The weakest part of the nasal bones that is more prone to fracture is their **distal anterior ends.**

Fracture of the nasal bones is commonly associated with septal fracture, e.g. **ski slope deformity,** or in association with fracture of the frontal process of the maxilla (Fig. 22.36).

The **isolated fracture of the nasal bones** occasionally takes place if a sufficient force was inflicted from a **frontolateral direction** specifically to these bones.

Clinically, the isolated fracture of the nasal bones is associated with clear unpleasant

Preoperative

Postoperative

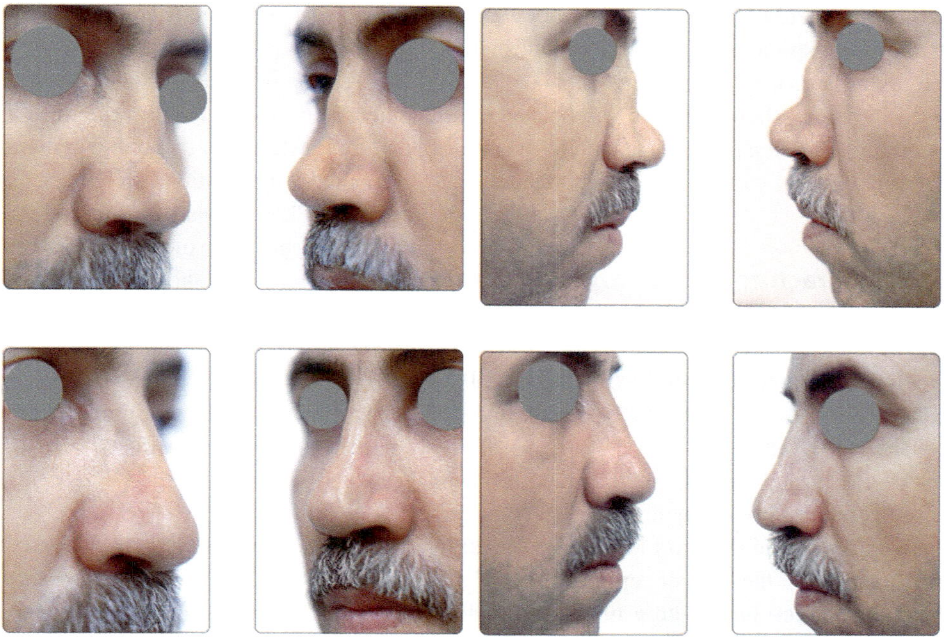

Fig. 22.35 Severe delayed saddling, after untreated septal hematoma and abscess

Preoperative

Postoperative

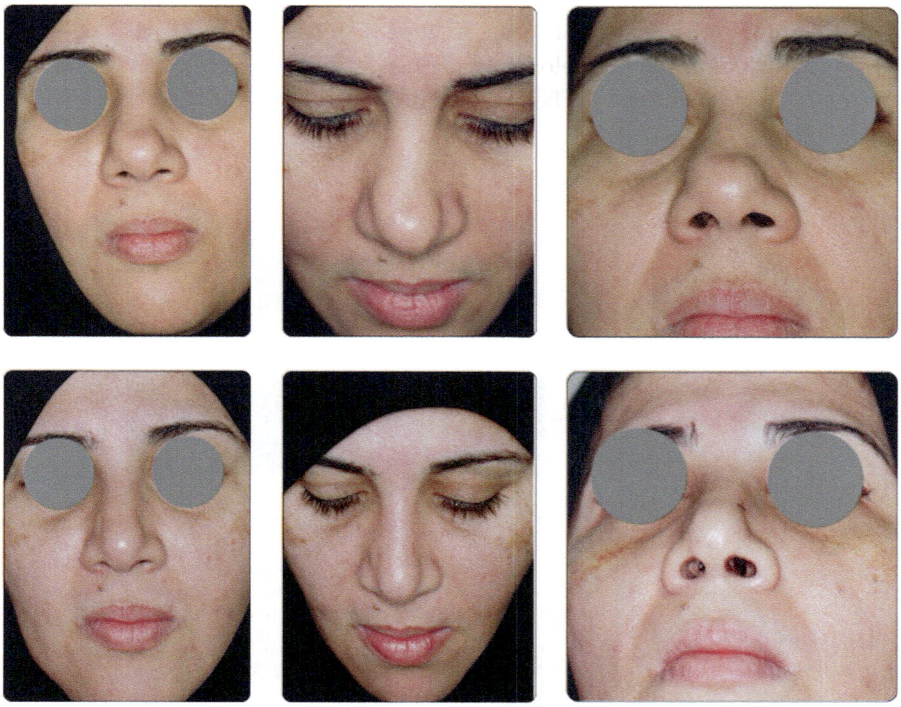

Fig. 22.36 Left ski slope deformity, exaggerated by vertical fracture of the cartilaginous septum

external irregularities of this bony dorsum, and **sharp bony spicules** of the broken bones add to the ugliness of the trauma (Fig. 22.37).

Ski slope deformity is associated with external depression that may extend to the area of the upper lateral cartilage on the affected side.

22.4.3 Fracture of the Frontal Process of Maxilla

Fracture of the frontal process of the maxillary bone results from a **direct lateral trauma** with **considerable force**.

As the frontal process of the maxilla is the base of the nasal bony pyramid, when fractured, the whole pyramid **deviates** to the **opposite side**. This results in the **classic appearance of the crooked broken nose** with a **bruising mark at the base of the traumatized side.** This is to be differentiated from causes of unilateral inherited blue discoloration of the lower eyelid (Fig. 22.38).

A confusing situation may happen if these individuals, with inherited discoloration, present with a history of trauma and the bony pyramid is deviated to the opposite side, as part of a facial asymmetry.

Trauma is not a considerable one, and usually, there is no bleeding from the nose following the trauma. Although the bony pyramid may have deviated, on palpation it feels quite smooth, with no pain depressions or sharp edges.

Classically, an old untreated fracture of the frontal process of the maxilla has a clinical trial of **crookedness, wide bony base and a large-sized lower lateral cartilage.**

Fracture of the frontal process of the maxilla may be associated with **other fractures,** e.g. **nasal bones** and **septum**.

22.4.4 The Aesthetic Management of the Fractured Nose

In order to achieve the best aesthetic results while performing rhinoplasty in a fractured nose, **all four areas of the nose have to be considered:**

i. The frontolateral walls;
ii. The medial wall;
iii. The bony pyramid and midvault;
iv. The alar base.

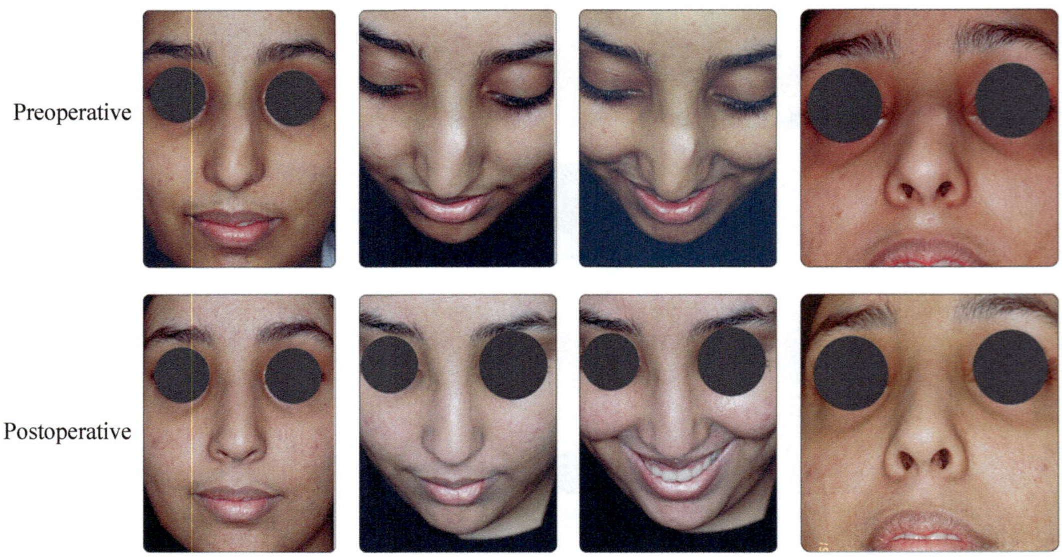

Fig. 22.37 Isolated fracture of the nasal bones. The base of the boney pyramid made by the frontal process of the maxilla remained intact

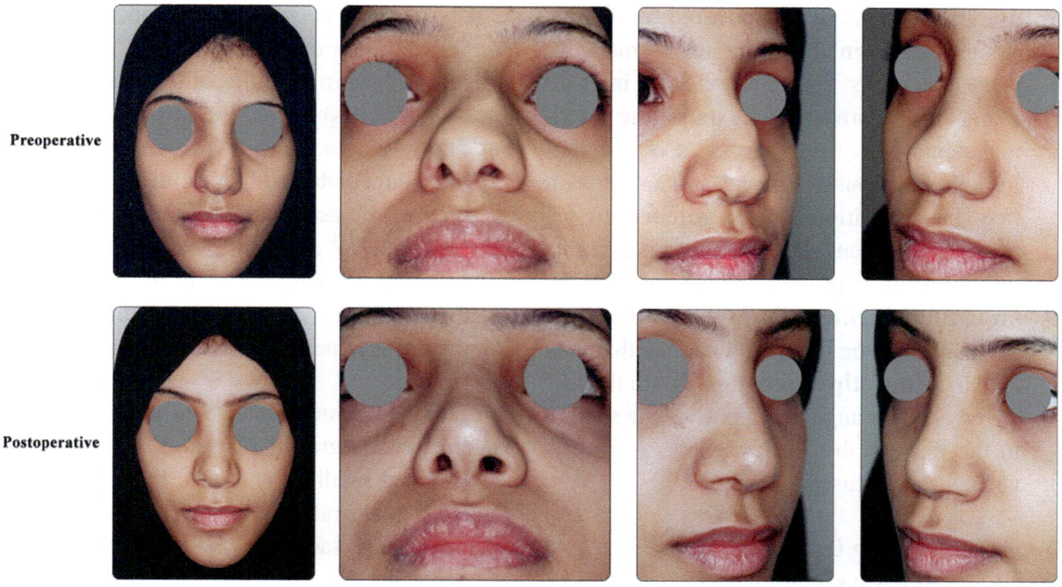

Fig. 22.38 Fracture of the frontal processes of maxillae

Dealing with bony deformities alone may have a satisfactory result, but not the best aesthetic achievement.

22.4.4.1 Management of the Fractured Septum

Although correcting the fractured bony pyramid is the ultimate goal of surgery that achieves the impressive aesthetic result and patient satisfaction, **successful management of the traumatic septum is an essential basis for a stable and better aesthetic result.**

The most important rule in septoplasty as part of the aesthetic process is that the procedure must be targeted to the aesthetic purpose. It **should not** be a routine septoplasty, e.g. correction of the caudal deviation to equalize the sizes of nasal apertures or correction of the higher deviation that causes a unilateral bulge of the lateral crus.

Meticulous dissection, conservative attitude and wise decisions are the gold standards of management.

The traumatic nasal septum may have different clinical presentations:

The Laterally Displaced Broken Distal Segment

This is the most common type of septal trauma. The distal segment is best managed by meticulously dissecting and then replacing it with the midline. The proximal cartilaginous septum is acutely angled with the distal segment, or it may be separated from it by an area of tough fibrous tissue.

In many cases, it is not very easy to continue dissecting the mucoperichondrial layer from the distal broken segment to the main proximal cartilaginous septum.

There are two situations in these conditions:

i. The **distal broken segment** is **continuous with the proximal segment:**

   In these conditions, the mucoperichondrium is dissected off the broken **distal** segment gradually till the proximal septum is reached. At this point, the cartilage of the distal segment is incised longitudinally at the location of the angle. The distal segment is thus **totally separated**. The mucoperichondrium of the **proximal septum** is then dissected as if it is a second septum.

ii. The **distal segment** is **separated by fibrous tissue** area from the proximal segment: In these conditions, a **second external incision** is made to approach and explore the proximal septum.
In both situations, the distal broken segment may be **repositioned and stitched to** the proximal segment. If it was not manageable in any useful way, then it may be **partially or totally sacrificed**. Excision of the distal segment must be done with care as this may lead to a **supratip depression** due to the loss of the anterior angular support of the septum to the floor of the weak triangle. A graft is needed to fill this depression.

Duplication of the Distal Segment

This is almost always an irregularly formed piece of cartilage that distorts the shape of the nasal aperture and has **no aesthetic**, **supportive** or **functional contribution. Total excision** is usually the fate of these duplicates. They may be used as **grafts**.

Excess Redundant Skin

There is almost always extensively stretched and thickened skin on the dislocated side of the broken septum, even in the absence of a duplicated cartilage.

This is secondary to post-traumatic fibrosis of damaged tissues and hematomas. The resulting thick skin of the columella distorts the shape of the nasal aperture. A judgment **trim of the excess skin** in conjunction with adjusting the underlying caudal septum, and nasal spine is necessary for the aesthetics of the columella and the nasal aperture.

Traumatic Dislocation, Fracture and Deviation

Dislocation off the maxillary groove may take place in a distally broken segment of the quadrilateral cartilage of the septum.

Traumatic fracture deviation is located at the high level of the septal cartilage or bony parts. Both are quite essential in stabilizing the three-dimensional shape of the traumatized weakened nose.

Any hasty or unwise decision of removing of destabilizing part of the septum may lead to total collapse or severe saddling of the nasal dorsum.

Saddling

(1) The immediate saddling is dealt with at the time of the accidental, or surgical trauma is corrected by attempting to replace the lost cartilage submucosally at the location of depression, i.e. near the two fixing points of the nasal bones and the anterior nasal spine.

Failing to achieve that, then a crushed cartilaginous dorsal graft is placed.

(2) Delayed saddling is treated by the appropriate dorsal graft. Depending on the size and degree of saddling, the type of graft is decided.

Grafts may be taken from the nasal septum. Cases of severe saddling that need a large graft, e.g. costal cartilage.

These cases are almost always associated with a wide base of the bony pyramid and a large lower third of the nose. Lateral osteotomies are necessary in order to aesthetically match the size of the base to that of the dorsal graft.

22.4.4.2 Management of the Fractured Bony Pyramid

The management of fractured nasal bones, frontal process of the maxilla or both is closely similar.

Isolated fracture of the nasal bones may sometimes be simpler and less complicated.

There are important considerations in performing rhinoplasty on a fractured bony pyramid:

Isolated Nasal Bone Fracture

i. **Irregularities in** the area of the nasal bones are only at the summit of the bony pyramid, and may only need to be rasped and smoothed down. No further management is needed.
ii. **Ski slope deformity** is usually associated with an external depression that extends the area of the upper lateral cartilage on the same

side. Augmentation of **cartilaginous graft** is necessary to elevate the depression.

Fracture of Frontal Process of the Maxilla

Fracture of the frontal process of the maxilla severely distorts the aesthetics of the bony pyramid. The nose is deviated or crooked. The bony base is usually wide.

Associated deformities may include the nasal septum. The latter may consequently affect the aesthetics of the nasal apertures and domes.

Osteotomies are necessary to readjust the bony pyramid to the straight midline position. This usually reduces the size of the bony pyramid to an aesthetically better shape.

Proportionate reduction of the size of the lower third of the nose avoids the trumpet shape deformity.

Reduction surgery therefore may be needed for the lower third of the nose, in the form of alar resection, defatting and cephalic resection of lateral crurae.

Areas of Prominences and Defects

The broken parts of the bony pyramid may project and produce hump-like protrusions or irregular and sometimes sharp bony spicules. These have to be smoothened down.

On the other hand, areas of defects are compensated by suitable grafts.

22.5 Part V: Secondary Rhinoplasty

Secondary or revision rhinoplasty is a situation, where a second or more surgery is thought to be required for the nose due to unacceptable aesthetic results of the primary one or more surgeries. This is usually not a very pleasant situation both for the patient and the surgeon.

There are two main challenges in these situations:

22.5.1 Surgical Challenges

There are variable degrees of definite aesthetic problems in these noses that need to be seen.

22.5.2 Psychological Challenges

Both the surgeons and the patients are in a definite but different state of psychological situation.

The surgeons are not quite as happy to deal with the cases of secondary rhinoplasty, even if they are their own. Patients' psychology varies from being calm, content and full of confidence in their doctor to the other extreme of discontent, anger, cynical, difficult to please or even aggressive and abusive.

On the other hand, problems in the nose may not be that easy or predictable to resolve against the changing level of patient satisfaction and expectations.

There are some rare but definite unusual situations where patients may try to deceive, abuse or even blackmail their original doctors in different ways.

- Patients may hide the fact that they underwent second or more failed surgeries by a different surgeon.
- Patients may deny an accident, trauma or assault to their noses.

In all of these conditions, patients should be met with a welcoming and understanding attitude. The doctor must be quite calm and prepared to listen as much as possible to the patient. He should be able to absorb all his concerns and worries and be prepared for a wide range of patient presentations.

After listening to what the patient has to say, the doctor must have a clear plan and system for the history and clinical examination.

The best and shortest way to reassure the patient is to reach the exact diagnosis and have an almost clear plan for the management.

22.5.3 Matching the History with the Clinical Findings

One must not jump to conclusions and make early decisions, especially if it is not an easy straightforward case.

Plenty of time must be taken to think about the history, clinical findings and photographic assessment. All the facts are carefully collected and studied.

If all of the clinical facts match with the patient's history then decisions are clearly made. But if the clinical findings do not match with the history and photographic findings, then patients are seen again and their clinical conditions are reconsidered.

22.5.4 Management of Secondary Rhinoplasty

Management of secondary rhinoplasty includes the following steps:

I. Clinical assessment
II. Psychological assessment (discussed in the Psychology section)
III. Surgical strategy

22.5.4.1 Clinical Assessment

It is wise to make the full clinical assessment before making any definitive judgment on the patient's psychology. A clinical assessment gives grounds for both parties to discuss and discover each other.

The problems may be fairly manageable and the aesthetic goals are easily achievable. In these cases patient's worries and tension are quickly settled and feels happy. Originally his discontent is not quite severe. More complicated cases are discussed with further details according to each condition.

All four areas of rhinoplasty are considered in the clinical assessment, viz., the bony pyramid including midvaults, the frontolateral walls, the medial wall and the alar base.

The clinical assessment must include:

History and Psychological Assessment

Careful critical history is taken, although many times it is not very clear. The patient's age, sex and background are of considerable importance.

An adult mature person is easier to reason with than a young immature individual. However, sometimes maturity is the patient's nature rather than the age or sex.

The patient's cultural, educational and social backgrounds are all landmarks for the grounds of discussion.

The following basic questions are generally asked:

1. Why did you want to have the first surgery?
   What was the original problem?
   Do you have any pre-operative photographs?
2. When was the primary surgery?
3. How many surgeries did you have on your nose?
   The patient may deny a second surgery if you were the original surgeon.
4. What has changed after the original surgery?
5. Who is the surgeon of the primary surgery?
   Is there a report?
   He might be a well-known surgeon with a well-known or familiar technique.
6. Did you receive any injury or trauma to your nose?
7. What are the reason and the location of dissatisfaction, deformity and depression?
   How soon did they develop after surgery?
8. Did you have any nasal symptoms before surgery, e.g. nasal blockage, pain or discharge?
9. Do you have any new symptoms after the surgery, e.g. blockage, pain, dryness or bleeding?
   Have you heard any comments about your nose?
   Are you affected by these comments from friends and relatives?
10. What would you like to be done to your nose? (unreasonable expectations). Which areas do you wish to change or modify?

11. What is your present work or job? Are you planning to have a job that has more exposure?
12. The patient is asked as many questions as possible.
    This is a good test of the patient's psychological stability.
    Patients tend to deny or hide many facts, clinical or psychological.
13. You may ask the same question in many different ways. Different answers may be obtained for the same question.

Clinical Varieties of Secondary Rhinoplasty

Omitted Surgery

These are cases where surgery in one or more of the four areas was omitted, overlooked or forgotten. The previous surgeon did not explore or operate in these areas. Commonly neglected areas in the order of frequency are:

1. The nasal septum;
2. The alar base;
3. The bony pyramid and midvault;
4. The frontolateral walls.

Completed Surgery

One or more areas of rhinoplasty underwent full surgical exploration and procedure that completely achieved their aesthetic goals, i.e. reasonable acceptable or excellent result.

Uncompleted Surgery

One or more areas underwent full surgical exploration and procedure, yet the results are short of achieving the satisfactory aesthetic goal as the surgery was insufficient in one or more of the explored areas, e.g. insufficient reduction of the dorsal hump or alar base.

Faulty Surgery

One or more areas underwent full surgical exploration and the procedure was fully carried out, yet the outcome result is unsatisfactory due to **immediate faulty technique** or **delayed faulty result,** e.g. unequal or too high osteotomies, overzealous resection of hump or alar base.

Delayed faulty results may be caused by one or more of the following factors:

- Erratic long-term healing process;
- Erratic and uneven graft resorption, rejection or infection;
- Accidental trauma;
- Untreated neighboring deformities, e.g. septal deviation or osteotomies;
- Immediate or delayed post-operative infection.

Clinical Examination of the Four Areas of the Nose

According to the type of surgery each of the four areas of rhinoplasty is meticulously examined. Patients may have the following clinical presentation:

Frontolateral Walls

According to the type of surgery performed, the patient may be present with the following:

- Over projection of the nasal tip, having had too long or bulky tip graft (faulty technique) (Fig. 22.39);
- Depressed tip after overzealous resection of middle crural cartilages (faulty technique);
- Insufficient tip projection;
- Unequal projection of the two sides of the nasal tip;
- Insufficient reduction of the size or bulk of the frontolateral walls.

Medial Wall

Attention is paid to the two structures of the medial wall:

The Columella

Omitted or faulty surgical management of the columella is addressed, e.g. protrusion, hanging or bifid columella.

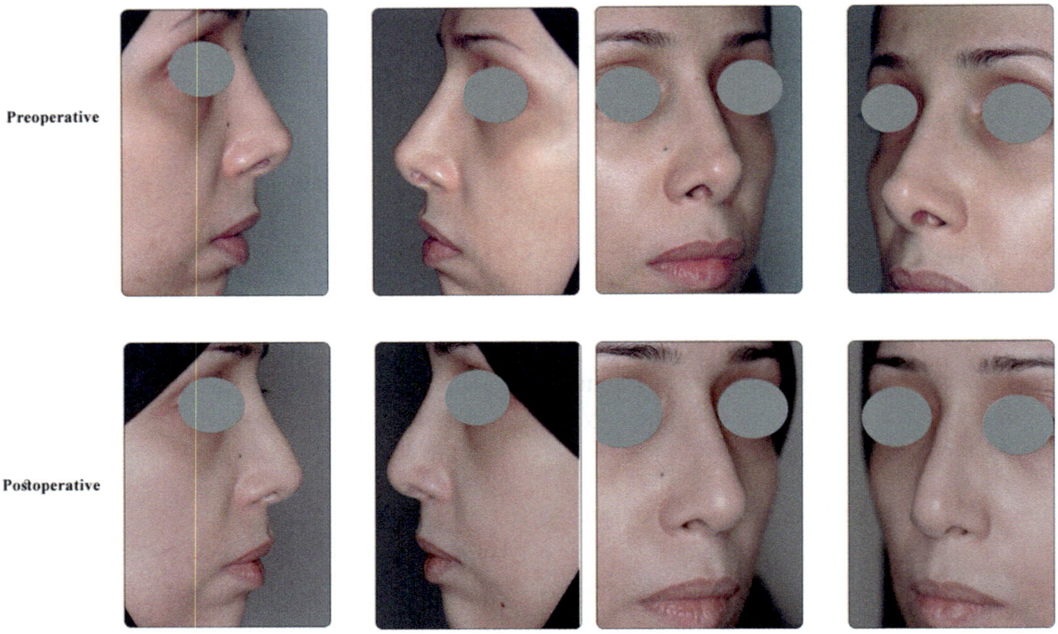

Fig. 22.39 Over projection of the nasal tip, after using a large-sized tip graft

The Nasal Septum

Septal contribution to nasal aesthetics is frequently not very well appreciated or underestimated and therefore overlooked.

It is a major mistake to avoid, overlook or have the false sensation of taking a shortcut by omitting septal surgery in rhinoplasty.

Faulty, incomplete or omitted septal surgery has one or more of the following consequences:

i. Nasal dorsum:
   High nasal dorsum, residual hump, supratip elevation and parrot beak deformities. One or more of these unaesthetic consequences may result from an incomplete dorsal reduction of the cartilaginous septum.
ii. Nasolabial area:
   - Acute nasolabial angle and residual plunging tip or vice versa, i.e. fullness and wide nasolabial angle with tight lip secondary to long caudal septum with a large anterior nasal spine.
   - Prolonged caudal septum may result in:
     – Protruding columella and hanging columella;
     – Lateral bulge of the medial crurae that may be unilateral or bilateral resulting in unequal nasal openings (Fig. 22.40);
iii. Deviation of the nose may never be corrected without correction of the septal deviation (Figs. 22.40 and 22.41).
iv. Unilateral bulge of one of the nasal tip domes.

The Bony Pyramid and Midvault

According to the type of surgery performed the patient may present with:

- Surprisingly, the most common findings in secondary rhinoplasty are faulty, incomplete or omitted medialization of the sidewalls of the bony pyramid after resection of the osteocartilaginous hump. There is a wide base and open roof deformity (Fig. 22.42).

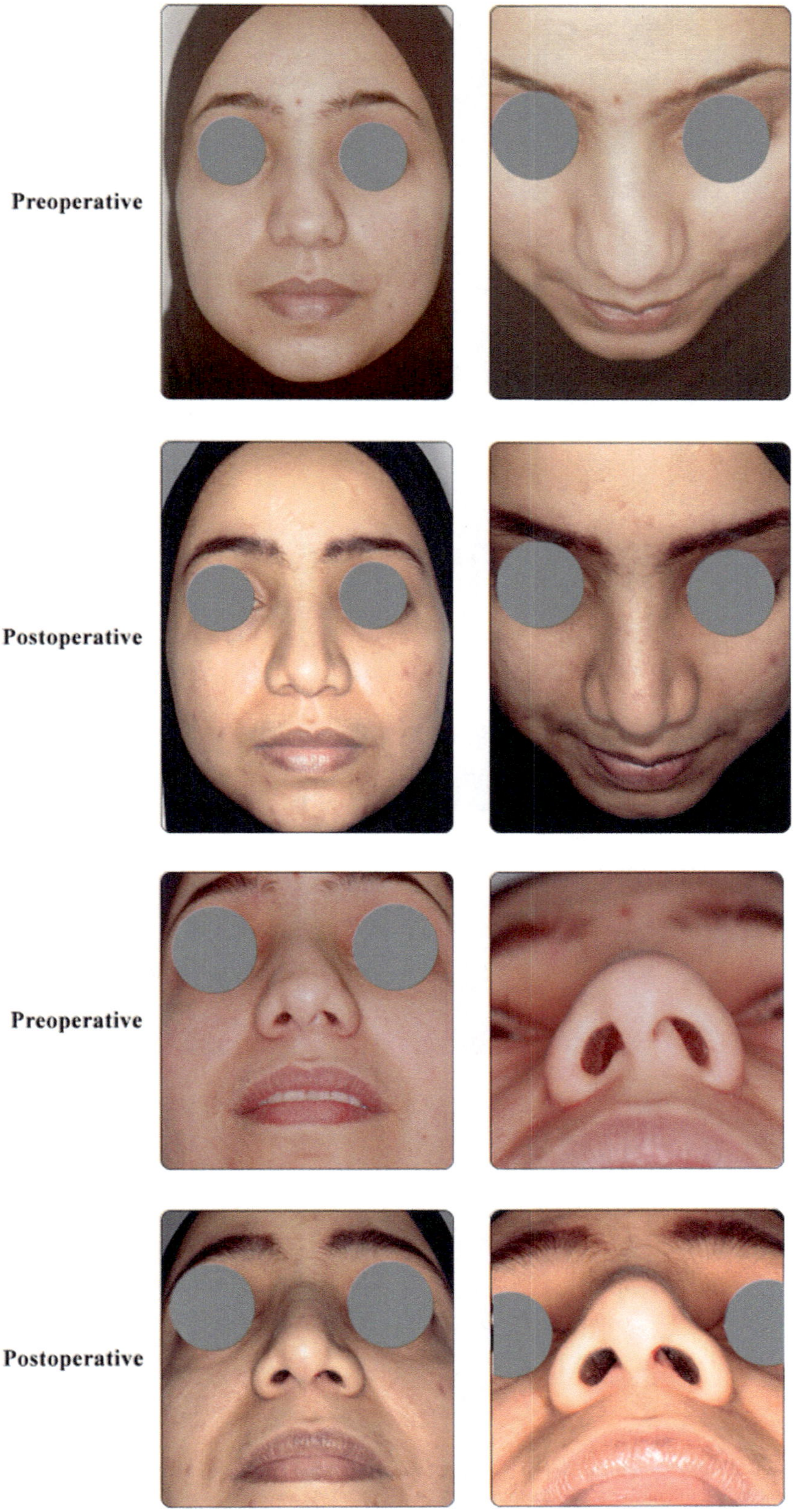

Fig. 22.40 Omitted septoplasty in primary surgery, with a consequent bulge of the left lateral crus and supratip depression. The dislocated caudal septum, distorting the left nasal aperture, which looks smaller than the right

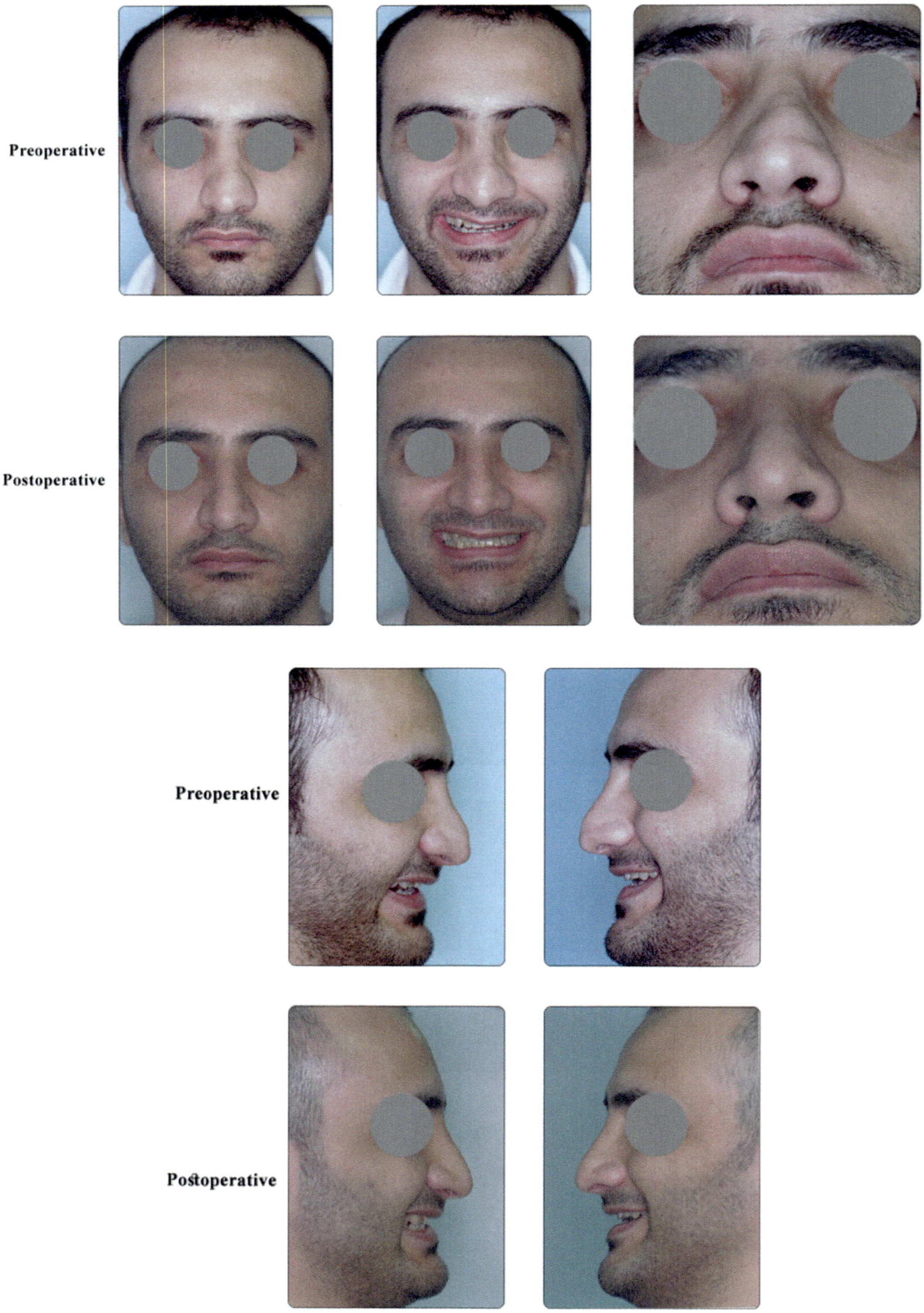

Fig. 22.41 Omitted Bony Pyramidal, Septal and Nasal Fat Surgeries. Pre-operative asymmetrical smile and sliding tip which is at a lower level than the nasal dorsum

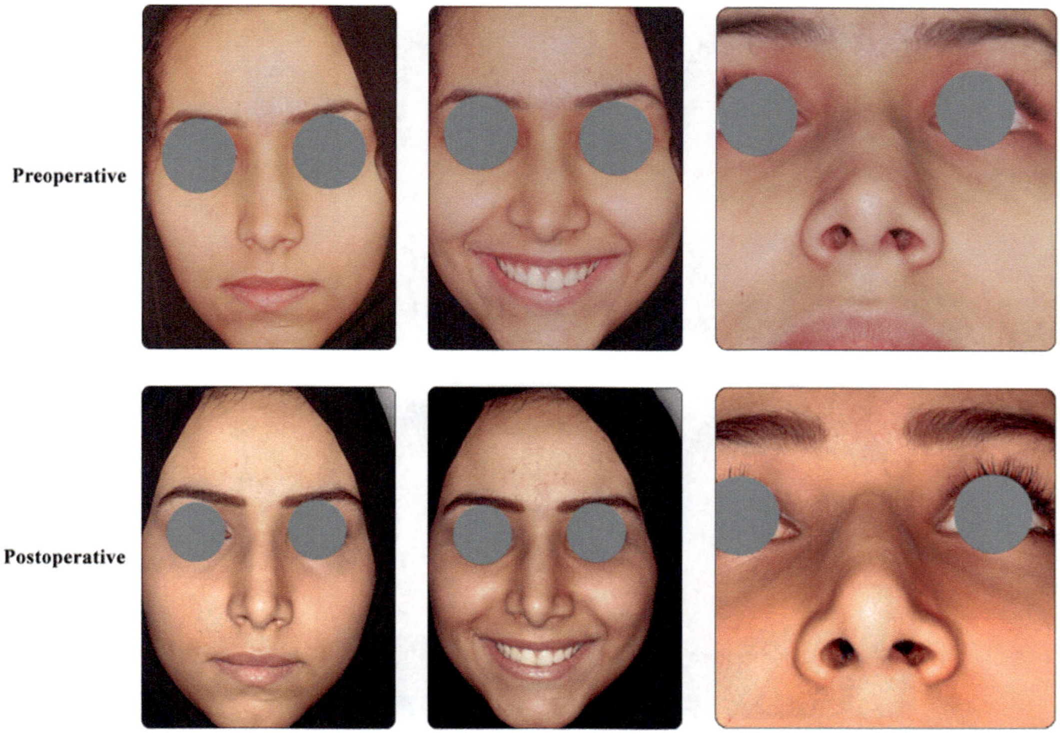

Fig. 22.42 Incomplete medialization of the right side of the boney pyramid. Left caudal deviation due to omitted septal surgery

- Insufficient reduction of the osteocartilaginous hump, i.e. residual hump and high nasal dorsum.
- Overzealous reduction of the hump with the low dorsum of the upper half of the nose.
- Oblique bony pyramid due to
  - Uncorrected septal deviation;
  - Incomplete lateral osteotomies;
  - Incomplete medialization of one side of the bony walls;
  - Maxillary asymmetry.
- Depressed one side of the bony pyramid or one side of the upper lateral cartilages, i.e. midvault.
- Areas of protrusions or depressions on the nasal dorsum or sidewalls.
- Delayed complications, weeks, months or even years after the primary surgery. Trauma may cause direct deformity or hematoma that may be infected.

Alar Base

- Unequal nasal openings (Fig. 22.43);
- Residual wide alar base (Fig. 22.44);
- Lateral angulation of one or both nasal openings (faulty technique) (Fig. 22.45);
- Vestibular stenosis (faulty technique);
- Unpleasant scars at the alar base that are unsightly located away from the alar groove or rim-sill folds;
- Grooving of the alar wound due to omitted subdermal closing stitches (Fig. 22.46);
- Stepping of alar scar if the incision was away from the alar groove (Fig. 22.47).

22.5.5 Acceptance and Plans for Surgery

Having taken the history, examined the patient and studied the photographs, the condition

Preoperative

Postoperative

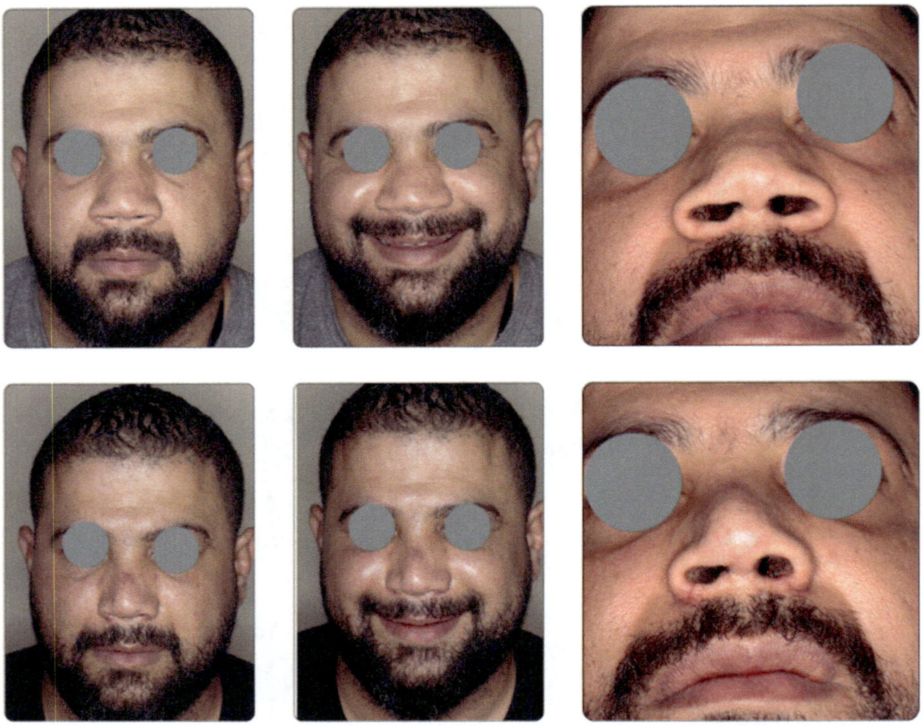

Fig. 22.43 Wide nasal apertures and deformed right flat triangle

Fig. 22.44 Omitted alar base reduction in the primary surgery

Preoperative

Postoperative

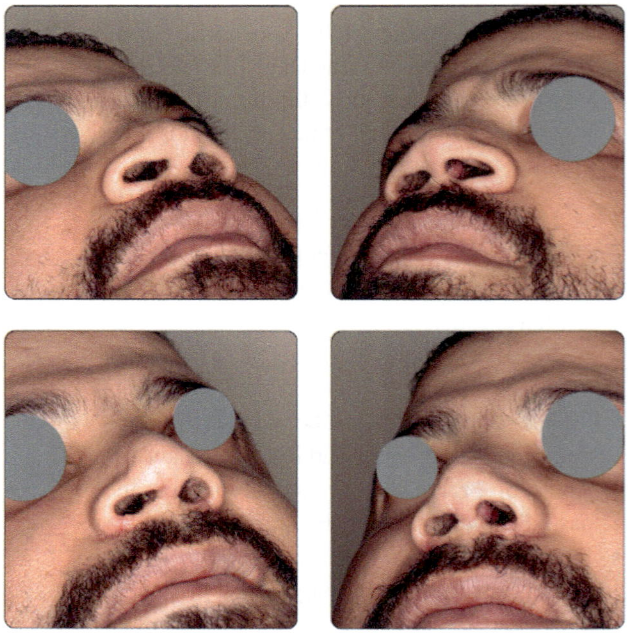

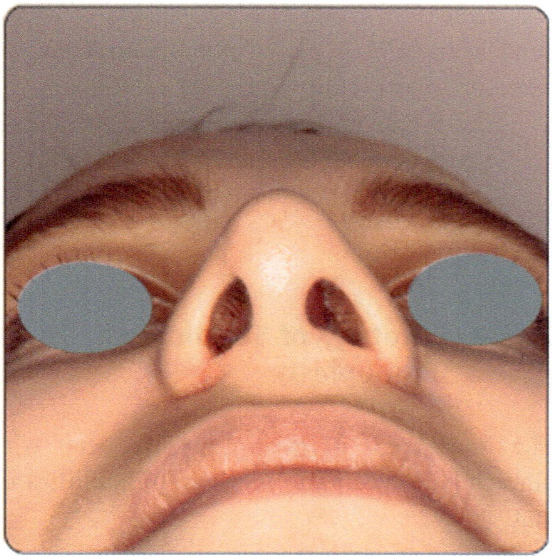

Fig. 22.45 Left angulation of the left nasal opening

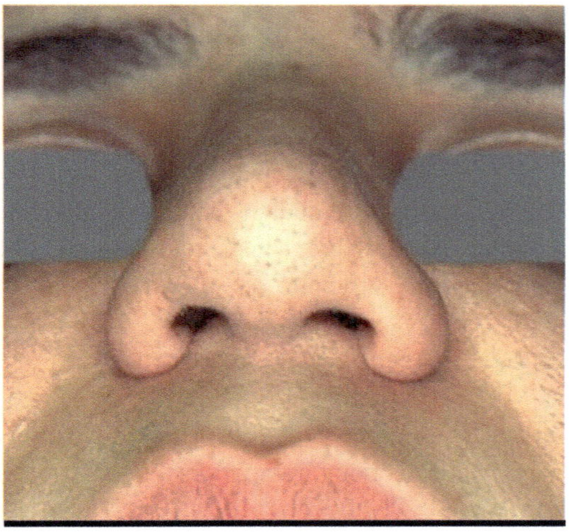

Fig. 22.46 Grooving of the alar wound; omitted subdermal stitches and wrongly placed skin stitches

becomes clear with the possible solution plans. Only then the surgeon may decide to take on the case and proceed with the surgery.

Patients are torn between the disappointments of previous surgery and the dreams of high expectations. These are associated with a mixed feeling of anxiety, fear and cynicism.

Patients must be clearly informed about the anticipated plans and outcomes of surgery. The expected results are based on clinical facts.

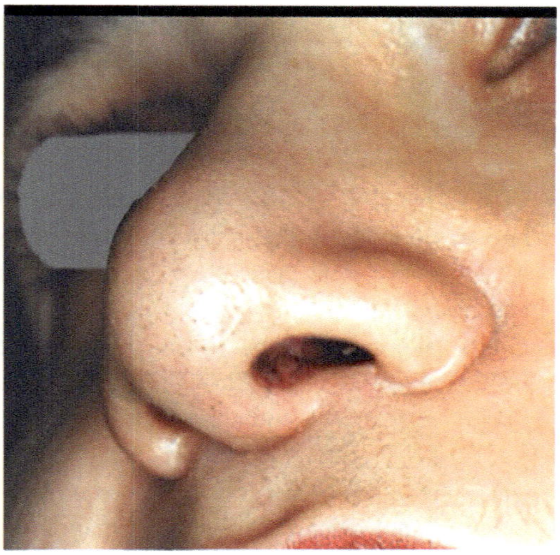

Fig. 22.47 Stepping of the left alar wound. The incision is above the posterior alar groove

Patients are clearly informed about the realistic expected results rather than the unrealistic dreams and high expectations.

22.5.6 Guidelines for Surgery in Secondary Rhinoplasty

On planning to operate on a patient for the second or third time, one must be aware of certain factors in the operated noses that are quite different from freshly unoperated ones.

These are mainly due to the **changing nature of the tissues** after healing and **the time** that takes for these tissues to heal and settle.

22.5.6.1 Timing of Surgery

As a general rule, secondary rhinoplasty is better delayed for at least six months to one year from the primary surgery.

There may be some exceptions to this rule, e.g.

- Nasal injury that causes obvious distortion of tissues;
- Grafts that clearly move out of place;
- Infection and abscess formation;
- Areas that are omitted, forgotten or overlooked.

Revision for the second, third or more time may need to be further deferred for two or more years.

Reasons for delaying the surgery are:

- Tissues of the nose **take a long time to heal and settle** to their final shapes. Certain areas take a longer time than others, e.g. nasal tip and nasofrontal area.
- Grafts take a long time to adapt and settle inside the nasal tissues. During this time grafts may change in size and shape.

There are varying degrees of graft resorption, so they may not reach the actual size before one year. Conchal and costal cartilage grafts, on the other hand, may change in shape, e.g. they may curve or bend, as well as resorption. Tissue reaction may be severe or mild, resulting in immediate or delayed rejections.

- Patient's psychology: it may take some time for the patient to settle on the realities and facts of the condition. Time is necessary to be prepared for the realistic outcomes of the revision surgery.
- Time is also needed for the surgeon to properly study, prepare and plan for the surgery.

22.5.6.2 Conservative Attitude

The long-term healing process affects all tissues in many ways.

(a) All tissues are toughened, especially the skin, subdermis and cartilage. Surgical planes are not as easy to reach and dissect.

The skin is thick, scarred and heals poorly. The subdermal planes are no longer soft easily dissected connective tissue layer; they are rather fibrosed and variably thick, sticky and tough.

Cartilages are fibrosed, broken and not as malleable. They will not comply with the different surgical techniques as the primary cartilages.

(b) Bones after primary osteotomies are of different shapes and locations.

(c) Grafts are surrounded by tissues fibrosis. Septal and lateral cartilaginous grafts have varying degrees of resorption.

Conchal and costal cartilaginous grafts tend to bend, especially if placed without trimming of perichondrium or crushing.

(d) Tissue reaction and rejection especially if foreign material is used. This may take place even many years after the primary surgery.

22.5.7 Strategy of Secondary Rhinoplasty

The **four areas** of rhinoplasty are dealt with differently according to the **four possibilities** so that

22.5.7.1 Omitted Areas

Omitted areas in precious surgeries are dealt with in the same way as the primary surgery, e.g. septal surgery, bony pyramid or alar base surgery.

22.5.7.2 Areas of the Completed Surgery

These areas are untouched as technically and aesthetically they are satisfactory to both the patient and the surgeon.

22.5.7.3 Areas of the Uncompleted Surgery

Surgery in these areas is completed, e.g. further reduction of the bony hump, dorsal height or alar base.

22.5.7.4 Areas of Faulty Surgery

These areas are dealt with in a very conservative way (vid supra).

No formal and full exploration is made, so the following is made:

- Resorption of any distorted tissues, e.g. bony wall cartilage or graft;
- Resection of any extra bone formation or tissue protrusions;
- Areas of depression are grafted. Only autogenous grafts are used. Other heterogenous grafts carry a high risk of being either rejected or infected.

- Surgery to adjacent unoperated areas may help to improve the faulty area, e.g.
- Correction of an omitted septal deviation may have positive effects on nasal deviation and aesthetics of the nasolabial area and aperture size (vid supra).
- Surgery on omitted lower lateral cartilages improves the aesthetics of the nasal tip.
- Osteotomies improve the aesthetics of alar base.
- Alar base surgery has a positive effect on the overall appearance of the nose.

22.5.7.5 Areas of Omitted Surgery

These areas are explored and dealt with as in the same techniques of primary surgery.

In summary, a successful secondary rhinoplasty depends mainly on the virtue of "patience" which will take both the surgeon and the patient through a careful detailed history and then clinical and photographic assessment.

Timing of surgery, conservative attitude and systemic approach are the mainstay for satisfactory and successful results.

GPSR Compliance

The European Union's (EU) General Product Safety Regulation (GPSR) is a set of rules that requires consumer products to be safe and our obligations to ensure this.

If you have any concerns about our products, you can contact us on ProductSafety@springernature.com

In case Publisher is established outside the EU, the EU authorized representative is:

Springer Nature Customer Service Center GmbH
Europaplatz 3
69115 Heidelberg, Germany

Batch number: 10732799

Printed by Printforce, the Netherlands